UK paediatric advanced life support algorithm 2010

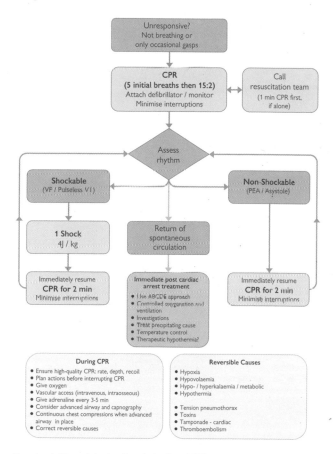

Unresponsive?
Not breathing or
only occasional gasps

CPR
(5 initial breaths then 15:2)
Attach defibrillator / monitor
Minimise interruptions

Call
resuscitation team
(1 min CPR first,
if alone)

Assess rhythm

Shockable
(VF / Pulseless VT)

Non-Shockable
(PEA / Asystole)

1 Shock
4J / kg

Return of
spontaneous
circulation

Immediately resume
CPR for 2 min
Minimise interruptions

Immediate post cardiac arrest treatment
- Use ABCDE approach
- Controlled oxygenation and ventilation
- Investigations
- Treat precipitating cause
- Temperature control
- Therapeutic hypothermia?

Immediately resume
CPR for 2 min
Minimise interruptions

During CPR
- Ensure high-quality CPR: rate, depth, recoil
- Plan actions before interrupting CPR
- Give oxygen
- Vascular access (intravenous, intraosseous)
- Give adrenaline every 3-5 min
- Consider advanced airway and capnography
- Continuous chest compressions when advanced airway in place
- Correct reversible causes

Reversible Causes
- Hypoxia
- Hypovolaemia
- Hypo- / hyperkalaemia / metabolic
- Hypothermia

- Tension pneumothorax
- Toxins
- Tamponade - cardiac
- Thromboembolism

Reproduced with permission from Resuscitation Council (UK).

OXFORD MEDICAL PUBLICATIONS

Oxford Handbook of
Tropical Medicine

Third edition

Published and forthcoming Oxford Handbooks

Oxford Handbook of Clinical Medicine 7/e (also available for PDAs)
Oxford Handbook of Clinical Specialties 7/e
Oxford Handbook of Acute Medicine 2/e
Oxford Handbook of Anaesthesia 2/e
Oxford Handbook of Applied Dental Sciences
Oxford Handbook of Cardiology
Oxford Handbook of Clinical Dentistry 4/e
Oxford Handbook of Clinical and Laboratory Investigation 2/e
Oxford Handbook of Clinical Diagnosis
Oxford Handbook of Clinical Haematology 2/e
Oxford Handbook of Clinical Immunology and Allergy 2/e
Oxford Handbook of Clinical Pharmacy
Oxford Handbook of Clinical Surgery 3/e
Oxford Handbook of Critical Care 2/e
Oxford Handbook of Dental Patient Care 2/e
Oxford Handbook of Dialysis 2/e
Oxford Handbook of Emergency Medicine 3/e
Oxford Handbook of Endocrinology and Diabetes
Oxford Handbook of ENT and Head and Neck Surgery
Oxford Handbook for the Foundation Programme
Oxford Handbook of Gastroenterology and Hepatology
Oxford Handbook of General Practice 2/e
Oxford Handbook of Genitourinary Medicine, HIV and AIDS
Oxford Handbook of Geriatric Medicine
Oxford Handbook of Medical Sciences
Oxford Handbook of Nephrology and Hypertension
Oxford Handbook of Nutrition and Dietetics
Oxford Handbook of Neurology
Oxford Handbook of Occupational Health
Oxford Handbook of Obstetrics and Gynaecology
Oxford Handbook of Oncology 2/e
Oxford Handbook of Ophthalmology
Oxford Handbook of Palliative Care
Oxford Handbook of Practical Drug Therapy
Oxford Handbook of Pre-Hospital Care
Oxford Handbook of Psychiatry
Oxford Handbook of Public Health Practice 2/e
Oxford Handbook of Rehabilitation Medicine
Oxford Handbook of Respiratory Medicine
Oxford Handbook of Rheumatology 2/e
Oxford Handbook of Sport and Exercise Medicine
Oxford Handbook of Tropical Medicine 2/e
Oxford Handbook of Urology

Oxford Handbook of
Tropical
Medicine

Third edition

Michael Eddleston
Wellcome Trust Career Development Fellow,
University of Edinburgh, *and*
Specialist Registrar in Clinical Pharmacology,
Scottish Poisons Information Bureau,
Royal Infirmary of Edinburgh

Robert Davidson
Consultant Physician, Northwick Park Hospital, *and*
Honorary Senior Lecturer, Imperial College School of
Medicine, London

Andrew Brent
Specialist Registrar in Infectious Diseases,
Oxford, *and* Wellcome Trust Fellow in
Clinical Tropical Medicine, Imperial College, London

Robert Wilkinson
Wellcome Trust Senior Fellow in Clinical
Tropical Medicine, *and* Professor of Infectious Diseases,
Imperial College, London, MRC Programme Leader,
National Institute for Medical Research, London, *and*
Hon Associate Professor, University of Cape Town.

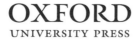

OXFORD
UNIVERSITY PRESS

OXFORD
UNIVERSITY PRESS

Great Clarendon Street, Oxford OX2 6DP

Oxford University Press is a department of the University of Oxford.
It furthers the University's objective of excellence in research, scholarship,
and education by publishing worldwide in

Oxford New York

Auckland Cape Town Dar es Salaam Hong Kong Karachi
Kuala Lumpur Madrid Melbourne Mexico City Nairobi
New Delhi Shanghai Taipei Toronto

With offices in

Argentina Austria Brazil Chile Czech Republic France Greece
Guatemala Hungary Italy Japan Poland Portugal Singapore
South Korea Switzerland Thailand Turkey Ukraine Vietnam

Oxford is a registered trade mark of Oxford University Press
in the UK and in certain other countries

Published in the United States
by Oxford University Press Inc., New York

© Oxford University Press, 2008

The moral rights of the authors have been asserted
Database right Oxford University Press (maker)

First published 1999
Second edition 2005
Third edition 2008
Reprinted 2009, 2010, 2011 with corrections

British Library Cataloguing in Publication Data
Data available

Library of Congress Cataloging in Publication Data
Data available

Typeset by Newgen Imaging Systems (P) Ltd., Chennai, India
Printed in China
on acid-free paper by
Asia Pacific Offset

ISBN 978–0–19–920409–0 (flexicover)

10 9 8 7 6 5

Foreword

Tropical Medicine — the old

This year, the Royal Society of Tropical Medicine and Hygiene (RSTM&H), that most durable promoter of the speciality of tropical medicine, celebrated its centenary in locations as diverse as Peru, Gambia, Malaysia and Bangladesh. The discipline of Tropical Medicine was probably a British invention, attributable to Joseph Chamberlain, Secretary of State for the Colonies at the turn of the 19/20th centuries. The concept was inspired by the research and teaching of the admirable Patrick Manson ('father of tropical medicine') but its ulterior motive was to maintain the health and activity of expatriates stationed in tropical colonies such as the 'white man's grave' that was West Africa.

Tropical Medicine — the new

Fortunately, tropical medicine quickly refocused on the welfare of the indigenous inhabitants of these countries and, as portrayed variously in Fred Zinnemann's movie 'The Nun's Story' (1959) and Graham Greene's novel 'A Burnt-out case' (1974), it became the uniquely colourful, exciting and humanitarian medical speciality. It did not deserve historian Roy Porter's amusing but disparaging verdict: 'In the modern epic of health, a hero's part has often been assigned to tropical medicine, the branch of the microbiological revolution bearing fruit in the Third World: intrepid doctors going off to the steaming jungles and overcoming some of the most lethal diseases besetting mankind.' (The Greatest Benefit to Mankind. A medical history of humanity from antiquity to the present. London: Harper-Collins 1997, p462). Yet there is something about that last lancinating phrase that reminds me of so many tropicalists I have known, not least the original medical student editors of the Oxford Handbook of Tropical Medicine (OHTM), Michael Eddleston and Stephen Pierini.

What is Tropical Medicine and what are tropical diseases?

Tropical diseases were defined by Manson in his classic work 'Tropical Diseases. A Manual of the Diseases of Warm Climates' (1898) as those 'occurring only, or which from one circumstance or another are specially prevalent, in warm climates'. One such 'circumstance' was and is the gripping poverty of financial and other resources that defines so many tropical environments, both rural and urban. This speciality must be broad to encompass all the necessary skills and experience needed to meet its special challenges: the zoology of vectors and reservoirs, hygiene, anthropology, economics, epidemiology and demographics as well as the mainstream medical sciences.

Should 'tropical medicine' be renamed 'medicine in the tropics'?

This was furiously debated by the RSTM&H a few years ago, but the motion: 'Tropical Medicine as a formal discipline is dead and should be buried' was comprehensively rejected (Trans Roy Soc Trop Med Hyg

1997;91:372-5). However, in the wider world, India, home to Calcutta's 19th century School of Tropical Medicine, no longer distinguishes it from general internal medicine. When the organisation of European Schools of Tropical Medicine (TropMed Europe) met in Addis Ababa in 1997, we were persuaded by our African colleagues that the term 'tropical medicine' still had patronising colonial overtones and should be replaced by 'international medicine' although this decision was never implemented. Such discussions will continue and may be interpreted as evidence of the vitality and sustained relevance of the discipline.

A new edition of the Oxford Handbook of Tropical Medicine

The increasing popularity of OHTM supports the view that tropical medicine is still important and interesting. Wherever I travel, I find this book exactly where it should be: sticking out of pockets or open and being consulted at the bedside in dispensaries, clinics, hospitals and in the field. Now emergent in a magnificent third edition, OHTM just goes on improving, maturing, and expanding. There are substantial and authoritative chapters on all the major classical tropical diseases and a broad coverage of those many neglected conditions that, while failing to kill multi-millions each year, still cause untold human misery and deserve our attention.

Tricks of the tropical medicine trade

Some practical knowledge can be learned only through first hand experience of working in the rural tropics. How to preserve insulin in the coolest place in an African hut lacking any sort of refrigeration? How to dry a thick blood film quickly in a very humid climate, again without mains electricity? The quickest technique for staining a malaria film in an emergency? How to check the pH of stains and buffers? How to weigh patients and monitor their fluid balance at the most peripheral levels of the health service? How to keep flies off open wounds? How to overcome upper airways obstruction without resorting to a bloody tracheotomy? How to check the polarity of earthed electric sockets in the ward and the sideroom laboratory and why this might be important?

Further reading

For readers who want more detail about some of the fascinating entities, many useful websites are provided. Or why not look at the companion Oxford Handbook of Expedition and Wilderness Medicine (due to publish 2008) or, if you have the means to view a CDRom, even the Oxford Textbook of Medicine?

OTM3e — an excellent read

Sampling OHTM3e will give you answers to many questions but, much more than that, it will prove an enjoyable experience that will stimulate enthusiasm for the still lustrous speciality of Tropical Medicine, however it is defined. Congratulations to the concertante group of editors: Eddleston, Davidson, Brent and Wilkinson; and to the orchestra of many able contributors!

David A. Warrell
Oxford
October 2007

Preface

Introduction

The 1st edition of the *Oxford Handbook of Tropical Medicine* (1999) was the work of Michael Eddleston and Stephen Pierini, both junior doctors at the time. It filled a gap between handbooks of clinical medicine, which were unsuitable for use in resource-poor settings, and WHO guidelines, which were appropriate but not available in a collected format. For the 2nd edition (2005), Robert Davidson and Robert Wilkinson became co-editors, and international experts contributed sections. For this 3rd edition, Andrew Brent joined the team as co-editor, and the multi-contributor format has been kept. As well as the four editors, 48 international experts have brought their wealth of tropical medical experience to this new, expanded edition. New sections have been added, reflecting the fact that medicine in the tropics is not just 'tropical medicine' in the old-fashioned sense of parasitic and infectious diseases, and fresh illustrations have been included. Guidelines from the WHO and other sources have been incorporated where possible.

We have tried to make this edition wiser as well as more comprehensive. Several sections now have 'Paediatric' boxes, highlighting special features in children, and 'Public health' boxes, with important information on disease control and prevention. At the same time, we have tried to restrict the length so it might remain affordable in most countries and pocket-sized.

Making this book specific to your local areas — a request

Clinical medicine differs in different environments and it is impossible to write a handbook which will be ideal for all continents and both urban and rural settings. However, we feel that there is enough in common across the tropics for a book like this to be useful to doctors, medical assistants, and nurses, supplying them with advice and guidance, often drawn up by the WHO. Readers will have to be critical and selective, deciding what is relevant for their own circumstances and facilities. The blank spaces and pages have been left to allow each reader to make notes, adapting the book to his or her circumstances. We expect the reader to attack the algorithms with pencils, changing them to reflect their experience of local practice. We wish to stimulate, not prescribe.

We ask that readers send us back comments and criticisms so that we may improve the book in future editions. You can send your comments to us via the OUP website: *http://www.oup.co.uk/isbn/0-19-852509-5*.

Royalties

All royalties from the sale of this book are donated to TALC (Teaching Aids at Low Cost, PO Box 49, St Albans, Herts, AL1 5TX, UK; *http://www.talcuk.org*; Email: *info@talcuk.org*). TALC is a charity whose mission is to provide essential books and training materials at the lowest possible cost for health workers in the poorest settings.

Acknowledgements

The editors would like to thank the following for their contributions to the text.

John Williams, for checking the laboratory aspects of the book; Millie Davis, for checking the drug recommendations and doses; and David Warrell, for the writing of the foreword.

Contents

Colour plates

Contributors

Jo Adu,
Renal Unit,
Queen Elizabeth Hospital,
Edgbaston, UK.
Chapter 9

Theresa Allain,
Department of Care of the
Elderly, Southmead Hospital,
Bristol, UK.
Chapter 12

Stephen Allen,
Department of Paediatrics,
School of Medicine, Swansea
University, Swansea, UK.
Chapter 1

Tania Araujo-Jorge,
Laboratory of Cell Biology,
Oswaldo Cruz Institute,
Rio de Janeiro, Brazil.
**Chapter 18
(Chagas' disease)**

Imelda Bates,
Disease Control Strategy
Group, Liverpool School of
Tropical Medicine,
Liverpool, UK.
Chapter 11

Tony Berendt,
Bone Infection Unit,
Nuffield Orthopaedic Centre,
Oxford, UK.
Chapter 15

Margaret Callan,
Division of Medicine,
Imperial College, Chelsea and
Westminster Hospital,
London, UK.
**Chapter 18 (infectious
mononucleosis)**

Francois Chappuis,
Médecins sans Frontières, and
Travel and Migration Medicine
Unit, Department of Community
Medicine, Geneva University
Hospitals Geneva, Switzerland.
**Chapter 18 (African
trypanosomiasis)**

Cecilia Chung,
Division of Rheumatology,
Vanderbilt University School of
Medicine, Nashville, USA.
**Chapter 18 (rheumatoid
arthritis, osteoarthritis, and SLE)**

David Dance,
Health Protection Agency
(South West), Derriford, UK.
Chapter 18 (plague, melioidosis)

Mildred Davis,
Chesterfield, Derbyshire, UK

Andrew Dawson,
South Asian Clinical Toxicology
Research Collaboration, University
of Peradeniya, Peradeniya, Sri Lanka

Nick Day,
Wellcome-Mahidol-Oxford
Tropical Medicine Research
Programme, Faculty of Tropical
Medicine, Mahidol University,
Bangkok, Thailand.
Chapter 2

Jeremy Farrar,
University of Oxford Clinical
Research Unit, Hospital for Tropical
Diseases, Ho Chi Minh City, Vietnam.
**Chapter 10,
Chapter 18 (influenza)**

Sara Ghorashian,
Department of Haematology,
Royal Free Hospital, London, UK.
Chapter 11

Sally Hamour,
Renal Unit, Royal Free Hospital,
London, UK.
Chapter 9

Stan Houston,
Departments of Medicine &
Public Health Science, University
of Alberta, Edmonton, Canada.
Chapter 4, Chapter 18
(prevention of infection in the
health care setting)

Michael Jacobs,
Division of Infection & Immunity,
University College Medical
School, London, UK.
Chapter 18 (sepsis,
arboviruses, VHF)

Beate Kampmann,
Academic Department of
Paediatrics, and Wellcome
Trust Centre for Research in
Clinical Tropical Medicine,
Imperial College, London, UK.
Chapter 5

Ike Lagunju,
Department of Paediatrics,
University College Hospital,
University of Ibadan,
Ibadan, Nigeria.
Chapter 1, Chapter 5
(paediatric acute respiratory
infections)

Bongani Mayosi,
Department of Medicine,
Groote Schuur Hospital and
University of Cape Town,
Cape Town, South Africa.
Chapter 8

Graeme Meintjes,
Division of Infectious Diseases
and HIV Medicine, GF Jooste
Hospital and University of
Cape Town, Cape Town,
South Africa.
Chapter 3

Marc Mendelson,
Division of Infectious Diseases
and HIV Medicine, Groote
Schuur Hospital and University of
Cape Town, Cape Town,
South Africa.
Chapter 7

Marc Nicol,
Institute of Child Health,
Red Cross Children's Hospital
and University of Cape Town,
Rondebosch, South Africa.
Chapter 18 (rickettsial
infections, brucellosis)

Andy Parrish,
Department of Medicine,
Cecilia Makiwane Hospital and
Walter Sisulu University,
East London, South Africa.
Chapter 3

Chris Parry,
Centre for Tropical Microbiology,
School of Infection and Host
Defence, University of Liverpool,
Liverpool, UK.
Chapter 18 (typhoid)

Vikram Patel,
Nutrition and Public Health
Intervention Research Unit,
London School of Hygiene &
Tropical Medicine, and Sangath
Centre, Goa, India.
Chapter 19

Mary Penny,
Instituto de Investigacion
Nutricional, Lima, Peru.
Chapter 6

Andrew Pollard,
Department of Paediatrics,
University of Oxford, Oxford, UK.
Chapter 22

Terence Ryan,
Green College, Oxford, UK.
Chapter 14

Matthew Snape,
Oxford Vaccine Group,
Department of Paediatrics,
University of Oxford,
Oxford, UK.
Chapter 22

Olugbemiro Sodeinde,
Department of Paediatrics,
University College Hospital,
University of Ibadan, Ibadan,
Nigeria.
Chapter 1

Jehangir Sorabjee,
Department of Medicine,
Bombay Hospital Institute of
Medical Sciences, and
University of Mumbai,
Mumbai, India.
Chapter 5

Mike Stein,
Division of Clinical
Pharmacology, Vanderbilt
University School of Medicine,
Nashville, USA.
**Chapter 18 (rheumatoid
arthritis, osteoarthritis,
and SLE)**

Yupin Suputtamongkol,
Division of Infectious Diseases
and Tropical Medicine, Faculty
of Medicine, Siriraj Hospital
and Mahidol University,
Bangkok, Thailand.
**Chapter 18
(leptospirosis)**

Jenny Thompson,
Nuffield Department of
Anaesthetics, John Radcliffe
Hospital, Oxford, UK.
Chapter 20

Andrew Tomkins,
Centre for International Health
and Development, Institute of
Child Health, University College,
London, UK.
Chapter 17

Kemi Tongo,
Department of Paediatrics,
University College Hospital,
University of Ibadan, Ibadan, Nigeria.
Chapter 1

David Warrell,
Centre for Tropical Medicine,
University of Oxford, Oxford, UK.
**Chapter 18 (relapsing fevers),
Chapter 21**

Douglas Wilkinson,
Nuffield Department of Anaesthetics,
John Radcliffe Hospital, Oxford, UK.
Chapter 20

John Williams,
Department of Infectious and
Tropical Diseases, London School
of Hygiene and Tropical Medicine,
London, UK

Henrietta Williams,
Melbourne Sexual Health Centre,
and School of Population Health,
University of Melbourne,
Melbourne, Australia
Chapter 16,

David Yorston,
Tennent Institute of Ophthalmology,
Gartnavel Hospital, Glasgow, UK.
Chapter 13

Syed Mohd Akramuz Zaman,
MRC Laboratories, Banjul, Gambia.
Chapter 18 (measles)

Symbols and abbreviations

±	with or without
=>	implies
≥	more than or equal to
>	more than
≤	less than or equal to
<	less than
↑	raised
↓	lowered
→	leading to
%	percent
~	approximately
+ve	positive
−ve	negative
1°	primary
2°	secondary
ABG	arterial blood gases
ACE	angiotensin-converting enzyme
ACPR	adequate clinical and parasitological response
ACS	acute confusional state
ACT	artemisinin-based combination therapy
ACTH	adrenocorticotrophic hormone
ADA	adenosine deaminase
ADLA	acute dermatolymphangioadenitis
AF	atrial fibrillation
AFL	acute filarial lymphangitis
AHA	autoimmune haemolytic anaemia
AIDS	acquired immunodeficiency syndrome
ALA	amoebic liver abscess
ALL	acute lymphoblastic leukaemia
ALS	advanced life support
ALT	alanine transferase
ANA	anti-nuclear antibodies
AML	acute myeloblastic leukaemia
ANCA	anti-neutrophil cytoplasmic antibody
ANS	autonomic nervous system

APBA	allergic bronchopulmonary aspergillosis
APKD	autosomal dominant polycystic kidney disease
APTT	activated partial thromboplastin time
ARB	angiotensin receptor blocker
ARF	acute renal failure
ARDS	acute respiratory distress syndrome
ARI	acute respiratory infection
ART	antiretroviral therapy
ARV	antiretroviral
ASOT	anti-streptolysin O titre
ATLS	advanced trauma life support
ATN	acute tubular necrosis
AV	atrio-ventricular
AXR	abdominal X-ray (plain)
BCC	basal cell carcinoma
BCG	Bacille Calmette Guerin
bd	bis die (twice a day)
BL	Burkitt's lymphoma
BLS	basic life support
BMI	body mass index
BP	blood pressure
BPM	beats per minute
BV	bacterial vaginosis
CA	carcinoma
CABG	coronary artery bypass graft
CAH	chronic active hepatitis
Cal	calorie
CAP	community-acquired pneumonia
CBD	common bile duct
CCF	congestive cardiac failure
CDAD	*Clostridium difficile* associated diarrhoea
CDC	Centers for Disease Control and Prevention, Atlanta, USA
CF	complement fixation
CF	cystic fibrosis
CFA	circulating filarial antigens
CIN	cervical intraepithelial neoplasia
CK	creatinine kinase
CKD	chronic kidney disease
CK-MB	creatinine kinase cardiac isoenzyme
CL	cutaneous leishmaniasis

CLAT	cryptococcal latex agglutination test
CLL	chronic lymphocytic leukaemia
CLO	columnar-lined oesophagus
CM	cerebral malaria
CMI	cell-mediated immunity
CML	chronic myeloid leukaemia
CMV	cytomegalovirus
CNS	central nervous system
COPD	chronic obstructive pulmonary disease
CPR	cardiopulmonary resuscitation
Cr	creatinine
CRF	chronic renal failure
CRP	C reactive protein
CRT	capillary refill time
CSF	cerebrospinal fluid
CSW	commercial sex workers
CT	computerized tomography
CVA	cerebrovascular accident (stroke)
CVP	central venous pressure
CVS	cardiovascular system
CXR	chest X-ray
DAEC	diffuse-adherent *E.coli*
DCL	damage control laparotomy
D&V	diarrhoea and vomiting
DCL	disseminated cutaneous leishmaniasis
DCT	direct Coomb's test
DEC	diethylcarbamazine
DF	dengue fever
DHA	dihydroartemisinin
DHF	dengue haemorrhagic fever
DIC	disseminated intravascular coagulation
DILS	diffuse inflammatory lymphocytosis syndrome
DIP	distal interphalangeal joint
DM	diabetes mellitus
DMARD	disease–modifying anti-rheumatoid drug
DNA	deoxyribonucleic acid
DOTS	directly observed treatment strategy
DPL	diagnostic peritoneal lavage
dsDNA	double stranded DNA
DSS	dengue shock syndrome

DT	diphtheria toxoid
DTP	diphtheria toxoid, pertussis, and tetanus toxoid
DVT	deep vein thrombi
dxm	dexamethasone
EAEC	enteroaggregative *E.coli*
EBV	Epstein-Barr virus
ECF	extracellular fluid
ECG	electrocardiogram
EEV	equine encephalitis virus
EHEC	enterohaemorrhagic *E.coli*
EIA	enzyme immunoassay
EIEC	enteroinvasive *E.coli*
ELISA	enzyme linked immunosorbant assay
EPEC	enteropathogenic *E.coli*
EPI	Expanded Programme on Immunization
ERCP	endoscopic retrograde cholangiopancreatography
ES	encephalopathic syndrome
ESR	erythrocyte sedimentation rate
ETAT	emergency triage and assesement
ETEC	enterotoxigenic *E.coli*
ETF	early treatment failure
F	female
FACS	fluorescence-activated cell sorter
FB	foreign body
FBC	full blood count
FCPD	fibrocalculous pancreatic diabetes
FDC	fixed drug combination
FDP	fibrinogen degradation product
Fe	iron
FEV_1	forced expiratory volume in first second
FFP	fresh frozen plasma
FHx	family history
FOB	faecal occult blood
FSGS	focal segmental glomeruloscerosis
FTA	fluorescent treponemal antigen test
G^+	Gram-stain positive
GAM	global acute malnutrition
GBS	Guillain-Barre syndrome
GCS	Glasgow coma scale
GFR	glomerular filtration rate

γGT	gamma glutamyl-transaminase
GH	growth hormone
GI	gastrointestinal
GMP	good manufacturing practice
GN	glomerulonephritis
GORD	gastro-oesophageal reflux disease
G6PD	glucose-6-phosphate dehydrogenase
GTN	glyceryl trinitrate
GTT	glucose tolerance test
GU	genitourinary
GWVI	genital wart virus infection
HA	haemagglutinin
HAART	highly active antiretroviral therapy
HAT	human African trypanosomiasis
HAV	hepatitis A virus
Hb	haemoglobin
HBeAg	hepatitis B virus e antigen
HBIG	hyperimmune hepatitis B immunoglobulin
HBsAg	hepatitis B virus surface antigen
HBV	hepatitis B virus
HCC	hepatocellular carcinoma
HCV	hepatitis C virus
HCW	health care worker
HDN	haemorrhagic disease of the newborn
HDV	hepatitis D virus
HEV	hepatitits E virus
HF	haemorrhagic fever
HHV-8	human herpes virus-8 (KSHV)
Hib	*Haemophilus influenzae* type b
HIV	human immunodeficiency virus
HL	Hodgkin's lymphoma
HLA	human lymphocyte antigen
HMMA	4-hydroxy-3-methoxymandelic acid
HMS	hyperreactive malarial splenomegaly
HOCM	hypertrophic obstructive cardiomyopathy
HONK	hyperglycaemic hyperosmolar non-ketotic coma
HPV	human papilloma virus
h	hour(s)
HRS	hepatorenal syndrome
HSV	herpes simplex virus

HT	hypertension
HTLV	human T-cell lymphotrophic virus
HUS	haemolytic uraemic syndrome
Hx	history
IBD	inflammatory bowel disease
ICP	intracranial pressure
ID	intradermal
IDD	iodine deficiency
IDDM	insulin-dependent diabetes mellitus
IF	immunofluorescence
IHD	ischaemic heart disease
IMCI	integrated management of childhood illness
IM	infectious mononucleosis
IM	intramuscular
INH	isoniazid
INR	international normalized ratio
IPT	intermittent presumptive treatment
IRIS	immune reconstitution inflammatory syndrome
ITU	intensive therapy unit
IUD	intrauterine device
IV	intravenous
JVP	jugular venous pressure
K^+	potassium ions
KCCT	kaolin cephalin clotting time
kJ	kilojoule
KMC	kangaroo mother care
KOH	potassium hydroxide
KS	Kaposi sarcoma
KSHV	Kaposi sarcoma-associated herpes virus
LAP	Lower abdominal pain
LBBB	left bundle branch block
LBRF	louse borne relapsing fever
LBW	low birth weight
LCF	late clinical failure
LD	lymphocyte depleted
LDH	lactate dehydrogenase
LFT	liver function test
LGV	lymphogranuloma venereum
Li^+	lithium ions
LIF	left iliac fossa

LIP	lymphocytic interstitial pneumonitis
LN	lymph node
LP	lymphocyte predominant
LP	lumbar puncture
LPF	late parasitological failure
LTB	laryngotracheobronchitis
LRTI	lower respiratory tract infection
LV	left ventricle
LVF	left ventricular failure
M	male
MAC	mycobacterium avium complex
MALT	mucosa-associated lymphoid tissue
max	maximum
MC	mucosal leishmaniasis
MCH (C)	mean corpuscular haemoglobin (concentration)
MCP	metacarpophalangeal joint
MCV	mean cell volume
MDGs	Millenium development goals
MDR	multi-drug resistant
Mg^{2+}	magnesium ions
MI	myocardial infarction
min	minutes
mmHg	millimetres of mercury
mmol	millimol
MMR	measles, mumps, and rubella (vaccine)
MND	motor neurone disease
MODY	maturity onset diabetes of the young
mosmol	milliosmol
MR	measles and rubella (vaccine)
MR	modified release
MRDM	malnutrition-related diabetes mellitus
MRI	magnetic resonance imaging
MRSA	methicillin-resistant *Staph aureus*
MSM	men who have sex with men
MST	morphine sulphate
MTCT	mother to child transmission
mths	months
MUAC	mid-upper arm circumference
NA	neuraminidase
Na^+	sodium ions

NCHS	National Centre for Health Statistics
ND	notifiable disease (WHO)
NG	nasogastric
NGT	nasogastric tube
NGU	non-gonococcal urethritis
NHL	non-Hodgkin's lymphoma
NIDDM	non-insulin-dependent diabetes mellitus
NNRTI	non-nucleoside reverse transciptase inhibitor
NS	nodular sclerosing
NSAID	non-steroidal anti-inflammatory drug
NTs	non-typhi salmonella
N&V	nausea and/or vomiting
O_2	oxygen
OA	osteoarthritis
OCP	oral contraceptive pill
od	omni die (once daily)
OHL	oral hairy leukoplakia
OI	opportunistic infection
O/P	outpatient
ORS	oral rehydration solution
ORT	oral rehydration treatment
OTM	Oxford Textbook of Medicine
$PaCO_2$	partial pressure of carbon dioxide in arterial blood
PAIR	percutaneous aspiration-injection-reaspiration
PAM	primary amoebic meningoencephalitis
PAN	polyarteritis nodosa
PBC	primary biliary cirrhosis
PCI	percutaneous coronary intervention
PCP	pneumocystis pneumonia due to *Pneumocystis jiroveci* (previously known as *Pneumocystis carinii*)
PCR	polymerase chain reaction
PCV	packed cell volume
PDPD	protein deficient pancreatic diabetes
PE	pulmonary embolism
PEFR	peak expiratory flow rate
PEL	primary effusion lymphoma
PEP	post-exposure prophylaxis
pg	picogram
PGL	persistent generalized lymphadenopathy
PHT	portal hypertension

PI	protease inhibitor
PID	pelvic inflammatory disease
PIM	post-infective malabsorption
PKD	polycystic kidney disease
pLDH	parasite lactate dehydrogenase
PML	progressive multifocal leukoencephalopathy
PMN	polymorphonuclear leukocyte (neutrophil)
PNS	peripheral nervous system
PO	per os (by mouth)
PO_4	phosphate
PPD	protein purified derivative
PR	per rectum (by the rectum)
PT	prothrombin time
PTB	pulmonary tuberculosis
PTH	parathyroid hormone
PTT	partial thromboplastin time
PUD	peptic ulcer disease
PV	per vaginam (by the vagina)
PVD	peripheral vascular disease
QBC	quantitative buffy coat
qds	quater die sumendus (to be taken 4 times a day)
q2h/q4h	every 2 hours/4 hours
RA	rheumatoid arthritis
RBBB	right bundle branch block
RBC	red blood cell
RD	respiratory distress
RDA	recommended daily allowances
RDT	rapid diagnostic test
RES	reticuloendothelial system
RF	rheumatic fever
RHF	right heart failure
RIF	right iliac fossa
RIG	rabies immunoglobulin
RNA	ribonucleic acid
RPR	rapid plasma reagin test for syphilis
RR	respiratory rate
RSV	respiratory syncytial virus
RUQ	right upper quadrant
RUTF	ready-to-use therapeutic food
RV	right ventricular

RVF	right ventricular failure
RVVC	recurrent vulvo-vaginal candidiasis
SAH	subarachnoid haemorrhage
SAM	severe acute malnutrition
SARS	severe acute respiratory syndrome
SBE	subacute bacterial endocarditis
SBP	spontaneous bacterial peritonitis
SC	subcutaneous
SCC	squamous cell carcinoma
SDTM	specially diluted therapeutic milk
SE	south east
SG	specific gravity
SIADH	syndrome of inappropriate ADH secretion
SIN	squamous intra-epithelial neoplasia
SLE	systemic lupus erythematosus
SOL	space-occupying lesion
SOP	standard operating procedure
SP	sulfadoxine-pyrimethamine
SSPE	subacute sclerosing panencephalitis
STI	sexually transmitted disease
SVC	superior vena cava
TB	tuberculosis
TBM	tuberculosis meningitis
TBRF	tick borne relapsing fever
Td	tetanus toxoid and low-dose diphtheria toxoid (vaccine)
tds	ter die sumendus (to be taken 3 times a day)
TEN	toxic epidermal necrolysis
TFT	thyroid function test
TIA	transient ischaemic attack
TIMI	thrombolysis in myocardial infarction
TIBC	total iron binding capacity
TIPS	transjugular intrahepatic portosystemic shunting
TLC	total lymphocyte count
TPE	tropical pulmonary eosinophilia
TPHA	*Treponema pallidum* haemagglutination assay
TSH	thyroid-stimulating hormone
TSS	tropical splenomegaly syndrome
TST	tuberculin skin test
TT	tetanus toxoid (vaccine)
TTI	transfusion transmissible infection

TTP	thrombotic thrombocytopaenic purpura
TURP	transurethral resection of the prostate
UC	ulcerative colitis
U&E	urea and electrolytes
URT	upper respiratory tract
URTI	upper respiratory tract infection
USS	ultrasound scan
UTI	urinary tract infection
UV	ultraviolet
VCT	voluntary consent and testing
VDRL	venereal disease research laboratory test for syphilis
VF	ventricular fibrillation
VHF	viral haemorrhagic fever
VL	visceral leishmaniasis
VMA	vanillyl mandelic acid
VSD	ventriculo-septal defect
VT	ventricular tachycardia
VZV	varicella-zoster virus
WBC	white blood cell
WCC	white cell count
WHO	World Health Organization
wks	weeks
XDR TB	extensively drug-resistant tuberculosis
YF	yellow fever
yrs	years
ZN	Ziehl–Neelsen

Management of the sick child

Section editors   **Ike Lagunju**
                       Kemi Tongo
                       Olugbemiro Sodeinde
                       Stephen Allen

Introduction

Every year >10 million children die (4 million in the first month of life). Deaths in hospitals often occur within the first 24 h of admission, so very sick children should be identified on arrival and appropriate treatment instituted. Emergency triage and treatment (ETAT) is a rapid screening process to identify children who require immediate treatment to avert death and long-term morbidity. Treatment of sick children must never be on a 'first come, first served' basis.

Among presentations to health-care facilities, children often outnumber adults. In many low-resource settings, there is no paediatrician and sick children are managed by non-specialists.

WHO/UNICEF developed a model of integrated management of childhood illness (IMCI) — see box. This syndromic approach to the triage and assessment of a sick child has successfully been used in low-resource settings. WHO also has online publications for the management of children at the first referral level (see box).

Integrated management of childhood illness (IMCI)

(http://www.who.int/child-adolescent-health/integr.htm)

Of the >10 million deaths/yr that occur in children <5 years, 70% are caused by acute respiratory infections, diarrhoea, measles, and malaria, with or without malnutrition. Most children present with clinical features of more than one diagnosis — a single diagnosis is therefore often impossible.

IMCI uses a syndromic approach, combining management of individual diseases with nutrition, immunization, and maternal health. It aims to improve the skills of health care workers (HCWs).

'Danger signs' are first identified. Children are then assigned defined clinical syndromes on the basis of simple questions to the mother and a basic clinical examination; more than one syndrome may be assigned. The severity of each syndrome is defined and management instituted: either urgent referral to a secondary care facility, treatment, and advice, or advice to the parent/caregiver for home management.

IMCI is targeted at HCWs in health centres and outpatient departments of small hospitals. This can be extended to include community health workers, shopkeepers, and pharmacists, who are often the first port of call for medical advice. ICMI has improved heath-care seeking behaviour, rational prescribing, immunization coverage, and availability of basic equipment, and has also reduced costs. Bigger reductions in mortality should result from combining IMCI with key programmes such as the WHO ARI and ORT case management strategies.

WHO online paediatric publications

Management of the child with a serious infection or severe malnutrition: guidelines for care at the first referral level in developing countries — (*www.who.int/child-adolescent-health/publications/ CHILD_HEALTH/WHO_FCH_CAH_00.1.htm*)

Pocket book of hospital care for children: guidelines for the management of common illnesses with limited resources — (*www.who.int/child-adolescent-health/New_Publications/CHILD_HEALTH/ PB/00.PB_full.pdf*)

Emergency triage assessment

Immediately on presentation to a health facility (i.e. *before* joining a queue), children should be rapidly triaged to:

- Those with emergency signs who require immediate treatment to prevent death.
- Those with priority signs who should be assessed and treated without delay.
- Non-urgent cases that have neither emergency nor priority signs. These follow the regular queue of non-urgent patients.

Triage should be carried out at the first point of contact; this may be at the outpatient clinic, the emergency room, or even in a hospital paediatric ward. All children must be assessed for these signs (as outlined on page 6) *before* any routine procedures like registration and weighing.

Emergency signs

- Central cyanosis.
- Severe respiratory distress.
- Obstructed breathing.
- Altered level of consciousness.
- Convulsions.
- Signs of shock.
- Signs of severe dehydration in a child with diarrhoea.

All children with emergency signs require immediate treatment to avert death (see 🕮 p 8–13).

Priority signs

- Any sick child aged <2 months.
- Visible severe wasting; oedema affecting both feet.
- High fever: temperature >38.5°C.
- Irritability, restlessness, lethargy.
- Severe palmar pallor.
- Major burns.
- Any respiratory distress.
- Child with urgent referral note from the health facility.
- Trauma or urgent surgical condition.
- Poisoning.
- Severe pain.

All children with priority signs require immediate assessment and treatment.

Signs of severe respiratory distress

- Lower chest wall indrawing (Fig. 1.1).
- Grunting.
- Inability to speak, drink, or feed due to respiratory distress.
- Head nodding/use of accessory muscles of respiration.

Other signs of respiratory distress

- Fast breathing — ≥60 breaths/minute in infants aged <2 months; ≥50/minute in children aged 2–11 months; ≥40/minute in children aged 12 months to 5 years.
- Nasal flaring.

Signs of obstructed breathing

- Stridor.   • Inability to speak.
- Weak cough.   • Splinted chest.

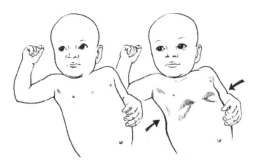

Fig. 1.1 Lower chest wall indrawing: with inspiration the lower chest wall moves in. (Note the distinction between lower chest wall *indrawing* and *intercostal recession*, in which the soft tissue between the ribs is sucked inwards on inspiration. Although intercostal recession may occur in respiratory distress, alone, it is not a sign of severe respiratory distress.) (Reproduced with permission of the WHO.)

Assessment for emergency and priority signs

Follow these steps to quickly determine if there are any emergency or priority signs:

- *Assess airway and breathing*
  Look, feel, and listen for chest movement, exhaled air, and breath sounds by placing your ear close to the child's nostrils. Check for respiratory distress and signs of airway obstruction (see box p 5). Check the tongue and buccal mucosa for central cyanosis.
  Note: do not move neck if cervical injury is possible e.g. following trauma. Instead, use the jaw thrust manoeuvre to open the airway if needed.

- *Assess circulation for signs of shock*
  Check if child's hands are cold. Assess capillary refill time (CRT) by applying pressure to whiten the nail of the thumb or big toe for 3 seconds. Release the pressure and note how long it takes the nail bed to refill and to turn pink; a CRT ≥3 seconds is usually a sign of shock or dehydration. Check the pulse: if the radial pulse is not palpable, feel for the brachial or femoral pulse in the infant, or the carotid pulse in older children. In shock, central pulses may be weak and rapid or absent.

- *Assess for coma, convulsions, or other abnormal mental status*
  Check if the child is continually irritable, restless, lethargic, or convulsing. Rapidly assess level of consciousness using AVPU scale (see box opposite) or Blantyre Coma score (📖 p 41).

- *Assess for severe dehydration if the child has diarrhoea*
  Check with mother if the child's eyes are unusually sunken. Assess skin turgor by pinching the skin of the abdomen halfway between the umbilicus and the flank. Pinch for 1 second and then observe how the skin returns — >2 sec implies marked loss of skin turgor (see diagram 📖 p 249). Severe dehydration is defined as ≥2 of the following: lethargy or unconsciousness; sunken eyes; marked loss of skin turgor; inability to drink or drinking poorly.

- *Assess for signs of severe malnutrition*
  Examine for severe muscle wasting, especially around the ribs, shoulders, arms, buttocks, and thighs. Examine for bilateral pedal oedema ± other signs of kwashiorkor.

- *Assess for severe anaemia*
  Compare the colour of the child's palm with yours: if the skin is very pale or so pale that it looks white, the child has severe palmar pallor.

- *Identify all sick infants <2 months old*

- *Assess for a major burn*

- *Identify all children referred from another health facility*

Signs of shock

- Cold hands.
- CRT >3 seconds.
- Fast, weak pulse.

Also note

- Anuria.
- Hypotension — a late sign in children.
- Altered level of consciousness.
- Acidotic (Kussmaul) breathing 2° to poor tissue perfusion.

AVPU scale

The AVPU scale is a quick and approximate way of rating a person's level of consciousness:

A — Alert
V — Responds to verbal commands
P — Responds to painful stimulus. Press down firmly on the middle fingernail with a pen, or rub your knuckles on the sternum
U — Unconscious

Emergency management of the sick child

If emergency signs are present, call for help and give emergency treatment:

Airway & breathing

- The presence of severe respiratory distress, obstructed breathing, or central cyanosis is an emergency.
- Is there a history or evidence of foreign body aspiration? If so, manage as for a choking child (opposite page).

If foreign body aspiration NOT suspected ▶ manage airway:
- Remove any foreign body from the mouth.
- Clear secretions from oropharynx (use suction if available).
- Open airway using head tilt and chin lift: in infants the 'tilt' should be to the neutral position to avoid obstruction of the airway due to hyperextension. In older children, tilt the head to the 'sniffing' position.

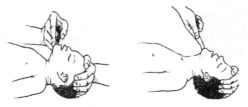

Fig. 1.2 (A) Neutral position in infants (B) 'Sniffing' position in older child. (Reproduced with permission of the WHO.)

- If inadequate or no spontaneous respiratory effort, ventilate using bag and mask. Aim to give 40–60 breaths per minute in neonates and a slower rate in older children. If there is also cardiac arrest requiring chest compressions, use a ratio of 90 compressions coordinated with 30 breaths/minute (3 compressions and 1 breath every 2 seconds) in neonates. In older children, give external cardiac massage at a rate of 100/minute with 2 breaths after every 15 compressions (ratio 15 compressions to 2 breaths).
- Where facilities and expertise exist, endotracheal intubation should be performed as soon as possible. However, attempted endotracheal intubation by the inexperienced must not compromise adequate ventilation by bag and mask.
- Give oxygen and ensure child is warm.
- If wheeze is present, give nebulized salbutamol.

NOTE: Unlike in adults, most arrests in young children are 1° respiratory arrests ± 2° cardiac arrest. As a result, adequate ventilation alone is sufficient to maintain cardiac output in most cases, while the cause of the arrest is identified and treated.

Foreign body aspiration/choking child

- If the child has an effective cough, encourage her to cough and continually reassess for clinical deterioration or relief of the obstruction.
- If NO effective cough, or there is severe respiratory distress, obstructed breathing, or central cyanosis, manage as for choking child.

For infants

- Give 5 back slaps using the heel of the hand as shown in Fig. 1.3.
- If obstruction persists, give 5 chest thrusts using 2 fingers (Fig. 1.3).
- If obstruction persists, check the infant's mouth for any obstruction that can be removed.
- If obstruction still persists, repeat this sequence, starting with back slaps.

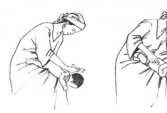

Fig. 1.3 Back slaps and chest thrusts to relieve airway obstruction in a choking infant. (Reproduced with permission of the WHO.)

For children ≥1 year

- Give 5 back slaps with the heel of the hand.
- If obstruction persists, perform the Heimlich manoeuvre (Fig. 1.4); stand behind the child and form a fist below the sternum with one hand; place the other hand over the fist and pull both hands backwards and upwards. Repeat this manoeuvre 5 times.
- If obstruction persists, check the child's mouth for any obstruction that can be removed.
- If obstruction still persist, repeat this sequence starting with back slaps.

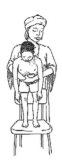

Fig. 1.4 Heimlich's manoeuvre in a choking older child. (Reproduced with permission of the WHO.)

Circulation

- Shock (identified by cold hands plus either CRT >3 seconds or a fast, weak pulse) is an emergency.
- Stop any bleeding; look for severe palmar pallor => severe anaemia.
- Give oxygen.
- Ensure child is warm.
- Insert IV line (and take blood for Hb/haematocrit and crossmatch).
- If unable to establish peripheral IV access quickly, insert external jugular or intraosseous line (Fig 1.5, 📖 p 12).
- Fluid resuscitate according to guidelines below and nutritional status.

Management of shock in children who are NOT severely malnourished

▶ **Fluid resuscitate rapidly:**
- Infuse 20 ml/kg bolus of normal saline or Ringer's lactate as rapidly as possible, then reassess.
- If no improvement, give a second 20 ml/kg fluid bolus as rapidly as possible, then reassess.
- If still no improvement, give a third 20 ml/kg bolus as rapidly as possible.

▶ **If still no improvement after 3rd bolus:**
- *If shock caused by profuse diarrhoea* — give 20 ml/kg normal saline or Ringer's lactate over 30 minutes.
- *If shock not caused by profuse diarrhoea* — give 20 ml/kg blood over 30 minutes.
- Reassess after fourth infusion; if still no improvement, further management is guided by the working diagnosis.

▶ **If improvement occurs at any stage** (pulse slower, CRT faster):
- *For infants <12 months* give 70 ml/kg Ringer's lactate or normal saline over 5 h.
- *For children aged 1–5 years* give 70 ml/kg Ringer's lactate or normal saline over 2 ½ h.

▶ **Reassess the child every 1–2 h:**
- Modify the infusion rate according to the clinical response.
- Give ORS solution (📖 p 251) 5 ml/kg/h as soon as child can drink.
- Reassess and classify dehydration after 6 h (infants) or after 3 h (older children). Follow appropriate treatment plan A, B, or C for dehydration (see Chapter 6).

Intraosseous needle insertion

Intraosseous infusion is a quick, safe, and reliable method of giving fluid (including blood) and drugs in an emergency when it is not possible to establish peripheral venous access. The usual site of insertion is the proximal tibia:

- Place padding under the child's knee so that it is flexed ~30° from the straight position with the heel resting on the bed /examination table.
- Identify the insertion site 1–2 cm below the tibial tuberosity, midway between the anterior ridge of the tibia and its medial edge.
- Use a dedicated intraosseous or bone marrow aspiration needle (15–18 gauge or, if not available, 21 gauge); if neither available, a large bore hypodermic or butterfly needle may be used in young children.
- Clean the skin with antiseptic solution.
- Stabilize the leg by grasping the thigh and knee above and lateral to the cannulation site with the non-dominant hand, taking care to keep this hand away from the cannulation site to avoid needlestick injury.
- Using aseptic technique, insert the needle with the point angled slightly away from the joint space and the bevel pointing towards the foot.
- Advance the needle using a gentle but firm, twisting or drilling motion, until there is a sudden decrease in resistance as it enters the marrow cavity; the needle should sit firmly in the bone.
- Remove the stylet, attach a syringe, aspirate ~1 ml marrow contents (looks like blood) and flush with normal saline to confirm the needle is in the marrow cavity. Blood from the marrow aspirate may also be sent for full blood count, biochemistry, malaria slide, and crossmatch.
- Apply dressing and secure needle in place. It is now ready to use.
- Stop the intraosseous infusion as soon as venous access is available.

Contraindications: infection at the site of insertion; fracture of the bone.

Alternative sites of insertion:

- Distal *femur*, 2 cm above the lateral condyle (~1–2 cm proximal to the superior border of the patella), slightly lateral to the anterior ridge.

Distal tibia, ~1–2 cm proximal to the medial malleolus in the centre of the bone.

Management of shock in children with severe malnutrition

- Signs of shock and dehydration are less reliable in children with severe malnutrition. These children are at risk of fluid overload and death from heart failure.

▶ **Resuscitate with IV fluids as follows only if the child is lethargic or unconscious:**

- Weigh the child (or estimate weight) to calculate fluid requirements.
- Record pulse and respiratory rate.
- Assess and treat hypoglycaemia (see below).

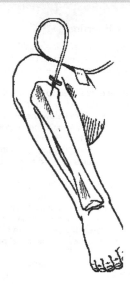

Fig. 1.5 Introaosseous needle insertion. (Reproduced with permission of the WHO.)

- Infuse 15 ml/kg IV fluid over 1 hour. Use (in order of preference) Ringer's lactate with 5% glucose, or half-normal saline with 5% glucose, or half-strength Darrow's solution with 5% glucose. Use Ringer's lactate if none of these are available.
- Monitor pulse and respiratory rate every 5–10 minutes.
- *If child deteriorates during IV rehydration (respiratory rate increases by 5/min or heart rate by 15/min), stop the infusion.*

▶ **If there are signs of improvement** (pulse & respiratory rates fall):
- Repeat 15 ml/kg IV bolus over 1 hour.
- Then switch to oral or NG rehydration with ReSoMal (📖 p 251) 10 ml/kg/h up to 10 h.

▶ **If there are still no signs of improvement:**
- Assume the child has septic shock.
- Give maintenance IV fluids (4 ml/kg/hr) while waiting for blood.
- Transfuse 10 ml/kg fresh whole blood slowly over 3 h; give packed cells if in heart failure.
- Start frequent small feeds with F-75 or alternative low lactose and low osmolarity preparation (📖 Chapter 17).

▶ **In all cases, proceed to full assessment and management of severe malnutrition, including broad-spectrum antibiotic therapy (Chapter 6).**

Children with severe anaemia and shock

▶ **Do not delay fluid resuscitation — resuscitate as required per guidelines above while awaiting blood for transfusion.**

- Obtain blood for Hb/haematocrit, crossmatch (+ malaria slide in endemic areas) in all children with severe palmar pallor.
- If Hb<4 g/dl/haematocrit <12%, or Hb result not available quickly and clinical signs of severe anaemia, substitute saline/Ringer's solution with 20–30 ml/kg blood in the above guidelines.
- *In the presence of very severe palmar pallor and shock,* consider urgent transfusion with O negative blood.

Coma and convulsions

- **The presence of coma or convulsions is an emergency.**

▶ **Manage airway** (see 📖 p 8)

▶ **If convulsing:**

- Give diazepam 0.5 mg/kg rectally.
- If still convulsing after 10 minutes, give a 2nd dose of diazepam 0.5 mg/kg rectally, or diazepam 0.25 mg/kg IV.
- If still convulsing after a further 10 mins, give paraldehyde 0.3–0.4 ml/kg rectally, or phenobarbital 15 mg/kg IV or IM (in infants <2 weeks old, give phenobarbital 20 mg/kg).
- To prevent aspiration, avoid oral medications until the convulsions have terminated and the child is alert.

▶ **If unconscious:**

- Position in the left lateral 'recovery' position. If head or neck trauma is suspected, stabilize the neck first and keep the child lying on the back.
- Tepid sponge if high fever.
- Assess and treat hypoglycaemia (see below).

Hypoglycaemia

▶ **Assess and treat hypoglycaemia:**

- *If lethargic or unconscious,* measure blood glucose. If unable to measure glucose quickly, or if blood glucose <2.5 mmol/l in a well nourished child (<3 mmol/l in severe malnutrition), give 5 ml/kg 10% glucose rapidly IV.
- *If alert,* treat hypoglycaemia with 10 ml/kg milk or 10% glucose by mouth or NG tube.

Hydration & nutritional status

▶ **Treat shock** if present (📖 p 10).

▶ **Assess and treat dehydration** as outlined in Chapter 6.

▶ **Assess and treat severe malnutrition** as outlined in Chapter 17.

Further assessment and diagnosis

After triage assessment for emergency and priority signs, complete clinical assessment. The most common acute problems in children are:
- Lethargy, altered level of consciousness, or convulsions.
- Cough, wheeze, or difficulty breathing.
- Diarrhoea.
- Fever.

Common problems that present less acutely include:
- Chronic cough (≥30 days).
- Fever lasting >7 days.

The major differential diagnoses for each of these clinical presentations are summarized below.

Causes of lethargy, impaired consciousness, or convulsions
1. Meningitis — Chapter 10.
2. Cerebral malaria — Chapter 2.
3. Febrile convulsions (see box).
4. Hypoglycaemia (see box).
5. Head injury — Chapter 10.
6. Poisoning/overdose — Chapter 21.
7. Sepsis (unlikely to cause convulsions unless meningitis).
8. Shock (unlikely to cause convulsions).
9. Acute glomerulonephritis with encephalopathy — Chapter 9.
10. Diabetic ketoacidosis — Chapter 12.

Causes of difficulty breathing ± cough
1. Pneumonia — Chapter 5.
2. Severe anaemia.
3. Malaria — Chapter 2.
4. Cardiac failure — Chapter 8.
5. Congenital heart disease (see box).
6. Inhaled foreign body — see earlier.
7. Tuberculosis — Chapter 4.
8. Pertussis — Chapter 5.

Causes of wheeze
1. Asthma — Chapter 5.
2. Bronchiolitis — Chapter 5.
3. Viral upper respiratory tract infection.
4. Pneumonia — Chapter 5.
5. Inhaled foreign body — see before.

Febrile convulsions

- occur in children aged 6 months — 6 years.
- typically a generalized tonic or tonic-clonic seizure lasting 1–2 minutes during a febrile illness.
- generally benign.
- may be a family history.
- in a minority of children they recur in the same or a subsequent illness.

A more serious cause (e.g. meningitis, cerebral malaria, encephalitis, brain abscess) suggested by:
- prolonged seizures (>30 minutes).
- multiple or focal seizures.
- age <6 months.

When in doubt, perform full septic screen including LP.

Causes of diarrhoea — see Chapter 6
1. Infections — viral, bacterial, and parasitic.
2. Malabsorption.
3. Severe malnutrition.
4. Antibiotic related diarrhoea.
5. Intussusception (see box).

Causes of fever without localizing signs
In most children with fever, the cause is apparent clinically. Examine the upper airways (viral URTI, otitis media, tonsillitis) and joints (septic arthritis) as well as the major systems (pneumonia, meningitis). Examine skin for infection or a rash (e.g. measles).

In the absence of localizing signs, a few common illnesses should be considered:
1. Malaria — Chapter 2.
2. Sepsis — bacteraemia/septicaemia (see box).
3. Urinary tract infection.
4. Typhoid.

Causes of chronic cough
1. Tuberculosis — Chapter 4.
2. Asthma — Chapter 5.
3. Persistent infection e.g. Pertussis — Chapter 5.
4. Inhaled foreign body — Chapter 5.
5. Bronchiectasis — Chapter 5.
6. Lung abscess — Chapter 5.
7. Recurrent pneumonia or HIV-associated lung disease — Chapter 3.
8. Recurrent aspiration.

Differential diagnosis of fever lasting >7 days
Diagnosis is often difficult. Many children will have already been empirically treated and diagnostic facilities may be limited. A detailed clinical assessment is essential. Causes will vary in different regions. A carefully considered trial of treatment for the most likely cause may be necessary if a secure diagnosis cannot be made.

Consider
- Partly treated, drug-resistant malaria.
- Occult abscess (e.g. subphrenic, psoas, retroperitoneal, lung).
- Typhoid and non-typhi *Salmonella* infection (see box).
- Infective endocarditis — Chapter 8.
- Rheumatic fever — Chapter 8.
- Tuberculosis — Chapter 4.
- Brucellosis (in endemic areas) — Chapter 18.
- Visceral leishmaniasis (in endemic areas) — Chapter 18.

Intussusception

- Invagination of one part of the intestine into the lumen of the adjoining bowel.
- Important cause of intestinal obstruction in children aged 2 mths –5 yrs (peak incidence 4–10 mths).
- Classically presents with recurrent, colicky, abdominal pain, vomiting, and bloody 'redcurrant jelly' stool; may palpate a sausage-shaped abdominal mass.
- AXR may show a soft tissue mass displacing loops of bowel; barium enema, a filling defect; and ultrasound scan, a 'target lesion'.
- Urgent intervention can prevent bowel ischaemia and perforation: reduce intussusception with air/contrast enema; if this fails, operate.
- Treat shock, sepsis, or electrolyte derangement.

Bacteraemia & septicaemia

- Common among children in the tropics.
- Under-diagnosed where there are no facilities for blood culture.
- Often there is a focus of infection (e.g. pneumonia, meningitis, soft tissue infection), but may occur without a focus, or a focus may develop later.
- Typhoid and non-typhoid Salmonella infections are a cause of sepsis without localizing signs; a similar syndrome may occur with many other organisms, especially in children with severe malnutrition or HIV.
- All children with sepsis should be admitted and started on empiric antibiotics (ideally after blood cultures), during investigations. Choose broad-spectrum antibiotics if the cause is unknown.
- Note that malaria is often accompanied by bacterial sepsis.

Non-typhi Salmonella (NTS) infection

- NTS infections are a common cause of childhood bacteraemia. Risk factors include malnutrition, malaria, HIV, and sickle cell disease.
- Children typically present with sub-acute or prolonged fever without localizing signs, but focal signs and/or diarrhoea occur; splenomegally is common.
- Some 1st line antibiotics (e.g. penicillin) do not cover NTS. Treatment is with chloramphenicol, co-trimoxazole, or ampicillin, but multi-drug resistance is an increasing problem. Alternatives are ciprofloxacin (resistance emerging) or ceftriaxone.

The sick young infant

Infants less <2 mth old are vulnerable, and their illnesses may rapidly progress to death. All sick young infants should, therefore, be given priority attention, even in the absence of emergency signs.

Assessment of the sick young infant

Symptoms and signs of illness in young infants are often subtle and non-specific and more than one illness may co-exist.

- **Check for the danger signs** (see box) — these indicate possible septicaemia, pneumonia, or meningitis requiring immediate treatment.

Danger signs in young infants

- Reduced activity or lethargy.
- Poor feeding.
- Vomiting.
- Convulsions — usually subtle or focal.
- Bloody diarrhoea.
- Fever (axillary temp >37.5°C, or rectal >38°C) — less common in this age group but may indicate serious bacterial infection.
- Hypothermia (axillary <35.5°C or rectal <36°C).
- Pallor, jaundice, or cyanosis.
- Tachypnoea (respiratory rate ≥60 breaths/minute).
- Severe chest wall indrawing (minimal intercostal indrawing may be normal in young infants in absence of other respiratory signs).
- Nasal flaring and grunting.
- Apnoeic episodes or irregular respiration.
- Bulging/tense fontanelle when not crying.

- **Check for focal signs of infection,** including joint/ limb swelling, reduced limb movement, or tenderness (osteomyelitis or septic arthritis); peri-umbilical hyperaemia ± purulent discharge; purulent ear discharge; skin infection. Suspect meningitis if child has convulsions, is irritable with high pitched cry, or bulging/tense anterior fontanelle. *Note:* neck stiffness is an unusual or late sign of meningitis in young infants.
- **Check for feeding problems and weight**: Check if sucking well and adequate weight for age. Refusal of feeds or inability to suck may be due to sepsis, cardiac or respiratory problems, or oral thrush. In an infant who feeds well but has low weight for age, look for underlying problems such as metabolic disorders or congenital heart disease.
- **Check for signs of dehydration** (📖 p 249). Inadequate intake, excessive fluid loss from diarrhoea, vomiting or tachypnoea may result in dehydration. Diarrhoea is uncommon in breastfed infants of this age group except as a sign of sepsis.
- **Check immunization status**: ensure that child is up to date with immunization according to the national schedule.
- **Check for** congenital malformations.

Emergency treatment of the sick young infant

Establish regular respiration and heart rate and reverse cyanosis. Resuscitation is usually successful if promptly performed:

Airway: ensure patent airway by careful suctioning and correct positioning of the neck: place a towel ~2.5 cm thick under the shoulders to allow the neck to drop to a neutral position or just minimal extension with chin lift; do not hyperextend the neck (Fig. 1.6).

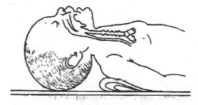

Fig. 1.6 Correct position of the neck for ventilation. (Reproduced with permission of the WHO.)

Breathing: look, feel, and listen for 10 seconds. If breathing is irregular, shallow, or absent, commence bag and mask ventilation with oxygen, ensuring that the mask covers nose and mouth. Check pulse every 2 minutes. Use room air if oxygen is not available. If the child is breathing but cyanosed, give oxygen.

> Unlike in adults, most arrests in young infants are 1° respiratory arrests ± 2° cardiac arrest. As a result, adequate ventilation alone is sufficient to maintain cardiac output in most cases.

Circulation: check for brachial pulse for no longer than 10 seconds. If pulse rate <60/minute, absent, or not sure, commence chest compressions and combine with ventilation in cycles of 15 compressions to 2 breaths (30:2 if there is no assistance). Use two finger tips over lower third of sternum or both thumbs with hand encircling chest. Aim to achieve 100 compressions per minute.

Drugs: if there is no response after 2 minutes, administer intravenous or intraosseous adrenaline 0.1 ml/kg of 1:10,000 solution (10 µ/kg) and continue chest compressions and ventilation. This may be repeated after 3–5 minutes if there is no response.

General measures in the management of sick young infants

Young infants with signs of serious illness (📖 p 18) require admission to prevent complications and rapid deterioration. Treatment, including antibiotics (see box), will be directed at the specific clinical syndrome. In addition, all young infants require ongoing supportive care, which is crucial to their survival even after recovery from the acute illness.

Feeding: ensure continued regular feeding. Express breastmilk and give by NG tube if infant is unable to suck, or by cup and spoon as soon as infant is able to take oral feeds. Oral intake should be stopped if there is abdominal distention, severe vomiting, or respiratory distress. Treat hypoglycaemia with IV 10% dextrose 5 ml/kg or 10 ml/kg via nasogastric tube and continue regular feeds or IV fluids.

Fluid therapy: assess hydration status and give ORS or IV fluids according to WHO guidelines (Chapter 6).

Temperature control: keep infant dry and well dressed/wrapped including bonnet and booties. Maintain environmental temperature of at least 25°C. Avoid excessive exposure during examination and procedures as this may lead to chilling. Use incubators when available to allow easy observation with minimal handling of baby in addition to thermal control. Direct skin to skin care (Kangaroo mother care (KMC) see box) may be used when the infant is stable. If there is fever, reduce dressing and expose but do not give antipyretics.

Oxygen therapy

Indications for oxygen therapy include: central cyanosis, grunting, severe lower chest wall indrawing, and head nodding.

Treatment of convulsions

Neonates (<2 weeks old): IM phenobarbital 15 mg/kg stat; if convulsions persist, give further doses of 10 mg/kg to a maximum of 40 mg/kg and watch for apnoea; if maintenance is required, give 2.5–5.0 mg/kg/day PO. *Infants 2 weeks–2 months old:* rectal diazepam 0.1 mg/kg, repeated twice at 10 min intervals if convulsions persist. Rectal paraldehyde 0.3–0.4 ml/kg may be given instead of a 3rd dose of diazepam.

Monitoring

It is essential to observe infant at least every 6 h for improvement or deterioration.

Outpatient treatment

Infants with non-bloody diarrhoea and some or no signs of dehydration (📖 p 249), or poor weight gain due to feeding mismanagement may be treated as outpatients. However, the mother should be informed of danger signs that would prompt urgent review. Local bacterial infections without constitutional symptoms are common and may be treated on an outpatient basis, with follow-up at short intervals because of the risk of rapid progression to septicaemia. They include: omphalitis (*without* hyperaemia of surrounding skin), skin sepsis (if only a few skin pustules), paronychia, and mild conjunctivitis.

Antibiotic therapy of infections in young infants

Choice of antibiotics should be based on local data of prevailing organisms and antibiotic sensitivities.

Sepsis or pneumonia

Give ampicillin 50 mg/kg IV/IM tds* (or benzyl penicillin 50,000 U/kg qds*) plus gentamicin 7.5 mg/kg* IV/IM od. Cefotaxime 50 mg/kg IV/IM qds* or ceftriaxone 100 mg/kg IV/IM od*† are alternatives. If S. aureus infection suspected (e.g. nosocomial sepsis, soft tissue infection), give cloxacillin 50 mg/kg IV qds* or cefuroxime 25 mg/kg tds, plus gentamicin. Treat until child has remained well for four days.

Meningitis

Give ampicillin 50 mg/kg IV/IM tds*, plus either gentamicin 7.5 mg/kg* or chloramphenicol 25 mg/kg qds (avoid chloramphenicol in premature neonates). Treat for a minimum of 14 days, or 21 days if gram-negative bacterial meningitis proven or suspected. Alternatives are cefotaxime 50 mg/kg IV/IM qds* or ceftriaxone 100 mg/kg/ IV/IM od.*†

Focal bacterial infections

Cotrimoxazole, amoxicillin, or a cephalosporin.

Conjunctivitis

Teach the mother to clean the eyes with saline or clean water ± apply topical antibiotic — review the child after 2 days. **Ophthalmia neonatorum** (🕮 p 532, 609) is a severe, suppurative conjunctivitis, often with associated blepharitis, that occurs in neonates, particularly in the 1st week of life, and may cause permanent blindness if not treated. It is caused by N. gonorrhoea or C. trachomatis perinatally; other organisms include S. aureus. Gram stain of the discharge may demonstrate gram positive diplococci (N. gonorrhoea) — if so, give ceftriaxone 50 mg/kg IM as a single dose, treat the parents presumptively for N. gonorrhoea (🕮 p 609).

* Doses in first week of life as follows: ampicillin 50 mg/kg bd; benzylpenicillin 50,000U/kg bd; gentamicin 5 mg/kg od if normal birth weight, 3 mg/kg od if low birth weight; cefotaxime 50 mg/kg tds in term neonates, bd in premature neonates; cloxacillin 25–50 mg/kg bd.

† Avoid ceftriaxone in neonatal jaundice as the drug may displace bilirubin from albumin, increasing the risk of kernicterus.

Kangaroo mother care (KMC)

This is direct skin to skin care of the infant. The baby is placed naked (except for the nappy) directly on mother's bare chest, and strapped in place to get warmth while the mother goes about her regular activity. KMC is an alternative to an incubator and may reduce hospital stay, help early establishment of breastfeeding, and promote mother/child bonding. Close family members, including the father, can also provide KMC.

Low birth weight (LBW) & prematurity

LBW infants (birth weight <2500 g) may result from prematurity or intrauterine growth retardation. Infants 1750–2250 g and born after 34 weeks' gestation may be nursed with their mothers, with close supervision, in the nursery. Infants >2250 g may be sent home if there are no danger signs. Essential aspects of LBW care include:

Prevention of infection: wash hands with soap and water each time the infant is to be handled.

Temperature control: (see above): maintain the infant's axillary temperature above 36.5°C.

Feeding: LBW babies are prone to hypoglycaemia and may not suck adequately. They should be breastfed within 1 hour of birth and may require additional expressed breast milk by cup and spoon. Mothers should be shown proper latching-on techniques.

Be alert for danger signs: promptly refer to the neonatal unit if present.

Monitor weight gain

Neonatal jaundice

Jaundice occurs in >50% neonates and is more common in LBW infants. Most jaundice is physiological. Jaundice may also be a sign of serious disease (e.g. infection; see box), especially if it occurs on day 1, is associated with fever, is deep (involves palms and soles), or lasts >14 days (>21 days if premature).

Severe jaundice may cause **kernicterus** (neurotoxicity). In its mild form, there is lethargy and reduced feeding. Severe kernicterus causes irritability, hypertonia, ± opisthotonos, and long-term neurological sequelae.

Investigations: total serum bilirubin and conjugated/unconjugated bilirubin, FBC, maternal and infant blood group, Coombs test, G6PD screen, thyroid function, syphilis serology; abdominal USS.

Management of jaundice:
- Ensure adequate hydration.
- Exclude serious causes (see box).
- Treat severe jaundice to prevent kernicterus — see box.
- *Phototherapy* reduces jaundice by using ultraviolet light to cause photodegradation of bilirubin in the skin; protect infant's eyes and beware dehydration, hypothermia, or hyperthermia; other complications include diarrhoea and rash.
- *Exchange blood transfusion* may be required for severe jaundice: twice the infant's blood volume (i.e. 2 x 80 ml/kg) is exchanged for fresh donor blood in 10–20 ml aliquots via an umbilical vein catheter; there is a low but definite risk attached to the procedure.

Problems associated with low birth weight

- Poor thermal regulation.
- Feeding problems (inadequate intake, gastro-oesophageal reflux).
- Necrotizing enterocolitis.
- Neonatal jaundice.
- Metabolic problems (hypoglycaemia, acidosis, hypocalcaemia, fluid and electrolyte imbalance).
- Apnoea.
- Respiratory distress syndrome.
- Patent ductus arteriosus.
- Increased predisposition to infections.

Common causes of neonatal jaundice

Jaundice starting within 24 h of birth:
- Haemolysis (e.g. Rhesus or ABO incompatibility; G6PD or pyruvate kinase deficiency; congenital spherocytosis).
- Infection (TORCH* organisms).

Jaundice starting from day 2 to week 2 after birth:
- Physiological jaundice.
- Breast milk jaundice.
- Severe bruising.
- Infection.
- Haemolysis.

Jaundice persisting for >2 weeks after birth:
- Biliary atresia.
- Neonatal hepatitis.
- Haemolysis.
- Congenital hypothyroidism.
- Infection.
- May also be persistence of breast milk or physiological jaundice.

* Toxoplasma; others, incl. syphilis, VZV, measles; rubella; CMV; Herpes simplex.

Table 1.1 Indications for treatment of neonatal jaundice according to serum bilirubin concentration (WHO)

	Phototherapy				Exchange Transfusion			
	Healthy term baby		Preterm or risk factors		Healthy term baby		Preterm or risk factors	
	mg/dl	µmol/l	mg/dl	µmol/l	mg/dl	µmol/l	mg/dl	µmol/l
Day 1	Any visible jaundice				15	260	13	220
Day 2	15	260	13	220	25	425	15	260
Day 3	18	310	16	270	30	510	20	340
≥ Day 4	20	340	17	290	30	510	20	340

Hypothermia

Hypothermia (body temp <36°C) is a common problem of LBW infants, resulting from low environmental temperature or sepsis. It causes increased O_2 consumption and energy expenditure and reduced O_2 delivery to tissues.

Complications: include: hypoxia, acidosis, and hypoglycaemia; poor weight gain; increased capillary permeability; and respiratory distress.

Treatment: re-warm infant using warm clothing, incubator preheated to 35–36°C, heated mattress, or skin to skin care. Exclude sepsis.

Prevention: nurse infants in warm environments. Avoid wet clothes. Do not place infant on cold surfaces e.g. X-ray plates and weighing scales.

Apnoea

Apnoeic episodes are common in LBW infants and may be accompanied by bradycardia if prolonged. Gentle physical stimulation often stimulates breathing, but respiratory stimulants (caffeine or theophylline) and occasionally ventilatory support, may be required. Seek underlying causes: infection, hypoxia, metabolic derangement, anaemia, or subtle seizures.

Perinatal asphyxia

In perinatal asphyxia there is hypoxia, acidosis, and CO_2 accumulation around time of delivery, which may cause hypoxic-ischaemic encephalopathy. It accounts for much neonatal mortality and long-term morbidity, especially in low-resource settings. Largely preventable with improved obstetric care, prompt resuscitation, and supportive care of the neonate.

Assessment

Risk factors for the development of asphyxia are listed in the box.
Prenatal and intrapartum parameters can indicate asphyxia and the following are indicators of asphyxia at birth:
- Apgar scores <3 at 1 minute, <7 at 5 minutes.
- Resuscitation >10 min before spontaneous respiration established.
- Cord blood pH <7 or base excess >12 mmol/l.

Prevention

Monitoring the mother's condition in pregnancy and labour helps to predict infants at risk of asphyxia. However, some babies who present with birth asphyxia have not been exposed to any of the known risk factors. Everyone involved in the delivery of babies should be skilled in newborn resuscitation in order to reduce the morbidity and mortality associated with asphyxia.

Risk factors for perinatal asphyxia:

- *Maternal medical or obstetric factors*: hyper- or hypotension, heart failure, diabetes, severe anaemia, haemoglobinopathies, infections, respiratory illness (e.g. pneumonia, asthma), smoking, alcoholism, pre-eclampsia/eclampsia, primigravidity or grandmultiparity, induction of labour, sedation, analgesia, prolonged rupture of membranes, prolonged labour.
- *Foetal factors*: multiple gestation, prematurity or post term, intra-uterine growth retardation or large for gestational age, intra-uterine infections, abnormal presentation, congenital abnormalities.
- *Placental factors*: abruptio placenta, placenta praevia, placental insufficiency, cord compression.

Complications of asphyxia and their management

Asphyxia may result in multi-organ dysfunction:
- *Respiratory system*: persistent pulmonary hypertension and respiratory distress syndrome. Ensure good oxygenation.
- *Cardiovascular system*: myocardial damage → poor cardiac output. Monitor capillary refill and BP. Avoid fluid overload and give inotropes if necessary.
- **Gastrointestinal system:** risk of necrotizing enterocolitis. Avoid enteral feeding in first 24–48 h (beware hypoglycaemia!). With introduction of feeds, avoid hyperosmolar feeds and stasis.
- **Metabolic**: hypoglycaemia or hyperglycaemia may worsen hypoxic damage to the brain. Hyponatraemia, hyperkalaemia, hypocalcaemia or acidosis may result; monitor blood glucose and electrolytes.
- **Renal function**: increased risk of urinary retention and renal failure. Monitor fluid intake, urine output, and urine specific gravity. Catheterize to differentiate between failure to produce or void urine.
- **Haematologic**: bone marrow suppression, neutrophil dysfunction, and coagulopathies. Monitor FBC and for evidence of bleeding.
- **Brain**: encephalopathy results from hypoxia, cerebral oedema, ↑ICP. Look for ↓reflexes, abnormal muscle tone, seizures, varying degrees of altered consciousness, and long-term neurological sequelae.
- **Other general measures**. Ensure thermoneutral environment, adequate calories, and hydration, and treat neonatal jaundice.

Neonatal tetanus

This frequently fatal but preventable condition remains common in some developing countries. *Clostridium tetani* usually gains access to the infant through the umbilical stump (due to poor hygiene or a tradition of applying dung to the stump) or through unsterile circumcision. In older children, entry may be due to ear piercing, scarifications, and other harmful traditional practices, or trauma. The pathogenesis of tetanus is described in Chapter 10.

Clinical features: neonatal tetanus usually presents between 2 and 14 days of age, but may occur later. Clinical features include:
- Refusal of feeds.
- Inability to open mouth.
- Excessive crying.
- Muscle rigidity and spasms — provoked and spontaneous.
- Fever.
- Intact consciousness.

Diagnosis: is mainly clinical.

Treatment
1. Muscle relaxants
   - Oral diazepam 5 mg/kg/day in divided doses via nasogastric tube.

For difficult to controlled spasms:
   - IV diazepam 0.1–0.3 mg/kg every 1–4 hrs titrated to spasm frequency.
   - IV midazolam 0.06 mg/kg/h is a suitable but expensive alternative.
   - IV magnesium sulphate may also be useful.
2. IM tetanus immune globulin 500 units or equine anti-tetanus serum 10,000 units single dose
3. Tetanus toxoid (in a different site) if >6 weeks old
4. Antibiotics
   - Metronidazole, procaine penicillin, or erythromycin.
   - Add broad-spectrum antibiotics if associated sepsis suspected.
5. Supportive care
   - Nutritional support.
   - Nurse in quiet, dark environment to prevent provoked spasms (but ensure adequate clinical supervision).
   - Ensure clear airway.
   - Ventilatory support if needed.

Poor prognostic factors
- Incubation period <7 days.
- Period of onset <24 h.
- Associated pneumonia.

Prevention of neonatal tetanus   PUBLIC HEALTH NOTE

- Maternal education.
- Maternal tetanus toxoid immunization.
- Hygienic delivery and cord care practices.
- Avoidance of harmful traditional practices.

Malaria

Section editor   **Nick Day**

Introduction

Malaria, a protozoan infection transmitted by anopheline mosquitoes, is the most important parasitic disease of humans. As many as 3 billion people in endemic areas are at risk of malaria and ~500 million clinical cases occur annually. Between 1 and 3 million die annually, largely African infants and young children. There are four human malaria parasite species (*Plasmodium falciparum*, *P. vivax*, *P. ovale*, and *P. malariae*), though occasionally other primate malaria species cause humans infections (e.g. *P. knowlesi* and *P. simium*). The manifestations of malaria vary greatly, not only from geographical region to region, village to village, but also from person to person. These differences are due to many factors and include mosquito biting and breeding habits, the infecting parasite species (*P. falciparum* resulting in the most severe forms of disease), the state of both genetic and acquired resistance of the host, and compliance with drug treatment.

Life cycle and transmission

The life cycle of the malarial parasite alternates between the sexual cycle in the invertebrate host (the female *Anopheles* mosquito) and the asexual cycle in the vertebrate host (in this case, human). Transmission occurs when the mosquito, requiring blood for the development of her eggs, bites the human host and injects motile sporozoites (see opposite) into the bloodstream which then invade hepatocytes, where they develop into liver schizonts. When each schizont ruptures, thousands of merozoites are released that invade red blood cells and initiate that part of the cycle responsible for all the clinical manifestations of the disease. Either immediately after release from the liver or (in the case of *P. falciparum*) after several asexual cycles, some parasites develop into longer-lived, morphologically distinct sexual forms (gametocytes). Male and female gametocytes ingested by mosquitoes taking a blood meal combine to form a zygote, which matures into an ookinete that encysts in the gut wall. There an oocyst develops, expanding by asexual division until it bursts releasing numerous sporozoites that migrate to the salivary glands to await inoculation into a human host when the mosquito next feeds.

Incubation periods

P. falciparum usually 7–14 days but may be longer (up to 6 weeks) in those with partial immunity or those on inadequate prophylaxis. *P. vivax* 12–17 days and *P. ovale* 15–18 days but may relapse many months or even years later as a result of the reactivation of a dormant form in the liver called the hypnozoite; *P. malariae*, which has no hypnozoite form, has an average incubation period of between 18 and 40 days.

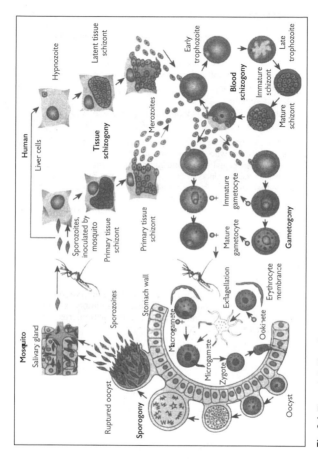

Fig. 2.1 The malaria life cycle.

Epidemiology

Malarial transmission depends upon a number of factors including:

a)   mosquito longevity (lifespan).
b)   the ambient temperature (shortens the cycle in the mosquito).
c)   population density of both mosquito and humans.
d)   the mosquito's human-biting habit.
e)   the host immune response.
f)   whether the drugs used in treatment have any activity against gametocytes.

In endemic areas, transmission may be measured using the parasite rate (% of the population who are positive for malarial parasites on blood film) or the spleen rate (% of population with splenomegaly), although the latter is less reliable since an enlarged spleen may be a result of other diseases. Neither method, however, reflects the clinical impact of mortality or morbidity of the disease on a given population.

Two distinct patterns of malarial transmission emerge which represent extremes:

• Stable malaria, where there is intense all year round transmission. The disease predominantly affects young children and pregnant women. Adults might be positive on blood film but are rarely ill with malaria.
• Unstable malaria, which affects all ages and occurs in areas of seasonal or low transmission.

Malaria control in stable areas is problematic, since interventions that ↓ transmission, but do not eradicate the disease, may impair the development of naturally acquired immunity in the population, resulting in a pattern of unstable disease.

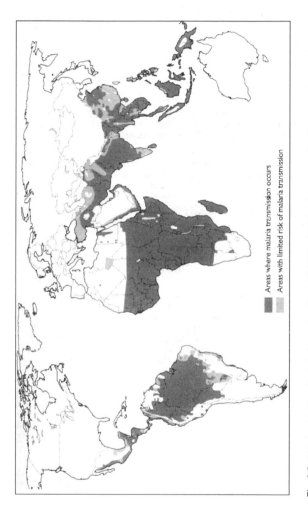

Fig. 2.2 Global endemicity of malaria. (Reproduced from WHO World Malaria Report 2005 (*http://rbm.who.int/wmr2005/*) with permission.)

Protection against malaria

Many innate factors of resistance against infection were first identified in falciparum malaria. Acquired resistance to malaria is slow to develop and the immune mechanisms involved are still unclear.

Innate immunity: Falciparum malaria remains the best example of a selective agent that results in genetic polymorphisms in the host that might provide partial protection against severe disease. Certain genetic variants of the red cell, notably sickle cell trait, glucose 6-phosphate dehydrogenase (G6PD)-deficiency, thalassaemia trait, and ovalocytosis, may partially protect against severe disease. The lack of Duffy antigen (the receptor for merozoites of *P. vivax*) on red cells in most West Africans may account for their protection against this infection.

Acquired immunity: is believed to require repeated exposure to malarial infection, possibly with differing genetic variants of the parasite. In areas of stable transmission, neonates are usually protected by maternal antibodies for the first 6 months or so of life, followed by a period of increased susceptibility during which it is thought that immunity to severe disease is slowly acquired ('**antidisease immunity**'). Depending upon the level of transmission, **antiparasite immunity** appears later, at ~10 yrs of age, when the parasite rate may be as high as 50%. Adults tend to get less severe bouts of disease but when they do, parasite densities are generally lower than in children. Without reinfection, immunity wanes after about 5 yrs. Pregnancy, severe illness, and surgery may also lead to ↓ immunity.

HIV infection: It is becoming increasingly apparent that a complex interaction exists between HIV infection and malaria. Malaria increases viral loads in HIV-positive individuals, and there is evidence that HIV increases both the incidence of malaria (in areas of stable transmission) and the occurrence of severe malaria complications (in areas of unstable transmission). In pregnancy, HIV predisposes the mother to malaria infection and the newborn to congenital malaria. HIV also exacerbates the birthweight reduction associated with malaria in pregnancy.

Complications of malaria

Falciparum malaria

- Falciparum malaria may progress to severe disease and death (malignant tertian malaria). In endemic areas where parasites persist after treatment or patients are soon reinfected, anaemia is common and further attacks, due to recrudescence of blood forms, may occur.
- In some countries, 30% of patients with falciparum malaria develop symptomatic *P. vivax* infection within 2 months without re-exposure to parasites, implying an initial mixed infection.

The benign malarias

- *P. vivax*: a rare complication of *P. vivax* infection is splenic rupture (mortality 80%). It results from acute enlargement with or without trauma and presents with sudden and persistent abdominal pain, guarding, fever, shock, and a lowered haemocrit.
- Relapses: *P. vivax* and *P. ovale* may relapse from 30 days to 5 yrs after initial infection despite treatment which eliminates all blood forms. This is due to latent liver hypnozoites undergoing schizogony and re-entering the blood stream — a true relapse (as opposed to recrudescence).
- *P. malariae*: persistent parasites may cause recurrent fevers when the infection recrudesces even decades following 1° infection. The fevers decrease in frequency and severity over time. Anaemia and splenomegaly may occur.

Clinical features

P. falciparum infection, if treated promptly and appropriately, generally follows a relatively mild course. However, without effective therapy it can become life-threatening, especially in young children and non-immune adults. By contrast, *P. ovale, P. malaria,* and *P. vivax* infection rarely result in severe disease or death except rarely with splenic rupture. Chronic infection or infection of pregnant women with these 'benign' species may lead to marked morbidity e.g. anaemia and reduced birth weight.

Two important features distinguish falciparum infection from benign malarias and account for the differences in severity: only falciparum malaria results in high parasite densities in the blood and only falciparum demonstrates 'sequestration' in the microvasculature of red cells containing mature parasites. Sequestration results mainly from cytoadherence of parasitized red cells to endothelial cells in the post capillary venules of critical organs including the brain, although other factors such as decreased deformability of both parasitized and unparasitized red cells, autoagglutination of parasitized cells, and adherence of unparasitized to parasitized red cells (rosetting) may play a role.

Acute malaria

The clinical presentation of acute malaria in adults with rigors is well known. There is usually a history of travel to or residence in an endemic area. Even the best compliance with the most effective antimalarial chemoprophylaxis cannot exclude malaria. There may be a prodromal period of tiredness and aching. The features of a classical paroxysm are:

- An abrupt onset of an initial 'cold stage' associated with a dramatic rigor (paroxysm) in which the patient visibly shakes.
- An ensuing 'hot stage' during which the patient may have a temperature >40°C, be restless and excitable, and vomit or convulse.
- Finally, the sweating stage, during which the patient's temperature returns to normal (defervesces) and sleep may ensue.

Such a paroxysm can last 6–10 h; a prolonged asymptomatic period may follow lasting 38–42 h in the case of vivax and ovale malaria ('tertian' fever) and 62–66 h in *P. malariae* infections ('quartan' fever).

In falciparum malaria, the periodicity of fever is be less predictable and the fever may be continuous. There may be an accompanying headache, cough, myalgia (flu-like symptoms), diarrhoea, and mild jaundice.

Malaria is rarely, if ever, the cause of lymphadenopathy, pharyngitis, or a rash, and alternative diagnoses need to be considered for these symptoms. In children, malaria may be non-specific and misleading with fever, early cough, D&V, anaemia, and hypoglycaemia. Jaundice, pulmonary oedema, and renal failure are much rarer in children than adults, although progression to other severe complications is usually faster (1–2 days) in children.

Chronic malaria

The persistence of low-level parasitaemia in the blood may lead to 'chronic' malaria. Symptoms include recurrent acute attacks of malaria, anaemia, hepatosplenomegaly, diarrhoea, weight loss, and increased incidence of other infections. Chronic malaria may resolve, with the onset of partial immunity, or progress, with 2° complications:

Burkitt's lymphoma is a childhood tumour common in areas of high falciparum malaria transmission. It is thought to be due to impaired T-cell immunity associated with repeated malaria infections and is strongly associated with Epstein–Barr virus infection.

Hyperreactive malarial splenomegaly (formerly called tropical splenomegaly syndrome) may develop with recurrent infections. It is characterized by massive splenomegaly, profound anaemia, 2° bacterial infections, fever, and jaundice. There is hypersplenism with pancytopenia, hypergammaglobulinaemia, and a lymphocytic infiltrate in the liver. There is a marked elevation of serum IgM. Although malarial parasites are seldom found in the blood, the condition responds to prolonged courses of antimalarial prophylaxis.

Quartan malarial nephropathy. *P. malariae* infection appears to be a cause of nephrotic syndrome, particularly in West and East Africa. Malarial antigens are found in the renal glomerular basement membrane. The condition unfortunately does not respond to antimalarial treatment, glucocorticoids, or cytotoxic drugs.

Pregnancy

Pregnancy increases the risk of contracting falciparum malaria in all levels of endemicity.

- In areas of high, stable transmission, despite higher parasite burdens, most infections are asymptomatic, but result in a reduction in birth weight with a consequent increase in infant morbidity and mortality. The effect is greater in primagravidae and (independently) in younger women.
- In areas of unstable transmission, pregnancy causes more severe disease, particularly anaemia, hypoglycaemia, and acute pulmonary oedema. Foetal distress, premature labour, and stillbirth occur and low birth weight is common. In severe malaria, foetal death is the usual outcome.
- *P. vivax* malaria in pregnancy is also associated with a reduction in birth weight, though to a lesser extent than *P. falciparum*. The effect is greater in multigravidae than primagravidae.

Congenital malaria has a very variable incidence. In some high transmission areas, parasitaemia in the newborn is >50%, but symptomatic disease rare.

Severe malaria (see WHO criteria opposite)

Severe malaria often manifests as a serious multisystem disease. The onset of severe disease can be rapid, with death (particularly in children) occurring in a matter of hours. In travellers from endemic regions, it is most frequently observed when the diagnosis of malaria is made late and treatment delayed.

Cerebral malaria (CM): is the most important complication of falciparum malaria and has a ~20% treated mortality. It most often occurs in non-immune adults and in children. CM is 'unrousable coma in the presence of peripheral parasitaemia where other causes of encephalopathy have been excluded'. However, any alteration in consciousness in the context of falciparum malaria should be taken seriously. Neck rigidity and photophobia are not usually seen and Kernig's sign is –ve. There may be one or more of: diffuse cerebral dysfunction with coma, generalized convulsions (~50%), focal neurological signs, and brainstem signs such as abnormal doll's eye or oculovestibular reflexes. Retinal haemorrhages are seen in ~15% of cases, increasing to ~40% if pupillary dilatation and indirect ophthalmoscopy are used. Neurological sequelae are found in ~5% of survivors (10% in children) and include hemiparesis, cerebellar ataxia, cortical blindness, hypotonia, and mental retardation. In children, CM carries a 10–40% mortality, most deaths occurring within the first 24 h.

Reduced GCS may follow a febrile convulsion in a child or be caused by hypoglycaemia, which must be excluded. Malarial convulsions can occur at any temperature and post-ictal coma may last several hours. In deep coma, abnormalities of posture and muscle tone are frequently seen. For young children use the Blantyre Coma Scale (shown opposite) to grade the coma.

Respiratory distress (RD): is manifest by rapid, laboured breathing, sometimes with abnormal rhythms of respiration. In children, there may be intercostal recession, use of the accessory muscles of respiration and nasal flaring, which is sometimes difficult to differentiate from an acute respiratory infection. RD in patients with malaria may be the result of a number of pathologies:

- In most cases, particularly in children, RD represents respiratory compensation for a profound metabolic acidosis. Severe metabolic acidosis (BE <–12) is associated with an 8-fold ↑ risk of death in children.
- Acute respiratory distress syndrome (ARDS) caused by direct alveolar capillary damage by parasites and neutrophils worsened by hypoalbuminaemia and iatrogenic fluid overload.
- A lung infection because of the immunosuppression caused by malaria.
- Air hunger as a result of severe anaemia.

Each requires different treatment.

WHO criteria for severe malaria

One or more of the following clinical or laboratory features:
Clinical manifestations:
- Prostration.
- Impaired consciousness.
- Respiratory distress (acidotic breathing).
- Multiple convulsions.
- Circulatory collapse.
- Pulmonary oedema (radiological).
- Abnormal bleeding.
- Jaundice.
- Haemoglobinuria.

Laboratory tests:
- Severe anaemia.
- Hypoglycaemia.
- Acidosis.
- Renal impairment.
- Hyperlactataemia.
- Hyperparasitaemia.

Taken from *WHO Guidelines for the Treatment of Malaria*, WHO, 2006.

Also see *Trans R Soc Trop Med Hyg* 2000; **94(Suppl. 1)**: 1–90

Blantyre Coma Scale

To obtain 'coma score' add the scores from each section.
Best motor response
• Localizes painful stimulus*	2
• Withdraws limb from painful stimulus**	1
• No response or inappropriate response	0

Best verbal response
• Cries appropriately with painful stimulus, or if verbal, speaks	2
• Moan or abnormal cry with painful stimulus	1
• No vocal response to painful stimulus	0

Eye movements
• Watches or follows (e.g. mother's face)	1
• Fails to watch or follow	0

* pressure with blunt end of pencil on sternum/supraorbital ridge

** pressure with horizontal pencil on nail bed of finger or toe

Anaemia: all patients with malaria sustain some fall in Hb level. The anaemia is normocytic. Severe anaemia with a haematocrit <15% (or Hb <5 g/dl) in the presence of parasitaemia >10,000/ul (about 0.2% of cells infected) is a common presentation in African children. Pallor, breathlessness, gallop rhythm, RD, pulmonary oedema, and neurological signs are common features of severe anaemia. Anaemia is exacerbated by 2° bacterial infections, haemorrhage, and pregnancy. Hyperparasitaemia and/or G6PD deficiency can result in massive intravascular haemolysis. In children, repeated episodes of otherwise uncomplicated malaria may lead to chronic normochromic anaemia with dyserythropoietic changes in the bone marrow.

Jaundice: is common in adult patients and results from a number of mechanisms including haemolysis, hepatocellular damage, and cholestasis. Both unconjugated and conjugated bilirubin may be >50 μmol/l (3.0 mg/dl). Clinical signs of liver failure are unusual unless there is concomitant viral hepatitis.

Renal impairment: may be pre-renal or renal in origin, usually occurs in adults, and is characterized by a ↑ serum Cr (>265 μmol/l or 3 mg/dl) and ↑ urea, with oliguria (<400 ml urine/24 h in an adult) or anuria due to acute tubular necrosis. Renal impairment may occur at the time of maximal parasitaemia or even when the parasites have been cleared. In some cases, there is polyuria. Renal failure in malaria has a poor prognosis (~45% die).

Blackwater fever: is massive haemoglobinuria (the urine becomes very dark) in the context of malaria. The cause is incompletely characterized but in some cases it follows treatment with quinine or treatment or prophylaxis with oxidant drugs such as primaquine. It is more common in patients with G6PD deficiency or other red cell enzyme deficiencies (e.g. pyruvate kinase). In colonial times, blackwater fever was more common and the mortality much higher.

Hypoglycaemia: (whole blood glucose <2.2 mmol/l, 40 mg/dl) may be due to impaired liver function or quinine/quinidine-induced hyperinsulinaemia (pregnant women are particularly prone). It presents with anxiety, sweating, breathlessness, dilated pupils, oliguria, hypothermia, tachycardia, and light-headedness, eventually leading to decreased consciousness, convulsions, and coma. However, it can easily be missed in patients with disturbed conscious level. In a fasting adult, hepatic glycogen stores last ~2 days; in a child ~12 h. Hence, hypoglycaemia is common in 1–3 yr olds (especially those with CM, hyperparasitaemia, or convulsions). Hypoglycaemia indicates a poor prognosis and is a risk factor for neurological sequelae. It is not associated with signs of malnutrition.

Indicators of a poor prognosis

Clinical
- Marked agitation.
- Hyperventilation (respiratory distress).
- Hypothermia (<36.5°C).
- Deep coma.
- Repeated convulsions.
- Bleeding.
- Anuria.
- Haemodynamic shock.

Laboratory
- Blood film showing hyperparasitemia >100,000/µl (about 2% of cells infected).
- Blood film showing >20% of parasites to be 'late stages' (pigment-containing trophozoites and schizonts).
- Blood film showing >5% of neutrophils with visible pigment.
- Hypoglycaemia (<2.2 mmol/l).
- Hyperlactataemia (>5 mmol/l).
- Acidosis (arterial pH <7.3, serum HCO_3 <15 mmol/l).
- Elevated serum creatinine (>265 µmol/l).
- Elevated total bilirubin >50 µmol/l.
- Leucocytosis (>12,000/µl).
- Severe anaemia (PCV <15%).
- Coagulopathy.
  - Decreased platelet count (<50,000/µl).
  - Prolonged prothrombin time.
  - Decreased fibrinogen (<200 mg/dl).

Lactic acidosis: pH <7.3 or ↑ plasma and CSF lactate levels (plasma >5 mmol/l) and a low plasma HCO_3^- (<15 mmol/l) carry a poor prognosis in both adults and children. Acidosis is a major contributor to RD, especially in children.

Fluid and electrolyte disturbances: hypovolaemia and dehydration are thought to be common, although recently this has become controversial. Low Na^+, Cl^-, PO_4^-, Ca_2^+, Mg_2^+ and endocrine dysfunction also occur, but seldom have major clinical implications except in the severely ill.

Acute respiratory distress syndrome: carries a 50% mortality and may occur at a time when the patient is otherwise improving. Excessive fluid replacement exacerbates this complication and is suggested by ↑ respiratory rate (exclude aspiration or acidosis). Predisposing causes include hyperparasitaemia, renal failure, and pregnancy (may occur suddenly after delivery). Hypoxia may cause convulsions and death within a few hours.

Shock (algid malaria): cold, clammy cyanotic skin; weak rapid pulses; prolonged capillary refill time in children (>3 s); supine systolic BP <70 mmHg (<50 mmHg in children) suggests circulatory collapse. Shock in malaria is commonly associated with 2° bacterial infection, metabolic acidosis, pulmonary oedema, dehydration, or a gastrointestinal bleed.

Disseminated intravascular coagulation (DIC): is due to pathological activation of the coagulation cascade. DIC may manifest with bleeding gums, epistaxis, petechiae, haematemesis, and/or melaena with significant blood loss. DIC occurs in <10% of patients but is more common in non-immune people (especially travellers). Blood film shows thrombocytopenia and schistocytes (damaged red cells). There is ↑ prothrombin time (PT) and ↓ plasma fibrinogen.

Hyperparasitaemia: a parasite density >100,000 parasites/µl (about 2% of cells infected) is associated with ↑ mortality, although non-immune patients may die with much lower counts and in highly endemic areas individuals may tolerate greater densities without accompanying clinical features. Parasitaemias of >500,000 parasites/µl is associated with a 50% case fatality.

Gastrointestinal symptoms: are common in children. Nausea, vomiting, abdominal pain, and diarrhoea without blood or pus are frequently seen. Persistent vomiting requires urgent parenteral drug administration.

Secondary infection: with septicaemia, pneumonia (e.g. following aspiration), urinary tract infection (following catheterization) and postpartum sepsis are common. Gram negative septicaemia may occur without any focus of infection.

Differential diagnosis

Differential diagnosis of malaria

Malaria is a great mimic and must enter the differential diagnosis of several clinical presentations.

- The presentation of fever needs to be differentiated from other endemic diseases such as typhoid and rickettsial infections, viral illnesses such as dengue fever and influenza, brucellosis, and respiratory and urinary tract infections. Less common causes of tropical fevers include leishmaniasis, trypanosomiasis, and relapsing fevers.
- The coma of CM needs to be differentiated from meningitis (including tuberculous meningitis), encephalitis, enteric fevers, trypanosomiasis, brain abscess, and other causes of coma.
- The anaemia of malaria can be confused with other common causes of haemolytic anaemia in the tropics such as that due to the haemoglobinopathies. The anaemia of malaria must be differentiated from that of iron, folate, or vitamin B_{12} deficiency.
- The renal failure of malaria must be distinguished from massive intravascular haemolysis, sickle cell disease, leptospirosis, snake envenoming, use of traditional herbal medicines, and chronic renal disease resulting from glomerulonephritis and hypertension.
- The jaundice and hepatomegaly of malaria must be distinguished from that of viral hepatitis (A, B, and E, cytomegalovirus and Epstein–Barr virus infections), leptospirosis, yellow fever, biliary disease, and drug-induced disease including alcohol.

Clinical diagnosis on its own is notoriously inaccurate in the diagnosis of malaria and a blood film is desirable. However, in areas of stable transmission with high population parasite rates this can be very non-specific. If in doubt, presumptive antibiotic treatment should be given alongside antimalarial drugs.

Laboratory diagnosis

Blood films

The diagnosis of malaria requires identification of parasites in smears of blood. See blood film diagrams and thick/thin film methodology.

Maintain a high index of suspicion and carry out at ≥3 blood films. Infection may exceptionally occur via transfusion, needlestick injury, intravenous drug abuse, and during brief airport stopovers in endemic areas or when infected mosquitoes 'alight' from airplane flights from endemic areas and bite individuals ('airport' malaria). In falciparum malaria, the presence of schizonts in peripheral blood samples may indicate severe infection as these forms would normally sequester.

Pitfalls of blood films

- A single negative film does not exclude malaria. Repeat on 3 occasions at intervals. Blood films do not have to be taken at times of fever spikes. The patient may have been partially treated, suppressing patent infection. Malaria prophylaxis should be stopped whilst investigating for active infection.
- In endemic areas, a positive film does not prove that malaria is responsible for the current symptoms.
- Correlation between parasite density and disease severity may be poor — patients with a low parasitaemia may be very ill, whilst semi-immunes may harbour high parasitaemias with relatively few symptoms.
- Platelets, cell fragments, and impurities in the stain can be mistaken for malarial parasites.

Non-blood film malaria diagnostic tests

Currently available tests include dipstick antigen capture tests (e.g. Paracheck, ParaSight F, Malaria PF Test, OptiMAL test), phagocyte malarial pigment, quantitative buffy coat (QBC) method, PCR and serodiagnosis (only to be used exceptionally and in retrospect).

Rapid dipstick methods

- Paracheck, ParaSight F, and Malaria PF Test antigen capture tests use a monoclonal antibody to detect the histidine-rich protein II of *P. falciparum*. These are useful in those who have not had malaria before and require minimal expertise. However, they are expensive, not quantitative, and detect only the presence of *P. falciparum*.
- The OptiMAL® test detects parasite rather than human lactate dehydrogenase — hence pLDH. This test can distinguish *P. falciparum* from non-falciparum malaria infections.
- PCR is very useful in epidemiological studies.

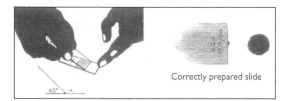

Fig. 2.3 Preparing blood film.

1. Clean the tip of the patient's left index finger.
2. Pierce the pulp of the fingertip with a sterile lancet or needle.
3. Squeeze the finger until a droplet of blood forms and place it onto the middle of a clean slide (holding the slide by the edges). This is for the thin film.
4. Place a further 3 droplets of blood onto the slide at a point to one side of the first droplet. These are for the thick film.
5. Using a second clean slide as a spreader, touch the first, small drop with the edge and allow the blood to run along its edge. With the spreading slide at 45°, push the spreader forwards slowly, ensuring even contact, so that the blood is spread as a thin film over the surface of the slide. (See Fig. 2.3)
6. Using the corner of the spreading slide, amalgamate the 3 drops of blood on the other half of the slide into a single small, denser film about 1 cm in diameter.
7. Label the slide with a pencil and allow to dry horizontally.

Problems: Badly positioned blood droplets, too much or too little blood, using a greasy slide, a chipped edge of the spreader slide.

Staining: (consult a laboratory manual for more details)

Giemsa stain: may be used for both films but is costly and difficult to do. It should be filtered before use. Thin films must first be fixed in anhydrous methanol then dipped in 10% Giemsa for 20–30 mins; thick films in 5% solution for 30 mins.

Field's stain: uses 2 solutions, A and B, that are cheaper and more suited to rapid bulk staining. For thick films, dip dried slides into solution A for 5 secs, avoiding agitation. Wash in tap water (preferably neutral pH) for 5 secs, then dip into solution B for 3 secs. Wash again in water for 5 secs, then allow to dry vertically. The centre of the film may not be stained, but optimal parasite staining occurs at the edges of the film. For thin films, use solution B before solution A.

Leishman's stain: may be used for thin films. 0.5 ml stain is added to each horizontal film, left for 30 secs, then 1.5 ml of buffered water added and left for 8 min. The slide is then washed in tap water.

Blood film identification of malarial parasites

1. Are there one or more red-stained chromatin dots and blue cytoplasm?
   YES — go to 2. NO — what you see is not a parasite.
2. Are the size and shape correct for a malaria parasite?
   YES — go to 3. NO — what you see is not a malaria parasite.
3. Is there malaria pigment in the cell?
   YES — go to 7. NO — go to 4.
4. Does the parasite have one chromatin dot attached to blue cytoplasm in the form of a regular ring in the cytoplasm?
   YES — this is a trophozoite. NO — go to 5.
5. Does the parasite have one chromatin dot attached to blue cytoplasm in the form of a small solid or regular ring or with a vacuole?
   YES — this is a trophozoite. NO — go to 6.
6. Is the parasite with one chromatin dot irregular or fragmented?
   YES — this is a trophozoite. NO — go to 8.
7. Does the parasite with malaria pigment have one chromatin dot?
   YES — go to 8. NO — go to 9.
8. Does the parasite have a vacuole or is it fragmented in some way?
   YES — this is probably a late trophozoite stage. NO — go to 11.
9. Does the parasite have 2 chromatin dots attached to a ring and have a vacuole?
   YES — this is a trophozoite. NO — go to 10.
10. Does the parasite have between 2 and 32 chromatin dots and pigment?
    YES — this is a schizont.
11. Is the parasite rounded or 'banana-shaped'?
    Rounded — go to 12. Banana-shaped — go to 14.
12. Does the rounded parasite have clearly stained chromatin and a deep blue cytoplasm?
    YES — this is a female gametocyte. NO — go to 13.
13. Does the rounded parasite have a reddish overall colour, so that the chromatin is indistinct?
    YES — this is a male gametocyte.
14. Does the 'banana-shaped' parasite have densely stained blue cytoplasm and bright red chromatin?
    YES — this is a female gametocyte. NO — go to 15.
15. Does the 'banana-shaped' parasite have a reddish overall colour, so that the chromatin is indistinct?
    YES — this is a male gametocyte.

From: WHO (1991) *Basic malaria microscopy — learner's guide*, WHO, Geneva.

	Early trophozoite (ring form)	Mature trophozoite
Plasmodium vivax	Thick rings, 1/3 – 1/2 the diameter of the red cell 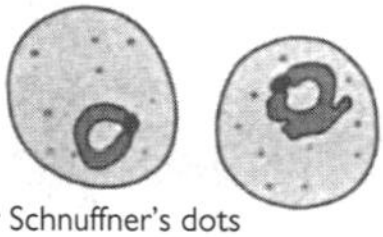 A few Schnuffner's dots Accolé (Shoulder) forms and double dots less common than with *P. falciparum*	Ameboid rings, 1/2 – 2/3 the diameter of the red cell Pale blue or lilac parasite with prominent central valuole 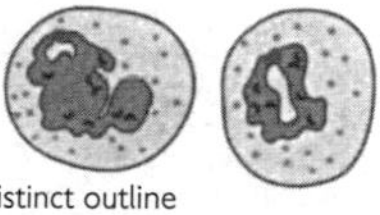 Indistinct outline Scattered fine yellowish-brown pigment granules or rods
Plasmodium ovale	Thick, compact rings, 1/3 – 1/2 the diameter of the red cell 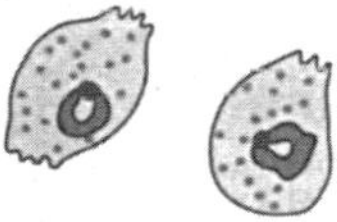 Numerous Schuffner's dots but paler than with *P. vivax*	Thick rings, less irregular than those of *P. vivax*, 1/3 – 1/2 the diameter of the red cell 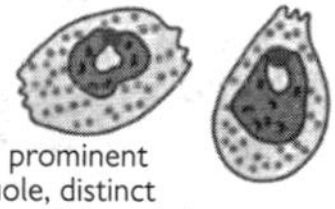 Less prominent vacuole, distinct outline Yellowish brown pigment which is coarser and darker than that of *P. vivax* Schuffner's dots prominent
Plasmodium falciparum	Delicate rings, 1/6 – 1/4 the diameter of the red cell 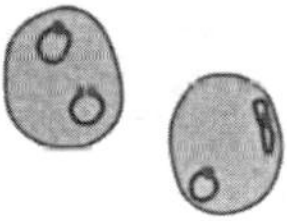 Double dots and Accolé forms common	Fairly delicate rings, 1/3 – 1/2 the diameter of the red cell 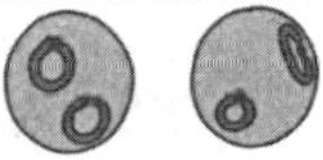 Red-mauve stippling (Maurer's dots or clefts) may be present Mature trophozoites are less often present in peripheral blood than ring forms
Plasmodium malariae	Small, thick, compact rings Small chromatin dot which may be inside the ring 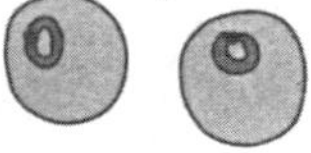 Double dots and Accolé forms rare	Ameboid form more compact than *P. vivax* Sometimes angular or band forms 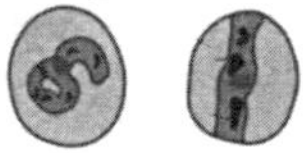 Heavy, dark-yellow-brown pigment No stippling unless overstained

Fig. 2.4 Diagrams of malarial blood cells. (Reproduced with permission from Bain BJ (1995) *Blood cells. A practical guide.* Blackwell Science, Oxford).

	Early trophozoite (ring form)	Mature trophozoite
Plasmodium vivax	Thick rings, 1/3 – 1/2 the diameter of the red cell 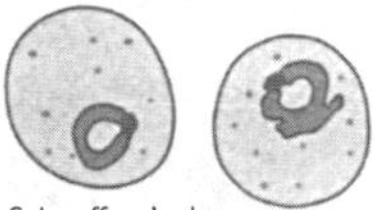 A few Schnuffner's dots Accolé (Shoulder) forms and double dots less common than with *P. falciparum*	Ameboid rings, 1/2 – 2/3 the diameter of the red cell Pale blue or lilac parasite with prominent central valuole 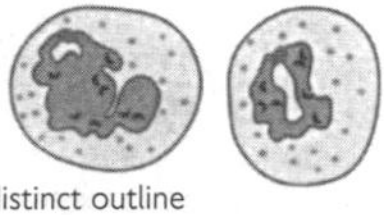 Indistinct outline Scattered fine yellowish-brown pigment granules or rods
Plasmodium ovale	Thick, compact rings, 1/3 – 1/2 the diameter of the red cell 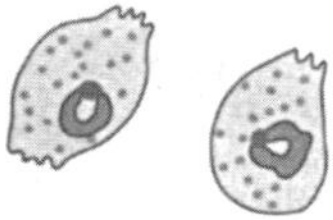 Numerous Schuffner's dots but paler than with *P. vivax*	Thick rings, less irregular than those of *P. vivax*, 1/3 – 1/2 the diameter of the red cell 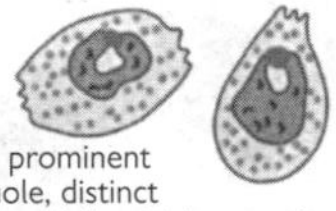 Less prominent vacuole, distinct outline Yellowish brown pigment which is coarser and darker than that of *P. vivax* Schuffner's dots prominent
Plasmodium falciparum	Delicate rings, 1/6 – 1/4 the diameter of the red cell 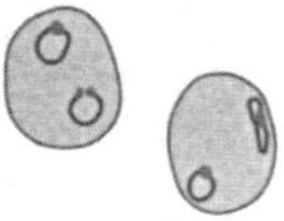 Double dots and Accolé forms common	Fairly delicate rings, 1/3 – 1/2 the diameter of the red cell 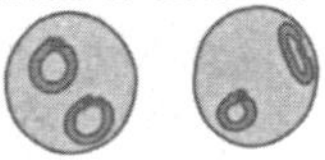 Red-mauve stippling (Maurer's dots or clefts) may be present Mature trophozoites are less often present in peripheral blood than ring forms
Plasmodium malariae	Small, thick, compact rings Small chromatin dot which may be inside the ring 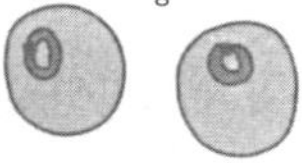 Double dots and Accolé forms rare	Ameboid form more compact than *P. vivax* Sometimes angular or band forms 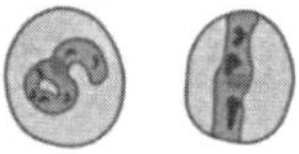 Heavy, dark-yellow-brown pigment No stippling unless ovestained

Fig. 2.4 *Continued* Diagrams of malarial blood cells. (Reproduced with permission from Bain BJ (1995) *Blood cells. A practical guide.* Blackwell Science, Oxford).

	Early schizont	Late schizont
Plasmodium vivax	Rounded or irregular Ameboid Loose central mass of fine yellowish-brown pigment 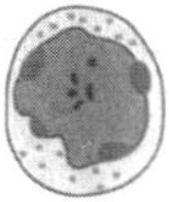 Schizont almost fills cell Schuffner's dots	12–24 (usually 16–24) medium-sized merozoites 1–2 clumps of peripheral pigment 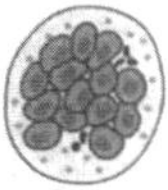 Schizont almost fills cell Schuffner's dots
Plasmodium ovale	Round, compact Darkish brown pigment, heavier and coarser than that of *P. vivax* 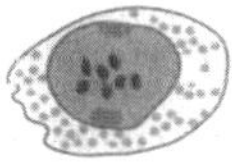 Schuffner's dots	6–12 (usually 8) large merozoites arranged irregularly like a bunch of grapes 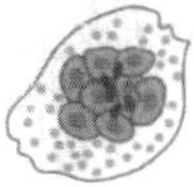 Central pigment Schuffner's dots
Plasmodium falciparum	Not usually seen in blood Very small, ameboid Scattered light-brown to black pigment	Not usually seen in blood 8–32 (usually few) very small merozoites; grouped irregularly Peripheral clump of coarse dark brown pigment
Plasmodium malariae	Compact, round, fills red cell 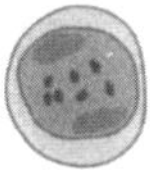 Coarse dark yellow-brown pigment	6–12 (usually 8–10) large merozoites, arranged symmetrically, often in a rosette or daisy head formation 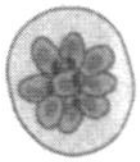 Central coarse dark yellowish-brown pigment

Fig. 2.4 *Continued* Diagrams of malarial blood cells. (Reproduced with permission from Bain BJ (1995) Blood cells. A practical guide. Blackwell Science, Oxford).

General management

Decide whether the patient has falciparum malaria or a benign malaria. If there are signs of severe falciparum infection, do not wait for laboratory confirmation. Weigh the patient and start treatment immediately.

Basic rules

- In many instances, especially in endemic areas, uncomplicated malaria can be treated on an outpatient basis.
- Await blood film results for uncomplicated malaria.
- Advise patients to return promptly if symptoms worsen or do not improve within 48 h.
- Beware of sending home patients who have mild symptoms but high levels of parasitaemia since they may deteriorate rapidly.

All patients will require antimalarial chemotherapy

Antimalarial treatment with appropriate antimalarial drugs should be started immediately. Choose the drug regimen bearing in mind likely compliance and side-effects, local resistance, and costs — see next page. Take into account the locally recommended chemotherapy.

Many patients will need antipyretics and analgesics

If fever causes distress or the child is prone to febrile convulsions, an antipyretic should be given orally or by suppository. In two studies, paracetamol has been shown to prolong parasite clearance, though the clinical significance of this is unclear. Several studies demonstrated a greater antipyretic effect with ibuprofen, which should be considered if there are no contraindications. Avoid aspirin in children — both because of Reye's syndrome and because aspirin can exacerbate acidosis. For hyperpyrexia, begin tepid sponging and fanning quickly to ↓ the likelihood of febrile convulsions. Consider giving intramuscular antipyretics.

Management

1. Assess the Airway, Breathing, and Circulation and intervene where necessary. Record vital signs: temperature, pulse, BP respiratory rate and capillary refill time (in children).

2. Obtain good quality venous access and take blood for investigations including blood film, haemoglobin or haematocrit, blood glucose, blood group and crossmatch. If available, do blood culture, biochemistry (electrolytes, renal and liver function), arterial blood gases analysis, and coagulation studies.

WHO Guidelines for the Treatment of Malaria 2006

The WHO guidelines encompass all of the recent important developments in the treatment of malaria, both uncomplicated and severe. The guideline development process was strictly evidence-based, and the resulting book is a valuable resource on all aspects of treatment. The guidelines discuss in detail two major recent developments in antimalarial therapy:

1. The wide acceptance and recommendation of artemisinin-based combination therapy (ACT) as the treatment of choice for uncomplicated falciparum malaria. The main clinical advantages of ACTs are a rapid therapeutic response and rapid initial reduction in the parasite biomass; in addition, they reduce the chance of drug resistance emerging and spreading and may — through their gametocytocidal effect — interfere with transmission.

2. The recommendation that artesunate, the most rapidly acting parenteral antimalarial, is now the drug of choice in preference to quinine for the treatment of severe malaria in low transmission areas and in the second and third trimesters of pregnancy, and a drug of choice alongside quinine in high transmission areas and in the first trimester of pregnancy.

The complete guidelines can be downloaded as a PDF from the WHO website on:
www.who.int/malaria/docs/TreatmentGuidelines2006.pdf

3. Treat hypoglycaemia if present. Give 50% dextrose 50 ml (children: 10% dextrose 5 ml/kg) by slow IV bolus if hypoglycaemic (blood glucose <2.2 mmol). Follow this with 10% dextrose infusion (0.1 ml/kg/hr). Monitor blood glucose levels 4 to 6 hourly, especially following infusion of quinine.

4. Weigh patient and initiate antimalarial therapy — see next page.

5. Consider empirical broad-spectrum antibiotic therapy if hypotensive or suspicion of bacterial infection (in Kenya bacteraemia occurs in 8 to 12% of children with severe malaria).

6. Lumbar puncture Patients with ↓ levels of consciousness should have a lumbar puncture to exclude bacterial meningitis. If there is concern about raised intracranial pressure, this can be delayed but antibiotic cover should be given.

7. Assess hydration Consider urinary catheterization and central venous line to monitor the central venous pressure. Rehydration may be required, particularly if diarrhoea and vomiting are present. Aggressive fluid resuscitation in children with severe malaria may be indicated but is controversial. Adults with severe falciparum malaria usually require 1–3 L of isotonic saline over the first 24 h — however, avoid overhydration.

8. Monitor renal output and BP hourly, and aim to keep central venous pressure (if available) in the low–normal range.

9. Blood transfusion with pathogen-free, compatible fresh blood or packed cells should be considered in patients with a haematocrit <15% or Hb <5 g/dl. Transfusion should be given urgently in children with a Hb <4 g/dl or a Hb <5 g/dl with respiratory distress or acidosis or parasitaemia >10%; in such cases, give blood 10 ml/kg over 30 mins, then a further 10 ml/kg over 2–3 h without diuretics. In DIC, fresh blood, clotting factors (FFP), and/or platelets should be given as required.

10. Exchange transfusion can be considered in some situations, especially parasitaemias >30%, although it has not been subject to a randomized controlled trial.

11. Dialysis if the patient is oliguric and develops renal failure — haemofiltration or haemodialysis may be indicated. Peritoneal dialysis should be used if these are unavailable but is less effective.

12. Oxygen and mechanical ventilation may be required for patients with respiratory distress or significantly raised ICP. If distress is due to pulmonary oedema, the patient should be nursed at 45° and IV diuretics given. Haemofiltration may be used if available.

13. Inotropes such as dopamine may be given through a central line if hypotension does not respond to volume expansion. Adrenaline should be avoided as it can exacerbate acidosis.

Cerebral malaria

Treat as above with the following additional specific measures:
- Nurse the patient on her side to avoid aspiration of vomit. Turn every two hours.
- The patient should be catheterized and have temperature, heart and respiratory rates, BP, and fluid balance measured regularly.
- Consciousness must be assessed regularly with the Glasgow or Blantyre Coma Scales.
- Hypoglycaemia must be treated promptly but is very difficult to detect in an unconscious patient. Blood sugar should be actively monitored at least 4–6 hourly and whenever there is any deterioration in the patient's clinical condition.
- If convulsions arise — be alert since they may be subtle — treat with diazepam 0.30 mg/kg (up to a maximum of 10 mg in adults) by slow IV injection. An alternative is diazepam 0.5 mg/kg rectally. Hypoglycaemia must be sought and treated if present.
- Avoid corticosteroids, mannitol, or other ancillary agents for cerebral oedema since they are of no proven benefit.

Antimalarial chemotherapy

There have been recent major changes in the treatment of malaria, particularly the use of artemisinin-based combination therapies (ACTs) for the treatment of uncomplicated falciparum malaria and the emergence of parenteral artesunate as the drug of choice for severe malaria. Resistance to many antimalarial drugs is an increasing problem worldwide and it is important to have up-to-date information on local resistance patterns. Chloroquine, for example, can no longer be used to treat falciparum malaria in most parts of the world. At the time of writing (2007) there is no clinically apparent resistance to the artemisinin derivatives, though resistance to the partner drugs in the ACT combinations is a major problem in many areas.

Artemisinin-based combination therapies (ACTs)

Combination therapy is the simultaneous use of two or more blood schizonticidal agents with independent modes of action. The aim is to reduce the spread of resistance, with the two components protecting each other. This principle has been widely applied in the treatment of HIV/AIDS and TB. In ACTs, one of these agents is an artemisinin derivative, the most rapidly acting class of antimalarial. This ensures a rapid fall in parasitaemia, reducing the total number of parasites at risk of developing resistance. Artemisinin derivatives are also gametocytocidal and thus may reduce malaria transmission.

Partial courses of ACTs should not be given, even when patients are considered to be semi-immune or the diagnosis is uncertain — this may encourage the development of resistance.

Treatment of uncomplicated *P. falciparum* malaria

- In the treatment of uncomplicated malaria, the aim is to reduce the parasitaemia as quickly as possible and to prevent recrudescence of the infection. Antimalarial drugs are given orally if tolerated. If the species is unknown or there is mixed infection, treat as falciparum malaria.
- ACTs are now the recommended treatment of choice for uncomplicated falciparum malaria worldwide. Monotherapy is specifically discouraged.
- Be aware of local patterns of resistance, particularly to the artemisinin derivative partner drug. These will influence the first-line ACT for the area.
- Treatment failures within 14 days of receiving an ACT should be treated with a second-line antimalarial (see below).
- Treatment failures (recurrent parasitaemia) after 14 days can be retreated with the original first-line ACT. However, retreatment with mefloquine within 28 days is associated with an ↑ risk of neuropsychiatric disorder, so if the first-line ACT was artesunate + mefloquine, a second-line antimalarial should be given.

Treatment of the benign malarias

- The standard recommended treatment remains chloroquine 25 mg base/kg divided over 3 days (e.g. 10 mg base/kg followed by 5 mg base/kg at 6 h, 24 h, and 36 h).
- The hypnozoite stages of *P. ovale* and *P. vivax* are not affected by blood scizonticides such as chloroquine, so to prevent relapses and effect a 'radical cure', the liver schizonticide, primaquine, must be given as well (0.25 mg base/kg daily (0.375–0.5 mg base/kg daily in SE Asia and Oceania where relatively primaquine-resistant strains occur)). *P. malariae* does not produce hypnozoite forms.
- Primaquine is an oxidant and causes haemolysis in G6PD-deficient individuals. Screening is generally unavailable, but in areas where mild G6PD deficiency is the common variant, primaquine in weekly doses of 0.75 mg base/kg for 8 weeks is better tolerated. Primaquine should not be given in severe G6PD deficiency. It should also not be given to pregnant women.
- Chloroquine-resistant *P. vivax* is increasingly a problem (particularly in Oceania, Indonesia, and Peru), and can be treated with amodiaquine 10 mg base/kg daily for 3 days, combined with primaquine.

The benign malarias are susceptible to all ACTs (the exception being *P. vivax* and artesunate + sulfadoxine-pyrimethamine(SP), since *P. vivax* responds poorly to SP monotherapy in many areas). Primaquine would still be required for radical cure.

Radical cures and primaquine

- Treatment with a blood schizontocidal drug, such as quinine, will not eliminate parasites from the liver. Therefore, patients infected with *P. vivax* or *P. ovale* are also given primaquine to kill the liver hypnozoites and prevent recrudescence later. *P. malariae* does not produce persistent liver forms.
- Since primaquine is also gametocidal, it is sometimes given to patients infected with *P. falciparum* in non-endemic regions. This prevents the blood gametocytes being taken up by local mosquitoes and possibly initiating local foci of infections.
- A major drawback is primaquine's ability to cause severe intravascular haemolysis in patients with G6PD deficiency. Weekly doses of 45 mg for up to 8 weeks are better tolerated in such patients than daily doses of 15 mg for 14–21 days.
- Relatively primaquine-resistant strains of *P. vivax* have been reported (in the Pacific region) that require at least 6 mg/kg total dose (~2 × normal dose).

Currently recommended ACTs

Artemether + lumefantrine (Co-artem®, Riamet®): fixed-dose combination (artemether 20 mg/lumefantrine 120 mg in each tablet) suitable for use in areas of multidrug resistance (SE Asia) as well as worldwide. Six doses over 3 days. Should be taken with milk or fat-containing food. Now recommended for children ≥5 kg.

Adult dose: (body wt >35 kg): 4 tablets at 0 h, 8 h, 24 h, 36 h, 48 h, and 60 h. *Paediatric dose*: reduce the number of tablets at each dose: body wt 25–34 kg, 3 tablets per dose; 15–24 kg, 2 per dose; 5–14 kg, 1 per dose.

Artesunate + mefloquine: the prototype ACT, with a fixed-dose combination under development. Suitable for use in areas of multidrug resistance (SE Asia); effective elsewhere but expensive. Currently available as separate scored artesunate (50 mg) and mefloquine (250 mg base) tablets. 3 day course.

Adult dose (>13 yrs): artesunate 200 mg on days 1, 2, and 3; mefloquine 1000 mg on day 2 and 500 mg on day 3.

Paediatric doses: 7–13 yrs, artesunate 100 mg on days 1, 2, and 3, mefloquine 500 mg on day 2 and 250 mg on day 3; 1–6 yrs: artesunate 50 mg on days 1, 2, and 3, mefloquine 250 mg on day 2; 5–11 months: artesunate 25 mg (1/2 tablet) on days 1, 2, and 3; mefloquine 125 mg (1/2 tablet) day 2.

Artesunate + sulfadoxine-pyrimethamine (SP): currently available as separate scored artesunate (50 mg) and SP (500/25 mg) tablets. Only suitable for areas where SP monotherapy 28-day cure rates exceed 80%. Useful in some parts of Africa but these are diminishing rapidly.

Adult dose (>13 yrs): artesunate 200 mg on days 1, 2 and 3; SP 3 tablets (1500/75 mg) on day 1.

Paediatric doses: 7–13 yrs, artesunate 100 mg on days 1, 2, and 3, SP 2 tablets (1000/50 mg) on day 1; 1–6 yrs: artesunate 50 mg on days 1, 2, and 3, SP 1 tablet (500/25 mg) on day 1; 5–11 months: artesunate 1/2 tablet (25 mg) on days 1, 2, and 3, SP 1/2 tablet (250/12.5 mg) on day 1.

Artesunate + amodiaquine: now available as a fixed-dose combination (each adult tablet contains artesunate/amodiaquine 100/270 mg, paediatric tablet 25/67.5 mg). Only suitable for areas where amodiaquine monotherapy 28-day cure rates exceed 80% (mainly West Africa).

Adult dose (>13 yrs): 2 adult tablets once daily for 3 days.

Paediatric doses: 7–13 yrs, 1 adult tablet once daily for 3 days; 1–7 yrs, 2 paediatric tablets once daily for 3 days; <1 yr, 1 paediatric tablet once daily for 3 days (not officially recommended for infants <24 months).

ACTs under development

Dihydroartemisinin (DHA) + piperaquine (Artekin©) is a promising fixed-dose combination, already used in Cambodia and Vietnam. It is suitable for treating multidrug-resistant malaria, cheap, and should be available soon in a GMP formulation. Artesunate + pyronaridine and artesunate + chlorproguanil-dapsone combinations are also under development.

Non-artemisinin based combination therapies

SP + chloroquine is not recommended as resistance to both components is already widespread and no synergy has been demonstrated. SP + amodiaquine in areas of parasite sensitivity may be more effective than either drug alone but less rapidly acting than ACTs. Therefore only recommended when ACTs are unavailable.

Second-line antimalarials for falciparum malaria

Used in cases of treatment failure <14 days after receiving an ACT.
In order of preference they are:
1. an alternative ACT known to be effective in the region (generally a 3-day course).
2. artesunate (2 mg/kg od) plus either tetracycline (4 mg/kg q6 h) or doxycycline (3.5 mg/kg od) or clindamycin (10 mg/kg q12 h).
3. quinine (10 mg salt/kg q8 h) plus either tetracycline (4 mg/kg q6 h) or doxycycline (3.5 mg/kg od) or clindamycin (10 mg/kg q12 h).

Regimens 2 and 3 should be given for 7 days. The quinine regimens are poorly tolerated and adherence is often poor. Doxycycline and tetracycline should not be used in pregnancy or in children under 8 yrs.

Pregnant women

- *First trimester:* quinine and clindamycin (see doses above) given for 7 days. If clindamycin is unavailable, give quinine monotherapy. Use an ACT if it is the only effective treatment available.
- *Second and third trimesters:* an ACT that is known to be effective in the region, or artesunate + clindamycin (7 days) or quinine + clindamycin (7 days).

Treatment of severe malaria

Severe malaria is a medical emergency. Full doses of parenteral antimalarial therapy should be started immediately and continued until the patient is well enough to take oral follow-on treatment (see below). The options are:

1. Artesunate 2.4 mg/kg IV or IM at 0 h, 12 h, 24 h, then once daily. Artesunate is the WHO recommended therapy in low transmission or non-malaria endemic areas, and a recommended therapy in high transmission areas.

- In a multi-country study of severe malaria, IV artesunate was associated with a 35% relative reduction in mortality compared with IV quinine.
- The currently available formulation of artesunate is non-GMP, although it is this formulation that has demonstrated superior efficacy over quinine in low transmission areas. A GMP formulation is being developed.

2. Quinine 20 mg salt/kg loading dose on admission, then 10 mg salt/kg q8 h thereafter, each dose given by rate-controlled IV infusion over 4 h or by divided IM injection. It is a WHO recommended therapy in high transmission areas.

- For IV infusion, quinine must be diluted in 5–10 ml/kg body weight of dextrose or saline solution. For IM use, quinine should be diluted in normal saline to 60 mg salt/ml and half the dose given in each anterior thigh. IM injection can cause abscess formation and has been associated with the development of tetanus.
- Quinine is associated with severe hyperinsulinaemic hypoglycaemia, particularly in pregnant women.
- In acute renal failure or hepatic dysfunction, the dose should be reduced by one third after 48 h to prevent accumulation and resulting toxicity. Dose adjustment in renal failure is unnecessary if the patient is receiving haemofiltration or haemodialysis.
- The first dose can be reduced to 10 mg salt/kg if there is certainty that the patient has received adequate pre-treatment with quinine before presentation. If in doubt, give the loading dose.

3. Artemether IM into the anterior thigh 3.2 mg/kg then 1.6 mg/kg per day. Artemether absorption from IM injection is erratic, especially in very ill patients. It is a WHO recommended therapy in high transmission areas.

4. Quinidine If the other, recommended, parenteral antimalarials are unavailable (e.g. in the USA), the anti-arrhythmic drug quinidine (an enantiomer of quinine) may be used. Give 15 mg base/kg infused IV over 4 h, followed by 7.5 mg base/kg over 4 h q8 h. Cardiac monitoring is required. Dose adjustments are necessary in renal failure and hepatic impairment as for quinine. Convert to oral therapy as soon as possible.

Pregnancy

Give the parenteral antimalarial used locally for severe malaria in full doses. Because quinine causes severe recurrent hypoglycaemia, where available, artesunate is the first choice and artemether the second choice in the 2nd and 3rd trimesters. As little evidence is available in the 1st trimester, artesunate, quinine, and artemether may all be considered options.

Pre-referral treatment

Rectal artesunate is well absorbed and is an option to buy time and prevent progression of severe disease while referral to a health care facility capable of giving parenteral treatment is made. Quinine can also be given intrarectally in such circumstances.

Follow-on treatment

Following initial parenteral therapy, when the patient is well enough to take oral medication, an oral antimalarial should be given to complete treatment and prevent recrudescence. Complete 7 days' treatment with an oral formulation of the parenteral drug + 7 days of doxycycline or clindamycin (in children and pregnant women). Alternatively, a standard full course of oral ACT can be given.

Chemoprophylaxis

Chemoprophylaxis against malaria rarely provides full protection and measures should be taken at all times to reduce the number of mosquito bites. Use insect repellents containing DEET (10 to 50%) or picardin (7%), and sleep under insecticide-treated bed nets in areas where mosquitoes bite indoors at night. Individuals should be aware of malarial symptoms, which may be non-specific, and report early for a blood film if malaria is suspected.

Travellers to malarial areas: should preferably begin prophylaxis 1 week (2–3 weeks in the case of mefloquine) before arrival, and must continue for 4 weeks after departure, except in the cases of atovaquone-proguanil and primaquine where prophylaxis may be commenced the day before entry into a malarious area and ended 7 days after return from a malarious area.

Any febrile illness occurring within 1 year of travel could be malaria. For long-term, non-immune residents there is a balance between the risks of infection and the side-effects of chemoprophylaxis. It may be possible to target prophylaxis during the transmission season alone.

Malaria endemic areas: antimalarial prophylaxis is not logistically or financially feasible. Intermittent presumptive treatment (IPT) is an alternative which shows some promise and may work at least partly through its prophylactic effects.

Drugs used in prophylaxis

Atovaquone-proguanil, mefloquine, doxycycline, and primaquine can all be used as prophylaxis throughout the malaria endemic world, whereas the usefulness of chloroquine and proguanil has been severely restricted by resistance.

1. *Atovaquone-proguanil (Malarone®):* well-tolerated, once-daily, fixed-dose combination effective against all types of malaria, including multidrug-resistant falciparum malaria. Should be taken with food and a milky drink to improve absorption. There is insufficient data to recommend its use in pregnancy, and it is very expensive.

Dose: adult daily dose 250/100 mg; 3.75/1.5 mg/kg in children <13 yrs.

2. Mefloquine: now a favoured drug for the prophylaxis of malaria in many areas where chloroquine resistance is present.

Nausea, dizziness, and vivid dreams are common side-effects, and approximately 1 in 10,000 recipients develops an acute reversible neuro-psychiatric reaction. Mefloquine is not recommended in neonates but has been used for prophylaxis in pregnancy.

Dose: 250 mg PO weekly in adults & children >45 kg (62.5 mg weekly in children 6–16 kg; 125 mg for 16–25 kg, 187.5 mg for 25–45 kg).

3. Doxycycline: useful as an alternate to mefloquine.

Dose: 1.5 mg/kg PO once daily, up to a max of 100 mg. Do not use in children <8 yrs and in pregnant and lactating women.

4. Primaquine: has proven in adults to be effective and safe against drug resistant *P. falciparum* and *P. vivax*. Should be taken with food to reduce gastrointestinal side-effects. Should not be given to G6PD-deficient individuals or pregnant women.

Dose: 0.5 mg base/kg or 30 mg, daily adult dose.

5. Proguanil: used for prophylaxis in pregnant women and non-immune people in areas of low risk only. It is more commonly used in combination with chloroquine (see below). Of limited use now due to resistance.

Dose: 200 mg PO daily in adults, including pregnant women. Children <12 wks 25 mg/day; 12 wks–1 yr 50 mg/day; 1–4 yrs 75 mg/day; 5–8 yrs 100 mg/day, and 9–14 yrs 150 mg/day.

A folic acid supplement should be taken during pregnancy.

6. Chloroquine: is used in combination with proguanil in low-risk areas, in pregnant women, and in individuals who cannot tolerate other antimalarials. It is not effective against most *P. falciparum* strains worldwide and resistance in *P. vivax* is also increasing.

Dose: 300 mg (as base) PO weekly in adults, including pregnant women. Children require 5 mg/kg weekly.

See *http://www.rbm.who.int/wmr2005/html/map5.htm*
for information on areas with resistant malaria.

Monitoring antimalarial drug resistance

With the rapid recent spread of drug resistance, there is an increased need to monitor the current levels of resistance to provide evidence to inform the choice of antimalarial drug therapy and ensure proper management of clinical cases. The monitoring systems available include:

1. Therapeutic efficacy testing: the WHO have developed a protocol for in vivo testing of the efficacy of antimalarial drugs against *P. falciparum* in the field (*www.who.int/malaria/docs/ProtocolWHO.pdf*). It is a simple one arm trial, with the treatment outcomes classified into:

Early treatment failure (ETF)
- Development of danger signs or severe malaria on days 1 to 3 in the presence of parasitaemia.
- Parasitaemia on day 2 higher than the day 0 count irrespective of axillary temperature.
- Parasitaemia on day 3 with axillary temperature ≥37.5°C.
- Parasitaemia on day 3 that is ≥25% of count on day 0.

Late clinical failure (LCF)
- Development of danger signs or severe malaria after day 3 in the presence of parasitaemia, without previously meeting any ETF criteria.
- Presence of parasitaemia and axillary temperature ≥ 37.5°C on any day from day 4 to day 28, without previously meeting any ETF criteria.

Late parasitological failure (LPF)
- Presence of parasitaemia on any day from day 7 to day 28 and axillary temperature <37.5°C, without previously meeting any of the criteria of ETF or LCF.

Adequate clinical and parasitological response (ACPR)
- Absence of parasitaemia on day 28 irrespective of axillary temperature without previously meeting any of the criteria of ETC or LCF or LPF.
- 'Clinical failure' can be summarized as ETF + LCF.
- 'Total failure' can be summarized as ETF + LCF + LPF.

2. In vitro resistance tests: technologically demanding and limited by exclusion of host factors and parasite factors unrelated to resistance. These tests are useful for providing additional information to support clinical efficacy data.

3. Molecular markers: if the molecular basis for resistance is known, these techniques can provide early warning of the presence of resistance to a range of antimalarial tests in a parasite population and guide therapeutic choices in epidemic situations. They do not always correlate well with therapeutic efficacy.

Malaria control   **PUBLIC HEALTH NOTE**

The three main limbs of malaria control are:
1. Effective antimalarial drug treatment, particularly with ACTs which may reduce transmission through their gametocytocidal effect.
2. Vector control by insecticide spraying, particularly indoor, and larval control (draining stagnant water, removing litter and debris that retain water and provide a mosquito breeding ground, and use of larvicides and larvivorous fish).
3. Personal protection with insecticide-impregnated materials such as bed nets and curtains.

Education of the population on the importance and practical application of all three of these is a pre-requisite for success.

The resources to apply these principles have benefited through major investment from e.g. Global Fund for HIV/AIDS, Malaria & Tuberculosis, the Roll Back Malaria Initiative, and the President's Malaria Initiative. Unfortunately, eradication is not yet feasible because of the huge number of infected individuals, the ecological success of the vectors, the continued widespread use of ineffective drugs, and the under-resourced health care and public health infrastructure in many parts of the tropical world. The current aims are to reduce morbidity, prevent mortality, and reduce socio-economic loss. There have been some successes: malaria incidence has been greatly reduced in some areas of unstable transmission, such as Vietnam, Thailand, and South Africa; and in East and West Africa, widespread deployment of insecticide-treated bed nets has been shown to reduce mortality.

A malaria vaccine has been the holy grail of malaria researchers for decades, but while there have been major recent advances, an effective, deployable vaccine is still a long way off. Further research is needed into the biology of the vector and the parasite and their interaction with the human host, the pathophysiology of the disease process, and the socio-cultural factors that determine health-seeking behaviour and compliance with drug regimens. In particular, there is an urgent need to discover and develop novel classes of antimalarial drug if we are not to face a malaria control catastrophe if and when the parasite develops resistance to the artemisinin derivatives.

HIV/AIDS

Section editors   **Graeme A Meintjes**
                      Andy G Parrish

HIV infection/AIDS

The human immunodeficiency viruses are the cause of the acquired immunodeficiency syndrome (AIDS) global pandemic.

Epidemiology

The first AIDS cases were recognized in the USA in 1981 and it is estimated that to date >25 million people have died as a result of HIV infection worldwide. An estimated 40 million people are living with HIV infection worldwide: 38 million adults and 2 million children <15 years old. 60% of those with HIV infection live in sub-saharan Africa, where 7% of the adult population is HIV infected. Seroprevalence rates among pregnant women are 30–40% in certain southern African nations. There are also rapidly growing HIV epidemics in eastern Europe and in central and east Asia.

HIV-1 accounts for most cases in the global pandemic; HIV-2 infection is found mainly in West Africa and people from that region. It has 40–60% genetic homology with HIV-1. It is less transmissible and is associated with a slower rate of CD4 and clinical decline. Many patients with HIV-2 are co-infected with HIV-1. 3rd generation ELISAs will diagnose both HIV-1 and 2 whereas earlier generation ELISAs and some of the rapid tests only diagnose HIV-1. HIV-1 viral load assays will not detect HIV-2. HIV-2 is intrinsically resistant to the non-nucleoside reverse transcriptase inhibitors (NNRTIs) and may carry pre-existing protease inhibitor (PI) mutations.

Transmission

Potentially infectious bodily fluids are: blood, serous effusions, cerebrospinal fluid, semen, vaginal fluid, and breast milk. Urine, vomitus, and saliva are non-infectious unless they are contaminated with blood. The virus survives poorly in the environment: no cases of environmental transmission are documented.

The main routes of HIV transmission are:

- Unprotected sexual intercourse (both heterosexual and homosexual). STIs, particularly those that cause genital ulceration, increase the risk of sexual transmission. In the developing world, heterosexual intercourse is the major mode of transmission for adults.
- Mother to child transmission (the highest risk is at the time of delivery, but transmission may also occur during the pregnancy or via breast milk). In the absence of preventative strategies, the risk of transmission in non-breastfeeding populations is 15–30%, but increases to 20–45% in breastfeeding women.
- Receipt of infected blood products (screening of blood products minimizes this risk).
- Injections or treatments with unsterile needles, syringes, surgical apparatus, or skin-piercing instruments.
- Needlestick injuries to health care workers. The risk is estimated to be 0.3% if no post-exposure prophylaxis is administered.

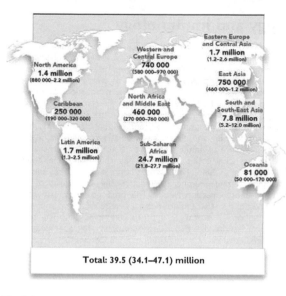

Fig. 3.1 Adults and Children estimated to be living with HIV in 2006.
Source UNAIDS and WHO.

Virology and immunology

Once HIV infects a human it attaches to and enters immune cells that bear the CD4 protein on their surface — mainly CD4 T-lymphocytes and macrophages. Within these cells, the virus replicates using viral enzymes such as reverse transcriptase and protease as well as hijacking human cellular mechanisms for RNA and protein production. During this process, copies of viral DNA are inserted into the chromosomal DNA of the host cell. Billions of new HIV particles are formed daily in this way in an infected person. The immune system responds by destroying the formed viruses, keeping the circulating virus at a constant or 'setpoint'. This results in a state of immune activation that persists for many years, during which the CD4 count slowly declines from the normal count of 500–1400 cells/mm^3. CD4 T-lymphocytes coordinate the body's immune response and, as their numbers fall during the late stages of AIDS, profound immunosuppression results. This predisposes the patient to a variety of infections that would not normally cause disease in an immuno-competent person — so-called 'opportunistic' infections. The specific opportunistic infections that occur depend on both the geographical area and the patient's degree of immunosuppression. Certain tumours, caused by viruses, are more common in AIDS patients: lymphomas (due to EBV) and Kaposi sarcoma (herpesvirus KSHV or HHV-8). AIDS-related conditions usually occur when the CD4 is <200 cells/mm^3.

There is no vaccine and no cure for the viral infection itself. Good therapies have been developed, however, for many of the opportunistic infections. Combination antiretroviral treatment (ART) can control viral replication and allow a considerable restoration of immune function that can last for many years.

Clinical phases of HIV infection

HIV infection progresses from a seroconversion illness soon after infection through a long asymptomatic period to symptomatic disease and AIDS.

Acute retroviral illness

An acute retroviral illness occurs in about 50% of patients 2–5 weeks after infection. It lasts from 3 to 21 days. It is similar to infectious mononucleosis with variable signs and symptoms that include malaise, fever, sore throat, myalgia, anorexia, arthralgia, headache, diarrhoea, nausea, generalized lymphadenopathy, and a maculo-papular eruption involving the trunk and arms. Rare complications include aseptic meningoencephalitis and mono/polyneuritis. Atypical lymphocytes may be seen in the blood film. There may be significant temporary immunosuppression during the acute infection with opportunistic infections having been reported during this period.

Asymptomatic HIV infection

An asymptomatic stage, during which the body's immune system attempts to control the virus, follows seroconversion. The virus itself is not latent at this stage but is in balance with the immune system. Billions of virus particles are produced and destroyed each day. The only sign of infection during this period may be generalized lymphadenopathy, probably due to HIV. The asymptomatic stage varies in length but ends when immune system dysfunction produces symptoms.

Symptomatic HIV infection

Symptoms occur as the immune system's function becomes compromised. These are initially mild, such as skin rashes and recurrent throat infections, but later the patient suffers from opportunistic infections, as well as the direct effects of HIV itself. Weight loss, weakness, and loss of functional capacity are common. Opportunistic infections attack multiple systems. Certain opportunistic infections become more common as the CD4 count falls, and this is reflected in the WHO's staging system.

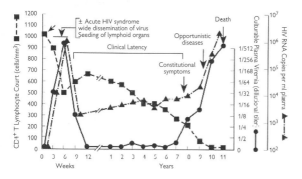

Fig. 3.2 Course of HIV infection in adults (Adapted with permission from G. Pantaleo et al. The immuno pathogenesis of human immunodeficiency virus infection, N Engl J Med, 1993, **328(5)**: 327–35.)

WHO clinical staging system for HIV infection and disease

This staging system was developed for epidemiological purposes. It is useful for estimating progression of HIV-related immunosuppression and making decisions about the need for co-trimoxazole prophylaxis and starting or switching ART. The presence of any of these manifestations in a previously healthy adult should suggest HIV infection. Any suspicion of HIV infection should be confirmed by laboratory tests.

The stages are (see box):

1 — asymptomatic
2 — mild symptoms
3 — advanced
4 — severe

In the absence of ART, the average time course from infection to AIDS is 9 years. Some patients are rapid progressors and may develop AIDS just a few years after infection. Typically, these patients have high viral load setpoints with rapid CD4 decline. Other patients may be slow progressors with slow CD4 and clinical decline. Opportunistic infections, in particular TB, may accelerate HIV disease by causing an increase in viral replication and the viral setpoint. HIV wasting syndrome is defined as weight loss of >10%, plus either unexplained diarrhoea (lasting >1 month) or chronic weakness and unexplained fever for >1 month.

WHO clinical staging system (2006)

Clinical stage 1
Asymptomatic
Persistent generalized lymphadenopathy (PGL)

Clinical stage 2
Weight loss <10% of body weight
Minor mucocutaneous lesions (seborrhoeic dermatitis, papular pruritic eruptions, fungal nail infection, recurrent oral ulceration, angular cheilitis)
Herpes Zoster
Recurrent upper respiratory tract infections

Clinical stage 3
Weight loss >10% of body weight
Unexplained chronic diarrhoea for >1 month
Unexplained prolonged fever for >1 month
Oral candidiasis, chronic vaginal candida
Oral hairy leukoplakia
Pulmonary TB
Severe bacterial infections (pneumonia, pyomyositis, empyema)
Acute necrotizing ulcerative oral disease
Unexplained anaemia (<8 g/dl), neutropaenia (<0.5 × 10^9/L) and/or chronic thrombocytopenia (< 50 × 10^9/L)

Clinical stage 4
HIV wasting syndrome
Pneumocystis jiroveci pneumonia (PCP)
CNS toxoplasmosis
Chronic cryptosporidiosis
Chronic isosporiasis
Cryptococcosis (extrapulmonary)
Cytomegalovirus (CMV) infection (retinitis or other organs)
Chronic HSV infection of >1 mth or visceral
Progressive multifocal leukoencephalopathy (PML)
Candidiasis of the oesophagus, trachea, bronchi, or lungs
Disseminated non-tuberculous mycobacterial infection
Recurrent septicaemia including non-typhoid *Salmonella*
Extrapulmonary TB
Lymphoma (cerebral or B cell non-Hodgkin)
Kaposi sarcoma (KS)
HIV encephalopathy
Invasive cervical cancer
Recurrent severe bacterial pneumonia
Disseminated mycosis (histoplasmosis or coccidiomycosis)
Atypical disseminated leishmaniasis
Symptomatic HIV nephropathy or cardiomyopathy

Laboratory tests in HIV infection

There are three main purposes for which HIV antibody testing is performed:

- Transfusion/transplant safety: screening of donated blood and organs to prevent HIV transmission.
- Surveillance: unlinked and anonymous testing to monitor prevalence and trends in HIV infection in a given population.
- Diagnosis of HIV infection: voluntary testing of serum from asymptomatic persons or from persons with clinical signs and symptoms suggestive of HIV infection or AIDS.

Screening requires sensitive tests that will pick up all contaminated blood/organs. By contrast diagnosis requires high specificity so that there are few false positives. The diagnosis of HIV can be made by the detection of HIV itself or the detection of antibodies to HIV.
Tests for virus are:

- HIV viral RNA PCR.
- Integrated HIV viral DNA.
- P24 antigen ELISA.
- Tests for antibodies to the virus.
- 1st, 2nd, 3rd generation ELISA.
- Rapid tests (point-of-care tests employ ELISA methodology; they have been shown to have sensitivity and specificity similar to ELISA).
- Western Blot.
- 4th generation combo-ELISA able to detect antibodies and p24.

All tests have a '*window period*' (the interval during initial infection between the patient becoming infected and the test becoming positive). Important window periods are: HIV RNA PCR, 10 days; P24 antigen, 17 days; 3rd generation ELISA, 22 days. Antibody tests are positive in virtually 100% of patients by 3 months, unless post-exposure prophylaxis was taken that may delay seroconversion.

Diagnostic tests for HIV infection should never be considered as positive, and the patient informed, until they have been confirmed by a second assay. The WHO recommends two tests be used to diagnose HIV in the clinical setting. The first screening test may be an ELISA or a rapid test and should have a high sensitivity to avoid false negatives. The second confirmatory test should be a second ELISA, a second rapid test, or a Western blot. The second test should have high specificity to avoid false positives. Two separate blood specimens should be used. A flow chart for the use of rapid tests in the diagnosis of HIV is shown in Fig. 3.3. The second rapid test should use different antigen specificity or a different platform.

HIV viral load: (copies/ml) determines the amount of virus circulating in blood. A higher viral load correlates with more rapid progression.

CD4 count: is measured by FACS. It is used to assess the degree of immunosuppression and decide on the need for prophylaxis and ART.

ALGORITHM FOR USE OF RAPID HIV TESTS IN TESTING
AND COUNSELLING SERVICES

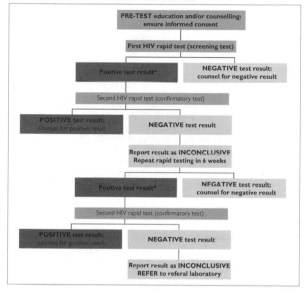

Fig. 3.3 Rapid HIVtests: guidelines for use in HIV testing and counselling services
in resource-constrained settings (Source: WHO, 2001).

Voluntary consent and testing (VCT)

Before being tested for HIV, patients should receive pre-test counselling and should consent to the test. This respects their rights and prepares them for the result. It has been demonstrated to modify subsequent risk-taking behaviour, thereby reducing further transmission.

Pre-test counselling

Pre-test counselling should include:
- The assurance of confidentiality.
- Exploration of the patient's knowledge and beliefs regarding HIV.
- Education around HIV, its transmission, prevention, clinical course, and treatment. Discuss the 'window period'.
- Discussion regarding benefits of testing (prophylaxis, ART, prevention of transmission to sexual partner).
- Exploration of consequences of positive and negative test. Discuss patient's support systems and coping strategies.
- Discussion of issues of disclosure of positive result and obligation to inform sexual partners.
- Documentation of consent (written or verbal).
- Arrangement of follow-up for result.

Post-test counselling

Post-test counselling for a positive result ideally should consist of two or more sessions. Many patients will be in a state of shock when first told the result and 'information overload' should be avoided in the first session. The session(s) should:
- Include feedback about the result, preferably with a written copy.
- Allow expression of emotions and dicussion about them.
- Identify immediate concerns and plans.
- Identify supports and include discussion of disclosure, especially to sexual partner.
- Include talk about safe sex and other risk reduction, healthy lifestyle, treatment, and prophylaxis of opportunistic infections and ART.
- Arrange follow-up and/or referral.
- If necessary, offer psychological or psychiatric referral, since some patients become depressed after a positive result.

If the result is negative, post-test counselling should focus on a discussion of the 'window period' and the need for a repeat test in 3 months and re-inforce prevention messages. The emphasis should be on the person staying negative.

Management of asymptomatic HIV infection

Counselling

The general purpose is to promote and maintain the maximum possible level of psychological and physical health among infected people, their partners and relatives, and caregivers. It has two aims:

- To support the ability of infected persons and those who care for them to cope with the stresses of HIV/AIDS.
- To prevent the transmission of HIV to others.

Medical management of asymptomatic persons with HIV has the following aims:

- Early detection of HIV-associated disease and treatment.
- Primary prophylaxis when indicated.
- Determination of the appropriate time to start antiretroviral therapy.

Knowledge of the CD4 count assists in interpretation of symptoms and when to initiate primary prophylaxis and antiretroviral therapy. Frequency of visits should increase as CD4 count falls.

On history, in high TB incidence settings, specifically ask about TB symptoms (cough, night sweats, and weight loss).

Physical examination should include:

- General: weight loss, fever.
- Neurological system: peripheral neuropathy, cognitive disorders.
- Skin changes: herpes zoster, herpes simplex, folliculitis, tinea, KS, pruritus, seborrhoeic dermatitis, psoriasis.
- Oral cavity: thrush, hairy leukoplakia, gingivitis, KS, lymphoma.
- Eyes: perform fundoscopy, especially if visual symptoms.
- Lymph nodes (see section on lymphadenopathy below).
- Lungs: check for consolidation and crepitations.
- Abdominal examination: hepatosplenomegaly.
- Genitalia: chancre, ulcers.
- Anus: ulcers, warts.

Tests to assess the degree of immunodeficiency may be considered in asymptomatic patients:

- Total lymphocyte count (poor marker).
- CD4 lymphocyte count.

Total lymphocyte count fluctuates greatly due to concurrent infections — it is only a crude guide to CD4 status and degree of immune deficiency. CD4 count is the best indicator of the immediate prognosis. Rate of CD4 decline indicates longer-term prognosis. Serial viral RNA measurements prior to initiating ART add very little to management. Other investigations should be directed by clinical problems.

Drug therapy: primary prophylaxis and administration of vaccines is valuable. Local prevalence of the following infections will determine whether primary prophylaxis or vaccination should be offered: TB, pneumocystis pneumonia, toxoplasmosis, pneumococcal pneumonia.

Symptomatic HIV infection

Acute fevers

When an HIV-infected patient presents with a febrile illness, the differential diagnosis is wide and investigations should be directed by history and examination. Infections that are common in a geographical location will often be more frequent and severe in the HIV-infected population. There are also distinctive geographical patterns for HIV-related opportunistic infections (e.g. penicilliosis frequent in parts of SE Asia and China). Always consider TB as a cause of systemic illness in an HIV-infected person.

History: Duration of symptoms, localizing symptoms (cough, dyspnoea, focal pain, headache, diarrhoea or dysentery, dysuria, genital discharge), weight loss, night sweats, travel history.

Examination: Do serial weights, feel for lymphadenopathy (see below), elicit signs of pneumonia, examine the ears, nose, and throat, and look for skin rashes, oral ulcers, and neck stiffness.

Investigations: to consider:
- CRP (↑ CRP suggests OI rather than HIV wasting syndrome).
- CD4 (influences differential diagnosis).
- Blood culture.
- Urine microscopy and culture.
- Stool microscopy and culture (if the patient has diarrhoea).
- Sputum and other specimens (e.g. induced sputum or urine) for TB microscopy and culture.
- Needle aspiration of nodes >2 cm.
- Malaria smears in endemic areas or traveller from endemic area.
- Bone marrow biopsy if pancytopaenic.
- Lumbar puncture if headaches (to exclude bacterial, cryptococcal, and tuberculous meningitis).
- Aspirate effusions for bacterial and TB microscopy and culture.
- Skin biopsy if patients have a disseminated rash.
- Chest radiograph.
- Ultrasound abdomen and pericardium (abdominal nodes, pericardial effusion, splenic lesions, ascites suggest TB in endemic areas and, less commonly, fungal infection or lymphoma).

In patients with acute illness and fever it is usually necessary to distinguish between viral illness (accompanied by symptoms of coryza, pharyngitis, or tracheobroncitis with normal CRP and WCC) or bacterial sepsis e.g.:
- Sinusitis.
- Pneumonia.
- Urinary tract infection.
- Meningitis (cryptococcal meningitis and TBM may also present acutely).
- Diarrhoea or dysentry (shigella, salmonella, campylobacter).
- Pyomyositis or septic arthritis.
- PID or other STI.
- Other septicaemiac illnesses (non-typhoidal *Salmonella* septicaemias, staphylococcal septicaemias and others).
- Consider malaria in endemic areas or returning travellers.

Subacute and chronic fevers

The following should be considered:

- *Tuberculosis* — pulmonary and/or extrapulmonary (the most common cause of HIV-related morbidity and mortality in the developing world). HIV-infected patients are frequently smear-negative and may have atypical chest radiograph changes. In endemic areas, if the diagnosis of TB is strongly suspected clinically or radiologically but smears are negative, it is sometimes necessary to commence empiric TB treatment with close follow-up to prevent further clinical decline before the diagnosis can be microbiologically proven.
- *Fungal infections* (cryptococcosis, histoplasmosis, penicilliosis, and others — vary according to geographical location).
- PCP (accompanied by dry cough and exertional dyspnoea).
- Non-tuberculous mycobacterial infection (disseminated mycobacterium avium complex is the most common).
- Nocardiosis.
- Bacillary angiomatosis (systemic bartonella infection with characteristic angiomatous nodules on the skin).
- Malignancies (lymphoma, disseminated Kaposi sarcoma).
- Pyogenic bacterial collections (empyema, intra-abdominal).
- Cytomegalovirus (CMV) infection.
- Enteric pathogens (e.g. isosporiasis and cryptosporidiosis, usually with diarrhoea and/or vomiting).
- Leishmaniasis in endemic areas.
- HIV wasting syndrome (seldom the cause of a fever on its own and seldom results in rapid weight loss).

Remember that immune reconstitution inflammatory syndrome may present with fever after ART is started (see below). Non-infective causes of fever to consider are DVT and drug fever.

Lymphadenopathy

- TB.
- Syphilis (papulosquamous rash ± recent genital ulcer).
- Fungal (histoplasmosis, cryptococcosis).
- Malignancy: KS (not necessarily associated with cutaneous KS), lymphoma.
- Dermatological conditions — seborrhoeic dermatitis, chronic pyoderma.
- Local infection that might explain the lymphadenopathy.

Persistent generalized lymphadenopathy (PGL) of HIV itself is common. It is defined as follows:

1. >3 separate lymph node groups affected.
2. At least 2 nodes >1.5 cm in diameter at each site.
3. Duration of >1 month.
4. No local infection that might explain the lymphadenopathy.

It is important to exclude the causes above. If nodes are rapidly enlarging or assymetrical or there are systemic signs, a lymph node must be biopsied to exclude TB, lymphoma, KS, and fungal infection.

Wasting syndrome and malnutrition

Documenting weight loss is essential — clinical impressions are often wrong, so weigh all patients at every outpatient visit and record the weight in a prominent place in the case notes. Causes of weight loss include poor diet (loss of income), chronic infections such as TB, and chronic diarrhoea. Poor appetite is less commonly recognized as remediable and there is often an iatrogenic contribution (iron tablets, multiple courses of unnecessary antibiotics such as erythromycin and metronidazole, and even milk-based nutritional supplements in individuals with lactose intolerance).

Nutrition: Nutritional advice is anxiously sought after, and freely given by health care workers. Unfortunately, the evidence base for much of this advice is scanty and it is often inappropriate to the socio-economic status of the patient. Finding malnutrition should prompt a vigorous search for its cause — usually TB or chronic diarrhoea (or both). Treat the cause and, if appropriate and feasible, consider starting ART. Affordable local diets with sufficient protein, carbohydrates, vitamins, and trace elements are part of the holistic management of all malnourished patients. In patients who are not malnourished, there is no convincing evidence that changing diet is clinically beneficial.

Multivitamins: Patients who are malnourished or clinically hypovitaminotic will benefit from replacement therapy. Most multivitamin preparations contain only recommended daily allowances of vitamins and are thus inappropriate for the correction of severe deficiencies — use single agents in appropriate doses e.g. nicotinamide for pellagra, thiamine for beri-beri, ascorbic acid for scurvy (doses see Chapter 17). If the individual components are unavailable, it may be necessary to treat by giving 10 or more multivitamin tablets daily, which is safe as long as the product contains only water-soluble vitamins in RDA quantities. In adult patients who are neither malnourished nor hypovitaminotic, supplemental vitamins are of unclear value. However, mild hypovitaminosis is difficult to exclude clinically, and so it is reasonable to consider widespread supplementation in the hope that it may retard disease progression.

Nutritional supplements and drug interactions: The number of medications given to individuals on ART creates considerable potential for drug interactions; throwing nutritional and herbal supplements into the mix may complicate matters further. The simplest advice for individuals on ART is to avoid nutritional supplements unless these are clearly innocuous. Relatively well-documented interactions are between St John's Wort and protease inhibitors and nevirapine, and garlic supplements in patients on saquinavir. Other potential difficulties concern alteration in absorption — antacid containing medications and didanosine, and all ART and activated charcoal, which is sometimes sold as a 'detoxifier'.

Skin and oral disease

Herpes zoster

A vesicular eruption typically in a dermatomal distribution. If started within 72 h of the onset of blistering, aciclovir (800 mg 5x daily for 7 d) or valaciclovir (1 g tds for 7 d) may shorten duration and ↓ risk of post herpetic neuralgia. Zoster involving the eye should be treated with topical aciclovir ophthalmic ointment — if possible, refer to ophthalmologist. Give analgesia e.g. paracetamol 1 g qds ± amitriptyline 10–25 mg nocte; occasionally opiates may be required.

Itchy rashes

Pruritic rashes are common. Consider treating for scabies even if distribution not typical as treatment is cheap and safe. Drug reactions are also common (see below) but in the absence of a clear drug aetiology, generalized itchy, fine, papular eruptions may be due to the so-called papular dermatitis of HIV ('itchy bump disease'.) This may respond to topical 0.1% betamethasone (1% hydrocortisone for the face.)

Crusted (Norwegian) scabies

A severe, hyperkeratotic form of scabies seen in immunocompromised persons. There is extensive crusting in areas accessible to scratching, with sparing of areas less easily reached, such as the middle of the back; the scalp is usually involved. Treatment —see 📖 p 545.

Drug rashes

Drug rashes vary from mild papular eruptions to Stevens–Johnson syndrome. Common causes include co-trimoxazole, anti-TB drugs, phenytoin, carbamazepine, and NNRTIs, but practically any drug can be involved. Check carefully for the presence of fever, new adenopathy, facial swelling, mucosal involvement, eosinophilia, or raised liver enzymes. The presence of one or more of these features is an absolute indication to stop all therapy. Do not be tempted to use drugs to treat a drug-induced skin disease — once the drug is stopped it will improve with time and supportive measures. In patients with only mild reactions (none of the above danger signs present), it may be reasonable to consider continuing 'essential' drugs (e.g. NNRTIs, co-trimoxazole) under close supervision.

Gingivostomatitis

This may be due to Candida or Herpes simplex (Chapter 16). *Major aphthous ulceration* is a disabling polymicrobial gingivostomatitis with extensive ulceration and necrosis. Consider topical therapy (e.g. povidone iodine mouthwashes) and oral amoxicillin plus metronidazole; in refractory cases with persistent ulceration, biopsy to exclude TB and syphilis. Persistent symptoms without an easily identifiable cause are an indication for considering antiretroviral therapy if this is available. In its absence, judicious corticosteroid use may induce a modest response.

Vaginal candidiasis

📖 See Chapter 16

Respiratory disease

Community acquired pneumonia

Presentation is usually acute (hours to days) with fever, pleuritic chest pain, and cough → purulent sputum. Clinical signs may be fewer with ↓ immunity, making diagnosis more difficult; classical lobar consolidation becomes less common. The differential diagnosis includes atypical TB or PCP. Therapy should be guided by local medication availability and resistance patterns but, in general, ill immunosuppressed patients should be treated with a parenteral agent with good gram-positive cover, such as a third generation cephalosporin (e.g. ceftriaxone 1 g od) or, if not available, ampicillin 1 g 6 hourly. If there is poor response within 48 h, add doxycycline 100 mg od and intensify the search for TB. Parenteral therapy can be changed to oral once there is clinical response.

Pneumocystis pneumonia (PCP)

Symptoms of dry cough and increasing dyspnoea have usually been present for days to a week or longer. There are usually few signs in the presence of quite marked hypoxia (cyanosis and tachypoea). CXR shows a diffuse interstitial infiltrate without effusion or adenopathy. Sputum induced by 10 minutes of nebulization with hypertonic saline may be positive on microscopy and, in dedicated hands, this procedure is as successful as bronchoscopy and lavage. Therapy is usually initiated on clinical and radiographic grounds in the absence of laboratory confirmation. Treatment is with co-trimoxazole (trimethoprim/sulphamethoxazole 80/400 mg) 4 tablets qds for 21 days (if <60 kg — the majority of adult patients — reduce to 3 tablets tds; see 🕮 p. 120 for paediatric doses); ↑ K⁺ and ↑ creatinine are recognized side-effects. If hypoxic, consider adding prednisone (40 mg bd for 5 days; then 40 mg od for 5 days; then 20 mg od for 10 days). Response is not always very dramatic and some patients may take > a week to start to settle. After treatment, give 2° prophylaxis with co-trimoxazole 80/400 2 tablets od (adult dose; may be reduced to 1 tablet od to improve tolerance).

Chronic cough

When associated with weight loss and other respiratory symptoms, chronic cough should prompt a search for an underlying chest infection, usually TB. The differential is quite wide in the absence of other systemic features and should include extrinsic bronchial compression from lymphadenopathy (TB, lymphoma, Kaposi sarcoma) and parenchymal lung diseases presenting atypically, without major clinical or radiological manifestations (e.g. pneumocystis and lymphocytic interstitial pneumonitis (LIP)). Pulmonary KS is an important although uncommon possibility, typically presenting with nodular opacities with hilar adenopathy with pleural effusion that may be confused with pulmonary TB. Look carefully for evidence of skin or oral Kaposi lesions which are often, although not invariably, present. Remember that HIV-infected people can also suffer from all the diseases of HIV-negative patients, so consider late onset asthma, drug side-effects (e.g. angiotensin converting enzyme inhibitors) and foreign bodies.

Table 3.1 Respiratory infection in HIV-infected people

Feature	Community-acquired pneumonia	Pulmonary tuberculosis	Pneumocystis pneumonia
Duration of symptoms	Hours to days	Days to weeks	Days to weeks
Loss of weight	If present, due to something else	Usually present	If present, due to something else
Purulent sputum	Occurs in only half of patients	Occurs in only one third of patients	Very rare — small amounts of white sputum occasionally
Chest pain	Poor discriminator, although the chest discomfort in pneumocystis is classically described as central and non-pleuritic		
Hypoxia	Variable	Uncommon unless severe disease	Quite commonly present at presentation
Respiratory signs	Variable	Often unimpressive	Usually unimpressive
Chest X-ray	May show lobar pattern	Typically hilar and upper mediastinal adenopathy with lower zone non-cavitating infiltrate	Diffuse bilateral infiltrate. Effusion or adenopathy make the diagnosis unlikely (but consider dual pathology)
Serum lactate dehydrogenase	Only helpful in discriminating between pneumocystis and suspected viral pneumonias		
Sputum induction	Rarely diagnostic	Helpful	Helpful
Fine–needle node aspiration		Frequently diagnostic	

Gastrointestinal disease

Gastroenteritis

Try the mnemonic: '**HERS**' is more acute — **H**ydration, **E**lectrolyte **R**eplacement, and consider **S**epticaemia; **HIS** is chronic — **H**istory, **I**nvestigations, and **S**tart ART if possible.

When history short, or in acute deterioration, determine hydration status (pulse and blood pressure lying and sitting, urine-specific gravity, and laboratory measurement of K^+, Na^+, urea, and creatinine concentrations). Signs of dehydration can be misleading in marasmus as patients commonly have sunken eyes and reduced skin turgor. If sufficiently dehydrated to require IV therapy, give 5% dextrose-saline, 1 litre 4–6 hourly adjusted according to clinical response. As most patients are hypokalaemic, start replacement with IV K^+ 20–40 mmol in each litre, unless the patient is anuric at presentation, in which case wait for a laboratory K^+ result. Oral K^+ may exacerbate nausea and vomiting. In *febrile patients* who have colitis (bloody diarrhoea with abdominal tenderness on palpation over the colon) or who do not respond to fluid resuscitation, gram-negative septicaemia is a possibility; consider either a quinolone or a third generation cephalosporin with activity against *Salmonella* and *Shigella*. If possible, take blood for culture before giving antibiotics.

Chronic diarrhoea

Diarrhoea can wax and wane, creating the illusion of response to symptomatic therapy and antibiotic cocktails. A review of weight charts usually reveals a trend. Enquire about milk and dairy intake, as occasional patients develop lactose intolerance.

Investigation: stool microscopy (looking for ova and parasites) and culture, ± *C. difficile* toxin. The majority of organisms identified (e.g. *cryptosporidium*) respond poorly if at all to specific medical therapy, and the general approach should be to assess for ART, as improvement in immunity usually cures the diarrhoea. Isosporiasis may respond to co-trimoxazole 80/400 two tablets qds for 3 weeks. There is also limited evidence for the efficacy of albendazole 400 mg bd for a month in patients with *microsporidium*. Home-based safe water systems (plastic container, chlorine tablets) may help reduce episodes of diarrhoea in counties without safe water supplies. Consider gastrointestinal TB and treat as appropriate.

Abdominal pain

In HIV-infected people, acute abdominal pain often presents a diagnostic dilemma. The usual differential of an acute abdomen is applicable, and the recovery rate after surgery is similar to that of HIV-uninfected people. Also consider:

- *Salmonella typhi* and its complications.
- Abdominal TB (often but not always associated with ascites and retroperitoneal adenopathy. The finding of splenic hypodensities on ultrasound is strongly suggestive of this condition.)
- CMV infection is often associated with vasculitis and episodic severe pain. Negative IgG CMV serology makes the diagnosis less likely.

- Herbal enema usage.
- 'Pus anywhere' — subphrenic abscess, PID-associated pelvic collections, psoas abscess.
- Neuropathic pain — zoster without the rash yet (it appears the next day, or may never develop but dermatomal distribution is suggestive).
- Gastritis related to medication.
- Pyelonephritis and cystitis (check the urine).
- Pancreatitis (due to CMV, TB, or drugs e.g. co-trimoxazole, D4T, DDI, and possibly 3TC).

Odynophagia and dysphagia

Oral causes: Candida infection is the usual cause; apart from the usual white plaques it can also present as ulceration, erythema, and circumoral dermatitis or angular cheilitis. Topical antifungals are usually effective — e.g. nystatin 100,000 units swirled around in the mouth every 6 h for a week. Other choices include clotrimazole or amphotericin lozenges.

Major aphthous ulceration (see ☐ p 83) may be due to polymicrobial bacterial infection and is sometimes associated with perineal disease.

Herpetic ulcers (due to Herpes simplex virus) have a typical clinical appearance and are usually self-limiting; aciclovir 400 mg 5x daily or valaciclovir 500 mg bd for 5 days may help; analgesia important.

Oesophageal causes: Pain or discomfort localized to the chest or lower neck is more likely due to an oesophageal cause. Candida is the most common cause and is most confidently diagnosed in the presence of associated oral plaques, although it can sometimes be present without this. This requires systemic therapy with fluconazole 200 mg PO od for 10–14 days. Ketoconazole is a cheaper alternative (200 mg/day) but is an enzyme inhibitor that reduces cortisol synthesis and may precipitate adrenal crisis; its absorption is also erratic in hypochlorhydric patients. Severe discomfort may make swallowing tablets impossible, necessitating parenteral treatment with amphotericin 0.5–1 mg/kg/day IV for 7 days (IV fluconazole is an alternative). If no visible thrush or no response to systemic anti-fungal therapy (fluconazole for 3 weeks), then oesophago-scopy is usually indicated, and may establish a diagnosis of CMV or herpes oesophagitis.

Perianal pathology

Perianal pathology is often very painful. Apart from *Candida* infection, non-specific painful ulceration is common. Consider STIs and check syphilis serology. Investigations depend on individual clinical presentation and available resources. Consider early treatment with specific therapy for herpes infection (e.g. aciclovir or valaciclovir) or a trial of antibiotics which include anaerobic cover (e.g. co-amoxiclav) for particularly infected looking lesions. Results of superficial pus swabs are seldom informative. In refractory cases or if there is evidence of fistula formation, a biopsy may reveal treatable disease e.g. TB. Topical therapies for pain are usually available, but vary and are seldom evidence-based.

Liver disease

Asymptomatic liver enzyme rises are quite common in HIV-infected people, often reflecting systemic illness or drug reactions. Minor rises of transaminases with drug therapy (e.g. anti-tuberculous medication) in an asymptomatic patient should be managed by repetition of the test a week later; if there is no clear trend to increase, then continue therapy. Elevation of transaminases >4x normal, or if there are signs of acute liver disease, should be managed as acute hepatitis.

Acute hepatitis

This is commonly due to hepatitis B infection, although CMV, herpes simplex, and hepatitis A are sometimes responsible. Hepatitis B morbidity and mortality may be greater in patients co-infected with HIV, but it is unclear if there is a more rapid progression to AIDS. Patients started on ART may also develop an immune reconstitution response to quiescent viral hepatitis, which is theoretically partially ameliorated by using drugs with activity against hepatitis B and C (e.g. 3TC.) Unfortunately, hepatitis B resistance to antiviral monotherapy develops rapidly. An ART combination containing both tenofovir and 3TC is preferable in HBV co-infected patients.

Drug-induced hepatitis

Common causes are TB drugs and ART, but almost any drug can be responsible. Principles of management are early recognition (also consider hepatitis B or C flare as part of IRIS); assessment of severity; and evaluation of the importance of the drug to the patient's treatment. Because the recognition of drug-induced hepatitis is often delayed, patients often present with severe liver dysfunction, and it is usually advisable to stop all medication initially — especially if liver enzyme rise is >5x upper limit of normal, or if there is fever, ↑ WCC, or an associated rash. ddI, d4T, and nevirapine are particularly well associated with hepatitis, so once the patient has settled clinically and biochemically, regimens that avoid these agents should be considered.

HIV cholangiopathy

Patients with late-stage HIV disease may develop right upper quadrant discomfort and an obstructive LFT profile. In the absence of gallstones (ultrasound), low-grade cholangitis should be considered; this may progress to resemble sclerosing cholangitis on ERCP. A wide range of potential pathogens (e.g. salmonella, toxoplasma, CMV, and cryptosporidium) have been implicated, but response to specific therapy is generally poor. Consider ART.

Hepatomegaly
- cardiac causes (cardiomyopathies, pericardial disease).
- infections, viral and TB, malaria, leishmaniasis.
- infiltrates (e.g. lymphoma).
- medication-associated steatohepatitis and malnutrition.

Cardiac disease

HIV-associated cardiomyopathy

This is usually due to HIV *per se* but cardiotropic viruses and opportunistic infections may also be implicated. Cardiac histology shows a myocarditis. It is important to exclude alternative (e.g. nutritional) causes. It typically presents with dilated cardiomyopathy and heart failure and a CD4 count <100/mm^3. There are case reports of improvement in myocardial function with ART. Associated cardiac failure should be treated.

Pericardial disease

Pericardial effusions may be tuberculous, bacterial, fungal, malignant (Kaposi, lymphoma), or idiopathic. In high-incidence TB settings in Africa, 86–100% of pericardial effusions in HIV-infected people are tuberculous. Diagnosis is confirmed by cardiac ultrasound ± pericardiocentesis. A presumptive diagnosis of tuberculous pericarditis may be made without pericardiocentesis in high-incidence settings and/or in patients in whom there is a high clinical suspicion of TB. Pericardiocentesis is, however, indicated in patients who present septic (to exclude pyogenic infection) and in cardiac tamponade.

Vascular disease

Vasculitis of the aorta and its large branches giving rise to narrowing. Aneurysmal dilatation is rare but well described in HIV. Pulmonary hypertension is more common and generally carries a poor prognosis. The incidence of coronary artery disease is increased in patients on protease inhibitors due to their adverse effect on lipid and glucose metabolism.

Renal disease

Acute renal failure due to sepsis and/or dehydration is common in patients with opportunistic infections; renal function usually normalizes with appropriate treatment and rehydration but may take 1–2 weeks following acute tubular necrosis and temporary dialysis may be required.

HIV-associated nephropathy

HIV-associated nephropathy manifests initially with proteinuria which may evolve to nephrotic syndrome and progressive renal dysfunction evolving to endstage renal failure over several months. Patients are typically not oedematous nor hypertensive because the condition is salt-wasting. Histology shows focal segmental glomerulosclerosis (FSGS) as well as tubular disease. The pathology results from direct infection of renal endothelial cells by HIV. Treatment includes ACE inhibitors and ART. ART may stabilize or improve milder cases but, if patients have lost significant renal function, the condition progresses despite ART.

Other forms of glomerulonephritis, such as post-infectious, may also occur in HIV-infected individuals. Thus, it is always preferable to confirm the diagnosis with renal biopsy if available. An immune complex mediated nephritis, distinct from FSGS, has been described in association with HIV.

Neurological disease

Chronic headache

Chronic headache should always be taken seriously in HIV-infected people. Fever and meningeal irritation may be absent in lymphocytic meningitides, and frontal lobe mass lesions may have little in the way of lateralizing signs until late. Consider:

- Common chronic meningitides (TB, cryptococcosis, syphilis).
- Sinusitis ± subdural empyema.
- Space-occupying lesions (toxoplasmosis, tuberculoma, lymphoma).
- Drugs (co-trimoxazole can rarely → sterile meningitis; zidovudine and efavirenz cause various CNS symptoms, including headache).

Meningitis

Any patient with HIV and a new headache or unexplained fever should be considered to have meningitis. Signs of meningism may not be present so absence of neck stiffness does NOT exclude the diagnosis. The variability in physical signs and CSF findings reflect the degree of immunocompromise and pattern of the associated meningeal process.

Cryptococcal meningitis

This is due to infection by the capsulate yeast, *Cryptococcus neoformans*, which is carried by birds (especially pigeons) and excreted in avian faeces. Infection follows inhalation of the yeast, and in immunocompetent individuals is asymptomatic or accompanied by mild self-limiting respiratory symptoms. Although meningeal infection may rarely occur in the immunocompetent, it is much more common in immunosuppressed individuals, particularly those with HIV. Rarely disseminated cryptococcosis may occur, involving almost any organ including skin, mucosae, and bones.

Clinical features of cryptococcal: meningitis are usually insidious in onset, with headache, malaise, low-grade fever, ± altered mental state.

Diagnosis: There are often few cells in the CSF but India ink staining of CSF usually shows characteristic capsulated yeast cells (capsule appears as a clear halo around the yeast). The cryptococcal latex agglutination test (CLAT) is highly sensitive and specific for both blood and CSF.

Treatment: is for life unless immunity is restored with ART and consists of an initial intensive phase followed by long-term low-dose maintenance (so-called secondary prophylaxis). Give:

- Amphotericin B (amB, 0.7–1 mg/kg/day diluted in 200 ml 5% dextrose water and infused over four hours) for 10 days. Test doses are unnecessary and the addition of heparin and antihistamines adds little: severe allergic reactions in amphotericin-naïve patients are rare. AmB is best avoided in renal failure and attention should be given to adequate hydration (consider IV fluids). Monitor K^+ as life-threatening hypokalaemia is relatively common.
- Following 10 days' treatment with amphotericin, give fluconazole 400 mg od for 2 months. (In patients who are very well, it is reasonable to dispense with the amphotericin and proceed directly to the fluconazole 400 mg/d for two months, but the evidence from head-to-head trials that this is equivalent to initial amphotericin is scanty.)

- Thereafter, continue for life with fluconazole 200 mg per day.
- In patients with ongoing headache or drowsiness, consider repeat LP with CSF manometry: if pressure >30 cm CSF, remove sufficient CSF to reduce to <20 cm CSF. This often leads to quite dramatic symptomatic relief but may need to be repeated if symptoms recur.

Table 3.2 Differences between forms of meningitis in HIV infection

Feature	Pyogenic	Tuberculous	Cryptococcal
Symptom duration	Hours to days	Days to weeks	Days to weeks
Headache	Usually	Usually but not invariable	Usually but not invariable
Neck stiffness	Variable	Variable	Usually absent (80%)
Fever	Usually	Variable	Variable
Chest signs (and CXR)	Rare	May have features of pulmonary TB	Usually normal, but cryptococcal pulmonary disease possible
CSF opening pressure	Variable	Often raised, but an unreliable differentiator	
CSF glucose	Low	Usually low	Normal in 50%
CSF protein	Usually modestly elevated	Often markedly elevated	May be normal, but usually mildly elevated
Cell count	Usually moderately or extremely elevated	Usually modestly elevated	Normal in about one third of patients
Lymphocyte/neutrophil ratio	Predominantly neutrophils	Lymphocytes but may have an early neutrophil predominance	If any cells, usually lymphocytes
Gram stain	May show organisms	Negative	Negative; sometimes reported as 'fungal elements present'
Indian ink	Negative	Negative	Usually but not always positive
Cryptococcal CSF antigen test	Negative	Negative	Usually but not always positive (sensitivity 90–100%)
CSF culture	Often informative	Often positive, but takes some weeks	Usually unnecessary

Space-occupying lesions (SOL)

Brain SOLs present with one or more of headaches, focal neurological signs, or fits (📖 p 432). Careful neurological examination for focal signs and signs of ↑ICP is essential. Frontal lobe lesions may cause personality changes. Brain imaging (CT or MRI) and biopsy may help diagnosis, but in their absence diagnosis and management relies on judgements about the most probable cause, presence of associated disease elsewhere, and response to therapy. The most common finding on brain imaging is a contrast enhancing mass lesion with surrounding oedema. Multiple lesions in a patient with a CD4 count <50 are likely to be due to toxoplasmosis. Toxoplasmosis is less likely if the CD4 count is higher (>150), toxoplasma IgG is –ve, or patient is on co-trimoxazole prophylaxis. Single lesions with considerable basal contrast enhancement and an abnormal CXR (particularly hilar adenopathy, a chronic lower zone infiltrate, or a miliary pattern) suggest TB. Other causes include primary CNS lymphoma (rare), pyogenic brain abscess, cryptococcoma, and syphilis; consider neurocysticercosis in endemic areas.

Management: Where facilities allow, diagnosis treatment should be based on specific investigations including serology, imaging, CSF examination, and brain biopsy. In the absence of a specific diagnosis, the following is a pragmatic approach to management:

- If evidence of TB elsewhere (LNs, CXR, abdominal USS looking for splenic hypodensities or adenopathy), treat for TB initially.
- In the absence of features suggesting TB, treat for toxoplasmosis initially, as therapy is less arduous and response can be assessed within a week. (It is advisable not to give corticosteroids for focal cerebral oedema unless they are considered to be life-saving, as they will cause many patients to appear to respond both clinically and radiologically.)
- If there is no response to treatment for toxoplasmosis within 2 weeks, and no other diagnostic pointers, it is common practice then commence on therapy for TB, although where there is access to a neurosurgical service, consultation with a view to biopsy is desirable.
- In patients who respond partially, there is no simple answer. In general, it is usually preferable to treat for TB as well, but the previously listed differential diagnosis should be re-scrutinized at this stage.

Seizures

Causes include those common to HIV-uninfected people, but the high incidence of organic CNS pathology in HIV means careful attention should be given to the exclusion of SOLs and chronic meningitides. In patients with very low CD4 counts, HIV encephalopathy may itself cause seizures. Management of patients with seizures who require antiepileptics presents a few specific issues. Firstly, conventional antiepileptic doses need adjusting according to the reduced weight of many patients, bearing in mind that the liver induction due to other medications may counterbalance this. In patients in whom ART is being contemplated, the drug interactions with phenytoin and carbamazepine can be problematic and a switch to valproate is often justified, particularly if prescribers are unfamiliar with the magnitude and direction of the interactions.

Toxoplasmosis

Toxoplasma gondii is an obligate intracellular parasite. Cats are the definitive host. Transmission occurs by ingestion of food contaminated by oocytes from cat faeces or tissue cysts in undercooked meat from domesticated animals. Infection is common and usually asymptomatic in immunocompetent adults, but may cause a mononucleosis-like syndrome. Primary infection of women in the early stages of pregnancy results in foetal infection and serious congenital malformations. Latent infection may become reactivated in immunocompromised patients, causing severe disease involving lungs, heart, and chorioretina. Cerebral toxoplasmosis is a common manifestation in HIV/AIDS.

Clinical features: of cerebral toxoplasmosis include headache, focal neurological signs, altered mental state, and coma. Diffuse cerebral involvement presents with generalized CNS dysfunction without focal signs. Toxoplasma pneumonitis manifests as fever with cough and dyspnoea; chorioretinitis is uncommon.

Diagnosis: of cerebral toxoplasmosis is clinical, supported by serology and brain imaging (MRI or CT). Typically, it presents with multiple ring enhancing brain lesions on CT, CD4 count is usually <50 and *toxoplasma* IgG +ve. Brain biopsy may be helpful in atypical presentations.

Management

Conventional therapy is with pyrimethamine plus sulphadiazine (or clindamycin) for 6 weeks. Bone marrow suppression occurs with pyrimethamine (a folate antagonist), so folinic acid is also given:

- Pyrimethamine 200 mg PO loading dose, 50–75 mg PO od, *plus*
- Folinic acid 10 mg od (pyrimethamine is a folate antagonist), *plus*
- *either* Sulfadiazine 1–1.5 g PO qds
- *or* Clindamycin 600 mg PO qds

Maintenance therapy should then continue for life with pyrimethamine 25–50 mg PO od plus sulfadiazine 0.5–1 g qds od.

Alternative regimen The above regimen is both difficult to obtain and expensive and there is preliminary evidence that single-strength co-trimoxazole 80/400 four tablets bd for 4 weeks, followed by two tablets bd for 3 months, is adequate. Secondary prophylaxis after that should continue for life (or until immune reconstitution on ART) with two tablets od. Not all patients treated with co-trimoxazole will demonstrate a complete clinical response, particularly if there is an associated infarct.

HIV-associated dementia

HIV-associated dementia is a slow onset process characterized by motor apraxia and mental slowing with forgetfulness. It is important to identify it early as it is an indication for consideration for ART: they can arrest the process and may even reverse some of the changes. Standard mini-mental tests are designed to screen for the predominantly cortical lesions of Alzheimer's disease, so alternative screening tools that also evaluate subcortical function have been proposed. One scale (see table below) has been cross-culturally validated to some extent and consists of three components — a memory test, a psychomotor component, and a motor component. Sensitivity is ~80%, specificity 55–57%.

Table 3.3 Rapid screening test for HIV dementia*

Item	Description	Outcome	Score
Motor	Tap together finger and thumb of non-dominant hand as many times as possible in 5 seconds	>15 times in 5 sec	4
		11–14	3
		7–10	2
		3–6	1
		0–2	0
Psychomotor	Repeat the following sequence of placement of the non-dominant hand on a flat surface as often as possible in 10 seconds: 1. Clenched fist. 2. Open hand, palm down 3. Ulnar surface of open hand down	4 or more repeats	4
		3	3
		2	2
		1	1
		Cannot perform	0
Memory	Before doing the previous two components, give the patient four words to remember (dog, hat, bean, red) and after finishing the other components, ask what they were	Each word spontaneously recalled	1
		Each word recalled after prompting	0.5
Total score	Add together scores from each of the three components	Max 12. <10 should prompt more formal evaluation for dementia	

* Sacktor NC et al. The International HIV Dementia Scale: a new rapid screening test for HIV dementia. AIDS 2005; **19**:1367–74.

HIV encephalopathy and progressive multifocal leukoencephalopathy

HIV is a neurotropic virus that can cause a slowly progressive (months) dementing illness characterized by forgetfulness and minor motor apraxias. Vacuolar myelopathy is a variant where the cortical changes are preceded by a progressive spastic weakness. Always exclude Vitamin B12 deficiency in the latter. Progressive multifocal leukoencephalopathy (PML) is a white matter illness due to JC virus infection which presents with lateralizing neurology, and speech and cognition difficulties. ART is always worth attempting in dementing patients who have adequate home resources to ensure adherence. A response in PML less often occurs.

Psychosis

Common causes include acute situational stressors (reactions to learning HIV status, often in the face of inadequate counselling), opportunistic CNS infections (chronic meningitides, frontal space occupying lesions), severe opportunistic infections elsewhere, metabolic disorders (hyponatraemia, dehydration, and uraemia) and medications (e.g. efavirenz). Thiamine and niacin deficiencies are seldom considered and well worth treating empirically even if merely suspected (see Chapter 17). Vitamin B12 deficiency is another potential cause for abnormal mentation.

Use of neuroleptic agents in frail, thin HIV-positive patients should be cautious — often tiny doses (e.g. haloperidol 0.5 mg bd) may be quite adequate.

Stroke

The abrupt onset of focal neurological signs is a devastating event for young HIV-infected persons, particularly if the resultant disability impacts on activities of daily living and the ability to look after children. A proactive approach looking at modifiable risk factors is essential. Causes:
- Blood.
  - Hyperviscosity.
  - Disseminated intravascular coagulation.
  - Antiphospholipid antibody syndromes.
  - Acquired protein C, protein S, or antithrombin III deficiency.
  - Thrombotic thrombocytopenic purpura.
- Blood pressure — hypertension (e.g. due to HIV nephropathy) or hypotension (septicaemia, dehydration).
- Embolic — infective endocarditis related either to previous rheumatic heart disease or IV drug use.
- Vessel wall.
  - Infective vasculitis (meningitis — TB, syphilis, cryptococcal, CMV, herpes zoster, and even toxoplasmosis).
  - Autoimmune vasculitis.
  - Haemorrhage (mycotic aneurysm, intracerebral Kaposi).
  - HIV vasculopathy is considered possible but is poorly characterized.

Diagnosis: look for clinical signs of embolic source; FBC, blood film, U&E, ESR, or CRP, syphilis serology, total serum protein (?hyperviscosity), ± thrombophilia screen (PT, anticardiolipin antibodies, protein C, protein S, and antithrombin III levels); brain imaging (CT or MRI).

Management involves treatment of any identified underlying cause and counselling about the condition and expected prognosis, attention to nutrition (able to swallow, adequate hydration plan?), and urine and bowel care plans (decisions about catheter versus nappies/linen savers if incontinent.) In the absence of any identified remediable cause, it is common practice to give aspirin 75–150 mg od as secondary prophylaxis, although evidence of benefit in this patient population has not been established.

Peripheral neuropathy

Consider HIV neuropathy, medication (INH, stavudine, didanosine), CMV (initial perineal pain, associated CSF polymorph rise), nutritional deficiencies (thiamine, niacin, pyridoxine, vitamin B_{12}), and vasculitic neuropathy (stepwise progression.)

Acute and chronic inflammatory demyelinating polyneuropathies (*Guillain–Barre syndrome*) present in the same way as in HIV-uninfected people, and a few cells in the CSF should not exclude the diagnosis if the clinical picture is correct. Steroids are often given in the chronic form but, as with the acute form, are probably of little value, and in patients with the asymmetrical pure motor form may in fact do harm.

Mononeuropathies

The most common mononeuropathy is an isolated VIIth (Bell's palsy), but practically any cranial nerve can be involved. The natural history of a Bell's palsy is similar to that in HIV-uninfected people, with lack of clear evidence of benefit from either antivirals (e.g. aciclovir) or steroids. The importance is recognizing the lower motor neurone nature of the lesion, which makes intracranial pathology unlikely.

Paraparesis

Patients with weak legs can have any of the causes of peripheral neuropathy; also consider intrinsic cord disease if upper motor neurone signs are present. TB and syphilitic myeloradiculitis are sometimes associated with dermatomal pain at the level of the lesion, and CMV infection may classically present with lumbosacral pain.

Depression

Depression in HIV-infected people is under-recognized. It may be situational or due to medication, intercurrent illness, or organic brain disease. Depressed people adjust poorly to new disease and therapeutic challenges, and adherence may be affected. Antidepressant medication and protease inhibitors may interact; interactions with NNRTIs are rare.

Eye disease

- *HIV retinopathy* is usually aymptomatic, although minor visual symptoms may occur. Soft exudates without haemorrhage are seen.
- *CMV infection* of the eye yields a characteristic ophthalmoscopic appearance and can be managed relatively simply by intraocular gancyclovir injections under the supervision of an ophthalmologist.
- *Acute retinal necrosis* is a condition characterized by rapid, initially peripheral retinal damage thought to be due to HSV (sometimes CMV) infection. Prompt referral to an ophthalmologist is appropriate.
- *Toxoplasmosis* causes largish, yellow-white exudates, usually without haemorrhage. It may be a feature of more generalized disease, and therapy is the same as for the encephalitic form.

HIV-related malignancy

Kaposi sarcoma (KS)

This is a tumour of lymphatic endothelial cells, caused by the Kaposi sarcoma-associated herpesvirus (KSHV, also known as human herpesvirus-8, HHV-8), that presents with lesions of the skin, oral cavity, and, in some cases, the viscera. The incidence of KS in HIV-infected populations is closely related to background prevalence of KSHV and is very common in west Africa.

Clinical features: KS typically presents as single or multiple lesions that are papular or nodular and pigmented, appearing black on black skin and purple on pale skin. Early lesions, being small and macular, are often difficult to recognize. While mostly asymptomatic, the lesions may become painful or ulcerate. They occur on all parts of the body, not just the skin, and are rarely limited to one anatomical region. Lesions on the face, legs, and in the mouth are common. Visceral disease may occur without skin involvement: the only visible lesion may be in the mouth. Oral lesions are often not raised and are usually asymptomatic but may result in bleeding, pain, and dysphagia. KS commonly involves lymph nodes (producing lymphoedema), the GI tract (can result in bleeding and anaemia), and the lungs (dyspnoea, cough). Patients with extensive KS may have B-symptoms such as weight loss and fever.

Diagnosis: clinical in most cases; a punch biopsy otherwise shows characteristic histology. Pulmonary involvement gives rise to characteristic CXR changes (flame-shaped linear and nodular infiltrates spreading from the hila) and may be accompanied by a blood-stained pleural effusion. GIT and pulmonary involvement is confirmed on endoscopy.

Management: ART is the first line of therapy. Limited skin and oral disease may regress with ART alone. If there is progression on ART, chemotherapy is considered. Patients with visceral involvement or extensive disease (>25 lesions, lymphoedema) usually require ART plus chemotherapy from the start. The common regimen used in resource-limited settings consists of combinations of doxorubicin, bleomycin, and vincristine. Local treatment such as radiation or topical liquid nitrogen can be used for localized lesions.

Lymphoma

Common forms in HIV-infected people:
- Non-Hodgkins lymphoma (NHL).
- Primary CNS lymphoma.
- Primary effusion lymphoma (PEL).

NHL is 200–600 times more common than in the general population and is usually related to underlying oncogenic EBV infection. Lymphomas typically present with chronic symptoms including wasting, fever, and symptoms related to location of disease. Patients may have adenopathy and/or GIT, hepatic, pulmonary, bone marrow, and CNS involvement. Diagnosis is confirmed by lymph node excision biopsy, bone marrow biopsy, or biopsy of other involved organs. Immunoblastic or Burkitt's lymphoma are the most common histologies. Most are B cell in origin.

Management: Combination chemotherapy (e.g. CHOP — cyclophosphamide, adriamycin, vincristine and prednisone); ART prevents relapses.

Primary CNS lymphoma causes focal signs and SOLs on CT and is EBV related: a positive EBV PCR in CSF supports diagnosis. Prognosis is poor even with chemotherapy, radiotherapy, and ART.

PEL presents with lymphomatous serous effusions in the absence of mass lesions. It is related to KSHV. It is diagnosed by pleural biopsy. Treatment is with chemotherapy and ART.

Cervical cancer

HIV infection in women is associated with a higher rate of cervical squamous intra-epithelial neoplasia (SIN) and a modest increase in the risk of cervical cancer. This is closely related to infection with certain oncogenic types of HPV. Invasive cervical carcinoma is a WHO stage 4 condition. Women with HIV should be screened annually with Pap smears. If high-grade SIN is present, then colposcopy and biopsy is indicated. Cervical cancer is treated with surgery and/or radiotherapy.

Prevention of opportunistic infections

Table 3.4 Primary prophylaxis

Condition	Medication	When to stop	Efficacy
Pneumocystis	Co-trimoxazole 2 tabs od *	CD4 >200 on ART	NNT (mortality) = 15
Tuberculosis	INH 300 mg/d for 6 months if no clinical evidence of TB, positive tuberculin test, and well functioning TB programme	No good evidence of benefit beyond 6 months	
Pneumococcal infections	Pneumococcal vaccine of unclear value		

* Co-trimoxazole single strength contains 80 mg trimethoprim and 400 mg of Sulphamethoxazole. Dose may be reduced to 480 mg daily to improve tolerance.

Table 3.5 Secondary prophylaxis

Condition	Medication	When to stop	Efficacy
Cryptococcal meningitis	Fluconazole 200 mg od	On ART with CD4 >200	NNT = 2 per episode of CM prevented at one year
Toxoplasmosis	Co-trimoxazole 2 tabs od	On ART with CD4 > 200	
Tuberculosis	Not usually recommended		
Non-typhi *Salmonellae*	Ciprofloxacin 500 mg bd	After 4 weeks	
Candidiasis	Not recommended — resistance issues		
Pneumocystis	Co-trimoxazole 1 tab od	On ART with CD4 >200	
Mycobacterium avium complex	Ethambutol and either azithymycizn or clarithromycin — same as initial treatment	Stop when CD4 >100 for 6 mths and at least 12 mths of MAC treatment	
Leishmaniasis	Amphotericin or antimony		
Penicilliosis	Itraconazole		
Isosporiasis	Co-trimoxazole 2–4 tabs od		

Preparing patients for ART

Prior to ART being commenced, the patient should be medically and psychosocially prepared. The following issues need to be addressed:

- *Screen for opportunistic infections:* ask about chronic cough (>2 weeks), night sweats, and recent weight loss — if any of these present, investigate for TB. Ask about visual disturbances — if present, screen for CMV. Screen for peripheral neuropathy (symptoms and signs). Use the WHO clinical staging system to classify each patient (📖 p 72). Treatment for all active OI should be initiated before starting ART and patients should be on appropriate primary and secondary prophylaxis.
- *Baseline blood tests:* depending on availability, these should include: FBC, LFTs (ALT is a useful screen), creatinine, CD4 count, HIV viral load, VDRL, hepatitis B surface antigen, hepatitis C antibody.
- *Potential drug interactions:* ensure no significant drug interactions between drugs the patient is taking and the ART to be started. Adjustments of medication or doses may be required.

The following issues should be addressed in counselling before a patient commences ART:

- HIV transmission and disease progression.
- Safe sex and other prevention messages (provide condoms).
- Understanding of CD4 count (and viral load if available).
- Benefits of therapy (treatment is NOT a cure).
- Side-effects and monitoring of treatment.
- Adherence and resistance.
- Family disclosure.
- Integrating treatment into daily life.
- Drug interactions (including alternative therapies).
- Dealing with complications.

Other issues

- *Substance abuse* should be addressed (counselling and referral). It is preferable that patients abstain before ART is started.
- *Depression* should also be treated before staring ART (counselling ± antidepressants).
- Patients with food shortages should be referred for appropriate support if this is available.

Disclosure of HIV status: patients should be encouraged to disclose their status to sexual partners and household members. Non-disclosure compromises adherence. If possible, patients should bring in a treatment supporter (friend, partner, or family member) who can also be educated about HIV and ART and remind and motivate the patient about their therapy. Other adherence tools include alarms, pillboxes, tick sheets, and reminders sent by mobile phone.

Antiretroviral therapy (ART)

Antiretroviral drugs act by inhibiting various steps in the replication cycle of HIV. The non-nucleoside reverse transcriptase inhibitors (NNRTI) and the nucleoside/nucleotide reverse transciptase inhibitors (NRTI/NtRTI) inhibit the viral enzyme reverse transcriptase, whereas protease inhibitors inhibit the viral enzyme protease. It is standard practice to combine ≥3 antiretroviral drugs into a regimen sufficiently potent to inhibit all viral replication and thereby prevent the emergence of resistant mutants — this is known as highly active antiretroviral therapy (HAART or ART).

With ART, it is possible to suppress the viral load below the limit of detection (usually <50 copies/ml) for years, provided patients adhere correctly. This allows for the CD4 to recover — on average 75 cells/mm^3 in the 1st month and 75 cells/mm^3 per year thereafter. With the rise in CD4 count, patients experience immune restoration. Opportunistic infections occur with reduced incidence, some OI regress without specific therapy (e.g. *cryptosporidium*), and patients are generally able to stop preventative therapies when CD4 counts rise >200 cells/mm^3. This results in reduced progression to AIDS, improvement in quality of life, and prolonged survival.

Treatment is lifelong, and correct adherence with therapy is critical. Patients taking ART should be adequately counselled before starting therapy. Patients need to have full insight into their disease, the drugs, the need for strict adherence, the side-effects, and prevention. Missing doses leads to inadequate viral suppression that results in the selection of mutations in the virus that confer resistance to the drugs. This causes sequential loss of drugs in a regimen due to the development of resistance, and patients require a change of regimen to attain viral suppression again. Over time, it is possible for patients to develop resistance to all classes of antiretrovirals making viral suppression impossible (multi-drug resistant HIV).

Starting therapy

The WHO recommendations regarding when to start ART differ according to whether CD4 counts are available or not (see opposite). In general all patients with clinically advanced disease and/or CD4 <200 require ART initiation. AIDS-defining illnesses (except TB) are uncommon with a CD4 count >200/mm^3 whole blood.

In addition to the medical criteria, patients must be psychosocially ready to commence lifelong daily therapy. This involves addressing issues such as substance abuse, depression, disclosure, and family relationships before starting. It is also useful for the patient to have a treatment supporter from their household or a friend who can motivate and remind.

Indications for starting HAART: WHO guidelines

Table 3.6 CD4 criteria for the initiation of ART in adults and adolescents

CD4(CELLS/MM^3)^a	TREATMENT RECOMMENDATION^b
<200	Treat irrespective of clinical stage ^{c}
200–350	Consider treatment and initiate before CD4 count drops below 200 cells/mm$^{3\ c\ d\ e}$
>350	Do not initiate treatment

a CD4 cell count should be measured after stabilization of any intercurrent condition.

b CD4 cell count supplements clinical assessment and should therefore be used in combination with clinical staging in decision-making.

c A drop in the CD4 cell count below 200 cells/m^3 is associated with a significant increase in opportunistic infections and death.

d The initiation of ART is recommended for all patients with any WHO clinical stage 4 disease and some WHO clinical stage 3 conditions, notably pulmonary TB and severe bacterial infections.

e The initiation of ART is recommended in all HIV-infected pregnant women with WHO clinical stage 3 disease and CD4 <350 cells/mm^3.

Table 3.7 Recommendations for initiating ART in adults and adolescents in accordance with clinical stages and the availabilty of immunological markers

WHO CLINICAL STAGING	CD4 TESTING NOT AVAILABLE	CD4 TESTING AVAILABLE
1	Do not treat	Treat if CD4 count is below 200 cell/mm$^{3\ a}$
2	Do not Treat ^{b}	
3	Treat	Consider treatment if CD4 count is below 350 cell/mm$^{3\ a\ c\ d}$ CD4 count drops below 200 cells/mm$^{3\ e}$
4	Treat	Treat irrespective of CD4 cell count ^{a}

a CD4 cell count advisable to assist with determining need for immediate therapy for situations such as pulmonary TB and severe bacterial infections, which may occur at any CD4 level.

b A total lympocyte count (TLC) of 1200 cells/mm^3 or less can be substituted for the CD4 count when the latter is unavailable and mild HIV disease exists. It is not useful in asymptomatic patients. Thus, in the absence of CD4 cell counts and TLCs, patients with WHO adult clinical stage 2 should not be treated.

c The initiation of ART is recommended in all HIV-infected pregenant women with WHO clinical stage 3 disease and CD4 counts below 350 cells/mm^3.

d The initiation of ART is recommended in all HIV-infected patients with CD4 counts below 350 cells/mm^3 and pulmonary TB or severe bacterial infection.

e The precise CD4 cell level above 200/mm^3 at which ART should be started has not been established

World Health Organization. Antiretroviral therapy for HIV infection in adults and adolescents: recommendations for a public health approach. WHO: Geneva, 2006.

http://www.who.int/hiv/pub/guidelines/artadultguidelines.pdf

First-line therapy

First-line therapy involves three drugs (see boxes for abbreviations). Common choices are one of AZT/D4T/TDF/ABC + one of 3TC/FTC + one of EFV/NVP. The following simple rules help decide which drug combination to use:

- Avoid D4T in patients with severe pre-existing neuropathy, as D4T may cause drug-induced neuropathy.
- Avoid AZT in patients with anaemia/neutropaenia as AZT bone marrow suppression is more likely if pre-existing problems.
- Avoid TDF in patients with renal dysfunction.
- Never use D4T and AZT together as they are antagonistic.
- Avoid NVP in patients with underlying liver disease, those with CD4>250 in women or >400 in men (↑risk of hepatitis) and those on TB treatment (shared toxicities and drug interactions).
- Avoid EFV in women of child-bearing age if there is any risk of pregnancy (potentially teratogenic). One advantage of EFV is its compatability with TB therapy, so if it needs to be used in such women because they are on TB treatment they should be counselled regarding contraception and switched to NVP on completion of TB therapy.

Monitoring prior to ART: If patients do not yet meet the criteria for commencing ART, they should be followed up and assessed at intervals. The CD4 should be repeated at 6–12 month intervals. Prior to starting ART, the clinical staging and/or CD4 count are the best monitors.

Monitoring on ART: Monitor for — adherence to therapy (e.g. self-reporting, pill counts); adverse effects (clinically, FBC, LFTs); new opportunistic infections and IRIS; CD4 and viral load where available. Viral load is the best assay to monitor therapy. If the viral load is undetectable, CD4 lymphocyte counts rarely alter management except to guide when to discontinue prophylaxis for opportunistic infections.

Table 3.8 ART doses and adverse effects

Nucleoside reverse transcriptase inhibitors (NRTIs)		
Abacavir* (ABC)	300 mg bd	Hypersensitivity (may be fatal) in 4%: fever, rash, GI. **Do not rechallenge**.
Didanosine (DDI)	400 mg od (250 mg if <60 kg)	Take on empty stomach (1 h before or 2 h after food). Peripheral neuropathy, pancreatitis, GI; rarely lactic acidosis, hepatic steatosis.
Emtricitabine (FTC)	200 mg od	Minimal. Rarely lactic acidosis, hepatic steatosis.
Lamivudine* (3TC)	150 mg bd or 300 mg od[1]	Minimal. Rarely lactic acidosis, hepatic steatosis.
Stavudine* (D4T)	40 mg bd (30 mg if <60 kg)	Peripheral neuropathy, lipodystrophy, pancreatitis, lactic acidosis, hepatic steatosis.
Zalcitabine (DDC)	0.75 mg tds	Peripheral neuropathy, stomatitis, pancreatitis, lactic acidosis, hepatic steatosis.
Zidovudine* (AZT)	250–300 mg bd	Bone marrow suppression (↓ Hb, neutropae-nia), myopathy; rarely lactic acidosis, hepatic steatosis.

Nucleotide reverse transcriptase inhibitors (NtRTIs)

Tenofovir (TDF)	245 mg od	Asthenia, headache, GI; rarely renal insufficiency.

Non-nucleoside reverse transcriptase inhibitors (NNRTIs)

Efavirenz* (EFZ)	600 mg od[2]	CNS effects (advise to take at night), hepatitis; contraindicated in pregnancy.
Nevirapine* (NVP)	200 mg bd or 400 mg od	Initially 200 mg daily, ↑ to 200 mg bd or 400 mg od after 2 weeks. Rash, Stevens–Johnson syndrome, hepatitis.
Delavirdine* (DLV)	400 mg tds	Diarrhoea, itching, rash.

Protease inhibitors (PIs)

Where a boosted PI regimen is used (📖 p 111), the dose given in brackets is used.

Amprenavir (APV)	1200 mg bd [600 mg bd]	GI, rash, oral paraesthesia, lipodystrophy
Atazanavir (ATZ)	400 mg od [300 mg od]	Take with food. ↑ bilirubin, cardiac conduction defect (prolonged PR interval)
Fosamprenavir (FPV)	1400 mg bd [700 mg bd]	GI, rash, lipodystrophy (less than other PIs).
Indinavir* (IDV)	800 mg tds [800 mg bd]	Nephrolithiasis, GI, ↑ bilirubin, lipodystrophy. fluids by 2 L daily.
Lopinavir (LPV)	[400 mg bd]	Take with food. Only used in boosted PI regimen with ritonavir. Pancreatitis, GI.
Nelfinavir (NFV)	1250 mg bd or 750 mg tds	Take with food. Diarrhoea, ↑ transaminases, lipodystrophy.
Ritonavir (RTV)	600 mg bd	Take with food. GI, paraesthesia, hepatitis, transaminases, pancreatitis, lipodystrophy
Saquinavir (SQV)	1200 mg bd or 600 mg tds [1000 mg bd][3]	GI, headache, transaminases, lipodystrophy.

Combined preparations

Combivir®	1 tablet bd, contains AZT 300 mg + 3TC 150 mg
Trizivir®	1 tablet bd, contains AZT 300 mg + 3TC 150 mg + ABC 300 mg
Truvada®	1 tablet od, contains TDF 300 mg + FTC 200 mg
Kivexa®	1 tablet od, contains ABC 600 mg + 3TC 300 mg
Kaletra®	3 capsules bd; 1 capsule contains LPV 133.3 mg + RTV 33.3 mg

* Consistent CSF Penetration. [1]Reduce to 250 mg when combined with TDF. [2]Consider reducing dose to 400 mg if <40 kg. [3]Alternative boosted PI regimen: SQV 400 mg bd + RTV 400 mg bd.

Table adapted with permission from Pattman et al, Oxford Handbook of Genitourinary Medicine, HIV and AIDS, Oxford University Press 2005. All doses are for adults.

Switching treatment and second-line therapy

Treatment failure: can be virological (virus detected in plasma repeatedly), immunological (no CD4 response or CD4 decline), and/or clinical (new WHO stage 3 or 4 events). Consider changing to second-line regimen in the following settings:

- *Clinical failure (if CD4 count/viral load not available)*: development of new stage 3 or 4 events (excluding TB which may occur at any CD4 count) after 6 months on ART.
- *Immunological failure (CD4 count but not viral load available)*: ↓ CD4 count to pre-therapy baseline (or below); *or* 50% fall from the on-treatment peak value (if known); or persistent CD4 count below 50 cells/mm^3 after one year on ART.
- *Virological failure*: where viral loads are available this is the best guide to the need for switching. Patients should be switched when viral load is persistently above a certain threshold (e.g. >10,000 copies/ml) despite adequate adherence interventions.

Second-line therapy: will successfully re-suppress viral replication in the majority of patients. Second-line therapy includes a protease inhibitor and two NRTIs (at least one of which has not been used previously). The decision regarding which regimen to use will depend on what drugs were used in the first line, available alternatives, and the national programme, and may need to be discussed with an experienced physician. It is preferable to use a 'boosted PI' regimen in second-line therapy (see below).

Side-effects of antiretroviral therapy — usual suspects

Severe ART toxicities	Most likely candidates
Anaemia/neutropenia	Zidovudine (especially with co-trimoxazole)
Neuropathy	Stavudine, didanosine
Pancreatitis	Didanosine, stavudine
Hepatic steatosis	Stavudine, didanosine
Lactic acidosis	Stavudine, didanosine > zidovudine > other NRTIs
Hypersensitivity	Abacavir (life-threatening, don't rechallenge)
Renal impairment	Tenofovir
Stevens–Johnson syndrome	Nevirapine > efavirenz
Hypersensitivity hepatitis	Nevirapine > efavirenz. Also abacavir
Psychiatric	Efavirenz
Nephrolithiasis	Indinavir
Diarrhoea	Protease inhibitors
Hyperlipidaemia	Protease inhibitors
Lipoatrophy	Nucleoside analogues, stavudine > zidovudine
Lipodystrophy/insulin resistance	Protease inhibitors

Boosted PI regimens

Combining other PIs with a small dose of ritonavir significantly improves the PI's pharmacokinetic profile, 'boosting' its concentration. 'Boosted PI' regimens utilize this by combining ritonavir 100 mg bd with a second PI (e.g. Lopinavir 400 mg + Ritonavir 100 mg bd).

ART dose adjustments in renal impairment

The following table gives a simple summary of suggested ART dose adjustments in renal failure. (For a more detailed breakdown of ART doses by creatinine clearance readers are referred to more specialist texts.)

Table 3.9 ART dose adjustments in renal failure

Drug	Creatinine Clearance 10–50	Creatinine Clearance <10
Zidovudine	Unchanged	300 mg daily
Didanosine	>60 kg 200 mg daily	>60 kg 100 mg daily
	<60 kg 150 mg daily	<60 kg 75 mg daily
Lamivudine	150 mg daily	50 mg daily
Stavudine	>60 kg 20 mg	>60 kg 20 mg daily
	12-hourly,<60 kg	<60 kg 15 mg daily
	15 mg 12-hourly	
Abacavir	Unchanged	Unchanged
Tenofovir	AVOID	AVOID
Zalcitabine	0.75 mg 12-hourly	0.75 mg daily
PIs	Unchanged	Unchanged
NNRTIs	Unchanged	Unchanged

Sources: Bartlett JG. *Medical Care of Patients with HIV Infection* 2003 and *The Sanford Guide to Antimicrobial Therapy* 2003.

ART side-effects

The majority of patients commencing ART will experience side-effects, especially in the first few weeks. Most will be mild and resolve spontaneously e.g. abdominal discomfort, nausea and vomiting (DDI and AZT), diarrhoea (PIs), headaches and fatigue (AZT). Warn patients these may occur. Management then involves excluding serious side-effects (e.g. hepatitis if nausea or vomiting), reassurance, and symptomatic therapy (e.g. antiemetic). Other, more serious side-effects, may also occur however, with potentially life-threatening/long-term consequences:

Peripheral neuropathy: Usually due to D4T or DDI. Peripheral sensory neuropathy initially, but may progress to motor involvement. Patients first complain of pain and paraesthesia in the feet. Management: Exclude other causes; amitriptyline 25 mg nocte; consider switching drugs (e.g. D4T to AZT).

Hypersensitivity hepatitis and/or skin rash: NVP (and less commonly EFV) may cause this, usually within 3 months of starting treatment. Women, and particularly those with CD4 >250 mm^3 are most at risk. Hepatitis may be asymptomatic. In those with ↑ ALT and symptoms, or those asymptomatic but with ALT >200, ART should be stopped and only recommenced once ALT has normalized — NVP should then be switched to an alternative drug (e.g. EFV or PI). The rash is morbilliform or maculopapular but may progress to a Stevens–Johnson syndrome. If mild, drugs can be continued with close monitoring. However, if severe (extensive rash, angioedema, desquamation or blistering, any mucous membrane or systemic involvement, or associated hepatitis) drugs should be stopped and recommenced only when the rash has resolved — NVP should again be switched to EFV or a PI. In the case of life-threatening NVP hepatitis or rash it is best to avoid EFV in future regimens as cross-reactivity is described.

Mitochondrial toxicity: is the underlying mechanism for many NRTI side-effects — neuropathy, fatty liver, pancreatitis, hyperlactataemia/lactic acidosis. Combinations of D4T and DDI (the most significant causes) should therefore be avoided and are contraindicated in pregnancy.

Hyperlactataemia and lactic acidosis: NRTIs (D4T>DDI>AZT>others) may cause acidosis as a consequence of mitochondrial toxicity. Severe lactic acidosis carries a high mortality (>50% in some studies). About a quarter of patients on these drugs will have a mildly raised lactate and be asymptomatic with no adverse consequences. Symptomatic hyperlactataemia is heralded by abdominal discomfort, nausea and vomiting, and weight loss. It usually occurs after patients have been on ART for several months (median 9 months). In severe lactic acidosis, patients may present in a critical condition with Kussmaul breathing ± circulatory collapse. *Management*: Early detection of hyperlactataemia is critical. Check lactate and ABG in symptomatic patients. If lactate ↑ (normal venous lactate <2.5 mmol/l) drugs should be stopped and a safer combination started once lactate has normalized (usually takes 2–3 months); patients who are acidotic should be admitted for IV fluids and vitamins. Sepsis may mimic lactic acidosis so it is often prudent to add a broad-spectrum antibiotic.

Fatty liver: (steatohepatitis) is also caused by NRTIs and is commonly associated with hyperlactataemia. *Management* principles are similar. Patients present with RUQ discomfort, firm hepatomegaly, and ↑ LFTs.

Pancreatitis: is a complication of DDI > D4T. *Management* involves stopping ART, admission and treatment for acute pancreatitis. Once resolved, ART can be recommenced with a regimen excluding these 2 drugs.

Bone marrow suppression: AZT may cause anaemia and neutropaenia, usually in the first 3 months of therapy. Patients with underlying marrow compromise (e.g. nutritional or TB) are more at risk. *Management* involves blood transfusions and neutropenic support if required. AZT should be switched to an alternative drug (e.g. D4T), especially if Hb < 6.5 g/dl and neutrophil <500/mm^3.

Lipid and glucose abnormalities: PIs may → hypercholesterolaemia and glucose intolerance (risk factors for cardiovascular disease) and hyper-triglyceridaemia (which may → pancreatitis). Patients on PIs should have other cardiovascular risk factors addressed (e.g. stop smoking) and all should be advised on a low-fat diet. Hypertriglyceridaemia >10 mmol/l and hypercholesterolaemia >7.5 mmol/l should be treated with dietary intervention and fibrate and/or statin therapy.

Lipodystrophy: (fat redistribution) is a consequence of long-term ART therapy. NRTIs (D4T>AZT) result in lipoatrophy (loss of facial and limb fat) and PIs result in lipohypertrophy (central obesity and dorsocervical fat accumulation). *Management* involves switching to alternative agents if possible, but reversal is slow.

Renal disease: TDF is associated with renal dysfunction and Fanconi's syndrome (a tubular wasting syndrome of protein, phosphate, and other substances) in a minority of patients, particularly those with pre-existing renal dysfunction. IDV may result in renal stones, particularly if a good fluid intake is not maintained.

Abacavir hypersensitivity: occurs in ~4% patients. Clinical features include flu-like symptoms, rash, fever and hepatitis; may be life-threatening with continued use. *Management*: stop abacavir; do not re-challenge.

Teratogenicity: EFV is teratogenic (neural tube defects reported in animals and humans in relation to first trimester exposure).

Neuropsychiatric: side-effects also occur with EFV, including dizziness, inattention, nightmares, dysphoria, and occasionally acute psychosis. These side-effects occur early and resolve in the majority within a few weeks. Advise patients to take EFV at night.

AZT-induced myopathy: is described, usually after prolonged therapy.

ART metabolism and interactions

Drugs belonging to the NNRTI and PI classes have a number of important drug interactions that need to be considered. These result from the fact that they are substrates of the cytochrome P450 enzyme system in the liver and intestine. In addition, the PIs are generally inhibitors of these enzymes, nevirapine an inducer, and efavirenz may be an inducer or inhibitor. Exceptions do, however, occur. Drugs that are commonly involved in these interactions are:

- **Inducers:**
  - Carbamazepine, phenytoin, phenobarbital, rifampicin.
- **Inhibitors.**
  - Macrolides, cimetidine, azoles (e.g. fluconazole).
- **Substrates.**
  - Warfarin.
  - Carbamazepine, phenytoin, phenobarbitone.
  - Oral contraceptive.
  - Statins.
  - Benzodiazepines, especially midazolam.
  - Ergot alkaloids.
  - Macrolides.
  - Calcium channel blockers.
  - Azoles.

When prescribing other drugs with ART it is important to check for interactions. A useful source of ART drug interaction information is: *www.hiv-druginteractions.org*

Some combinations are contraindicated (e.g. ergotamine and PI) and in others, dose adjustments are required (e.g. warfarin and nevirapine guided by INR). The interactions may be bi-directional, for example, carbamazepine and nevirapine may reduce each other's levels. Other drug combinations share toxicities and should not be used together, for example, ganciclovir and AZT because both drugs are bone marrow suppressants.

NRTIs are not metabolized by the cytochrome P450 system but are excreted by the kidney. Certain interactions occur at this level e.g. tenofovir increases didanosine levels and thus toxicity. For this reason (and also because this combination is less potent than other NRTI combinations), these two drugs should preferably not be used together. If they are, the didanosine dose should be reduced. If renal function is impaired, it is important to reduce the dose of NRTI drugs (see table p 111).

Table 3.10 Common ART drug interactions and how to manage these

Interacting drugs	Effect	Management
Rifampicin and efavirenz	Rifampicin lowers efavirenz levels moderately (22%)	Standard-dose Efavirenz
Rifampicin and nevirapine	Rifampicin lowers nevirapine levels more substantially (37%) and these drugs have common toxicities	Preferably avoid nevirapine, but if it is started in patients on rifampicin do not use lead-in dose (i.e. commence treatment with 200 mg bd)
Rifampicin and kaletra	Marked reduction in lopinavir level (75%)	In patients on rifampicin, use kaletra 6 capsules bd (double dose) OR kaletra 3 capsules bd plus ritonavir 300 mg bd
NNRTI or PI and warfarin	Warfarin levels increased or reduced and thus INR control disturbed	Monitor INR closely when starting, switching, or stopping ART and adjust warfarin dose accordingly
Phenytion, phenobarbital, or carbamazepine and NNRTI	Bidirectional interaction: levels of both these anticonvulsants and the NNRTI are reduced	Avoid if possible — use amitriptyline rather than carbamazepine for neuropathic pain and valproate for epilepsy
Efavirenz and oral contraception	Levels of ethinyl oestradiol are increased	Avoid high-dose OC — low-dose oral or injectable contraceptive or IUD are alternatives A barrier method must be used.
PIs or nevirapine and oral contraceptives	Levels of ethinyl oestradiol are reduced	Avoid low-dose OC — high-dose oral or injectable contraceptive or IUD are alternatives. A barrier method must also be used.
PIs and midazolam or triazolam	Levels of benzodiazepines increased with risk of sedation	AVOID
PIs and ergot alkaloids	Substantial increases in levels of ergot alkaloids leading to vasospastic crises	AVOID

Immune reconstitution inflammatory syndrome (IRIS)

After ART is commenced, there is a rapid reduction in HIV viral load and a rise in CD4 count. This is accompanied by a restoration of pathogen-specific immunity. Immunopathological reactions in the days to months after starting ART may result as a consequence of immune dysregulation. This is often in response to a high burden of microbial antigen related to an OI that was present prior to ART. This is termed IRIS, for which the following case definition has been proposed:

• HIV-infected patient receiving ART with ↓ viral load and ↑ CD4 count (which may lag behind the fall in viral load) *plus*
• Clinical features consistent with inflammatory process *and*
• Clinical course not consistent with expected course of either a previously diagnosed OI or newly diagnosed OI or drug toxicity.

Several forms of IRIS are described:

• '*Unmasking*' IRIS — this describes an inflammatory and often atypical presentation of an OI soon after starting ART that was untreated prior to ART commencement.
• *Paradoxical reactions* — patients experience recurrence or worsening of OI symptoms and signs after starting ART despite being on appropriate OI treatment. The reaction here is thought to result from an immune response directed towards residual antigen.
• *Sarcoidosis and auto-immune diseases* (e.g. Grave's disease) are described as IRIS phenomena.
• Kaposi sarcoma may worsen with an increase in lesions or inflammation of existing lesions in 5% of patients (most KS lesions regress on ART).
• Reactions to inert foreign materials (e.g. tattoos).

IRIS most commonly occurs in association with OI such as TB, cryptococossis, MAC, CMV, and HBV. An example of a CMV 'unmasking' IRIS is a patient presenting with an inflammatory CMV uveitis after starting ART. TB paradoxical reactions are seen in up to 45% of patients starting ART while on TB treatment, manifesting as recurrence of fever and other TB symptoms, enlarging lymphadenopathy, or recurrent pulmonary infiltrates early after starting ART. Dermatological manifestations (e.g. flare of acne) are also seen.

Management: involves diagnosing the OI and excluding additional OIs or antimicrobial resistance. In most cases, ART and effective OI therapy should be continued. In certain severe cases, steroids (e.g. prednisone 1 mg/kg, duration dependent on response) should be considered. If the reaction is life-threatening (e.g. CNS involvement) and not responding to steroids, it may be necessary to interrupt ART.

Special aspects of paediatric HIV/AIDS

Diagnosis (WHO guidelines)

Early diagnosis is the key to effective management of HIV in children. HIV-infected adults should be encouraged to get their children tested, and in areas where the prevalence of paediatric HIV is more than a few per cent, HIV testing should become a routine part of inpatient care and not merely reserved for children with signs of advanced HIV/AIDS.

In children >18 months, diagnosis is as for adults (📖 p 74)

In children <18 months, diagnosis is based on:

- Positive virological test for HIV (HIV-RNA or HIV-DNA or ultrasensitive HIV p24 antigen), confirmed by a second virological test obtained from a separate sample taken >4 weeks after birth.
- Positive antibody testing is *not recommended* for definitive or confirmatory diagnosis of HIV infection in children until 18 months of age.
- However, *presumptive diagnosis* of severe HIV disease may be made if:
  - the infant is seropositive **and**
  - an AIDS-defining illness is present **or**
  - the infant has symptoms of 2 or more of the following: oral thrush, severe pneumonia, or severe sepsis.

Other factors supporting the diagnosis of severe HIV disease include:

- Maternal death due to (or advanced) HIV infection.
- % CD4 <20.

Confirmation of the diagnosis should be sought as soon as possible.

Effects on growth and development

Poor growth is one of the most sensitive indicators of HIV progression. From birth, HIV-infected infants are often smaller and have lower birth-weight than uninfected children born to HIV-infected women. Causes of poor growth include alterations in GI function, chronic or recurrent infections, alterations in metabolic and endocrine function, and side-effects of medication for HIV and OI. Pubertal delay is common, especially among boys. The use of effective ART leads to improvements in growth indices.

Prevention of opportunistic infections in children

Co-trimoxazole prophylaxis has been shown to halve all cause mortality, and is recommended for all HIV positive children. Primary isoniazid preventative therapy is also associated with an all-cause mortality benefit, although the optimal duration of therapy is unknown.

WHO clinical staging for HIV/AIDS in children with confirmed HIV infection (2006)

Clinical stage 1 Asymptomatic   PAEDIATRIC NOTE

Persistent generalized lymphadenopathy (PGL)

Clinical stage 2
Unexplained persistent hepatomegaly or parotid enlargement
Papular pruritic eruption, fungal nail infection
Recurrent oral ulceration, lineal gingival erythema
Herpes Zoster
Recurrent upper respiratory tract infections
Extensive wart virus or molluscum contyagiosum infection

Clinical stage 3
Unexplained moderate malnutrition not responding to therapy
Unexplained chronic diarrhoea for >14 days
Unexplained prolonged fever for >1 month
Persistent oral candidiasis beyond first 2 months of life
Oral hairy leukoplakia
Pulmonary and lymph node TB
Severe bacterial pneumonia
Symptomatic lymphoid interstitial pneumonitis
Acute necrotizing ulcerative oral disease
Unexplained anaemia (<8 g/dl), neutropaenia (<0.5 × 10⁹/L) and/or chronic thrombocytopenia (<50 × 10⁹/L)

Clinical stage 4
Unexplained severe wasting/malnutrition not responding to therapy
Pneumocystis jiroveci (*carinii*) pneumonia (PCP)
CNS toxoplasmosis (after 1 month of life)
Chronic cryptosporidiosis or isosporiasis
Cryptococcosis, extrapulmonary
Cytomegalovirus (CMV) infection with onset after 1 month of life
Chronic HSV infection of >1 month duration or involving viscera
Progressive multifocal leukoencephalopathy (PML)
Candidiasis of the oesophagus, trachea, bronchi, or lungs
Disseminated non-tuberculous mycobacterial infection
Recurrent severe bacterial infection, excluding pneumonia
Extrapulmonary TB
Lymphoma (cerebral or B cell non Hodgkin lymphoma)
Kaposi sarcoma
HIV encephalopathy
Disseminated mycosis (histoplasmosis or coccidiomycosis)
Symptomatic HIV nephropathy or cardiomyopathy

Therapy of opportunistic infections in children

Whilst many of the principles required to recognize, diagnose, and manage OI in children are similar to those in adults, there are important differences e.g. higher incidence of some opportunistic conditions in children and the problems posed by drug therapy. The notes on the following pages emphasize management and are not exhaustive. They are based on a comprehensive CDC review that is available for download free from: www.cdc.gov/mmwr/preview/mmwrhtml/rr5314a1.htm

Pneumocystis jiroveci pneumonia (PCP)

PCP is an important cause of ARI in children and the leading cause of ARI among children aged 2–6 months. Treatment of ARI in the latter group should always include PCP treatment; treat older children for PCP when suspected clinically.

- Trimethoprim-sulfamethoxazole (TMP/SMX) 15–20 mg/kg TMP plus 75–100 mg/kg SMX IV or PO daily in 3–4 divided doses for 21 days.
- Alternative therapies include:
  - Pentamidine 4 mg/kg IV od for 7–10 days followed by atovaquone for 14 days.
  - Atovaquone 15–20 mg/kg (max 750 mg) bd.
- Prednisolone (2 mg/kg for 5 days, 1 mg/kg for 5 days then 0.5 mg/kg for 5 days) should be added if paO2 <70 mmHg (<9.3 kPa) on room air.
- Lifelong secondary prophylaxis with TMP/SMX is recommended.

Toxoplasmosis

- Congenital: Treat for 6 months with pyrimethamine (2 mg/kg od for 2 days then 1 mg/kg od for 2–6 months, then 1 mg/kg 3x weekly) plus folinic acid 10 mg with each dose, plus sulfadiazine 50 mg/kg bd.
- Acquired: Treat for 6 weeks with pyrimethamine (2 mg/kg [max 50 mg] od for 3 days then 1 mg/kg [max 25 mg] od) plus sulphadiazine 25–50 mg/kg qds plus folinic acid 10–25 mg od.
- Clindamycin 5–7.5 mg/kg (max. 600 mg/dose) PO/IV qds can be substituted for sulphadiazine.
- Lifelong secondary prophylaxis is recommended.

Cryptosporidiosis

No consistently effective therapy exists and the best treatment is ART.

Microsporidiosis

The best treatment is ART, although albendazole 7.5 mg/kg (max 400 mg) bd is effective against all forms except Enterocytozoon bienusi.

Tuberculosis

- Standard quadruple therapy but treat PTB for 9 m and extrapulmonary TB for 12 m. Drug-resistant TB requires expert advice. See below for combination with ART.
- Adjunctive treatment with corticosteroids is recommended by some for CNS, pericardial, and substantial endobronchial disease.

Mycobacterium avium complex (MAC)

- At least two drugs should be given: clarithromycin 7.5–15 mg/kg (max. 500 mg) bd *plus* ethambutol 15–25 mg/kg (max. 1 g) od.
- In severe disease, rifabutin 10–20 mg/kg (max. 300 mg) can be added and azithromycin 10–12 mg/kg (max. 500 mg) od can be substituted for clarithromycin.

Candidiasis

- *Oropharyngeal*: Fluconazole 3–6 mg/kg (max 400 mg) od for 7–14 days *or* itraconazole 2.5 mg/kg (max 200–400 mg) bd. (Nystatin and clotrimazole preparations are less effective.)
- *Oesophageal*: As for oropharyngeal candidiasis but extend treatment for 21 days.
- *Invasive*: Ampotericin B (AmB) 0.5–1.5 mg/kg IV od until 2–3 weeks after last positive blood culture. If AmB is unavailable, fluconazole can be used at 5–6 mg/kg bd (max 800 mg/day).

Coccidiomycosis

- *Diffuse pulmonary or disseminated*: AmB 0.5–1.0 mg/kg IV od for several weeks, followed by chronic suppressive therapy with an azole.
- *Meningeal infection*: Fluconazole 5–6 mg/kg bd (max 800 mg/day) for several weeks followed by secondary prophylaxis.

Cytomegalovirus (CMV)

- *Congenital*: Ganciclovir 6 mg/kg IV bd for 6 weeks.
- *Retinitis & visceral disease*: Ganciclovir 5 mg/kg IV bd for 14–21 days followed by 5 mg/kg IV od 5–7 days per week as suppressive therapy. An alternative is foscarnet 60 mg/kg IV tds for 10–21 days then 90–120 mg/kg od for chronic suppression.

Cryptococcosis

- AmB 0.75–1.5 mg/kg IV od for at least 2 weeks *plus* flucytosine 25 mg/kg PO qds.
- If AmB unavailable, fluconazole 5–6 mg/kg bd (max 800 mg/day) can be used, although its efficacy in children is not documented.
- Chronic suppressive therapy with fluconazole should also be instituted.

Histoplasmosis

- *Mild*: Itraconazole 4–10 mg/kg bd (max 600 mg daily) IV/PO for 3 days, followed by 2–5 mg/kg (max 200 mg) bd for 12–16 weeks.
- *Severe and disseminated*: AmB 1 mg/kg IV od for 2–3 weeks followed by consolidation therapy as above.
- Lifelong secondary prophylaxis with itraconazole is recommended.

HSV

- *Neonatal*: Aciclovir 20 mg/kg IV tds for 21 days.
- *CNS*: Outside neonatal period acyclovir 10 mg/kg IV tds for 21 days.
- *Gingivostomatitis*: Aciclovir 5–10 mg/kg IV tds.
- *Genital herpes*: Aciclovir 20 mg/kg (max 400 mg) PO tds for 7–10 days.
- Foscarnet can be given for acyclovir-resistant disease. 2nd generation nucleoside analogues (valaciclovir, famcicolvir, penciclovir) are not fully evaluated in children.

VZV

- *Chickenpox*: Aciclovir 10 mg/kg IV tds for 7 days or until no new lesions. Oral acyclovir (20 mg/kg qds) should only be used for children with very mild disease or in those with normal or only slightly decreased CD4 counts.
- *Zoster*: Aciclovir 20 mg/kg PO qds for 7–10 days; consider IV acyclovir 10 mg/kg in severe immunodeficiency.

HCV

Interferon-alpha-2b *plus* ribavirin. Treatment is expensive and not available in most low-resource settings. Treat HCV genotype-1 infections for 48 weeks; genotypes 2 and 3 can be treated for 24 weeks.

HBV

- Interferon-alpha. Treat for 6 months if HBeAg +ve, 12 months if HBeAg −ve.
- The antiretrovirals lamivudine (3TC) and tenofovir (TDF) have activity against HBV. 3TC monotherapy can give rise to drug-resistant HBV and ideally should be combined in HBsAg +ve children but the data on TDF dosage in childhood are limited.

ART in children

The best way to reduce paediatric HIV is to reduce MTCT. However, ~1500 new infections occur daily in children <15 years, the majority in the developing world. HIV-infected children frequently become symptomatic, and 30% die in the first year of life. There is thus a need to provide antiretroviral therapy (ART) for HIV-infected infants and children.

When to start ART

The following are indications for starting ART in infants and children based on clinical stage of disease, CD4, and total lymphocyte count (see tables opposite):

- Stage 4 disease, irrespective of CD4 count. Treat and stabilize active OI first.
- Stage 3 disease. (If age >12 months and the stage 3 defining disease is TB, LIP, oral hairy leukoplakia, or thrombocytopenia, and the CD4 is above threshold, then ART could be deferred.)
- Stage 1 or 2 disease with CD4 or total lymphocyte count (TLC) below threshold for severe immunodeficiency (see table opposite).

General principles

- Use one formulation or a fixed-drug combination (FDC) if possible.
- Use syringes to accurately dose liquid formulations.
- Avoid large volumes of liquid drugs; switch to solids when possible.
- If solid paediatric formulations unavailable, adapt adult forms. Many tablets can be divided in half.
- Some adult FDCs (e.g. those contaning NVP) may underdose during induction and should be avoided during this phase.
- Avoid differing a.m. and p.m. regimens where possible.
- Weigh the child at each visit and adjust doses accordingly.
- If capsules or tablets are broken into food, ensure all food is eaten.

Recommended first-line ART regimens

- AZT + 3TC + NVP/EFV *or*
- D4T + 3TC + NVP/EFV *or*
- ABC + 3TC + NVP/EFV *or*
- Triple NRTI (to simplify drug interaction and toxicity) *or*
- AZT/d4T + 3TC + ABC.

The disadvantage of the triple NRTI combination is its lower virological potency in adults. The advantages are that it can be combined with TB treatment (see below), is non-teratogenic in pregnant adolescent girls, and when combined as a single pill can improve adherence. There is insufficient evidence to guide prescribing in infants who were exposed to the maternal or infant component of MTCT treatment or in infants exposed via breastfeeding. A particular concern is children exposed to single-dose NVP. WHO recommends that the above first-line regimens be used in the first instance.

Table 3.11 Recommendations for initiating ART in HIV-infected infants (WHO, 2006)

WHO paediatric stage	CD4 available?	Age-specific treatment recommendation	
		<12 months	≥12 months
Stage 4	N/A	Treat all, irrespective of availability of CD4 and age	
Stage 3	Yes	Treat all	Treat all, but CD4 guided if stage 3 defined by TB, LIP, oral hairy leukoplakia, or thrombocytopenia
	No		Treat all
Stage 2	Yes		CD4 guided
	No		TLC guided
Stage 1	Yes		CD4 guided
	No	Do not treat	

Table 3.12 CD4 and total lymphocyte count (TLC) criteria for severe immunodeficiency (WHO, 2006)

Marker	Age-specific recommendation to initiate ART			
	<12 months	12–35 months	36–59 months	≥5 years
% CD4	<25%	<20%	<15%	<15%
CD4 count	<1500/mm3	<750/mm3	<350/mm3	<200/mm3
TLC	<4000/mm3	<3000/mm3	<2500/mm3	<2000/mm3

Dosage of paediatric ART

This is a complex area because of a relative lack of pharmacological data and formulations appropriate to children. What is presented is derived from WHO guidelines (2006).[*] Readers are encouraged to seek specialist advice where possible. Where *body surface area* (BSA) has been used, this is calculated by the formula:

$$BSA = \frac{\sqrt{weight\ (kg) \times height\ (cm)}}{3600}$$

PAEDIATRIC NOTE

Lamivudine (3TC)	Target dose: 4 mg/kg (max150 mg) bd 2 mg/kg bd if <30 days old.
Stavudine (D4T)	Target dose: 1 mg/kg bd (<30 kg) 30 mg/dose bd if >30 kg Adults >60 kg: 40 mg bd recommended currently
Zidovudine (AZT)	Target dose for infants >6 weeks old: 180–240 mg/m^2 (max 300 mg) bd. Prevention of MTCT in infants: 4 mg/kg po bd; start within 12 h after birth and continue up to 6 weeks. IV alternative (until oral administration possible): 1.5 mg/kg qds, infused over 30 mins.
Abacavir (ABC)	Target dose: 8 mg/kg (max 300 mg) bd
Didanosine (DDI)	<3 months: 50 mg/m^2 bd 3 months to 12 years: 90–120 mg/m^2 bd Max dose >12 years or >60 kg: 200 mg/dose bd or 400 mg od
Efavirenz (EFV)	>40 kg: 600 mg od <40 kg: 19.5 mg/kg od (syrup) or 15 mg/kg od (capsule/tablet) Not currently recommended for children <3 years
Nevirapine (NVP)	Target maintenance dose 160–200 mg/m^2 bd (max 200 mg bd) Induction dose: for first 14 days give half maintenance dose od. (A mild rash may be observed during induction — defer escalation if necessary. A serious rash requires discontinuation.)
Saquinavir (SQV)	33 mg/kg tds (not licensed for use in children <16 years or <25 kg)
Nelfinavir (NFV)	<10 kg: ~75 mg/kg/dose bd ≥10 kg to 19.9 kg: ~60 mg/kg/dose bd ≥20 kg: maximum recommended 1250 mg/dose bd
Lopinavir/ ritonavir (LPV/r) co-formulation	*Lopinavir* target doses (children ≥6 months): 5–7.9 kg 16 mg/kg bd; 8–9.9 kg 14 mg/kg bd; 10–13.9 kg 12 mg/kg bd; 14–39.9 kg 10 mg/kg bd (equivalent to 300 mg/m2). *Ritonavir* target doses: 7–15 kg 3 mg/kg/dose bd; 15–40 kg 2.5 mg/kg/dose bd (equivalent to 75 mg/m^2) Maximum dose: 400 mg lopinavir + 100 mg ritonavir bd

* www.who.int/hiv/pub/guidelines/paediatric020907.pdf

ART toxicity in children

Overall, the spectrum of adverse events is similar to adults (see above). Hypersensitivity and hepatitis due to NVP are somewhat less frequent. Severe toxicities and potential drugs to switch to are listed in the table below (source WHO). In general, acute serious adverse reactions require discontinuation of all ART until the symptoms resolve. More chronic or subacute toxicities may be managed by withdrawing and then substituting the most likely offending drug (e.g. AZT-induced anaemia).

Drug	Toxicity	Suggested substitution
ABC	Hypersensitivity	AZT
AZT	Haematological toxicity	d4T or ABC
	Lactic acidosis	ABC
	Severe gastrointestinal intolerance	d4T or ABC
d4T	Lactic acidosis	ABC
	Peripheral neuropathy	AZT or ABC
	Pancreatitis	AZT or ABC
	Lipoatrophy/metabolic syndrome	ABC
EFZ	CNS toxicity	NVP
	Potential teratogenicty	
NVP	Acute hepatitis	EFZ
	Hypersensitivity	3rd NRTI or PI
	Stevens-Johnson syndrome	3rd NRTI or PI

Switching to second-line therapy due to treatment failure

Poor adherence or drug absorption and viral drug resistance can contribute to treatment failure. Prior to switching therapy, ensure that ≥24 weeks of treatment have been completed, adherence has been optimized, and the CD4 count has been measured at least twice. As far as possible exclude IRIS (📖 p 116) as a cause of clinical deterioration. The CD4 criteria to guide decision making on switching are as follows (see table on p 125 for age-related definitions of severe immunodeficiency):

- development of severe immunodeficiency after initial immune recovery.
- new progressive severe immunodeficiency, confirmed with at least one subsequent CD4 measurement.
- rapid decline to below threshold of severe immunodeficiency.

Recommended 2nd-line regimen: 2 RTIs plus boosted PI

Failed 1st line regimen	Preferred 2nd-line regimen		
2 NRTI + 1 NNRTI (AZT or D4T containing)	DDI + ABC		LPV/r
			or
2 NRTI + 1 NNRTI (ABC containing)	DDI + AZT	plus	SQV/r (if >25 kg)
			or
Triple NRTI	DDI + EFZ or NVP		NFV

Combining ART with TB treatment in children: special considerations

This is a complex area with little evidence to guide practice. Essentially:
- TB may be an indication for ART.
- The development of TB during ART may be a sign of ART failure.
- Alternatively, TB may become manifest ('umasking IRIS') or worsen ('paradoxical IRIS') during ART.
- Rifampicin-based therapy for TB complicates the choice of ART.

When to start ART

For WHO stage 4 disease and for stage 3 disease where no CD4 is available, ART should be commenced 2–8 weeks after starting TB therapy. If the response to TB in stage 3 disease is very good and the child is on co-trimoxazole prophylaxis, ART can be delayed. For stage 3 disease where the CD4 indicates mild or no immunodeficiency, ART can be deferred providing clinical response is satisfactory. If the CD4 indicates severe immunodeficiency, ART should be started.

Optimum drug regimens

WHO recommends either a triple *NRTI regime (AZT or d4T + 3TC + ABC) or two NRTI + NVP (<3 years) or EFZ (≥3 years).* In children already on such a regime, the advent of TB may herald treatment failure. If this is established, switching regimens may be required — specialist advice should ideally be sought. If the child is already on a PI-containing regimen, again expert advice will be required to determine the optimal salvage regimen in the clinical circumstances.

TB–IRIS

An alternative explanation for clinical deterioration of TB or the rapid appearance of TB during ART is TB–IRIS. This syndrome is even more poorly characterized in children than it is in adults, but typically occurs within weeks of starting ART. A pronounced inflammatory component is characteristic, as is the history of a previously good response to TB treatment. Wherever possible, ART should not be discontinued and the IRIS should be treated symptomatically. There is no hard evidence for the concurrent use of steroid therapy but this may be considered in children with severe and life-threatening forms of IRIS involving vital structures or the CNS (prednisolone 1.5 mg/kg per day).

Prevention

In the absence of a vaccine, primary prevention is the only method of controlling the AIDS pandemic. Strategies to control HIV infection should be aimed at the main methods of transmission: sexual, parenteral, and vertical.

Sexual

Changing high-risk sexual behaviour through health education could have a major effect on sexual HIV transmission. It would also have a marked effect on STI transmission. Creative educational approaches that respect cultural traditions are necessary to make the population aware of the dangers of HIV infection and AIDS, and to encourage protective measures. Several governments have now initiated such health education programmes. However, these programmes will have to be accompanied by approaches that influence the social determinants of risk, such as gender inequality, to enable those vulnerable to infection to protect themselves. It is increasingly recognized that male circumcision is an important additional HIV prevention intervention.

Blood transfusion

Screening of blood donations for HIV antibody may result in high benefit-to-cost ratio for the prevention of AIDS in populations with a high infection rate. Drawbacks are cost, logistics, and the lack of detectable HIV antibodies for 3–6 weeks (with 3rd generation ELISAs) after infection. Efforts to identify and exclude high-risk donors have proven to be difficult, but they may be important in decreasing the risk of HIV-infected sero-negative persons donating blood.

Injections

Prevention of infection through contaminated needles is feasible with the use of universal precautions. However, the use of disposable needles and syringes may be prohibitively expensive for some countries and health workers should be trained to give as few injections as possible and to sterilize reusable equipment. The risk of transmission after a needlestick injury may be reduced by antiretroviral post-exposure prophylaxis (see 📖 p 134).

Vertical

Most importantly, this involves the prevention of HIV infection in women of childbearing age and advice on contraception to HIV +ve women. See next page for details of prevention of MTCT.

Prevention of mother to child transmission (MTCT)

The cumulative risk of HIV transmission from mother to her child is 30–40% in the absence of preventive interventions. The following measures have been shown to substantially reduce this risk:

- *Formula feeding*: WHO recommends that, where the 1° causes of infant deaths are infectious disease and malnutrition, the standard advice to pregnant women (including those known to be HIV +ve) should be to breastfeed; where this is not the case, HIV +ve women are advised not to breastfeed but to use a safe feeding alternative for their babies. There may also be socio-cultural reasons why women choose to breastfeed. Formula feeding should only be considered in a setting where there is a reliable supply of both formula feed and safe water. If exclusive formula feeding cannot be guaranteed, then exclusive breastfeeding is advisable as it carries a lower risk of mother to child transmission than mixed breast and formula feeding.
- *Elective caesarian* section has been shown to reduce the risk of transmission, particularly in women with high viral loads, but is not practical as a routine procedure in most high-prevalence settings.
- *ART* to prevent transmission: Various regimens have been studied and utilized. In general, the following are the options:

1. **Single dose nevirapine** 200 mg to mother in labour and single dose to infant (2 mg/kg) within 72 h of delivery. This reduces transmission risk to ~8% provided mother does not breastfeed.

2. **Dual therapy** (e.g. AZT to mother from 28 weeks and to infant for 1 week, and single-dose nevirapine to mother and infant as above). This reduces the risk to ~2% provided the infant is not breastfed. There are other dual therapy options.

3. **Triple drug ART** starting in the second trimester reduces the risk to around 1%. Women for whom ART is indicated for their own health because of advanced HIV should be started on ART and continue ART after the pregnancy; those that receive it for prevention of MTCT alone should stop ART in the month after the pregnancy. On stopping ART, continue the NRTIs for 5–10 days after stopping nevirapine, because of the long half-life of nevirapine. Note that EFV and the combination of D4T+DDI are contraindicated in pregnancy. It is not advisable to commence nevirapine in women with CD4>250 because of higher risk of hepatotoxicity.

The use of single-dose nevirapine (options 1 and 2) carries the risk of causing NNRTI resistance in the mother and infected infant, and compromising future ART options. While ART is obviously the optimal form of MTCT prevention, resource and service limitations in many developing world settings result in one of the other options being chosen at a programme level.

Post-exposure prophylaxis (PEP) following needlestick injuries

Health care workers (HCW) are at risk of HIV infection if they sustain a needlestick injury with a needle that has been used in someone who is HIV infected. The estimated risk of infection is 0.3% per needlestick event. Injuries are regarded as high risk if the needle was in a vessel, the injury was deep, if there was visible blood on the needle, or if the source patient has a high viral load. Splash injuries with HIV-infected blood onto non-intact skin (e.g. dermatitis or open wound) or mucous membranes, including conjunctivae, may also result in HIV infection (estimated risk of transmission ~0.1%). Other fluids such as CSF and serous effusions are also potentially infectious. Following a significant exposure, the risk of transmission can be substantially reduced by taking PEP for 28 days (AZT monotherapy reduced risk by 81%).

Other infections that can be potentially transmitted in such circumstances are HBV, HCV, and syphilis.

Action that should be taken following a needlestick or splash injury:

- Local measures — prolonged washing with soap.
- ART PEP should start as soon as possible. This should be taken before the source patient's status is known. If the patient is HIV-uninfected, the PEP can be stopped. See table opposite for recommended regimens.
- Obtain consent from the source patient for HIV testing if status is unknown. Also test for hepatitis B and C and VDRL status (do the same tests for HCW — if the HCW is HIV positive, then PEP should NOT be prescribed).
- Counsel the HCW. Psychological support is necessary.
- Document details of the event and all investigations and management. This is critical for compensation of HCWs who seroconvert.
- If patient is HIV-seronegative, stop PEP unless it is clinically suspected that the patient has a seroconversion illness.
- If the patient is HIV-infected or the status is unknown, continue PEP for 28 days.
- In HCW on PEP regimens containing AZT, the Hb and neutrophil count should be checked at baseline and 2 weeks.
- The HCW should have an HIV ELISA test performed at 6 weeks, 3 months, and 6 months (PEP may delay seroconversion).
- The HCW should be advised to use condoms or abstain from sexual intercourse until seronegativity is documented.
- If the HCW is not Hepatitis B immunized and the source patient is Hepatitis B infected, then Hep B immunoglobulin and vaccination should be administered. HCWs who have been immunized but have inadequate antibody titres (<10 mIU/ml) may require booster vaccination.

If source patient is on ART and suspected to have drug resistance, then standard PEP should be instituted as soon as possible but modification in the regimen, based on likely resistance patterns, discussed with an expert.

Side-effects such as nausea are common with AZT and antiemetics may be required. It must be remembered that drugs used for PEP are potentially toxic. Thus, PEP should not be administered if the risk of infection is negligible.

Table 3.13 Recommended HIV PEP for percutaneous injuries

Exposure type[1]	HIV-infected source	HIV-infected source — high risk[2]	Source of unknown HIV status[3]	HIV negative
Less severe	2 drugs	3 drugs	No PEP*	No PEP
More severe	3 drugs	3 drugs	No PEP*	No PEP

2 drugs = AZT 300 mg bd + 3TC 150 mg bd for 28 days

3 drugs = AZT 300 mg bd + 3TC 150 mg bd for 28 days + lopinavir 133 mg/ritonavir 33 mg (Kaletra®) 3 capsules bd or an alternative PI.

[1]Less severe — solid needle, superficial injury; more severe — large-bore hollow needle, deep wound, visible blood on needle, needle in patient's vessel.

[2] High-risk source patient — patient with AIDS or acute seroconversion illness or who is known to have high viral load.

[3] Unknown source — e.g. needle from sharps container.

* In these settings, if source patient has risk factors for HIV infection or exposure to HIV-infected blood is likely, then 2 drug PEP should be considered. In areas with high HIV prevalence rates it would be advisable to prescribe PEP in such circumstances.

Guidelines are similar for splash injuries to non-intact skin or mucous membranes, but generally 2 drugs are used unless there is a large volume of blood from a high-risk patient. No PEP is required for a splash injury to intact skin.

Running an ART Clinic

Provision of ART in a clinical service that is well coordinated and prepared for this task is important for providing optimum patient care, ensuring patient follow-up and adherence, and achieving long-term success from the therapy for patients. The following are key components of a successful service:

- **Staffing** — medical, nursing, counselling, pharmacy, and clerical staff all form an important part of the service. Some clinical services are run by doctors, others by nurses with the doctor seeing complicated cases only.
- **Adequate counselling services** — often lay people who have been trained to be HIV and ART adherence counsellors play a very important part in the preparation of patients for ART. Being from the patients' community, speaking their language, and having time specifically for counselling, they can ensure the patient has a thorough knowledge of their disease and the treatment, and address any concerns.
- **Team work** — all members of the clinical team are important. The decision whether a patient is ready to commence ART, is best made collectively, with all members of the team contributing their insights as to the patient's medical and psychosocial readiness. A formal team meeting is useful for this.
- **A reliable drug supply is essential** — patients cannot afford to have the health service letting them down if they are adherent. The pharmacist in the clinic should play a role in educating patients regarding exactly how to take their medication and what side-effects they might expect.
- **Data collection and management** — Clerical staff play an important role in ensuring reliable and accurate data are collected and stored. Often those sponsoring ART programmes will require outcome data, and audit of clinic practice is important for quality of care assurance.
- Psychological, social worker, and nutritional input are also important.

Palliative care

Pain

Pain in late-stage HIV-positive patients is often multi-factorial, and treatment plans should recognize this. Common problems include painful peripheral neuropathies, post-zoster pain, pain related to disseminated KS involving a limb, HIV cholangiopathy, oral and perineal aphthous ulceration, and bedsores.

Start by attempting to address the cause e.g. treating bacterial pneumonia can control the chest pain associated with it. More commonly, the cause cannot be remedied, and attention should be given to appropriate analgesia. *Neuropathic pain* may respond to low-dose tricyclics — e.g. amitriptyline 10–25 mg nocte. The addition of carbamazepine 200 mg bd, working up to 400 mg bd may be of benefit (but note interaction with NNRTI and PIs). Patients with *musculoskeletal pain* may respond to NSAIDs e.g. ibuprofen 400 mg tds. In patients with less easily characterized pain, or where side-effects may be an issue, start with paracetamol 1 g qds. When control is inadequate with simple analgesics, codeine or tramadol can be added. Frequently, it is appropriate to move on to the use of oral morphine (📖 see p 676 for regimen). Give laxatives to prevent and treat opiate-induced constipation.

Chronic diarrhoea

Simple attention to nursing basics (gloves for attendants, disposable nappies for patients) may make a considerable impact. In patients unable to access ART, which often relieves chronic diarrhoea, consideration needs to be given to the use of antidiarrhoeals such as loperamide or diphenoxylate/atropine.

Dyspnoea

Patients with terminal pulmonary metastatic malignancy (e.g. Kaposi sarcoma) are often very dyspnoeic. Tapping a large effusion may cause some relief, as may supplementary oxygen via face mask or nasal prongs. Most severely ill patients with profound dyspnoea will, however, require judicious sedation with morphine.

Family support

Family support for late-stage HIV-positive individuals can be very helpful, but requires considerable counselling input. If breadwinners (e.g. a spouse) need to temporarily become care-givers, then short-term assistance with social grants can help. Time and effort spent on empowering and encouraging families can decrease hospital admissions.

Tuberculosis*

Section editor   **Stan Houston**

* This chapter is intended for use in conjunction with the relevant national TB programme manual

Current global situation and trends

Tuberculosis (TB) has been curable for more than 50 years, yet the global burden of morbidity and mortality due to TB continues to increase, the impact being greatest in sub-Saharan Africa. Approximately one-third of the world's population is infected with *Mycobacterium tuberculosis*, with nearly 9 million developing active TB and almost 2 million dying of TB each year. About 95% of cases occur in low-income countries and 75% are in the 15–50 age group. Both globally and within countries, there is a striking link between poverty and TB.

Modern TB treatment regimens of 6–8 months are highly effective in curing patients and preventing transmission. TB treatment is among the most cost-effective of all health interventions.

Several important developments have occurred in the past two decades:
- TB incidence has increased dramatically in communities highly endemic for HIV, particularly in Africa.
- Increasing drug resistance caused by deficiencies in TB treatment programmes, decreasing cure rates and complicating TB control.
- Expansion of 'DOTS' TB control programmes in much of the developing world, leading to stabilizing or declining incidence except in sub-Saharan Africa.

Lessons learned in TB treatment and control

- TB treatment and control is a core public health activity since identifying and curing infectious patients is the principal means by which we can reduce transmission and prevent new infections in the community.
- In stable political situations, the public sector has primary responsibility for ensuring the proper functioning of TB treatment and control, usually through the establishment of a National Tuberculosis Programme.
- TB treatment must be provided free of charge to patients.
- TB treatment and control must be integrated with the general health services of the community since that is where TB cases present.

Elements of the WHO 'DOTS' (directly observed therapy, short course) TB control strategy

- Sustained political commitment.
- *Microscopy*: case detection using sputum smear microscopy among symptomatic patients presenting to the health services.
- *SCC/DOT*: standardized short-course chemotherapy (SCC) using regimens of 6–8 months at least for all confirmed smear-positive cases. Good case management includes directly observed therapy (DOT) during the intensive phase for all new sputum-positive cases, during the continuation phase when rifampicin is used, and throughout a re-treatment regimen.
- *Drug supply*: establishment and maintenance of a system to supply all essential anti-TB drugs and to ensure no interruption in their availability.
- *Recording and reporting*: establishment and maintenance of a standardized recording and reporting system, allowing assessment of treatment results.

TB & public health   PUBLIC HEALTH NOTE

Impact: Globally, *M. tuberculosis* is the 2nd most common cause of death among all infectious agents.

TB control
1) Identification & cure of smear-positive pulmonary cases.
2) BCG in infants.
3) Poverty reduction; HIV prevention & treatment.

Key lessons of TB control
1) Application of the DOTS principles.
2) Treatment must be free to the patient.
3) The public health care sector must play a strong role.

Threats & obstacles to TB control
1) Failure of the programme to provide a sustainable diagnostic service, TB drugs, supervision of therapy, and outcome monitoring.
2) Drug resistance.
3) HIV and poverty.

Disease and pathogenesis

Microbiology

Mycobacteria are slender aerobic bacilli which are 'acid-fast' on Ziehl–Neelsen (ZN) staining. Members of the genus *Mycobacterium* which are of particular interest in the tropics include *M. leprae* and *M. ulcerans*, the causes of leprosy and Buruli ulcer (see Chapters 10 and 14). The *M. tuberculosis* complex comprises *M. tuberculosis, M. africanum*, and *M. bovis*: *M. africanum*, seen mainly in Africa, behaves clinically and epidemiologically like *M. tuberculosis*. *M. bovis* is a pathogen of cattle and other species of domestic and wild animals. Subsequent references to *M. tuberculosis* refer to the *M. tuberculosis* complex unless otherwise stated.

M. tuberculosis multiplies slowly so that up to 6 weeks are required for growth in culture. Correspondingly, disease due to *M. tuberculosis* tends to progress relatively slowly, and responds slowly to treatment.

Transmission

Individuals with active pulmonary TB produce airborne droplet nuclei containing infectious *M. tuberculosis* in the course of speaking, sneezing, and particularly coughing. Infection occurs when these are inhaled by a susceptible individual. Crowding, poor ventilation, and duration of exposure increase the risk of transmission. *M. bovis* can also be transmitted by the airborne route, but human infection often occurs through ingestion of unpasteurized milk from infected cows. Other sources of *M. tuberculosis* infection, except for handling TB cultures in the laboratory, are extremely rare.

TB infection

Aerosolized particles containing *M. tuberculosis* reach the alveoli where they initiate a non-specific response. The bacilli are ingested by macrophages and transported to regional lymph nodes. They may either be contained there or spread via the lymphatics or bloodstream to other organs. With the development of specific cell-mediated immunity, cytokines secreted by lymphocytes recruit and activate macrophages, which organize into the granulomas characteristic of TB, effectively walling in the organisms.

In immunocompetent hosts, the most common outcome of infection with *M. tuberculosis* is containment of the infection without the development of clinical illness. A granuloma can sometimes be seen on CXR; more commonly, the lesion is not detectable radiographically and a positive tuberculin skin test (TST) or T-cell-based assay is the only evidence of infection. A distinctive characteristic of *M. tuberculosis* is its ability to persist intracellularly in a quiescent state, within macrophages, retaining the ability to reactivate at a later time. This is known as 'latent tuberculous infection'.

Active TB disease

On average ~10% of immunocompetent adults infected with *M. tuberculosis* ultimately develop active TB. About half of this risk is concentrated in the first 1–2 years after infection, the other half is distributed over the remainder of the individual's lifetime. A number of factors greatly increase the risk of disease reactivation (see box).

In a minority of cases, infants or those with depressed cell-mediated immunity being at particular risk, 1° infection is not contained and symptomatic disease develops directly from 1° infection (progressive 1° TB).

Post primary TB occurs as a reactivation of latent infection, sometimes years after the 1° infection; sometimes, but not always, due to an identifiable immunosuppressive condition.

Patients, particularly those with HIV infection, can be reinfected with a new strain of *M. tuberculosis* after successful treatment of TB, but the proportion of TB cases attributable to this mechanism is unclear.

Risk factors for development of active TB disease in individuals infected with *M. tuberculosis*
- HIV — the most powerful known factor.
- Recent infection — the risk per year of developing active TB is much greater in the first 1–2 years after infection.
- Age — weakened immunity at the extremes of age.
- Malnutrition, including vitamin D deficiency.
- Diabetes mellitus.
- Silicosis or other types of lung fibrosis.
- Intercurrent infections (e.g. measles, visceral leishmaniasis).
- Toxic factors (e.g. alcohol and smoking).
- Poverty — probably many biologic mechanisms involved.
- Immune suppression (e.g. corticosteroid therapy, malignancy).
- 'Herd immunity' — members of populations with little historical exposure to TB appear to be more susceptible to disease.

Clinical features

The diagnostic resources available varies widely in different settings where TB is treated. This section mentions technologies such as TB culture and histologic examination of biopsies, which may be required for the diagnosis of extrapulmonary and other less common forms of TB. However, the majority of TB cases, especially those with the poorest prognosis and those most infectious to others, can be diagnosed with very basic resources, particularly smear microscopy.

TB in adults

One or more non-specific systemic symptoms — weight loss, anorexia, fever, night sweats, or malaise — are present in the majority of patients.

Pulmonary TB (PTB) is the most common presentation. It is also the most important epidemiologically since it is the form which is infectious to others. However, TB may affect any organ, leading to a variety of clinical presentations.

Pulmonary TB (PTB)

Involves the lung parenchyma. The great majority of patients have a cough, which is often productive. A cough of prolonged duration (>3 weeks) should always raise the suspicion of TB. Haemoptysis, chest pain, or breathlessness may also be present in some patients.

Physical examination is often normal or the findings non-specific. Some patients may look ill and wasted with a fever and tachycardia, but a few can appear surprisingly well. Chest examination may reveal localized crackles or findings of a pleural effusion. Finger clubbing suggests a diagnosis other than TB, such as lung cancer, bronchiectasis, or empyema but occasionally bronchiectasis may be 2° to lung damage from chronic or previous PTB.

Approximately 65% of PTB cases, somewhat less in the HIV-infected, are sputum smear positive. Smear-positive patients are most infectious (several times more likely to transmit TB than patients who are smear-negative, even if culture-positive) and also sickest (without treatment, their average mortality is considerably higher than that of smear-negative patients). A positive smear for acid-fast bacilli in a high TB prevalence area almost always indicates TB since M. tuberculosis occurs much more frequently than atypical mycobacteria in these settings.

Smear-negative PTB is relatively common but the diagnosis always involves a degree of uncertainty. Many of these patients will become smear-positive later if not treated. While under-diagnosis of smear-negative PTB is clearly undesirable, over-diagnosis also creates problems, by misusing the scarce resources of the TB programme, overlooking other treatable diagnoses, and undermining the programme's credibility in the community by reducing the success rate of treatment.

Complications of pulmonary TB: Acute complications include haemoptysis which is occasionally life-threatening, and pneumothorax. Chronic complications include post-TB bronchiectasis, extensive lung fibrosis, and aspergillomas (fungus balls) in residual cavities.

Pleural TB

An effusion can often be detected on physical examination and confirmed by X-ray and/or diagnostic aspiration. In TB endemic areas, in the absence of obvious alternative explanations such as heart failure, acute pneumonia, or malignancy, TB will be the most common cause of a 'straw-coloured' effusion. TB effusions are exudates (fluid protein >50% serum protein concentration) and contain increased lymphocytes but are seldom smear-positive for acid-fast bacilli. Many patients with pleural TB also have involvement of the pulmonary parenchyma. Hence, sputum examination should always be performed. Culture of pleural biopsy tissue is very sensitive and histology of a pleural biopsy usually shows granulomas.

TB lymphadenitis

Can involve any site, but cervical lymph nodes are most common. Nodes may initially be rubbery and non-tender, becoming matted or fluctuant, and sometimes discharging spontaneously through the skin to produce chronic sinuses with scar formation. The nodes have typically been present for weeks or months, and are seldom acutely inflamed, distinguishing them from most lymphadenopathy due to acute viral or bacterial infections. Paradoxically, they sometimes enlarge during anti-TB therapy. These characteristics, and the asymmetrical involvement, help to distinguish most cases of TB adenitis from the persistent generalized lymphadenopathy of HIV.

A needle aspiration is often smear-positive in HIV-infected patients, less frequently among HIV-negative lymph node TB patients. If the smear is negative, diagnosis can be confirmed by excision biopsy of a node, usually a minor procedure in adults, with histologic examination and/or culture.

Bone TB

Most commonly affects the spine (Pott's disease). Vertebral collapse may ultimately produce a characteristic angular deformity. Some patients develop features of spinal cord involvement. Paravertebral cold abscesses or psoas abscesses may accompany Pott's disease but do not generally require open surgical drainage.

The presence of a characteristic angular kyphosis or 'gibbus' in a TB-endemic area is virtually diagnostic of spinal TB. In the absence of this striking clinical finding, X-ray changes with intervertebral disc and adjacent bone involvement ± paravertebral soft tissue densities suggest an infectious aetiology, but cannot reliably distinguish between TB and other infections (e.g. brucellosis, staphylococal). If present, a cold abscess can be aspirated for ZN staining ± culture; most abscesses will be smear-negative. Imaging-guided biopsy of the infected disc or adjacent bone can provide a histologic or microbiologic diagnosis, but requires sophisticated resources. Spinal TB generally responds well to drug treatment. Occasionally, patients may present with rapidly progressive spinal cord compression and these patients may benefit from urgent surgery to decompress the spinal cord and stabilize the spine. If that is not available, strict bed rest should be used until the neurological features improve after several weeks of treatment. Exceptional patients with severe deformities or chronic neurologic compromise might benefit from neuro or orthopaedic surgery if available. With these exceptions, neurologic improvement or even complete recovery, albeit with persistent deformity, occurs with medical therapy alone in most patients. TB of other joints such as hip and knee generally requires synovial biopsy to distinguish TB from other chronic infections.

Miliary TB

Is an aggressive form of hematogenously disseminated TB more common in infants and the immune suppressed. Typically, there is a rather non-specific but progressive history of fever, malaise, and weight loss without other identifiable cause. Clinical suspicion is raised by a history of known or likely recent contact with infectious TB. Physical findings are commonly non-specific but can include hepatomegaly, mild splenomegaly, tachypnoea, and wasting.

A CXR demonstrating diffuse, tiny, nodular opacities is the clue to miliary TB and warrants initiation of TB treatment if the clinical picture is compatible. Occasionally, choroidal tubercles are visible on fundoscopy. Sputum smear examination and TST are often negative. If available, biopsy of liver, bone marrow, lymph nodes, or lung parenchyma may yield granulomata and/or acid-fast bacilli.

TB meningitis

More common in children and the immune suppressed. It presents as a progressive febrile illness which may be accompanied by headache, irritability, vomiting, and decreased consciousness, ultimately progressing to coma. The pace of illness is characteristically slower than in acute bacterial meningitis. Neck stiffness is variable, especially early in the course. Cranial nerve palsies (particularly III, IV, VI, and VIII) occur commonly, reflecting the basilar distribution of the inflammation. Seizures and focal neurologic deficits can also develop.

Diagnosis of TB meningitis rests on CSF examination. Typically, the CSF white blood count is increased with a lymphocytic predominance, the protein is elevated and glucose decreased, although all 3 abnormalities are not present in every case. CSF should also be examined to exclude cryptococcus if there is any possibility of HIV infection. CSF is rarely smear-positive for acid-fast bacilli; culture is positive in the majority.

A decision to start TB treatment must be made on the basis of clinical features, suggestive CSF abnormalities, and the absence of a likely alternative diagnosis, since delay in treatment is a major predictor of poor outcome. In some early cases, the diagnosis may be suggested when the clinical course and evolution of CSF findings on repeat examination over a few days are more typical of TB than of alternative diagnoses such as viral or bacterial infection. The available evidence and most expert opinion supports adjunctive therapy with corticosteroids at a suggested dose of prednisone 1 mg/kg/day for 1 month, then tapered over 2–4 weeks.

Intracranial tuberculomas (presenting as epilepsy or focal neurological deficit, and seen on brain scans) may accompany TB meningitis, or may develop in isolation or as part of disseminated (miliary) TB. Tuberculomas may also develop or enlarge 'paradoxically' during treatment of these forms of TB, and require prolonged courses of steroids along with TB treatment.

Abdominal TB

Gastrointestinal TB may present as abdominal pain, weight loss, diarrhoea or partial bowel obstruction with a history of fever. It can occur at any site in the GI tract, most commonly, the terminal ileum. The diagnosis is usually made from specimens taken at surgery or endoscopy; the histology resembles that of Crohn's disease. Often peritoneal tuberculosis supervenes after some time, increasing abdominal distension being the first sign. Peritoneal TB may be suspected on the basis of ascites without another obvious cause such as liver disease. The characteristics of the ascitic fluid are similar to those of TB pleural fluid (see above). The peritoneum has a characteristic appearance on direct inspection; culture and histology of a peritoneal biopsy, preferably taken at laparoscopy, is usually required for diagnosis. CT scans may show thickened terminal ileum, mesenteric lymph nodes, thickened contrast-enhancing peritoneum, and ascites. Oesophageal TB occurs occasionally, causing ulceration and strictures; mediastinal lymph nodes may compress or erode into the oesophagus, or cause a fistula to the trachea or bronchi.

Pericardial TB

Is often first suspected on the basis of globular enlargement of the cardiac silhouette on CXR in patients investigated for systemic and cardiorespiratory symptoms. It is more common in HIV-infected patients. Clinical features of tamponade (elevated jugular venous pressure, pulsus paradoxus, hypotension) may be present and a pericardial rub is occasionally noted. Ultrasound can readily confirm an effusion. Therapeutic pericardial aspiration for tamponade requires ultrasound or at least ECG control; pericardial fluid has the same characteristics as pleural fluid in TB (see above). In practice, the diagnosis must often be made by demonstrating the presence of an effusion in the absence of other likely aetiologies. The risk of tamponade and later constriction is reduced by adding corticosteroids for the first 6–12 weeks of TB treatment. The recommended adult dose is prednisone 60 mg/day tapered over up to 12 weeks.

Genitourinary TB

Can involve any part of the male or female genitourinary tract. Renal TB may present with dysuria, hematuria, and pain or a mass in the flank. The urinalysis typically shows pus cells, but routine culture is negative. Diagnosis usually requires TB culture of urine. TB of the uterus or adenexae presents as infertility, pelvic pain or mass, or bleeding. Epididymal swelling is the most common presentation of genital TB in males. Biopsy is usually required to distinguish TB from other possible causes, though imaging (CT scan) may be suggestive of TB.

TB in children

The probability of progression to disease following *M. tuberculosis* exposure is greater in infants and young children than in adults. Infants who develop TB have a high fatality rate without prompt treatment. By contrast, children in the 7 to 12 age range have the lowest risk, of any age group, of developing active TB.

Even where culture, X-ray, and other facilities are available, diagnosis of childhood TB is often very difficult. TB may be suspected clinically in the presence of persistent fever, malaise, and cough. A history of close contact with a smear-positive pulmonary TB patient makes TB more likely. A positive TST is suggestive of TB in a child with an unexplained illness, because the incidental or 'background' rate of TST positivity is expected to be low in this age group. Sputum-smear microscopy is usually negative in children with PTB. A CXR may show enlarged intra-thoracic lymph nodes with or without lung consolidation. Culture of specimens obtained by gastric lavage or sputum induction can improve the rate of confirmed diagnosis. Several scoring systems have been developed to rationalize the diagnosis of childhood TB — none has been validated, but they may provide a framework to guide the approach of the puzzled clinician. An example is given below.

Example of a scheme to aid diagnosis of TB in children*

1. Score chart for child with suspected TB

Score	0	1	3
Length of illness	<2 weeks	2–4 weeks	>4 weeks
Weight for age	>80%	60–80%	<60%
Family TB (past or present)	None	Reported by family	Proved sputum +ve

2. Score for other features if present

- Positive tuberculin skin test (TST)   3
- Large painless lymph nodes: firm, soft, and/or sinus in neck, axilla, and groin   3
- Unexplained fever, night sweats, no response to malaria treatment   2
- Malnutrition, not improving after 4 weeks   3

3. If the TOTAL score is 7 or more — treat for TB

- Treat children with a score less than 7 if:
  - CXR is characteristic of TB infection, or
  - The child does not respond to two 7-day courses of two different antibiotics.

* Dr Keith Edwards, University of Papua New Guinea, published in Crofton *et al.* (1997) *Clinical tuberculosis*, MacMillan.

Diagnosis

Sputum smears

Access to reliable, quality controlled sputum smear microscopy is a prerequisite to the establishment of a TB treatment programme. Three sputum samples should be examined microscopically in any patient who has been coughing for >2–3 weeks. When patients must travel some distance to the clinic, the 'spot-morning-spot' protocol can be used: the 1st specimen is collected and submitted at presentation, the 2nd is an early-morning sputum produced at home the next morning and submitted at a clinic visit that day, and the 3rd is produced and submitted during that clinic visit.

Chest X-ray

CXR is not routinely necessary for the diagnosis and management of TB. It is most useful in patients with undiagnosed chest symptoms who are repeatedly smear-negative and in identifying other findings such as pleural effusions or nodules. The interpretation of a CXR varies with the skill of the reader and even between skilled readers. A normal CXR makes PTB unlikely. However, a CXR cannot distinguish reliably between TB and other diseases or between changes of active and past, inactive TB. It does not predict infectiousness (as the sputum smear does), nor supply the definitive identification provided by culture.

Diagnosis of sputum smear-negative TB

Reassessment and repeat sputum examinations after 2–3 weeks, following a therapeutic trial of a broad-spectrum antibiotic, may clarify the diagnosis. CXR, interpreted with the cautions mentioned below, may help to estimate the likelihood of TB in suspects who remain smear-negative. Culture and sputum induction can increase sensitivity of diagnosis. Before diagnosing smear-negative PTB, consider alternative diagnoses such as:
- Pneumonia.
- Asthma.
- Chronic bronchitis.
- Non-TB respiratory complications of HIV infection.
- Bronchiectasis.
- Lung abscess.
- Lung cancer.

In some TB programmes, a decision to start treatment for smear-negative PTB can only be made by a doctor or individual with particular expertise in TB.

Tuberculin skin testing (TST)

This is a test for infection with M. tuberculosis; it cannot by itself be used to diagnose active TB. It relies on the fact that cell-mediated hypersensitivity typically develops within 8 weeks after infection with M. tuberculosis. Following intradermal injection of PPD (purified protein derivative), the diameter of skin induration (swelling, not redness) is measured at 48–72 h. Training and experience in interpreting skin test responses is critical to achieving accurate results. In most situations, 10 mm of induration to a standard tuberculin dose is the cut-off between negative and positive; 5 mm is considered positive in HIV-infected individuals. Both false negative and false positive TST results are relatively common (see box). The larger the area of induration, the less likely it is to be a false positive. New T-cell-based assays using blood samples eliminate most false positives encountered with the TST, but are costly, and their role in clinical practice is still being determined.

Uses of the TST

- Epidemiologic — determining prevalence or incidence of M. tuberculosis infection in a population or specific group e.g. health care workers.
- Diagnostic — to aid in assessing the likelihood of TB as the cause of a clinical illness. In high-prevalence countries, this use is largely limited to children because the 'background' prevalence of incidental TST positivity in the general population increases with age.
- Identification of candidates for 'chemoprophylaxis' (e.g. paediatric contacts of pulmonary TB patients, HIV-infected individuals).

A false positive TST can be caused by

- BCG: TST response following BCG is variable; BCG in infancy is unlikely to account for a strongly positive TST in adulthood.
- Exposure to environmental mycobacteria.
- Incorrect interpretation.

A false negative TST can be caused by

- Normal variation.
- Long interval since infection.
- Reduced cell-mediated immune response (HIV, old age, corticosteroid therapy, measles, malnutrition).
- Severe illness, including overwhelming TB.
- Incorrect TST technique or interpretation.

Treatment

Aims of treatment

- To cure the patient, preserve life, and prevent disability.
- To prevent transmission.
- To prevent development of resistant TB.

Principles of anti-TB therapy

- The right drugs: treatment must always include a minimum of 2 drugs to which the organism is sensitive.
- The right duration: generally 6–8 months for drug-sensitive TB.
- Assured adherence — the TB programme must ensure that each patient completes the full course of therapy.

Treatment supervision

Directly observed therapy ('DOT') was initially intended to mean observed swallowing of each dose by a health care worker. Because this may not be feasible in all settings, a range of alternative supervision strategies have been suggested, tried, and appear to have been successful, at least in small projects. Treatment supervisors have included teachers, employers, community-chosen volunteers, ex-TB patients, and, more controversially, family members. If any of these strategies for treatment supervision are used, there must be adequate provision for selection, training, and regular monitoring of the treatment supervisor, a reliable mechanism for delivery of drugs, proper record keeping, and rigorous monitoring of treatment outcomes.

Drug dosage and standard regimens (see box)

Standard TB treatment and duration appears to be effective regardless of disease site, although some authorities recommend prolonging the consolidation phase for TB meningitis and bone disease (up to 12 months total). Preferably, TB drugs should be provided in the form of fixed-dose combination (FDC) tablets which make monotherapy impossible and provide an extra defence against the development of drug resistance.

Most national TB programmes have a standard regimen and a re-treatment regimen — the latter for patients who have defaulted, failed treatment, or relapsed after initially successful treatment.

Anti-TB drug (abbreviation)	Recommended dose (mg/kg)	
	Once daily regimen	3×/week regimen
Isoniazid (H)	5	10
Rifampicin (R)	10	10
Pyrazinamide (Z)	25	35
Streptomycin (S)	15	15
Ethambutol (E)	15	30
Thiacetazone (T)	2.5	N/A

Anti-TB drugs

- *Isoniazid* (INH; 'H'): potent anti-TB activity. Main serious adverse effect is liver toxicity; can cause peripheral neuropathy.
- *Rifampicin* (rifampin in North America; 'R'): essential to the success of modern short course (<12 months) TB therapy. Major drug interactions with warfarin, anticonvulsants, oral contraceptives, some antiretrovirals, etc. Less commonly hepatotoxic than Z or H.
- *Pyrazinamide* ('Z'): 'sterilizing' activity allows treatment courses of 6 months. Contribution to 1st-line regimens limited largely to the first 2 months of therapy. May cause arthralgias; most hepatotoxic 1st line TB drug.
- *Ethambutol* ('E'): weak anti-TB agent; main role is prevention of resistance to other drugs. Main serious adverse effect is ocular toxicity, which is uncommon at recommended doses.
- *Thiacetazone* ('T'): weak anti-TB agent formerly used in conjunction with isoniazid in the continuation phase. Largely abandoned in high HIV-prevalence countries because of high rates of Stevens–Johnson syndrome in HIV-co-infected patients.
- *Streptomycin* ('S'): now limited to 2nd-line or re-treatment regimens because of the desire to avoid unnecessary injections in the HIV era. Ototoxicity (vertigo > hearing loss) and renal toxicity are the main adverse effects. The drug should be avoided or dosage adjusted carefully in renal dysfunction. Contraindicated in pregnancy.

Special groups

- Isoniazid causes peripheral neuropathy more commonly in **diabetic, malnourished, alcoholic, and pregnant** patients, and in those with pre-existing neuropathy including those with **HIV**. Give pyridoxine 10–15 mg/d to protect against peripheral neuropathy.
- **Women on oral contraceptives** must use another form of contraception (e.g. an IUD) during rifampicin therapy and for 4–8 weeks after stopping rifampicin.
- **Pregnancy**: TB drugs, except for streptomycin, may be used in pregnancy. Any theoretical risks to the foetus are much less than the risks from untreated TB.

First-line regimen (WHO) 2HRZE 4HR or 2HRZE 4H₃R₃

- Isoniazid, rifampicin, pyrazinamide, and ethambutol od for 2 months.
- Followed by a 'continuation phase' of isoniazid and rifampicin either od (4HR) or 3×/week (4H$_3$R$_3$) for 4 months.

First-line regimen (International Union Against Tuberculosis and Lung Disease) 2HRZE 6HE

- Isoniazid, rifampicin, pyrazinamide, and ethambutol od for 2 months.
- Followed by isoniazid and ethambutol od for 6 months.

This regimen has been shown to have somewhat lower efficacy and would be chosen mainly in situations where adequate supervision during the continuation phase was not deemed possible.

'Re-treatment regimen' (defaulters, treatment failure, relapse) 2HRZES 1HRZE 5H₃R₃E₃

- Isoniazid, rifampicin, pyrazinamide, ethambutol, and streptomycin od for 2 months.
- Followed by isoniazid, rifampicin, pyrazinamide, ethambutol od for 1 month.
- Then isoniazid, rifampicin, ethambutol 3×/week for 5 months.

It is increasingly recognized that this regimen is suboptimal in patients who have failed fully supervised first-line therapy, but at the moment, no fully satisfactory or generally accepted alternative exists for low-income country settings.

Monitoring treatment: sputum-positive patients should be monitored by sputum smear examination after 2 months of treatment and at least one other time prior to treatment completion. All other patients should be monitored clinically.

Education: regarding adverse drug reactions is essential. Of particular importance, every patient should be advised to present to a clinic or hospital immediately if jaundice is noted.

Treatment adherence: Good adherence is the most important determinant of successful treatment. As patients feel better after starting treatment, their motivation to continue therapy for many months is naturally likely to wane. It is the responsibility of the treating health care worker and the TB programme to ensure that patients complete TB therapy. The patient and community must be well informed and aware, specifically, of the risks of drug resistance. The relationship between the patient and programme or clinic staff is a major factor promoting adherence. Practical measures such as clinic hours which can accommodate working patients are very important. Individualized approaches to the specific problems of individual patients at increased risk of defaulting are the hallmark of a committed and successful programme staff. These could include help with transportation, nutritional support, addiction treatment, home visits, etc. Early identification and tracing of defaulters is an essential function of a TB programme.

A 'therapeutic trial' of treatment

A therapeutic trial is widely used in many settings to diagnose TB. This strategy has not been validated, is not recommended by WHO, and risks creating confusion in a TB programme. If a 'therapeutic trial' is to be used:

- All efforts to make a diagnosis should have been exhausted.
- An objective indicator (e.g. fever) of success and the planned trial duration (fever resolves within 14 days of starting treatment in most cases) should be established before starting the trial.
- Preferably, the drugs used for the trial should have antimycobacterial activity (isoniazid, ethambutol, and pyrazinamide) but not be effective against other infections (rifampicin and streptomycin).
- The trial patient should be clearly distinguished from other patients in the TB programme records.

TB and HIV

TB incidence has increased up to 6-fold in communities severely affected by the HIV pandemic. Up to 80% of TB patients in these settings are HIV +ve. Among patients with HIV infection, TB is the most common cause of death globally. The mechanism underlying the powerful interaction between these two diseases is the suppression, by HIV infection, of the cell-mediated immune response (CD4+ helper T-cells and macrophages) to TB.

Chemoprophylaxis or treatment of latent TB infection

The risk of developing active TB in the future, among HIV +ve, TST +ve individuals is markedly reduced by 'chemoprophylaxis' with isoniazid for 6–9 months. This benefit declines over time, especially if the patient lives in a community where the risk of re-infection is high. In practice, it has proven difficult to implement this intervention on a large scale in a low-income country. Any use of TB drugs must be strictly managed to avoid promoting resistance. Antiretrovirals are very effective in reducing the risk of TB in HIV +ve patients (by preventing CD4 decline).

HIV testing of TB patients: There is increasing agreement that all TB patients should be encouraged to undergo HIV testing. TB programmes should be prepared to offer testing and coordinate follow-up and support with the HIV programme.

Management of TB in HIV +ve patients

Most patients presenting with HIV-related TB do not know their HIV status. Some will have clinical features of HIV infection such as oral candidiasis, chronic diarrhoea, skin and hair changes, peripheral neuropathy, herpes zoster scars, etc. However, since TB can occur early during the course of HIV disease, these clinical features of HIV are more often absent.

Extrapulmonary TB is common in HIV +ve patients, particularly lymphadenopathy, pleural and pericardial effusions, miliary TB, and meningitis. However, PTB remains the most common form of disease.

The radiographic appearance of PTB in HIV-infected patients is often atypical, depending on the individual's degree of immune suppression. HIV +ve patients less commonly have upper lobe disease and cavities and, more commonly, have intrathoracic adenopathy, effusions, and miliary shadowing.

Diagnosis: Sputum smear microscopy remains the primary investigation, but is somewhat less sensitive in HIV +ve patients. If the smear is negative, the differential diagnosis of lung disease in the HIV +ve patient includes:

- Bacterial (most often pneumococcal) pneumonia: a short history and a response to antibiotic therapy is suggestive.
- *Pneumocystis jiroveci* pneumonia (PCP; previously known as *Pneumocystis carinii pneumonia*): characteristic features include severe dyspnoea and hypoxia, diffuse changes on X-ray, absence of effusions, and a response to high-dose co-trimoxazole therapy.
- Pulmonary Kaposi sarcoma: most patients have cutaneous or oral lesions.

Treatment regimens

TB drug treatment regimens are the same in HIV +ve and uninfected patients. Cure rates are similar provided standard rifampicin-containing regimens are used. Recurrence rates are higher in the HIV +ve, at least partly due to the increased rate of reinfection. Mortality during and after treatment is markedly increased among patients with HIV, mainly due to HIV-related causes other than TB.

Increasing numbers of patients in low-income countries have access to antiretroviral therapy (ART). Treatment with ART and TB drugs at the same time creates the potential for a variety of complex and challenging problems:

- Adverse effects which could be due to either TB or ART drugs and which could result in treatment interruption.
- Complex, clinically important drug interactions, particularly involving rifampicin and protease inhibitors.
- Immune reconstitution reactions (IRIS, see Chapter 3).

Knowledge in this area is evolving rapidly; participation of someone with current knowledge and expertise in HIV/TB management is highly desirable.

An immune reconstitution reaction (or immune reconstitution inflammatory syndrome, IRIS) is most likely to occur in a patient with a very low initial CD4 cell count or clinical evidence of profound immune suppression. It may occur days to months after the ART initiation. The mechanism is thought to involve an enhanced inflammatory reaction to a pre-existing opportunistic infection (especially TB) as cell-mediated immunity improves in response to ART. The reaction is usually characterized by fever and localized appearance or worsening of the opportunistic disease process e.g. enlarging lymph nodes or worsening pulmonary infiltrate. Treatment failure or a second complicating infectious process must be excluded as far as possible, before arriving at a diagnosis of IRIS. Corticosteroids (prednisolone 40–60 mg/day) are usually recommended for severe manifestations of IRIS.

Patients taking ART prior to the diagnosis of TB should continue on it when TB treatment is started, but may require modifications in the ART regimen to ensure compatibility with rifampicin. In patients not taking ART at the time of TB diagnosis, starting TB treatment is the first priority. In general, the indications for ART in TB patients are similar to those in patients without TB — patients with CD4 counts < 200 cells/mm3 or with clinical features of advanced HIV disease are eligible for ART. The timing of ART initiation, however, is unclear. Most experts would advise waiting 4–8 weeks after starting TB treatment.

A regimen consisting of efavirenz plus 2 nucleoside analogues (e.g. lamivudine and stavudine) if otherwise appropriate, is currently the best established regimen for patients receiving simultaneous ART and TB therapy which includes rifampicin. (*Note*: efavirenz is contraindicated in pregnancy.)

Patients receiving a non-rifampicin-containing continuation phase (HE) can be given any otherwise appropriate ART regimen.

HIV-infected TB patients should receive long-term prophylaxis with cotrimoxazole.

HIV & TB

In HIV +ve patients, by comparison with HIV −ve patients:
- The incidence of TB is markedly increased.
- The clinical & radiographic presentation may be different.
- TB treatment is the same and cure rates are similar.
- Recurrence is more frequent and mortality is more frequent.
- Concomitant ART complicates TB treatment substantially.

Paediatric TB   PAEDIATRIC NOTE

- Probably under-recognized.
- High case fatality, particularly in infants.
- Diagnosis commonly difficult and uncertain.
- Diagnostic clues: clinical.
  - History of close contact with smear +ve TB.
  - Unexplained fever, unresponsive to other therapy.
  - Unexplained, unresponsive weight loss.
  - Persistent lymphadenopathy.
- Diagnostic clues: lab & imaging.
  - +ve TST.
  - Intrathoracic adenopathy ± infiltrate on CXR.
  - Smear (culture more sensitive) of gastric aspirate or induced sputum.

TB and HIV drug interactions website:
http://www.cdc.gov/nchstp/tb/TB_HIV_Drugs/TOC.htm

Drug resistance and multi-drug resistant (MDR) TB

Development of **acquired drug resistance** in a TB patient requires 2 steps: 1) a random mutation in the TB bacillus conferring resistance to that drug, followed by 2) selection 'pressure' from the use of that drug. The resistant organisms will then replicate more rapidly than drug-sensitive organisms, unless suppressed by the use of one or more other effective TB drugs. Once an organism has acquired resistance, the resistant strain can be transmitted to another individual who will then have **primary drug resistance**, even if he or she has never taken TB drugs. Fundamentally, the cause of drug resistance is inadequate treatment due to a failure of the TB programme. Conversely, TB drug resistance is almost entirely preventable by a TB programme which assures adequate adherence to effective therapy.

The definition of MDR TB is resistance to isoniazid and rifampicin ± other drugs (see treatment, below).

Third-line anti-TB drugs; treatment of MDR TB

Recently, some programmes have implemented treatment of MDR TB. Treatment of MDR TB is much longer (>18 months), much more toxic, much more costly, and considerably less effective than treatment of drug-sensitive TB, re-emphasizing the critical importance of preventing resistance. MDR treatment should only be introduced in settings where a DOTS programme is established and demonstrating good outcomes. MDR TB treatment ('DOTS Plus') requires supervision of treatment for 18 months, specialized medical expertise, a well-structured programme and guidelines, appropriate laboratory and culture resources, and an assured supply of 3rd line drugs. Expert advice and drugs at reduced cost can be obtained through the WHO 'Green Light Committee' by programmes which meet its standards.

Suggested regimens for various patterns of drug resistance (assuming access to culture and sensitivity studies) can be found at:
http://www.cdc.gov/mmwr/preview/mmwrhtml/rr5211a1.htm#tab16 (table 16).

Extensively drug resistant (XDR) tuberculosis

XDR is defined as resistance to at least rifampicin and isoniazid plus resistance to any quinolone plus resistance to at least one injectable second line agent (capreomycin, amikacin, kanamycin). For some years, such strains have been known to exist in Asia, the Americas, and Europe. Of 17,000 TB isolates collected from around the world between 2000–2004, 2% of MDR strains were also XDR, being most frequently found in eastern Europe, western Asia and South Korea. Population-based data from the USA, Latvia, and South Korea revealed that 4%, 19%, and 15% of MDR strains, respectively, were XDR. A large outbreak of XDR-TB amongst HIV infected people recently occurred in South Africa that was associated with almost 100% mortality.

TB control programmes

TB control programmes require a structure, usually extending up to the national level, that coordinates programme elements such as regimens and protocols, training, drug supply, lab quality assurance, and monitoring of programme outcomes.

Smear-positive PTB patients are the main source of TB transmission. Detecting and curing infectious cases is the most effective means of reducing new infections.

The first priority of a TB programme is to achieve a high rate of treatment success, since treating cases badly can promote drug resistance. Once a TB programme is achieving good treatment outcomes (>85% treatment success), the next priority is to improve case finding. This activity must be integrated with the primary health care service since it depends upon recognition and appropriate investigation (mainly sputum smear examination) of symptomatic TB suspects presenting to 1° health care workers.

Bacille Calmette Guerin (BCG) is a live attenuated vaccine derived from *M bovis*. Protective efficacy ranges from 0 to 80% for reasons which remain controversial. BCG provides some protection against miliary TB and TB meningitis in children, and should be given at birth to all children in high TB-prevalence countries (except those with symptomatic HIV disease). BCG appears to have little or no impact on the overall incidence or transmission of TB in a community.

Household and close contacts of TB cases: symptomatic contacts should be sought out and investigated for active TB — a particularly efficient form of case finding. Chemoprophylaxis should be given to household contacts of smear-positive PTB patients aged <5 years after an assessment to rule out active TB.

In high HIV-prevalence countries, both HIV prevention and antiretroviral treatment are likely to reduce TB incidence. Ultimately, poverty reduction with improved housing and nutrition may be the most definitive TB control measures.

Prevention of TB transmission in the health care setting

See Chapter 18, 🕮 p 736.

Respiratory medicine

Section editors   **Jehangir S Sorabjee**

Beate Kampmann

(Acute respiratory infections)

Ike Lagunju

(Paediatric acute respiratory infections)

Symptoms of respiratory disease

Cough

An acute cough usually requires no investigation or treatment, but a persistent cough associated with phlegm, fever, dyspnoea, or chest pain warrants further investigation. A change in the pattern of any longstanding cough is significant, especially in smokers.

Common causes of cough

- Viral URTIs and LRTIs.
- Asthma (can be without wheezing).
- Pneumonia (including atypical pneumonias).
- TB (including involvement of mediastinal lymph nodes).
- Pleural effusion.
- Drugs — (ACE inhibitors and beta blockers).
- Gastro-oesophageal reflux disease(GORD).
- Chronic obstructive pulmonary disease (COPD).
- Acute or chronic sinusitis, with a post nasal drip.
- Tropical pulmonary eosinophilia (TPE).
- Bronchiectasis.

Nocturnal coughing is a feature of asthma, left ventricular failure, TPE, and GORD.

Most causes of cough can be diagnosed by physical examination, a blood count, ESR, spirometry, and a chest X-ray.

Haemoptysis

Haemoptysis should always be taken seriously and patients should be placed under close observation and investigated. Only a very careful history can differentiate haemoptysis from haematemesis, oropharyngeal bleeding, or a posterior epistaxis, and sometimes it needs to be witnessed to be sure. Patients with haemoptysis will continue to expectorate blood for 24 h after the acute event.

Severe haemoptysis is an emergency — maintain a clear airway, as patients die of aspiration rather than exsanguination.

Common causes of haemoptysis

TB, bronchiectasis, mitral stenosis, carcinoma of the bronchus, acute pneumonia, pulmonary embolism (with infarction), acute bronchitis.

Other causes of haemoptysis

- Infections: lung abscess, parasitic disease (e.g. paragonimiasis), fungal disease (e.g. aspergillosis), pleuro-pulmonary amoebiasis, leptospirosis.
- Trauma: lung contusions, foreign body aspiration, post endotracheal intubation or following aggressive endotracheal suctioning.
- Diffuse pulmonary parenchymal disease: Goodpastures syndrome, Wegeners granulomatosis, systemic vasculitides.
- Cardiovascular disease: pulmonary oedema, pulmonary hypertension, aortic aneurysm.
- Bleeding tendency: sepsis, DIC, snake bite, haemorrhagic fevers.

Dyspnoea/breathlessness

Look for anaemia, wheezing (may have both pulmonary and cardiac causes), signs of LVF, and note the pattern of breathing. In most instances, a CXR, ECG, and blood count will suffice to guide appropriate investigations and treatment. Distinguish dyspnoea from tachypnoea associated with voluntary hyperventilation, metabolic acidosis, and thyrotoxicosis.

Diagnosis

- **Pulmonary**: often associated with wheezing or chest pain — consider asthma, COPD, pleural effusions, pneumothorax, interstitial lung disease and pulmonary fibrosis, pulmonary embolism, pulmonary hypertension, severe and extensive pneumonia, interstitial pneumonia (e.g. *Legionella*, PCP, or CMV).
- **Cardiac**: often with paroxysmal nocturnal dyspnoea, orthopnoea, or ankle oedema — inability to lie flat is a crucial observation. LVF due to valvular or ischaemic heart disease or myocardial disease due to myocarditis or cardiomyopathy are the usual causes.
- **Diseases of the chest wall**: severe kyphoscoliosis, Guillan Barre syndrome, neurotoxic snake envenoming, myasthenia gravis, ankylosing spondylitis, hypokalemia, etc.
- **Anaemia**: if acute or if chronic and severe.

Wheeze/stridor

Wheezes are (generally expiratory) 'coo-ing' sounds coming from the larger airways. Wheezes may vary in pitch and intensity and can be heard at the mouth in some patients. A localized wheeze may be due to partial endobronchial obstruction. Stridor is a harsh sound heard in inspiration due to obstruction of the trachea or larynx by a foreign body or tumor.

Causes of wheezing

- All causes of airways obstruction — asthma, COPD (often exacerbated by infection or use of beta blockers).
- Left ventricular failure — peribronchial oedema causes bronchospasm and wheezing.
- Inhalation of toxic chemicals.
- Endobronchial obstruction from a tumour or foreign body (localized wheeze).

Multiple causes of a wheeze may exist in a single patient.

Pneumonia

Pneumonia kills ~3 million children per year in the developing world and affects adults of all ages. While pneumonia may occur as part of a severe systemic viral infection (esp. measles or influenza), most serious cases are bacterial. CXR or clinical findings do not reliably differentiate between bacterial or viral agents.

Aetiology

Many organisms are capable of causing pneumonia, depending on the patient's age, season of the year, and the presence of other diseases (see box). It is often impossible to obtain microbiological confirmation; hence the choice of antibiotics should always cover the most likely causes. Consider factors which help determine the likely cause and severity, and guide the patient's management. Also establish the immunization history of the patient.

- Where was the pneumonia acquired — community or hospital?
- Was the patient previously healthy (1° pneumonia)? or chronically ill (2° pneumonia)?
- Are risk factors for pneumonia present including: malnutrition, pregnancy, HIV infection, diabetes, underlying chronic disabilities impairing lung function (e.g. cerebral palsy), periods of unconsciousness (alcohol, epilepsy, surgical patients), absence of a functioning spleen (post-splenectomy or due to sickle cell disease).

Clinical features

- The patient is systemically ill with malaise, fever, anorexia, body aches, and headache. Delirium can occur in severe infections. In children, symptoms can be less specific and include abdominal pain, vomiting, refusal of feeds.
- Respiratory signs and symptoms include raised respiratory rate (note: this is age-dependent — see box), nasal flaring, intercostal and subcostal recession, tracheal tug, cough, sputum production, dyspnoea, pleural pain, and, rarely, haemoptysis. Chest movements might be reduced on the affected side; inspiratory crackles and pleural rub may be present on auscultation. After a few days, an effusion often occurs. Sputum is often initially scanty or absent, becoming purulent or blood-streaked later in the infection. Children tend to swallow their secretions/sputum, so the absence of sputum production does not exclude pneumonia.
- Lower lobe pneumonia with diaphragmatic pleurisy may mimic an acute abdomen — abdominal pain, ileus, rigidity.
- In the very young, elderly, or debilitated, there may be fewer signs. Look for raised respiratory rate and perform a careful chest examination.

Age	Organism
Neonates	Group B streptococcus Gram-negative organisms (*E. coli, Klebsiella*) Less common: CMV, HSV, *Chlamydia, Listeria, Bordetella pertussis*; also consider maternal infections
<5 years	*Streptococcus pneumoniae* *Haemophilus influenzae* Group A Streptococcus *Staphylococcus aureus* (severe), especially post measles infection *Bordetella pertussis* Viral: RSV, measles, influenza, adenovirus, parainfluenza (always check immunization history)
School age	*Streptococcus pneumoniae* *Mycoplasma, Chlamydia* Viral pneumonias as above
Adults	*Streptococcus pneumoniae* 'Atypical' organisms (*Mycoplasma, Chlamydia, Legionella*) *H. influenzae* Viral pneumonias: influenza, adenovirus, *Varicella zoster*

Guide to respiratory rates (RR)   **PAEDIATRIC NOTE**
in children of different ages

Always count RR for 1 min in calm circumstances, as crying will give a elevated RR

Age	Normal RR/min	Severe respiratory distress
Infants <2 months	40–30	>60
2–12 months	40–30	>50
12 months–5 yrs	30–25	>40
>5 yrs	25–20	>30

Community-acquired pneumonia (CAP)

In a previously healthy person with community-acquired pneumonia, the most likely pathogens are S. pneumoniae and, less often, atypical organisms. TB should also be considered, especially if the response to antibiotics is poor. Consider whether the patient is:

- Previously healthy or had chronic lung disease. The latter condition predisposes to colonization e.g. with H. influenzae.
- Generally debilitated, an alcoholic, or an intravenous drug abuser. These patients are commonly infected by gram-negative bacteria and also at increased risk of TB and pneumococcal infection.
- Aspiration pneumonia may occur in those who have alcohol or drug habits, or reduced conciousness (e.g. head injury or epilepsy). Mouth and gum flora from poor dental hygiene includes anaerobes — causing pneumonia which often progresses to a lung abscess (see below).

Common bacterial causes of CAP (see box p. 167)

- *Streptococcus pneumoniae*.
- *Haemophilus influenzae* type B occurs particularly in children <5 yrs old who often present with lobar pneumonia, pleural involvement, and an effusion. It also occurs in adults both as a primary infection and in previously damaged lungs. The onset is slower than the other bacteria. The pneumonia is often accompanied by infection elsewhere (e.g. meninges, epiglottis). The use of the Hib vaccine in the tropics should markedly reduce its incidence, if the vaccine can be afforded.
- *Staphylococcus aureus* can cause pneumonia in patients with pre-existing chronic or acute lung disease, particularly following viral infection, usually influenza or especially measles. Note that the influenza infection may be subclinical. Alternatively, haematogenous spread from a distant site of infection (e.g. skin, bones and joints, or heart) may produce pneumonia in a previously healthy lung. In these circumstances, S. aureus may be isolated from blood. It is always a serious condition with high fever and cyanosis; common complications include pulmonary abscess formation, cavitation, empyema.

A poor prognosis is associated with

- Presence of bacteraemia (e.g. the fatality rate increases from 5% in isolated S. pneumoniae pneumonia to 25–35% fatality rate when the bacillus is cultured from blood).
- Infections with S. aureus, H. influenzae, and gram −ve bacteria.
- Previous illness, either chronic (e.g. COPD, cardiac disease, malnutrition) or acute (influenza, measles).

Clinical features	Investigations
• Confusion/sepsis	• Blood urea >7 mmol/l
• Respiratory rate >30/min (Note: age-dependent see opposite)	• WCC <4 × 10^9/l or >30 × 10^9/l
	• Arterial PO$_2$ <8 kPA
• Diastolic BP <60 mmHg	• Serum albumin <25 g/l
• New atrial fibrillation	• Multilobe involvement

Pneumococcal pneumonia

Streptococcus pneumoniae causes 25–50% of ARIs in children admitted to hospital and >1 million deaths/yr in children. It is most common in crowded communities with poor living conditions. Adults with debilitating diseases (e.g. diabetes, HIV, alcoholism, asplenia, hypogammaglobinaemia) are at increased risk of pneumonia and invasive pneumococcal disease. *Streptococcus pneumoniae* has progressively become less sensitive to penicillin: >50% of pneumococcal isolates in some countries have reduced sensitivity to penicillin. Many isolates also have reduced sensitivity to other common antibiotics such as tetracycline. Currently, the prevalence of penicillin-resistant pneumococci in many parts of the developing world is unknown.

Transmission: person–person via droplet spread. Long-term nasopharyngeal carriers of *S. pneumoniae* are common. Local spread to ear or meninges (particularly after head trauma) can produce otitis media or meningitis.

Clinical features: sometimes following an URTI, there is a sudden onset of fever, rigors, malaise, headache, and myalgia. At the extremes of age, onset is often less clear — children show tachypnoea in addition to fever and cough, while the elderly may have little fever and present with confusion. Chest pain (pleuritic, sometimes referred to shoulder if diaphragm is involved) and cough (initially painful and dry → blood-tinged → purulent) commonly follow. Lower lobe involvement can result in abdominal pain and guarding. The WCC is often raised; leukopenia is a poor prognostic sign.

Complications: pneumococci in the lungs may spread directly to the pleura, where a reactive effusion may already be present, producing a complicated parapneumonic effusion or an empyema (see below). Haematogenous spread can result in infection of meninges, joints, eyes, or abscess formation in distant organs. Rare complications include: acute septicaemia in patients with underlying conditions, such as asplenia; endocarditis; peritonitis in patients with lowered immunity; and ascites (nephrotic syndrome, cirrhosis).

Diagnosis: mainly clinical; bacteria can be cultured from sputum or blood; or by aspiration of abscesses in distant organs.

Management: follow local guidelines if local antibiotic sensitivities are known. If not known, use empiric antibiotics (see box p. 173).

Prevention: protein-conjugate vaccines are increasingly used (see Chapter 22). Seek to improve underlying health problems e.g. smoking, untreated HIV infection.

Atypical pneumonia

'Atypical' organisms cause <10% of all pneumonias in developing countries. Of those, common causes are *Mycoplasma pneumoniae* and *Chlamydia pneumoniae*. Others include *C. trachomatis* and *C. psittaci, Coxiella burnetti, Legionella pneumophila*, and viruses such as influenza and adenovirus. These organisms are difficult to culture and diagnosis is clinical, supported by CXR, blood picture, serology, or nasopharyngeal aspirate (if available). Atypical pneumonia affects previously healthy individuals of all ages. Symptoms are dyspnoea, dry cough, fever, and malaise. Localizing features (pleuritic chest pain, splinting, and respiratory distress) are rare. The CXR often shows bilateral, fluffy infiltrates, and appears worse than the clinical signs would suggest; the WCC can be normal, but hyponatraemia, elevated liver transaminases, proteinuria, and renal impairment are common. The clinical course is normally benign; occasionally it is severe and requires ICU admission.

Legionnaires' disease

The importance of *Legionella pneumophila* in the tropics is unknown. It is transmitted by inhalation of aerosolized water droplets from air conditioning systems, water storage tanks, showerheads, and medical equipment such as nebulizers.

Clinical features: vary from subclinical or mild infections to severe pneumonia. In severe infection, after 2–10 days, there is abrupt high fever, rigors, myalgia, and headache followed by the onset of a dry cough, dyspnoea, and crackles on auscultation. The patient becomes very ill, appearing toxic, sometimes with delirium or diarrhoea. Complications include respiratory failure, pericarditis, myocarditis, and acute renal failure. CXR shows homogeneous shadowing, often basal initially, subsequently widespread with deterioration.

Diagnosis: gram –ve slender rods of variable length in biopsy or sputum samples; bacterial antigen in urine for first 1–3 weeks.

Management: erythromycin 0.5–1 g/6 h IV or PO (± rifampicin 600 mg bd, moxifloxacin 400 mg od, or ciprofloxacin 500 mg bd) for 2–3 weeks.

Prevention: treatment and maintenance of stored water and tanks to prevent bacterial colonization and spread.

Recurrent pneumonia

Defined as more than two episodes of pneumonia, it may be caused by:
• Localized respiratory disease — bronchiectasis, bronchial obstruction (foreign body, bronchial carcinoma, lymphadenopathy, bronchial stenosis), intrapulmonary sequestration.
• Generalized respiratory disease — COPD ± bronchiectasis, impaired local defences.
• Non-respiratory problem — recurrent aspiration, immunosuppression.
• Acquired immunodeficiency (recurrent pneumonia is a frequent finding in HIV-infected children).

Nosocomial pneumonia

Definition: pneumonia that occurs more than 48 h after admission to hospital.

Signs: development of fever, increased WCC, purulent sputum, lung infiltrate on CXR.

Risk factors: ITU patients, increasing age, obesity, smoking, long pre-operative stay, prolonged anaesthesia, intubation, abdominal/thoracic operations, plus risk factors for aspiration pneumonia (see below).

Aetiology

- Aspiration of nasopharyngeal secretions — particularly of Gram −ve bacteria and anaerobic bacteria that may colonize nasopharynx during hospital stay. Broad-spectrum antibiotics and serious illness predispose to such colonization.
- Inhalation of bacteria from contaminated instruments — such as ventilators, nebulizers, intubation and nasogastric tubes.
- Haematogenous spread — e.g. from abdominal infection, infected cannulae, or catheters left in situ for too long.

Prevention: prevent smoking pre-operatively, encourage early mobilization. Good hospital staff and respiratory equipment hygiene, and good general infection control measures should decrease the risk. Chest physiotherapy post-operatively may help decrease nosocomial pneumonia.

Aspiration pneumonia

Risk factors: impaired consciousness (e.g. alcoholics, epileptics), dysphagia, being bed-bound, neuromuscular diseases, decreased ability to clear bronchial secretions or cough after general anaesthesia or abdominal/thoracic surgery.

Aetiology

- In the community — anaerobes from oropharynx and teeth crevices (normally penicillin-sensitive).
- In hospital — aerobic bacteria become more important, particularly Gram −ve enterobacteria and *P. aeruginosa*.

It may be possible to diagnose anaerobic infection from a history of poor dental hygiene, aspiration, or impaired consciousness. In children, also consider gastro-oesophageal reflux and underlying neurological/neuro-muscular disorders. As the infection proceeds, tissue necrosis results in foul-smelling purulent discharge.

Management of pneumonia

- O_2 — monitor saturation whenever possible; use paediatric probes for children.
- Antimicrobials: see below and box.
- Analgesia for pleuritic pain.
- Fluids (IV if necessary) to rectify dehydration and maintain an adequate urine output (>1 ml/kg/hour). Remember that losses are increased if the patient is febrile. In children, calculate volume replacement carefully in ml/kg according to age and state of hydration. Hyponatraemia secondary to SIADH is a common feature of severe pneumonia.
- Bed rest. The patient should sit up rather than lie flat — except in cases of severe pneumonia where this may exhaust the patient.
- Physiotherapy is not recommended in the acute stage of pneumonia; useful when pleuritic pain has subsided.

Antimicrobial use: general points

- If the patient is very ill, obtain culture specimens then immediately begin empirical IV antibiotic therapy. Be aware of local guidelines and, if possible, seek advice from a senior colleague. Empiric antibiotic choice depends upon the clinical situation.
- Only give IV therapy if the patient is very ill, cannot swallow/vomits, or if the GI tract is not functioning. Use IV antibiotics sooner in very young children, as disease progresses more rapidly. It is often possible to switch to PO antibiotics after a few doses IV.
- Calculate antibiotic dosages according to weight in children.
- Antibiotics can be given for 3–7 days in mild pneumonia. For severe pneumonia, continue treatment according to the clinical response. In the presence of cavitation and abscesses, continue treatment for 3–4 weeks.
- Change the guidelines given in the box to reflect the most common pathogens and their antimicrobial sensitivities in your region.

Chest X-rays in pneumonia

CXRs are expensive and their interpretation subject to wide variation. Therefore, the value of an CXR for each patient should be carefully considered before ordering one. In particular:

- Is the diagnosis already clear from the clinical features?
- Will the CXR change the patient's management?

Note: CXR changes in pneumonia may take weeks to resolve following successful treatment and clinical improvement by the patient.

Table 5.1 Empiric treatment of pneumonia

Clinical picture	Likely organisms		Antibiotic
1. 1° CAP (mild to moderate)		**PO**	**IV**
	S. pneumoniae	Ax	A
	If 'atypical'	Add E	
2. 2° pneumonia			
• Previous lung disease (e.g. COPD)	S. pneumoniae H. influenzae	Co	Co + E or C + E
• If following flu, measles, or URTI	S. aureus	Add F to above regimen	
• Aspiration	S. pneumoniae, Klebsiella spp, anaerobes, Gram −ve organisms	P + M + G	
• Immunosuppression (e.g. leukaemia)	Pseudomonas spp	×	Cz + G
• Nosocomial (especially if 2° disease)	Gram −ve	×	Ct + G
• Sepsis elsewhere	Treat as for sepsis	×	F + G + M
3. **Severe pneumonia**	Widest possible range	×	Ct + E + G

Key to antimicrobials (dose indicated is for adults)

A	Ampicillin 500 mg q6 h IV
Ax	Amoxicillin 500 mg tds PO
C	Cefuroxime 750 mg q8 h IV
Co	Co-amoxiclav 1 tablet (500 mg/125 mg) tds PO or 1.2 g (1000 mg/200 mg) q8 h IV
Ct	Ceftriaxone 1–2 g od IV or cefotaxime 1 g q8 h IV
Cz	Ceftazidime 2 g q8 h IV
E	Erythromycin 500 mg qds PO or 500 mg q6 h slowly IV
F	Flucloxacillin 500 mg qds PO or 250–1000 mg q6 h slowly IV
G	Gentamicin 3–5 mg/kg od IV
M	Metronidazole 500 mg po q8 h (for up to 7 days)
P	Benzylpenicillin 1.2–1.8 g q6 h IV (dose may be increased)
X	Oral therapy is inappropriate in these situations
	A, Ax, and oral Co doses can be doubled in severe infections; the IV Co dose can be increased in frequency to q6 h.

Severe acute respiratory syndrome (SARS)

In 2002 and 2003 an unusual coronavirus was responsible for a large number of cases of a severe acute respiratory syndrome (SARS) which had a high morbidity and mortality and spread rapidly across continents from its origin in Guandong in China and Hong Kong.

Pathology

Coronaviruses commonly infect humans and cause the common cold. The coronavirus strain causing SARS was previously unknown in humans and was identified in civet cats and racoons from which human transmission occurred as a result of ingestion. Following droplet inhalation or ingestion, the coronavirus spreads to the bloodstream and urine and causes severe pulmonary inflammation characterized by desquamation of pneumocytes, hyaline membrane formation, and oxygenation failure (ARDS). Mortality occurs in approximately 10–20% of individuals, especially the elderly and those with pre-existing cardiovascular disease and diabetes.

Clinical features

Fever, cough, malaise, diarrhoea, myalgias, and headache occur after an incubation period of 2–7 days. In many patients, the chest X-ray shows infiltrates and patchy consolidation especially in the lower zones. As the illness progresses, X-ray shadowing worsens along with the development of ARDS and multi-organ dysfunction. Recovery may be slow and some patients develop pulmonary fibrosis as a sequelae.

Diagnosis is based on the clinical sequence of events and the appropriate setting. WHO criteria are regularly updated and should be studied. Cultures of SARS-CoV are not possible in routine laboratories and an RT-PCR may be useful on blood, urine, and sputum samples. Rising antibody titres may be of help but are generally valuable only in convalescence.

Management

No specific antiviral therapy, including ribavarin, is of value. Steroids have been tried on account of a postulated immunopathological mechanism but no benefit has been found. Supportive treatment in an ICU setting is the best option.

Paediatric specific acute respiratory infections

Epiglottitis

Epiglottitis is an acute bacterial infection of the epiglottis, aryepiglottic folds, and arytenoid cartilages. It occurs mainly in children aged 2–7 years and is almost always caused by *Haemophilus influenzae* type b (Hib). Following direct or haematogenous infection of the upper airway, there is rapid swelling and risk of airway obstruction. Hib conjugate vaccine substantially reduces the incidence of life-threatening infections. However, many EPI programmes do not include Hib immunization and severe disease also occurs where immunization coverage is low. In older individuals, *Streptococcus pneumoniae, Haemophilus parainfluenzae*, group A Streptococcus, and *Staphylococcus aureus* may cause a similar illness.

Clinical features: Typically starts suddenly and progresses rapidly. The affected child presents with sudden onset of high fever, sore throat, and muffled voice. Stridor, respiratory distress, and drooling of saliva follow. The child appears toxic, refuses to eat or drink, and prefers to sit upright, leaning forward in an effort to maintain patency of the airway. Other associated symptoms include loss of voice (aphonia) and dysphagia.

Diagnosis: Consider epiglottitis in any young child with compatible clinical presentation, esp. if not immunized against Hib. Visualization of a large, swollen, cherry-red epiglottis by direct laryngoscopy at the time of endotracheal intubation confirms the diagnosis.

Management: Epiglottitis is a medical emergency. The goals of management are prevention of airway obstruction and eradication of infection.

- Give humidified O_2.
- Make urgent arrangements for securing an artificial airway (preferably nasotracheal), irrespective of the severity of respiratory distress.
- Be prepared to perform a tracheostomy if endotracheal intubation fails.
- Until the airway has been secured do **NOT**:
  - *examine the throat* (reflex laryngeal spasm may cause complete airway obstruction).
  - *attempt venepuncture* (associated anxiety and pain may precipitate acute laryngeal spasm).
  - *send the child for an X-ray* (immediate intervention will be necessary if airway obstruction occurs).
- Once definitive airway secured, take samples for FBC and cultures of blood and epiglottic surface.
- Give antibiotics: IV ceftriaxone or IV ampicillin and chloramphenicol, for 7–10 days.

Note: adrenaline and corticosteroids are NOT effective in epiglottitis.

Once the airway is secured, most children improve rapidly with signs of improved oxygenation and respiratory effort. The epiglottitis resolves after a few days of antibiotics, and the patient can be weaned from the endotracheal or nasotracheal tube.

Differential diagnosis of acute upper airways obstruction in children   **PAEDIATRIC NOTE**

- viral croup (most common).
- bacterial tracheitis.
- measles tracheitis.
- epiglottitis.
- diphtheria.
- severe tonsillitis.
- infectious mononucleosis.
- laryngeal foreign body.
- smoke or steam inhalation.
- trauma.
- laryngomalacia (sub-acute, chronic or acute on chronic cause in infants).
- peritonsillar or retropharyngeal abscess.

Bacterial tracheitis

Presentation is similar to croup, but bacterial tracheitis may affect any age group and does not respond to croup treatment. Unlike epiglottitis, bacterial tracheitis rarely causes airway obstruction. Causes include *S. aureus*, group A streptococci, *H. influenzae, Moraxella catarrhalis*, *Klebsiella* species, other gram negatives, and anaerobes. There is diffuse inflammation of the larynx, trachea, and bronchi with formation of an adherent or semi-adherent mucopurulent membrane in the trachea.

Clinical features: include fever, bark-like/brassy cough, hoarseness, respiratory distress, stridor, and sepsis.

Diagnosis: is clinical supported by elevated WBC, CXR (which may show narrowing of trachea), and blood culture. Direct visualization and culture of purulent tracheal secretions by laryngotracheobronchoscopy is the only means of definitive diagnosis.

Treatment: involves airway management and administration of broad-spectrum antibiotics. Affected children may decompensate acutely with worsening respiratory distress and sepsis.

Acute laryngotracheobronchitis: croup

Laryngotracheobronchitis (LTB; croup) is the most common form of upper airway obstruction in childhood, usually occurring between 3 months and 5 years of age. The majority of cases are viral in origin. LTB initially affects the mucosa of the nose and nasopharynx, then spreads to involve larynx and bronchial tree. In young children, in whom the subglottic mucosa is loosely attached, inflammation causes submucosal oedema and narrowing of the airway.

Human parainfluenza viruses cause ~75% cases; other causes include adenoviruses, RSV, influenza, and measles.

Clinical features: LTB begins as a mild URTI with mild brassy cough, low-grade fever, and intermittent stridor. Over the ensuing few days, progressive compromise of the airway results in a characteristic sequence of symptoms and signs: coughing increases, stridor becomes continuous (± wheeze), and signs of respiratory distress develop, including nasal flaring, suprasternal, intercostal, and subcostal recession (lower chest wall indrawing), associated with a prolonged, laboured expiratory phase of respiration. Symptoms are characteristically worse at night. Crying and agitation aggravate symptoms and the child prefers to sit up in bed or be held upright. Examination reveals reduced breath sounds, wheezes, and crackles.

Most children improve spontaneously within 48–72 h but some progress to severe airway compromise and, therefore, require further intervention to avert death from respiratory failure. The croup score is useful for the initial assessment of the child, as well as the evaluation of the response to treatment.

Diagnosis: is clinical.

Management

Indications for admission are listed in the box opposite.

- Give humidified O_2.
- Give dexamethasone 150 mcg/kg IV/IM/PO or prednisolone 1–2 mg/kg PO or nebulized budesonide 2 mg stat; repeat at 12 h if necessary.
- Give IV fluids to children with moderate to severe respiratory distress.
- Ensure minimal disturbance as symptoms worsen on agitation.
- Observe closely for signs of worsening airway obstruction.
- If severe airway obstruction develops (cyanosis, air hunger, restlessness), consider nebulized adrenaline (give 400 mcg/kg up to max 5 mg, of 1 in 1000 (1 mg/ml) solution, repeated after 30 minutes if required), ± tracheostomy or nasotracheal intubation.

Note:

- Sedation is contraindicated in croup because it masks restlessness, which is one of the principal clinical indices of the severity of airway obstruction and the need for tracheostomy or nasotracheal intubation.
- Expectorants, bronchodilators, and antihistamines are not helpful in the management of croup.

Indications for admission in a child with croup include   PAEDIATRIC NOTE

- worsening stridor or respiratory distress.
- severe stridor at rest.
- hypoxia or cyanosis.
- restlessness, lethargy, or unconsciousness.

Managing milder episodes at home

Children with mild croup can be managed at home but must be watched closely for signs of worsening respiratory obstruction. Management is supportive. Cool mist inhalation may help: this can be achieved by placing the child in a bathroom filled with steam from the shower or by taking the child outdoors in the cool, night air.

Croup score   PAEDIATRIC NOTE

Clinical parameter	Score		
	1	2	3
Colour	Normal	Cyanosed in room air	Cyanosed on 40% O_2
Stridor	Absent	Inspiratory	Expiratory
Cough	Nil	Mild, brassy	Severe
Respiratory distress	Absent	Nasal flaring	Intercostal recession, indrawing
Air entry	Normal	Slightly reduced	Greatly reduced

A croup score of ≥6 is an indication for ICU care

Acute bronchiolitis

Acute bronchiolitis is common among children aged <2 years (peak 3–6 months). In >50% of cases it is caused by RSV; other causes include adenoviruses, parainfluenza virus, and *Mycoplasma*. The source of infection is usually an older child or adult with a minor respiratory illness. Risk factors for severe RSV bronchiolitis include low birth weight, overcrowding, exposure to tobacco smoke, and a family history of asthma. Exclusive breastfeeding offers some protection in infancy.

Clinical features: Characteristically begins as a URTI; the infant appears slightly unwell, with low-grade fever, a blocked nose, serous nasal discharge, cough and feeding difficulty. Within 24–48 h, the signs of airway obstruction appear with paroxysmal wheezy cough, dyspnoea, and irritability. Breast and bottle-feeding become difficult as the rapid respiratory rate does not give enough time for sucking and swallowing. Examination reveals tachypnoea, nasal flaring, intercostal and subcostal recession. The chest is hyper-resonant with obliteration of the cardiac dullness due to hyperinflation. Rhonchi and fine crepitations are heard on auscultation. The liver and spleen may be palpable due to hyperinflation. In mild cases, symptoms resolve over 1–3 days while severe cases may run a more protracted course.

Diagnosis: is primarily clinical, supported by CXR which may show hyperinflation (flattening of the diaphragm) ± associated pneumonia.

Management: is mainly supportive:
- All children with respiratory distress should be hospitalized.
- Keep propped up in bed (30–40° above horizontal).
- Give humidified O_2 via a nasal catheter.
- Ensure adequate fluid intake.
- Feed via NG tube.
- Wheezing may respond to nebulized salbutamol.

Note:
- Antibiotics are indicated for any associated pneumonia.
- Corticosteroids are of no benefit in the management of bronchiolitis.

Lymphocytic interstitial pneumonitis (LIP)

The HIV pandemic has made LIP a common respiratory disorder; it constitutes 22–75% of pulmonary disease in paediatric patients with HIV, but is uncommon in adults. LIP also occasionally occurs in EBV infection, HTLV infection, lymphoproliferative disorders, and autoimmune disease. Pathologically, there is a pleomorphic lung infiltrate of lymphocytes, plasma cells and immunoblasts, with activation of T cells and increased production of lymphokines.

Clinical features

May be asymptomatic in the early stages. Symptoms are usually progressive and include:

- Chronic cough.
- Dyspnoea.
- Parotid enlargement.
- Generalized lymphadenopathy.
- Hepatosplenomegaly.
- Digital clubbing.
- Wheezing.

± other features of the underlying immunosuppressive disease.

Diagnosis: is clinical, supported by CXR

- ABG may confirm hypoxia.
- CXR findings include bibasilar interstitial or small nodular infiltrates which coalesce into alveolar consolidation, widened mediastinum, and peri-hilar adenopathy.
- Serum LDH is often increased to 300–500 iu/L.
- Tests for underlying disease, especially HIV.

Differential diagnoses include varicella pneumonia, miliary TB, and metastatic carcinoma. Definitive diagnosis requires open lung biopsy which is rarely performed in view of its attendant complications.

Treatment

Asymptomatic children require no treatment but should be followed up for clinical and/or radiological signs of deterioration. For symptomatic children:

- O_2.
- Prednisolone 2 mg/kg PO daily; treat for 4 weeks then gradually taper dose. Long-term steroid therapy may be required if symptoms recur.
- Bronchodilators may be used to treat children with wheeze.
- Treat the underlying cause: anti-retroviral therapy for HIV infection.

Diphtheria

The Gram +ve bacterium *Corynebacterium diphtheriae* causes infection of the naso-pharynx and occasionally skin and mucous membranes. Its endotoxin has potentially fatal effects on the heart, kidney, and peripheral nerves. Death occurs in 75% without treatment, and in 5–10% despite treatment. Children <5 yrs and adults >40 yrs have a worse prognosis. Although its incidence is falling worldwide, it remains a significant problem in some developing countries where vaccination programmes are unavailable.

Transmission is by droplets or secretions from infected humans (the only reservoir). Incubation is 2–5 days. Patients are infectious for ~1 mth; however, some become carriers.

Clinical features

The incubation period is ~2–5 days (7 days for cutaneous diphtheria). The patient may present with general non-specific symptoms, including: fever and chills, malaise, sore throat, hoarseness and dysphagia, wheezing, nausea and vomiting, headache.

Local: mucosae are initially red and oedematous; this progresses to necrosis of epithelium. An inflammatory grey-white pseudo-membrane forms at the site of infection (commonly the tonsils and oropharynx); it is adherent and separates with bleeding. There is fever, malaise, sore throat (may cause dysphagia), cervical lymphadenopathy, and bad breath. The neck is often swollen with oedema and enlarged lymph nodes. Palatal paralysis by toxin produces a 'nasal' quality to the speech.

Tracheo-laryngeal: hoarsness, dry cough, and, rarely, airways obstruction.

Cutaneous: this is rare. There are pustules and ulcers with a grey membrane.

Systemic effects of toxin: myocarditis (10%), heart block (often >1 wk after acute infection; can cause death up to 8 wks after), murmurs, heart failure. Neuronal demyelination causes peripheral neuritis (often ~6 wks after initial illness), paralysis (soft palate, ocular, and intercostals muscles). There may be renal failure (tubular necrosis) and pneumonia.

Malignant diphtheria: indicates rapid spread of membranes, neck oedema and adenitis, stridor, and shock.

Diagnosis

Treat on suspicion — do not wait for confirmation. Arrange for throat swabs of membrane, ECG (look for ectopics, ST and T wave changes, RBBB, complete heart block), U&Es, FBC.

Treatment

Give antitoxin as soon as possible. A test dose of diluted diphtheria antitoxin should 1st be given intradermally to exclude hypersensitivity; then give 10,000–30,000 units IM for mild–moderate disease, and 40,000–100,000 for severe disease (for children <10 yrs give half this dose). For doses >40,000 units, give by IV infusion. Antitoxin is made from horse serum, so beware anaphylaxis which is rare but potentially fatal. Have adrenaline drawn up. Tracheostomy may be life-saving; do not delay if there are signs of respiratory distress. Give high-dose antibiotics IV (penicillin, erythromycin, cephalosporin, tetracycline are all effective).

Prevention

Routine childhood vaccination prevents disease. Recovering patients should also receive vaccine as a booster dose, as well as close contacts. Immunity can be assessed by the Shick test.

Causes of sore throat and tonsillar exudates

- *Streptococcus pyogenes* (sequelae are rheumatic heart disease and glomerulonephritis).
- Mild viral infections.
- *Corynebacterium diphtheriae*.
- *Epstein–Barr virus* — infectious mononucleosis.
- *Neisseria gonorrhoeae*.
- 2° syphilis.
- *Herpes simplex* virus — especially in AIDS patients.
- *Lassa virus*.
- *Fusobacterium necrophorum* (part of Lemierre syndrome).

Whooping cough

Bordetella pertussis commonly affects infants aged 2–4 yrs but can cause illness and death at any age. Vaccination has reduced the incidence but it is still a major problem in some countries.

Clinical features

The incubation period is 6–20 days. The first phase is indistinguishable from the common cold and lasts 1–2 weeks. Fever is not usually prominent.

Paroxysms of severe coughing with a 'whoop' are the classical feature. The 'whoop' is caused by forced inspiration against a partly-closed glottis and can cause cyanosis and hypoxic syncope. Infants <6 mths do not whoop but become apnoeic. The child commonly drools and vomits after coughing, and may become exhausted. Wheezing does not occur. After 1–3 weeks of whooping, a more tolerable chronic cough may persist for several weeks; adults and older children may have a chronic cough throughout.

Many cases are uncomplicated and self-limiting; however, illness can persist for weeks to months and result in bronchiectasis and malnutrition. Prolonged coughing may produce petechiae, conjunctival haemorrhages, and rectal prolapse. Death is usually due to severe infection, 2° pneumonia, or encephalopathy — reduced consciousness that is not due to hypoxia, seizures, or brain damage.

Diagnosis

Normally made clinically. The WCC shows a lymphocytosis. Culture is difficult — a per-nasal swab is taken.

Management

Erythromycin is recommended, but its effect in modifying whooping cough is weak. Nebulized beta-agonists and steroids are sometimes used but generally have little effect because wheezing is not a prominent feature.

Prevention

Routine immunization.

Pleural effusion

The presence of fluid in the pleural cavity. This is generally unilateral but may be bilateral.

- Exudates are inflammatory fluid collections caused by an underlying infective/inflammatory disease. They are generally unilateral; cellular pleocytosis is common, and protein content and fluid LDH levels are generally high. Exudates have a straw-coloured appearance and a high protein content (>50% of serum protein or >30 g/L).
- Transudates are serous fluid collections that occur as a result of passive flow across capillaries. They have a low protein content and are generally bilateral; cellular pleocytosis is minimal. All oedema-causing conditions — CCF, nephrotic syndrome, liver cell failure, anaemia, and hypoproteinaemia — may cause transudative pleural effusions.
- Chylothorax — the fluid appears milky on macroscopic appearance and has a high lipid content. It is caused by leakage from the thoracic duct due to damage by filariasis or a neoplastic process.
- Empyema — the fluid contains frank pus.
- Haemothorax — pure blood or heavily bloodstained fluid.

Clinical features: Pleuritic chest pain is usually present if the pleura is acutely inflamed — less common in TB (chronic inflammation). Patients are tachypnoeic and may be dyspnoeic. Chest wall expansion is impaired on the affected side and there is stony dullness to percussion with ↓ tactile fremitus and ↓or absent breath sounds. Signs are commonly detected at the bases posteriorly and in the mid-axillary line.

Diagnosis: The presence of fluid is confirmed by CXR or ultrasound. Aspiration of 50–100 ml is generally done for diagnosis but in patients with respiratory distress, 700–1000 ml is aspirated to relieve symptoms. Fluid is best withdrawn posteriorly with the patient leaning forward and the needle inserted one or two intercostal spaces below the upper level of dullness. Fluid should be sent for routine biochemical examination, pH, cytology, Gram and AFB staining, adenosine deaminase (ADA) and lactate dehydrogenase (LDH) levels, and appropriate cultures.

Management: Treat the cause of the effusion. Where the fluid is causing dyspnoea, repeated aspirations or chest tube insertion may be beneficial. Where recurrence is a problem, a pleurodesis may be performed.

Empyema

Pus in the pleural space is often a complication of a bacterial pneumonia, pulmonary TB, aspiration pneumonia, or rupture of a liver or lung abscess. A putrid odour indicates anaerobic bacterial infection. An empyema should be suspected in any patient with persistent (often high spiking) fever, with signs of fluid in the pleural space. Diagnosis is established by the aspiration of pus from the pleural space and the fluid obtained should be Gram stained and cultured. Broad-spectrum antibiotics (suitable choices: co-amoxiclav; ceftriaxone; cefotaxime) are indicated until the results of culture are obtained. Intercostal tube drainage or a decortication may be required if a prolonged course of IV antibiotics combined with repeated ultrasound guided aspiration fails. A fluid pH <7.1 or high LDH level (>60% of serum LDH or >1000) suggests an empyema is developing, and needs to be drained.

Causes of pleural effusion

Exudates:

- Tuberculosis.
- Lung cancer.
- Pneumonia.
- Mesothelioma.
- Collagen diseases.
- Sub diaphragmatic infections/abscesses.
- Metastatic carcinoma.
- Pulmonary embolism.
- Pancreatitis.

Transudates:

- Cardiac failure.
- Liver cell dysfunction especially when associated with ascites.
- Nephrotic syndrome.
- Anaemia and hypoproteinaemia.
- Pericardial disease.

Haemothorax:

- Trauma.
- Mesothelioma.
- Metastatic carcinoma.
- Vascular pleural adhesions.

Chylothorax:

- Filariasis.
- Lymphoma.
- Trauma to the thoracic duct.
- Metastatic carcinoma.

Diagnostic features of pleural effusions

- Exudates — protein >3.0 gms (with normal serum proteins), LDH >200 i.u., fluid:serum LDH ratio >0.6.
- Transudates — protein <3.0 gms, LDH <200, LDH ratio <0.6.
- Increased ADA levels suggests TB.
- Neutrophilia — bacterial pneumonias, empyemas.
- Lymphocytosis — TB, lymphomas, viral infections.
- Abnormal cytology — carcinomas, mesotheliomas.
- Low pleural fluid sugar — RA, infections, malignancies.

Lung abscess

This is a suppurative infection of the lung parenchyma. It is commonly caused by aspiration of mouth anaerobes and, less often, by blood-borne infection.

Clinical features

Patients present with a cough, fever with chills, chest pain, and haemoptysis. Gingivitis with poor dentition, the usual source of the bacteria, is often found. When the abscess communicates with a bronchus, copious quantities of purulent sputum, often blood-streaked, are expectorated. Clubbing develops rapidly and if the abscess ruptures into the pleural space, an empyema will result. Chronic abscesses with waxing and waning symptoms may result from inadequate antibiotic therapy.

Diagnosis

Characteristically, the CXR shows a rounded opacity with an air-fluid level. Multiple abscesses suggests a blood-borne infection e.g., infected pulmonary emboli or tricuspid endocarditis. Leukocytosis with raised ESR and CRP are typical. Blood and sputum cultures help in identification of the causative organism. If the abscess does not resolve on antibiotics, bronchoscopy may be performed to seek an endo-bronchial obstruction (foreign body, malignancy, bronchial adenoma).

Management

IV antibiotics are mandatory until fever and leukocytosis settles. Co-amoxiclav, clindamycin ceftriaxone, or cefuroxime are good initial choices and may be modified according to cultures. Metronidazole may be added for additional anaerobic cover and an antistaphylococcal antibiotic such as flucloxacillin may be used in the appropriate setting.

Causes of lung abscesses

Pulmonary aspiration: most occur in the right lung; aspiration while supine results in abscesses in apical segment of the lower lobe or posterior segment of the upper lobe. Often caused by anaerobes of gingival origin.

Bronchial obstruction: due to lung CA or inhaled foreign body. Caused by mixed anaerobes.

Bacteraemia/septicaemia: often multiple abscesses from sites such as right-sided endocarditis, infected IV cannulae, IV drug abuse. Common causes are *S. aureus*, *Streptococcus milleri*.

Primary infection with cavitation: TB or as a complication of severe pneumonia with *S. aureus*, *Klebsiella pneumoniae*, *Nocardia asteroides*.

Spread from subphrenic or hepatic abscess: produces 2° abscess, often in the right lower lobe. Due to *Entamoeba histolytica*, coliforms, *Streptococcus faecalis*.

Immunosuppression: such as malignancy, AIDS. Predisposes to unusual infections.

Cavitating lesions seen on CXR, mimicking abscesses, may be caused by TB; paragonimiasis; fungal infection; cavitating squamous cell CA; pulmonary infarction; Wegener's granulomatosis.

Fungal pulmonary infections

Some fungi can infect the lung after inhalation of their spores, which are found airborne and in soil and, in the case of histoplasmosis, bat faeces. Human–human transmission does not appear to be a problem. Accidental transmission may occur through the skin.

The infections depend on the immune status of the individual and the level of exposure. While many cases are asymptomatic, illness may present as:

- *Self-resolving pneumonitis* (acute pulmonary form): cough, chest pain, fever, joint pains, malaise, occasionally erythema nodosum or multiforme. Specific therapy may be required in addition to bed rest.
- *Localized cavitation*: may be asymptomatic and found on CXR for other reasons. No treatment is required. However, since they can be similar to lung tumours, they may be diagnosed only at surgery.
- *Persisting or spreading cavitation*: producing chest pain, cough, and sometimes haemoptysis (which can be heavy). Surgery and antifungal therapy may be required. These manifestations look similar to, and can be mistaken for, pulmonary TB.
- *Acute or chronic systemic dissemination*: to organs characteristic of each infection. Patients present with fever, often marked weight loss, skin lesions. If acute, there may be signs of lung disease and purpura due to thrombocytopenia. Disseminated disease is fatal in the absence of systemic antifungal therapy.

Moderate immunosuppression associated with diabetes predisposes to spreading cavitation in some infections. Immunosuppression or neoplasia predispose to acute disseminated disease. The elderly, pregnant women, and children are also at increased risk of disseminated disease.

Aspergillosis

Most infections are caused by *Aspergillus fumigatus*, *A. flavus*, or *A. niger* in predisposed hosts. The fungus is ubiquitous; infection and disease occur sporadically throughout the world.

Clinical forms and management

- *Allergic bronchopulmonary aspergillosis* (APBA): persistent endobronchial infection/colonization elicits a chronic Type 1 hypersensitivity response in atopic individuals. This produces asthma and, with time, a chronic cough (producing mucoid plugs) and dyspnoea. CXR may show shadowing in the peripheral fields. Eosinophilia is a feature. Manage with steroids. May lead to proximal bronchiectasis.
- *Aspergilloma*: a fungal ball that develops in a pre-existing cavity (commonly due to TB). Intermittent cough is often the only sign but haemoptysis may develop. If this is severe, the aspergilloma should be surgically excised. CT scan appearances are distinctive.
- *Invasive disease*: occurs in brain, kidney, liver, and skin of the severely immunocompromised (e.g. bone marrow transplant recipients). Attempt to reduce immunosuppression, if possible. Give amphotericin B 1–1.5 mg/kg IV od, to a total dose of 2–2.5 g. This is a toxic drug.

Diagnosis of Aspergillus infection

This is often difficult. Microscopic analysis of skin lesion scrapings, sputum, or pus for evidence of fungal infection. Serology (*Aspergillus* precipitins), specific fungal cultures. In disseminated disease, yeasts may be seen in Giemsa-stained bone marrow. Skin prick tests to *Aspergillus* and *Aspergillus* RAST test is useful in ABPA. In acute fungal lung infections, the radiographic appearances may give a clue, being typically more severe than expected from clinical examination. Isolated chronic lung lesions (mycetomas) may only be distinguished from lung tumours at surgery.

Histoplasmosis

This occurs in two forms and commonly affects HIV-infected patients:

- *Small-form* histoplasmosis (caused by *Histoplasma capsulatum* var. *capsulatum*) occurs in the Americas plus Africa and Asia. This gives acute or chronic pulmonary infections, pericarditis, or progressive disseminated histoplasmosis in immunocompromised individuals. Disseminated small-form histoplasmosis affects bone marrow, spleen, liver, lymph nodes, and skin (papules, ulcers). A chronic form in immunocompetent patients presents with persistent painful oral ulceration and/or hypoadrenalism. Complications include laryngeal ulceration, endocarditis, and meningitis.

- *Large-form* or African histoplasmosis (*H. capsulatum* var. *duboisii.*) occurs in central and west Africa. African histoplasmosis is either a focal disease affecting bone, skin, and lymph nodes or a progressive disseminated disease affecting mucosal surfaces, particularly the GI tract and lungs.

Blastomycosis

A systemic infection caused by *Blastomyces dermatitidis* that occurs in northern America, Africa, India, and Middle East. It causes chronic pulmonary or disseminated disease (involving both lung and skin of face and forearm). Skin lesions are commonly an initial single nodule, then crusted plaques, ulcers, and abscesses. Complications include lytic bone lesions (particularly axial skeleton) and GU tract disease (particularly epididymitis).

Coccidioidomycosis

A disease of semi-arid regions of the Americas, caused by the fungus *Coccidioides immitis*. It is inhaled into the distal airspaces, where it rounds up and divides to form a large spherule with thick outer wall. The clinical features are typically varied with dissemination occurring particularly to meninges, joints, and skin.

Paracoccidioidomycosis

A granulomatous disease caused by the fungus *Paracoccidioides brasiliensis*. It occurs sporadically in south and central America where it is the most common systemic mycosis. An acute form of the disease occurs in children and adults <30 yrs, while a chronic form is more common in 30–50 year olds, particularly agricultural workers living in endemic areas. The M:F ratio is ~10:1.

- *Acute form*: presents with generalized lymphadenopathy, moderate hepatosplenomegaly, fever, and weight loss over several months. The nodes are hard but may become fluctuant. Involvement of mesenteric and hepatic perihilar nodes may produce an appendicitis-like picture or obstructive jaundice. Complications include lytic bone lesions, small bowel disease, multiple mucocutaneous lesions (lymphatic/ haematogenous spread). Pulmonary involvement is uncommon. Immunosuppression can lead to severe superinfection (e.g. TB, cryptococcus, pneumonia).

- *Chronic disease*: normally presents with lung disease: dyspnoea, cough, (rarely haemoptysis and fever), with extensive involvement on CXR.

Mucocutaneous lesions are common on skin (face, limbs); painful lesions in the mouth, pharynx, or oesophagus inhibit eating, producing marked weight loss. *Other features*: ulcerated tongue, hypoadrenalism. Chronic inflammation and fibrosis may result in tracheal/laryngeal fibrosis, pulmonary fibrosis, and bowel obstruction due to enlarged lymph nodes. Tumours may arise in the skin or lung lesions.

Management of systemic fungal infections

Follow local guidelines
- Am B (increase daily dose from 0.6 mg/kg/day to of 1.0–1.5 mg/kg/day, as renal function permits) to a cumulative total of at least 15 mg/kg.

(Alternative: fluconazole 200–400 mg PO od for 6–18 months depending on specific fungus)
- Meningitis due to coccidioidomycosis requires fluconazole 400–600 mg PO od for 9–12 months.
- Surgery may be required for management of chronic sequelae in paracoccidioidomycosis.

Paragonimiasis (lung fluke disease)

A persistent lung disease, occurring widely around the globe, which is caused by >15 different species of *Paragonimus* trematodes.

Transmission

Humans are infected by eating undercooked freshwater crabs and crayfish infected with the metacercariae. The immature flukes burrow out of the human intestine into the peritoneum, where they mature and tunnel their way into the lungs. Here they cause inflammation, haemorrhage, and necrosis of the lung parenchyma. Adult flukes (stout, bean-shaped, ~1 cm long) live in cavities in proximity to airways. Ova are expelled either in expectorated sputum or in the faeces after being swallowed. Flukes that miss the lungs produce extrapulmonary symptoms (due to cysts, granulomas, and abscesses) in muscles, abdominal viscera, brain, genitalia.

Clinical features of paragonimiasis

Days–weeks after eating infected food, migration of the flukes within the peritoneal and pleural cavities causes signs of inflammatory and allergic responses — fever, rashes, urticaria, abdominal and chest pain or discomfort.

The classic feature of chronic pulmonary disease is a persistent cough with production of a thick brownish-red sputum (due to the presence of ova and flukes). The CXR has features often resembling TB, except that cavities are often basal. CXR changes may also include areas of consolidation and pleural effusions. Physical examination of the chest often reveals little and the patients appear quite well.

Aberrant migration of the flukes may produce signs of a cerebral SOL (epilepsy, raised ICP, psychiatric syndromes, meningeal irritation) or spinal SOL, necrosis of abdominal viscera, transitory subcutaneous swellings. Extrapulmonary disease may occur in the absence of pulmonary signs, but this is uncommon.

Diagnosis: presence of ova or adult flukes in the sputum, faeces, or effusion; serology.

Management: praziquantel 25 mg/kg PO tds for 2–3 days often produces rapid symptomatic improvement, although radiological changes may take some months to improve.

Treatment: of cerebral infection may result in neurological deterioration, in some cases producing seizures and coma. Beware of raised ICP due to dying parasites. Treat cautiously and consider using dexamethasone 4 mg IV q6 h as cover.

Prevention: improve health education to decrease consumption of undercooked crustaceans; mass treatment of persons in endemic areas.

Tropical pulmonary eosinophilia

This acute or chronic lung syndrome occurs in areas where Bancroftian filariasis is endemic. TPE is an amicrofilaraemic syndrome, resulting from hypersensitivity to microfilarial antigens. In most instances, the diagnosis is based on a therapeutic response to diethylcarbamazine (DEC).

Pathology

Culex mosquitoes carry the larvae that mature into adult worms of *Wurchereria bancrofti* and *Brugiya malayi* within lymphatics. Female worms discharge millions of microfilaria many of which are trapped and destroyed within the lungs eliciting an eosinophilic hypersensitivity reaction.

Clinical features

Young adults are generally affected. Nocturnal cough associated with wheezing may occur due to the nocturnal periodicity of microfilaraemia. Low-grade fever, malaise, and weight loss may occur. Wheezes and crackles are heard in severe or advanced cases, but in many patients respiratory examination is normal. Significant eosinophilia is typical with total eosinophil counts 3000–50,000/mm^3. Symptoms do not correlate with the degree of eosinophilia. Filarial serology is positive but is unhelpful in endemic areas. CXRs may be normal or show a reticulonodular appearance resembling milliary mottling. In long-standing cases, features of pulmonary fibrosis are seen. PFTs show a mixed restrictive and obstructive pattern with diffusion abnormalities prominent in longstanding cases.

Management

Diethylcarbamazine 5 mg/kg daily in three divided doses x 3 weeks. Patients who respond poorly should have a 2nd course of DEC for a longer duration.

Asthma

Asthma is a disorder of the airways caused by chronic inflammation and associated with reversible obstruction to the large or small airways. It is often precipitated by environmental triggers, on a background of genetic susceptibility. Triggers may be:

- Allergens e.g. dust, food, pets etc. in atopic individuals.
- Infections, especially viral in children e.g. RSV.
- Environmental or occupational pollutants such as smoke, automobile exhausts, and various industrial dusts.

Acute symptoms may be caused in any asthmatic individual on exposure to any of the above and may be worsened by beta-blocker therapy or use of NSAIDS

Pathology

Constant exposure to environmental triggers causes persistent mucosal inflammation. Asthmatic attacks occur due to:

- Bronchial hyper-responsiveness to cold dry air, pollen, fumes, and paints.
- Inflammatory bronchial wall oedema and intra-luminal mucus accumulation which cause airway narrowing, airflow obstruction, and distal air trapping.

Clinical features

Breathlessness, cough, and expiratory wheezing are the hallmarks. 'Chest tightness' is a common symptom. Symptoms may occur only during exercise or exposure to cold air. Wheezes are often low-pitched and heard only on forced expiration.

Diurnal variation is common, due to the circadian variation in endogenous cortisol production. Symptoms are generally worse on waking and, in severe cases, may cause nocturnal awakening with cough, chest tightness, and dyspnoea. Symptoms generally improve through the day and episodic exacerbations may be triggered by various stimuli and last minutes, hours, or days.

Diagnosis of asthma

This is based on characteristic clinical features. Measurement of variability in diurnal or stimulus-induced serial PEFR measurements is also useful. Astma is diagnosed when spirometry or peak expiratory flow rate (PEFR) shows >15% reduction in response to stimulus challenge e.g. 6–10 minutes of strenuous exercise; PEFR is <60% predicted or varies by >30%; or PEFR improves by >20% with bronchodilators or steroids.

Management

Identify and avoid all environmental and other triggers; relief of acute symptoms with β-agonist inhalers and suppression of chronic inflammatory airways hyper-reactivity with inhaled or oral steroids or leukotrine antagonists.

Aims of treatment

- Freedom from symptoms, especially nocturnal asthma.
- Lung functions within the normal range varying by <20% during 24 h.
- Normal quality of life.

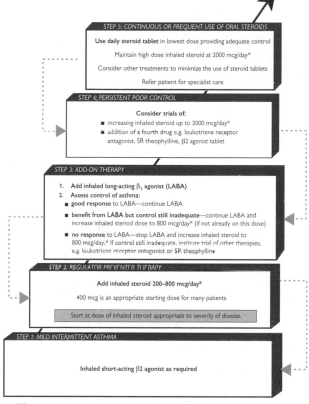

STEP 5: CONTINUOUS OR FREQUENT USE OF ORAL STEROIDS

Use daily steroid tablet in lowest dose providing adequate control

Maintain high dose inhaled steroid at 2000 mcg/day*

Consider other treatments to minimize the use of steroid tablets

Refer patient for specialist care

STEP 4: PERSISTENT POOR CONTROL

Consider trials of:
- increasing inhaled steroid up to 2000 mcg/day*
- addition of a fourth drug e.g. leukotriene receptor antagonist, SR theophylline, β2 agonist tablet

STEP 3: ADD-ON THERAPY

1. Add inhaled long-acting β₂ agonist (LABA)
2. Assess control of asthma:
   - **good response** to LABA—continue LABA
   - **benefit from LABA but control still inadequate**—continue LABA and increase inhaled steroid dose to 800 mcg/day* (if not already on this dose)
   - **no response** to LABA—stop LABA and increase inhaled steroid to 800 mcg/day.* If control still inadequate, institute trial of other therapies, e.g. leukotriene receptor antagonist or SR theophylline

STEP 2: REGULAR PREVENTER THERAPY

Add inhaled steroid 200–800 mcg/day*

400 mcg is an appropriate starting dose for many patients

Start at dose of inhaled steroid appropriate to severity of disease.

STEP 1: MILD INTERMITTENT ASTHMA

Inhaled short-acting β2 agonist as required

* BDP or equivalent

Fig. 5.1 Summary of stepwise management in adults. BDP = beclometasone dipropionate; LABA = long actibe beta agonist. Reproduced with kind permission from the British Thoracic Society, BMJ Group.

Acute severe asthma

Ascertain the recent best or predicted PEFR, the current medication, (especially that recently taken for relief of this attack), and the date of the last severe attack.

Features of severe asthma
- Cannot speak in whole sentences.
- Respiration >25 breaths/min.
- Pulse >110 beats/min.
- PEFR <50% of best or predicted.

Life-threatening asthma
- Silent chest, cyanosis or feeble respiratory effort.
- Bradycardia, dysrhythmia, or hypotension.
- Exhaustion, confusion, or coma.
- O_2 saturations <92%, PO_2 <8KPa(60 mmHg), PCO_2 normal or ↑, pH↓.
- PEFR <33% of best or predicted.
- Rule out airways obstruction due to a foreign body, epiglotitis, mediastinal masses.

Immediate management
1. Sit the patient up and give 40–60% O_2.
2. Give Salbutamol 5 mg or terbutaline 10 mg by O_2-driven nebulizer. Alternately, give 4–6 puffs via a spacer and repeat every 10–20 minutes.
3. Give hydrocortisone 100 mg iv or prednisolone 40–60 mg po.
4. Do ABGs, CXR, PEFR, oximetry.

If there is no improvement or there are signs of life-threatening asthma
1. Contact an anaesthetist about possible emergency intubation.
2. Add ipratropium 0.5 mg to the nebulized salbutamol.
3. Give aminophylline 5 mg per kg by iv infusion over 20 mins but avoid or use with great caution in patients already taking oral aminophylline.

If the patient is improving continue with
1. Oxygen 40–60% guided by O_2 saturations which should be >92%.
2. Prednisolone 40–60 mg per day or hydrocortisone 100 mg iv q6 h.
3. Salbutamol 5 mg nebulized q4–6 hourly and SOS.

If the patient is not improving
1. Continue with O_2 and steroids.
2. Nebulized salbutamol 5 mg up to every 15–30 mins until the bronchospasm is relieved.
3. Ipratropium 0.5 mg q 6 hourly.
4. Consider a continuous aminophylline infusion 750–1000 mg over 24 h (500 mcg/kg/hr); monitor blood concentrations if possible.

Monitoring response to therapy

1. PEFR 15–30 mins after treatment and at least q 6 hrly.
2. Maintain SaO_2>92% with supplemental oxygen.
3. Recheck ABG to monitor potential respiratory failure.

On discharge from hospital

- Patient stable on discharge medication for 24 h and have had their inhaler technique checked and recorded.
- PEFR >75% of best or predicted and PEFR diurnal variability <25% (no nocturnal dipping).
- Treatment initiated with high-dose inhaled steroids to cover tapering oral steroid therapy.
- Follow-up in one week or SOS.

Chronic obstructive pulmonary disease (COPD)

This is a chronic progressive disease of the airways and terminal alveoli that occurs in smokers, ex-smokers, and people exposed to smoke (e.g. people cooking food on open fire with poor ventilation). It is characterized by cough, sputum production, wheezing, and exertional dyspnoea.

Pathology

Inhalation of smoke elicits a neutrophil inflammatory response in the airways which overcomes the protective effects of pulmonary protease inhibitors and causes chronic bronchial inflammation and airway damage. Lung defences are impaired by smoke resulting in recurrent respiratory infections and bacterial colonization of the proximal airways. Bronchial mucosal gland hyperplasia and hypertrophy causes excessive mucus secretion and airway thickening and consequent narrowing. This gives rise to a chronic productive cough, often seasonal and worse in winters. Alveoli are particularly damaged in *emphysema*. This causes a loss of lung units and overdistention of the remaining alveoli, leading to compression of the terminal bronchioles and further airway obstruction.

Clinical features

Patients with COPD often experience chronic productive cough, recurrent respiratory infections, and/or exertional dyspnoea. Pulmonary function deteriorates after respiratory infections, and this may take weeks to recover. Minor respiratory infections may precipitate respiratory failure and necessitate hospitalization. Patients are often wheezy, tachypnoeic, and use accessory muscles of respiration during exacerbations. In advanced cases, patients may be plethoric, cyanosed, and show signs of right heart failure (cor pulmonale). Type I or Type II respiratory failure is common — confusion, drowsiness, and flapping tremor indicates CO_2 retention.

Management

Stopping smoking and reducing exposure to indoor cooking smoke is essential. Bronchodilators provide relief and are required regularly. A trial of prednisolone 30–40 mg per day should be given for 2–3 weeks and pre- and post-steroid lung functions obtained to establish whether the individual patient has steroid response. Chest physiotherapy helps in clearing mucus and may build respiratory muscle strength.

O_2 therapy should be closely monitored as some patients require the hypoxia to drive respiration and rapid correction of hypoxia with unmonitored high concentrations of oxygen may cause CO_2 retention and narcosis. Home and portable O_2 therapy helps many patients, and some require non-invasive ventilation with a BiPAP machine.

Advice to smokers regarding smoking cessation[*]

- *Preparation*: make a positive decision and list reasons for quitting. Get the support of family/friends. Set a target date. Have realistic expectations of the difficulty. Know that most relapses occur in the first week after quitting.
- *Switch brands*: to one that is distasteful and low in tar/nicotine prior to the target date.
- *Cut down the number of cigarettes*: smoke only half of each cigarette. Postpone the first cigarette of each day by 1 h. Smoke only during odd or even hrs of the day. Remember that cutting down is not a substitute for quitting.
- *Don't smoke automatically*: smoke only the cigarettes you really want. Don't empty ashtrays. Make yourself aware of each cigarette you smoke by using the opposite hand or putting the cigarettes in an unusual location.
- *Make smoking inconvenient*: buy one packet/cigarette at a time. Stop carrying them on your person.
- *Make smoking unpleasant*: only smoke alone, if accustomed to smoking in company. Whilst smoking, isolate yourself from others and focus on the negative effects of smoking. Collect all butts in a large glass container.
- *Prepare for the target day*: practise going without cigarettes. Think of quitting in terms of one day at a time.
- *On the day of quitting*: throw away all cigarettes and matches, and hide ashtrays and lighters. Make a list of things you want to buy, price them in terms of cigarettes and put the money aside to buy them. Keep very busy on the target day. Remind family/friends about the day. Buy yourself a treat or do something special.
- *Immediately after quitting*: develop a clean, fresh, non-smoking environment around you. Go to places where smoking is not allowed.
- *Avoid temptation*: avoid situations you associate with smoking; socialize only where smoking is not allowed.

[*]From *Dilworth* and *Baldwin* (2001) *Respiratory medicine specialist handbook, Harwood.*

Oxygen therapy

- If the patient has a PaO_2 <8 kPa on air, give a trial of oxygen at 2 l/min via a mask. Recheck ABG after 1 h.
- If there is no rise in $PaCO_2$, increase the oxygen to 4 l/min and recheck ABGs after another hour.
- If there is still no rise, the patient is not CO_2 retaining and may have oxygen therapy without risk.
- If CO_2 does rise, reduce oxygen delivery to the level before which CO_2 was retained.
- At this point, if available, it is worth considering non-invasive ventilation via mask (e.g. BiPAP).

Bronchiectasis

This condition is characterized by long-standing damage and dilatation of bronchi and bronchioles leading to inflammation and accumulation of infected mucus. Persistent infection within the bronchiectatic airways with *H. influenza*, *S. pneumoniae*, *M. catarrhalis*, or *Ps. aeuruginosa* causes the clinical symptoms.

Aetiology

Bronchiectasis may be localized as a result of a previous infection or generalized as occurs in congenital conditions e.g cystic fibrosis, Kartagener's syndrome, or hypogammaglobulinaemia. Most cases are 2° to pulmonary TB, TB lymph node disease, necrotizing pneumonias, whooping cough, foreign body inhalation, allergic bronchopulmonary aspergillosis (proximal bronchiectasis).

Clinical features of bronciectasis

Depending on the severity, patients may continuously produce mucoid or purulent sputum. Patients may be asymptomatic between acute exacerbations — when the individual coughs abundant purulent sputum. Fever, haemoptysis, and chest pain are often features, especially when infection spreads to the lung parenchyma producing bronchopneumonia. Chronic sinusitis and otitis media may be associated. Clubbing is prominent, expiratory crackles with occasional wheezes are heard in the lungs.

Complications

Recurrent episodes of pneumonia, hypoxia, and respiratory failure, massive haemoptysis, 2° amyloidosis, brain abscesses, and arthropathy.

Diagnosis

Largely based on the history and clinical features. Bronchiectetic cysts with fluid levels and 'tram lining' are seen on CXRs, but CXR underestimates the extent of bronchiectasis. Confirmation and disease extent is best gauged on a high-resolution CT scan. Airways obstruction and reversibility should be gauged by PFTs. Sputum should be cultured to choose appropriate antimicrobial therapy. Congenital syndromes should be excluded by sinus X-rays, sweat test, ECGs, and immunoglobulin levels.

Management

- Physiotherapy is useful at all times especially during acute exacerbations. Patients should be taught postural drainage and deep breathing/coughing exercises.
- Underlying conditions will require separate and continuous treatment. Focal disease with severe recurrent symptoms may be suitable for surgical resection — but CT often shows bronchiectasis is widespread and bilateral, which rules out surgery.
- Severe haemoptysis may require angiographic embolization or surgical resection.
- Airways obstruction requires bronchodilators and hydration.

- Antibiotics are indicated as soon as the patient is symptomatic with purulent sputum. Co-amoxiclav is a reasonable first choice and should be modified once cultures are available. Therapy should continue for 1–2 weeks.
- *Pseudomonas* colonization requires use of fluoroquinolones or IV ceftazidime or other aminoglycosides — depending on sensitivities.
- Patients should be given a prescription for 3 or 4 oral antibiotics (amoxicillin, erythromycin, chloramphenicol, doxycycline) and advised to rotate through them with each fresh infection.

Prevention

Hib, pneumococcal, and influenza vaccination. Early identification and treatment of TB and whooping cough.

Lung cancer

Carcinoma of the bronchus is a disease of smokers (>95% of cases) and is related to the quantity and duration of exposure to cigarette smoke. Most patients present too late for cure, and prevention by continuously emphasizing the danger of smoking is the best option.

Clinical features

Patients may have widely differing symptoms:

- *Pulmonary features*: persistent cough or alteration in the previous chronic cough; haemoptysis; chest pain; dyspnoea. Distal pneumonia, pleural effusions, localized wheezing, or stridor may be found.
- *Local/mediastinal invasion*: vocal cord paralysis, Horner's syndrome, SVC obstruction, chest wall invasion, bony pains, brachial plexus involvement, dysphagia, and pericardial effusion.
- *Metastatic spread*: symptoms and signs depend on the organ involved e.g. brain, liver, adrenal, skin, and bones (esp. ribs, spine, and femoral). Lymph node involvement is common esp. mediastinal, scalene, and supraclavicular.
- *Systemic symptoms*: fatigue, lassitude, anorexia, marked weight loss. Fever may occur without infection.
- *Endocrinopathies*: SIADH is common, as is hypercalcaemia from secretion of PTH-like substances or from bony metastases. Ectopic ACTH production, gynaecomastia, and testicular atrophy can also occur.
- *Others*: clubbing is common, occasionally severe, with hypertrophic pulmonary osteoarthropathy. Neuromuscular syndromes (e.g. Eaton Lambert syndrome) are rare.

Diagnosis

This is based on CXR or CT imaging which shows a mass, collapse/consolidation, or invasive disease; CT is also useful in staging the disease. Histology is obtained from a biopsy/cytology obtained via a bronchoscopy/BAL, FNAC, truecut CT guided biopsy or, in certain cases, a mini-thoracotomy. The yield from sputum cytology is low but non-invasive. Pleural fluid cytology is useful in patients with disseminated lung cancer and mesotheliomas.

Management

Surgery is often impossible because of extensive cancer or co-existant COPD caused by prolonged smoking. A small group of patients (<20%) with localized non-small cell disease may respond well to surgery. Palliative chemotherapy and radiotherapy both prolong life and improve complications such as haemoptysis, SVC obstruction, and recurrent pleural effusions. Patients with small cell cancer almost always have disseminated disease and surgery is not an option — palliative chemotherapy and radiotherapy can extend and improve quality of life and manage complications.

Prevention

Aggressive anti-smoking campaigns benefit patients and those exposed to passive smoke. Reduce chemicals and dust in the work environment.

Lung cancer: tumour types

- *Squamous cell carcinoma*: tumours with a medium rate of growth that often present with obstruction. Metastatic spread is common (80% of tumours at presentation).
- *Small-cell (oat-cell) carcinoma*: fast-growing tumours that often present with disseminated disease. They may secrete hormones.
- *Adenocarcinoma*: (includes bronchoalveolar cell carcinoma) the most common peripheral tumour, it may produce mucin and will surround associated bronchi, stenosing the lumen. May not be smoking-related.
- *Large-cell carcinoma*: large, necrotic, pleomorphic, mucin-producing tumours. They are frequently peripheral and locally invasive; while metastatic spread is common, survival rates post-surgery are good.
- *Carcinoid tumours*: a group of tumours that are unrelated to smoking and occur in a younger age group. They may be malignant and metastasize to distal organs. Most occur in proximal airways.
- *Metastases*: often from primaries in the breast, colon, kidney, prostate, and lung. Less often choriocarcinoma, testicular cancer, sarcomas, melanoma.
- *Mesotheliomas*: malignancies of the pleural space caused by exposure, often remote, to asbestos. Spread is local but rarely may metastatise.

Pulmonary embolism (PE)

Most pulmonary emboli occur as a result of migration of soft thrombi of recent onset from the deep veins of the leg or the pelvis. Embolism from mural intracardiac thrombi and right-sided endocarditis may also occur. Septic thrombophlebitis due to infected central lines is increasingly common and severe thrombotic disease due to congenital or acquired thrombogenic states (protein C, protein S, or antithrombin III deficiency, antiphospholipid antibody syndrome, etc.) may cause recurrent deep vein or other thrombosis and embolism or in situ pulmonary thrombosis.

Clinical features

Most patients will have minor and subacute symptoms with tachypnoea, mild dyspnoea, a cough, and occasionally low-grade fever. Pleuritic chest pain and haemoptysis indicate pulmonary infarction and represent larger degrees of embolism. In cases of massive pulmonary embolism, the patient has circulatory collapse and may die acutely. In patients with showers of low-grade emboli over many years, pulmonary hypertension and cor pulmonale may ensue.

Respiratory findings are sparse, and hypoxia with a normal CXR suggests the possibility of a PE (the other main cause of hypoxia with a normal CXR is PCP). A DVT may be present. Investigations: CXR, ECG, V/Q scan, CT pulmonary angiogram, Doppler ultrasound of the legs, and D-dimer levels. These tests are useful in both the confirmation and exclusion of DVTs and PEs.

Management

Initially, patients are anticoagulated with intravenous conventional heparin or with low molecular weight heparin. When PE is confirmed, oral anticoagulation with warfarin is commenced and a target INR of 2.5–3.0 is necessary for 48–72 h before heparin can be safely discontinued. In acute massive PE, thrombolysis with streptokinase is useful.

Pneumothorax

This condition is caused by the entry of air into the pleural space leading to collapse and sometimes compression of the underlying lung. When a rapid ongoing accumulation of air occurs with each bout of coughing (tension pneumothorax), there is severe cardiorespiratory compromise and relief of the tension pneumothorax is an emergency. A small or moderate pneumothorax may be sufficient to cause respiratory failure in a patient with pre-existing lung disease. Pneumothorax may be asymptomatic in an otherwise healthy patient.

Causes

- *Spontaneous pneumothorax*: Common in tall and thin men with no pre-existing lung disease. The chance of recurrence is 20% after the 1st episode and increases to 65% after the 2nd episode.
- *Secondary pneumothorax*: Occurs in patients with scars of previous TB or in patients with active TB, often cavitary. Also in patients with COPD, severe necrotizing lung infections such as staphylococcal pneumonia, aspiration pneumonias, and, in some cases of PCP.
- *Traumatic pneumothorax*: Occurs from penetrating external injuries e.g. stabbing or road traffic accident.
- *Iatrogenic pneumothorax*: May be a complication of central line insertion, transbronchial lung biopsy, or due to barotrauma caused by high-pressure mechanical ventilation.

Clinical features

Most patients will complain of sudden onset of pleuritic chest pain and dyspnoea. Hyper-resonance to percussion is accompanied by ↓ movement and ↓ or absent breath sounds on the affected side. Breathing is generally shallow on account of splinting due to pain. A patient with tension pneumothorax has features of mediastinal displacement away from the pneumothorax, with severe tachypnoea, dyspnoea (often with hypoxia), and cardiovascular instability.

Management

- Small pneumothoraces (CXR shows pneumothorax occupies <15% of hemithorax) in asymptomatic, otherwise healthy, individuals need no treatment other than observation. Follow-up X-rays should demonstrate gradual absorption of the pneumothorax. Small pneumothoraces in symptomatic patients or in patients with pre-existing lung disease require needle aspiration — possibly followed by a tube drain. Needle aspiration is suitable for iatrogenic pneumothoraces because these are unlikely to recur.
- Large pneumothoraces should be aspirated through the second intercostal space with a cannula and a syringe fitted to an underwater drain. If >2 litres of air is freely withdrawn it is likely that a bronchopleural fistula exists and an intercostal chest drain should be placed. Use the 5/6th intercostals space in the mid-axillary line.
- Pleurodesis may be required in patients whose pneumothorax fails to resolve despite 1–2 weeks of intercostal drainage and suction.

- A tension pneumothorax is a medical emergency and requires the immediate placement of a wide bore needle into the 2nd intercostal space on the affected side. Air usually bubbles out in a rush and the relief is immediate. Intercostal tube drainage should follow.

Pleurodesis

This procedure aims to cause sterile chemical inflammation of the pleura and obliteration of the pleural space as a result of subsequent adhesions and fibrosis. It is painful and adequate analgesia is a must. 20 ml of 1% lignocaine is diluted with saline to form a volume of 100 ml and this is inserted into the chest tube which is then clamped. The patient is placed on his back, side, and chest in order to disperse the anaesthesia and after this is drained off, 0.5 g of tetracycline dissolved in 30–50 mL normal saline or 20 ml of povidone-iodine 10% added to 80 mL normal saline is inserted into the chest drain and the procedure repeated. The solution is kept in the chest for 3–4 h and then drained off. The chest drain is maintained in situ till air ceases to bubble through it.

Diarrhoeal diseases

Section editor   **Mary E. Penny**

Introduction

Diarrhoea is the passage of abnormally loose or fluid stools more frequently than normal. Normal bowel habit varies, but recent onset >3 liquid/loose stools per day is considered abnormal.

Infective diarrhoea is the 3rd highest cause of death due to infection in the world, with ~1–2 million deaths each year; 80% deaths are in children under <2 yrs, most of these during and shortly after the introduction of complementary foods between 6–12 months. Micronutrient deficiencies, especially zinc deficiency, increase the incidence of infective diarrhoea. Breastfeeding, especially exclusive breastfeeding, confers significant protection. Repeated attacks of diarrhoea initiate a vicious cycle of malnutrition, reduced immunity, and more intestinal infections. Diarrhoea is a common symptom of HIV/AIDS.

An accurate history will give clues to the aetiology and severity of diarrhoea. Ask about previous episodes and current medication.

The treatment of most diarrhoeal episodes depends on treating and preventing dehydration regardless of the aetiology. Antimicrobials are only recommended for dysentery and cholera, and for severe episodes with laboratory diagnosis in certain vulnerable groups (see below). Anti-diarrhoeal agents should be avoided in young children.

Some key questions to be asked
- How long has the diarrhoea been present?
- Is there (or was there) fever or other systemic symptoms?
- What is the stool like — specifically is there blood (bright red or dark) and/or mucus?
- How frequent and abundant are the motions?
- Is there any abdominal pain — if so, where?
- Is there tenesmus (a sense of incomplete emptying following defecation)?
- Has the patient vomited — if so, how much, when, what?
- Has the patient lost weight?
- Have any household or close contacts had diarrhoea?
- What did they eat and drink in the 24 h before getting diarrhoea — anything unusual?
- If the diarrhoea is recurrent/remittent, is it related to any particular food or drink?
- Is anyone else in the family ill?
- Is there a history of recent travel? If so, where?
- Has the patient been exposed to malaria?
- Is the patient at risk of HIV infection?

In examining the patient, one should look for signs of dehydration and malnutrition, as well as for clues to determine the disease aetiology.

Classification of diarrhoea

Subdivide diarrhoeal diseases according to presence or not of blood in the stool, since the causes are generally different, but be aware that both shigellosis and Campylobacter infections may present as acute watery diarrhoea. Here we shall divide the diseases into acute diarrhoea with blood (dysentery) and acute diarrhoea without blood. Persistent diarrhoea lasts >14 days and additional diseases need to be considered — this condition is accorded a separate section.

Antimicrobial drugs

In the majority of cases, symptoms of diarrhoea improve with treatment of dehydration alone, without the need for antibiotics. Antimicrobial drugs may be beneficial in:
- *Bloody diarrhoea (dysentery) that does not improve after 3 days of rehydration therapy*: If a specific cause is found, it should be treated appropriately (see relevant section below). If no cause can be found, an antimicrobial effective against *Shigella* (e.g. ciprofloxacin) should be given.
- *Cholera with severe dehydration:* Any suspected case of cholera should be treated with an effective antimicrobial (e.g. azithromycin) and control agencies notified.
- *Laboratory-proven symptomatic cases of* G. intestinalis *infection:* that do not improve after 3 days of ORS therapy should be treated with an antimicrobial (e.g. tinidazole).
- *Laboratory-proven enteropathogenic* E. coli *infections:* respond to antibiotics (e.g. ciprofloxacin) and should be used in vulnerable hosts such as young babies.
- *Traveller's diarrhoea:* duration is reduced when treated with an antibiotic (e.g. ciprofloxacin).

Investigations

Most uncomplicated cases of diarrhoea can be managed without any laboratory tests. In a hospital setting or if diarrhoea continues beyond 2–3 days, do Hb, FBC, U&E, and glucose. Stool culture and microscopy are often requested but few centres can offer diagnostic tests for all enteropathogens; mixed infections are common; single-stool cultures are insufficient for some pathogens (e.g. *Giardia*, amoebae, *Shigella*); and results will often come back too late to influence management. Apart from investigation of outbreaks, surveillance, and research purposes, stool culture in uncomplicated cases should be limited to the exclusion of those pathogens for which antibiotic treatment is indicated (e.g. parasites, *Shigella* species, and *Vibrio cholerae*). If appropriate, do a blood film for malaria.

How to make a direct faecal smear

1. Write the patient's name on a clean slide. Place a drop of sterile saline in the centre of the left-hand side of the slide and place a drop of iodine in the centre of the right-hand side of the slide.
2. With a match or applicator, pick up a small portion of faeces (~2 mg — or about the size of a match head) and add it to the drop of saline. Repeat and add to the iodine. Mix the faeces with the drops to form suspensions.
3. Cover each drop with a coverslip.
4. Examine each drop with the ×10 objective or, for identification, with the higher-power objectives, searching in a systematic manner. When organisms are seen, switch to higher power for more detail.

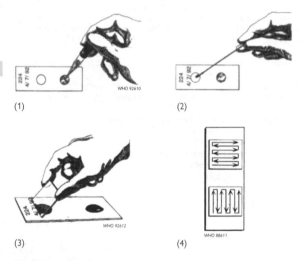

(1)   (2)

(3)   (4)

Fig. 6.1 How to make a direct faecal smear. (Reproduced with permission, from *Bench Aids for the Diagnosis of malaria*, 2nd edition, the WHO.)

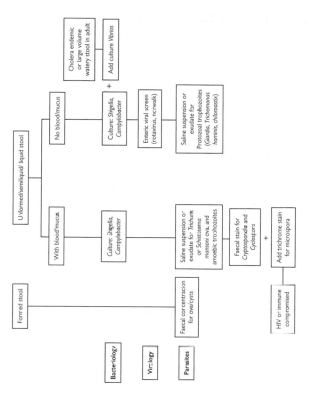

Fig. 6.2 Recommended diagnostic tests for enteropathogens depending on stool characteristics.

Acute diarrhoea with blood

The presence of blood in diarrhoea is called **dysentery** and usually signifies ulceration of the large bowel. The most common bacterial agents causing dysentery are *Shigella* (bacillary dysentery) and *Campylobacter*. Shigellosis can be a serious infection that progresses to complications and death. Dysentery should be treated on clinical diagnosis with antibiotics that cover *Shigella*. If no improvement after 48 h, antibiotics should be changed taking into account stool culture findings. If culture results are negative or unavailable, still change the antibiotic (e.g. from co-trimoxazole to nalidixic acid or ciprofloxacin, or from ciprofloxacin to azithromycin) on the basis of a lack of clinical response to initial therapy.

Bacillary dysentery (shigellosis)

Shigella dysenteriae, S. flexneri, S. boydii, and *S. sonneii* cause the disease known as bacillary dysentery, with the former two species responsible for most morbidity and mortality (which may reach 20% in untreated cases). The disease may occur both endemically and epidemically, with children most frequently affected. The incubation period in humans (the only natural host) is 1–5 days following direct person to person contact (often with asymptomatic excreters) or ingestion of contaminated water and food.

Clinical features: range from mild disease in which there is intermittent watery diarrhoea alone, to severe systemic complications. In severe cases, onset is usually rapid, with tenesmus, fever, and passage of frequent (up to 100/day ~every 15 minutes) bloody mucoid stools. *Intestinal complications* include: toxic megacolon, perforation, and protein-losing enteropathy. *Systemic complications* include: dehydration, hypoglycaemia, and electrolyte imbalance (particularly hyponatraemia), haemolytic-uraemic syndrome, convulsions (particularly in children, often before the onset of diarrhoea), Reiter's syndrome, thrombotic thrombocytopenic purpura, pneumonia. Invasive disease may give 'rose spots' — crops of 2–4 mm papules which fade on pressure, usually appearing on the upper abdomen and lower chest.

Diagnosis: the clinical distinction between bacillary and amoebic dysentery is usually impossible. Stool microscopy often shows leukocytes (pus cells) in shigellosis vs. haematophagus trophozoites in amoebic dysentery.

Management

Oral rehydration is sufficient for mild disease. In severe disease, ampicillin or trimethoprim (or co-trimoxazole) should be given, although resistance is common; quinolones (e.g. ciprofloxacin) are an alternative. Antimicrobial therapy should be tailored to the local sensitivity pattern if individual sensitivity of isolates is not possible.

Prevention: food and hand hygiene; no vaccine is currently available.

Reiter's syndrome

Classic Reiter's syndrome is a triad of urethritis, conjunctivitis and a seronegative, large joint, mono- or oligoarthritis, but it can also follow dysentery. *Associated features*: iritis, enthesopathy, keratoderma blenorrhagica, and circinate balanitis.

Infective causes of acute diarrhoea with blood (dysentery)

- Bacillary dysentery (shigellosis).
- Enterohaemorrhagic *E. coli.*
- *Campylobacter* enterocolitis.
- *Salmonella* enterocolitis.
- *Clostridium difficile* associated (pseudomembranous) colitis.
- *Yersinia* enterocolitis.
- Amoebic dysentery.
- *Balantidium coli* enterocolitis.
- Massive *Trichuris* infection.
- *S. mansoni* or *S. japonicum.*

All may also cause diarrhoea without blood. Non-infectious causes include IBD, colorectal cancer or polyps, ischaemic colitis.

Enterohaemorrhagic *E. coli* (EHEC) and haemolytic uraemic syndrome (HUS)

These bacteria produce vero cell cytotoxins similar to the toxin produced by *Shigella dysenteriae*. The most common EHEC is *E. coli* 0157. These bacteria have been associated with a number of outbreaks of inflammatory, haemorrhagic colitis, and haemolytic uraemic syndrome (HUS). Infections occur most frequently in the summer months. Contaminated food is the most common cause, particularly ground beef in hamburgers, or milk. Fruit, vegetables, and cider may be contaminated by animal faeces. Cross-contamination of meat products has been responsible for outbreaks.

Clinical features: the illness usually starts with watery diarrhoea, blood appearing after 2–3 days. Vomiting and abdominal tenderness are common (can mimic appendicitis, intussusception, or IBD). **HUS** is a life-threatening complication in 8–10% of children with *E. coli* 0157 infection, usually about a week after onset of diarrhoea. (Other causes include shigellosis and drugs.) HUS is characterized by a microangiopathic haemolytic anaemia, thrombocytopaenia, renal failure, and CNS involvement. Clinical features overlap with those of thrombotic thrombocytopaenic purpura (TTP) in which CNS involvement is much more common.

Diagnosis: stool culture diagnostic but not generally available. The presence of an outbreak and exposure risk often found in the history.

Management
1. Oral rehydration and supportive care.
2. Antibiotics are not indicated: they have been associated with increased duration and may increase the risk of HUS.
3. Antimotility drugs should be **avoided**.

Prevention: improve animal husbandry and slaughterhouse management to prevent contamination of meat with intestinal content; pasteurize dairy products; cook beef adequately; wash hands frequently with soap including after contact with farm animals or meat.

Campylobacter enterocolitis

C. jejuni (also *C. coli* and *C. lari*) cause epidemics in nurseries or paediatric wards and are common in the community in developing countries. Bacteria may be excreted in the faeces up to 3 weeks after the cessation of diarrhoea. *Campylobacter* sp. infect most mammals and birds and transmission may be by contact with animal or poultry excreta or contaminated food or water.

Clinical features: Episodes typically start with fever, abdominal pain, and watery diarrhoea. This may be followed by bloody diarrhoea, indistinguishable from *Shigella* and *Salmonella* infections. Abdominal pain may be prominent even after diarrhoea settles. The disease normally settles in 5–7 days. Severe, disseminated infection can occur in presence of malnutrition, liver disease, malignancy, diabetes, renal failure, and immunosuppression. Complications include bacteraemia, meningitis, deep abscesses, cholecystitis, reactive arthritis/Reiter's syndrome, and Guillain-Barré syndrome.

Diagnosis: Gram stain or dark-field microscopy of faecal smears shows curved gram-negative rods with 'gull wing' and 'S-shapes'; confirmed on culture. In severe disease, colonoscopy/biopsy may be needed.

Prevention: *Campylobacter* infection is an almost ubiquitous zoonosis. Prevention depends on breaking the chain of food and water contamination. No vaccine is currently available.

Yersinia enterocolitis

Yersinia enterocolitica is a rare cause of diarrhoea in the tropics. There may be low-grade fever, bloody diarrhoea, and abdominal pain affecting mainly children <5 yrs, plus nausea, vomiting, headache, or pharyngitis. Infection may spread to cause septicaemia; peritonitis; hepatic, renal, and splenic abscesses; pyomyositis; and osteomyelitis. These complications are more common in immunocompromised patients or those who are iron overloaded (e.g. haemochromatosis).

Diagnosis: culture from stool or other sites of infection.

Management of *Campylobacter* and *Yersinia* enterocolitis

Rehydration and supportive care are usually sufficient for *Campylobacter* and *Yersinia* infections. Severe disease may require antibiotics:

- **Campylobacter**: Use erythromycin; resistant strains (esp. *C. coli*) may need trimethoprim (or co-trimoxazole), ciprofloxacin, or azithromycin.
- **Yersinia**: In complicated disease, use one of the following: gentamicin, cefotaxime, ciprofloxacin, or doxycycline.

Salmonella **enterocolitis**

Salmonella typhimurium and *S. enteritidis* enterocolitis are an important public health problem in the developing world. Transmission is usually by ingestion of contaminated food (they survive freezing at −20°C). The organisms are common among wild and domestic animals. Reptiles kept as pets may also be a source of *Salmonella* infection. The incubation period is 24–48 h (up to 72 h); bacteria are then excreted in the faeces for up to 8 weeks following infection. More common in HIV infection.

Clinical features: range in severity according to the serotype involved. Two (often overlapping) clinical syndromes are seen:

- *Acute enterocolitis*: nausea and vomiting, headache, fever, and malaise, rapidly progressing to diarrhoea with cramping abdominal pains. Initially voluminous and watery, the stool changes to be bloody with mucus as the disease progresses. There may be LIF pain and rebound tenderness. Infrequently, ileal involvement is dominant with symptoms mimicking appendicitis. Toxic megacolon may complicate severe colitis.
- *Invasive salmonellosis*: bacteraemia rates of 8% have been recorded, with higher rates for certain serotypes. Predisposing factors are: extremes of age, immunosuppression, malignancy, gastric hypoacidity (e.g. antacid use), severe comorbidity, bartonellosis, HIV, malarial anaemia and sickle cell disease. Invasive salmonellosis is characterized by swinging fevers, rigors, and toxaemia accompanying the diarrhoea, or a typhoid-like illness characterized by sustained fever, splenomegaly, rose spots, and minimal diarrhoea. There may be metastatic spread to meninges (children <2 yrs old), bones and joints, lungs, heart valves and arteries, liver, spleen, ovaries, or kidneys. A reactive arthritis can occur. Patients with chronic schistosomiasis are prone to 2° *Salmonella* bacteraemia since the bacteria live within the worm and are protected from antibiotics.

Diagnosis: requires isolation of the bacteria from faecal or blood cultures. Sigmoidoscopy may be necessary in severely ill patients. *Salmonella typhi* and *S paratyphi* (📖 p 684) do not usually present with diarrhoea and should not be confused with enterocolitis due to non-typhi *Salmonellae*.

Management

- Rehydration and supportive care are usually sufficient.
- Most antibiotics do not shorten the diarrhoea and may prolong bacterial carriage.
- Treat patients with severe colitis and/or invasive disease, or in whom the risk of developing severe disease is high (e.g. neonates, immunosuppressed, and elderly), with ciprofloxacin 500 mg PO bd for 5 days.
- Chloramphenicol, amoxicillin, trimethoprim, or co-trimoxazole may be effective in systemic disease, but resistance is increasing. Cefotaxime/ceftriaxone still highly effective, where available.

Amoebic dysentery

Around 48 million people worldwide are infected by the protozoon *Entamoeba histolytica* and, although only about 10% are symptomatic, it is an important parasitic cause of death with an annual mortality of ~70,000. Severe infection occurs in pregnant women, very young children, the malnourished, and people on steroids. It is now recognized that most of those previously thought to have asymptomatic *E. histolytica* infection are actually infected with the related amoeba *E. dispar*, which is morphologically indistinguishable but non-pathogenic to humans.

Transmission: is usually through food and drink contaminated with human faeces; prevalence is highest where human faeces are used as fertilizer. Sexual transmission also occurs. Cysts are ingested and pass into the small and large intestine, dividing to form metacysts and trophozoites. As trophozoites pass through the colon they desiccate to form 'precysts' and then cysts. Mature cysts are evacuated in the stool and remain viable and infective for up to 2 months in cool, damp conditions. *E. histolytica* has the capacity to destroy almost any tissue in the body, with amoebic liver abscess being the most common extra-intestinal manifestation.

Clinical features: are related to the degree and location of tissue damage by trophozoites and range from an asymptomatic carrier state to fulminant colitis and invasive extra-intestinal disease (see box). Intestinal amoebiasis usually has an insidious onset with abdominal discomfort and diarrhoea becoming increasingly bloody and mucoid as severity increases. Rectosigmoid involvement is frequently associated with tenesmus. On palpation, there may be tenderness over the caecum, transverse, and sigmoid colon; if involved, the liver may be enlarged and tender. Colonoscopy may reveal hyperaemic, necrotic ulcers covered with a yellowish exudate, particularly in the region of the flexures. *Complications* include toxic megacolon and bowel perforation. Following repeated infection, an amoebic granuloma (amoeboma) may develop (most frequently at the caecum) where it may be palpable and mistaken for a malignant mass.

Diagnosis: is often difficult and relies on identification of *E. histolytica* cysts or trophozoites in the stool. Demonstration of cysts does not prove amoebiasis is cause of symptoms as *E. histolytica* cysts are macroscopically identical to common, non-pathogenic *E. dispar* cysts.

- Examine at least 3 stool samples for cysts using concentration and permanent stain techniques, preferably before administration of medications or contrast media since these interfere with amoebae recovery.
- A 'hot stool' (examined within 30 minutes) is required to look for trophozoites. Examine a wet mount preparation for motile amoebae. The presence of *E. histolytica* trophozoites containing ingested erythrocytes is diagnostic of amoebiasis.
- Techlab Entamoeba 11® is a faecal ELISA that will differentiate invasive *E. histolytica* cysts or trophozoites from those of *E. dispar*.
- *E. histolytica* serology useful in non-endemic areas.

Management
- Metronidazole 800 mg PO tds for 5 days, *followed by.*
- Diloxanide furoate 500 mg PO tds for 10 days.
- If there are signs of peritonism, add a broad-spectrum antibiotic.

- Metronidazole is effective against the trophozoites but because it has little effect on the cysts, treatment should be followed by a luminal amoebicide such as diloxanide or paromomycin.

Prevention: Ensure safe disposal of human faeces; prevent faecal contamination of water supplies. Filtering water with sand or diatomaceous earth is effective. Personal hygiene including handwashing.

Extra-intestinal amoebiasis

Following colonic invasion, trophozoites may travel in the portal circulation to the liver; further direct or haematogenous spread may occur to almost any tissue of the body. The most common form of extra-intestinal disease is amoebic liver abscess (ALA, 📖 p 286). ~10% ALA patients have diarrhoea; ~20% have a history of previous dysentery. Digestion of hepatocytes by trophozoites leads to foci of liver necrosis which coalesce to form abscesses containing reddish-brown 'anchovy sauce' fluid. This fluid is digested liver, not pus (WBC not seen on microscopy) and has no odour; it seldom contains visible amoebae. Rupture into the pericardium (esp. of left lobe abscesses) causes **pericardial amoebiasis**, often → cardiac tamponade and death; adequate pericardial drainage usually requires thoracotomy. ALA rupture through the diaphragm to form a bronchohepatic fistula and cause pleuro-pulmonary amoebiasis, with cough, dyspnoea, and expectoration of 'anchovy sauce' material. **Peritoneal amoebiasis** occurs due to colonic or ALA rupture, cutaneous amoebiasis due to **percutaneous rupture**, and **cerebral amoebiasis** due to haematogenous spread. All may occur without diarrhoea.

Diagnosis: is usually clinical ± demonstration of trophozoites (which may be scarce) in the affected tissue and/or in the stool. Amboebic serology is sensitive.

Management: Medical management as for amoebic dysentery. Liver abscess often aspirated to differentiate from bacterial liver abscess (fluid is pus, often foul-smelling; in bacterial liver abscess, drainage or aspiration is important for cure). In ALA, drainage or aspiration of abscess is indicated if poor response to medical therapy or high risk of rupture (especially for abscess in left lobe of liver).

Balantidium enterocolitis

Balantidium coli is a rare protozoal pathogen of humans. It exists in cyst and trophozoite forms; cysts are responsible for faeco-oral transmission. Trophozoites invade intestinal mucosa producing inflammation and ulceration. Clinical features resemble amoebic colitis and include:
- Asymptomatic carrier state (80%).
- Acute dysentery that may be associated with nausea, abdominal pain, and weight loss. This is potentially fatal.
- Chronic diarrhoea, frequently without blood.

Diagnosis: rests upon identification of the trophozoite in the faeces.

Management: Symptomatic plus rehydration. Tetracycline 500 mg PO qds for 10 days in severe disease. (Alternatives: ampicillin, metronidazole.)

Trichuriasis (whipworm)

Thought to infect ~25% of the world's population, *Trichuris trichiura* are 3–4 cm long and colonize the colon and rectum after ingestion of faecally contaminated soil.

Life cycle: ingested eggs hatch in the small intestine releasing larvae which mature in the villi for ~1 week before colonizing the caecum and colorectum. Released eggs pass out in the stool and can resist low temperatures, but not desiccation. The time from ingestion to appearance of eggs in the faeces is 60–70 days. Heavy infection is most common in children.

Clinical features: are often absent in mild infections. However, co-infection with *Ascaris lumbricoides* or hookworms is common and may result in abdominal distension, flatulence, RIF pain, vomiting, and weight loss. Heavy worm burden can result in lower GI haemorrhage, mucopurulent stool, dysentery ± rectal prolapse (worms usually seen attached to prolapsed mucosa), and growth retardation. Massive worm burdens may cause a protein-losing enteropathy, severe anaemia, and finger clubbing. 2° infection with *E. histolytica* or *B. coli* can aggravate mucosal ulceration and exacerbate dysentery.

Diagnosis: is by detection of eggs in the stool (>30,000/g stool = heavy infection = several hundred adult worms). There may be anaemia, hypo-albuminaemia, and eosinophilia. Proctoscopy may reveal worms attached to a reddened, ulcerated rectal mucosa. AXR can show changes similar to those seen in Crohn's disease.

Management: mebendazole 500 mg or albendazole 400 mg, both PO once, are equally effective, although there may be regional differences in albendazole sensitivity. 3-day courses may be used for heavy infections.

Prevention: control is as for other soil-transmitted helminths.

Clostridium difficile associated diarrhoea (CDAD) & colitis

This condition (also known as antibiotic-associated colitis and pseudomembranous colitis) is caused by infection with *C. difficile* following disruption of the normal bowel flora by antibiotic therapy. It is an important cause of hospital acquired diarrhoea.

Clinical features: are due to the production of toxins and vary from the asymptomatic to severe colitis with toxic megacolon. Disease severity probably depends on a combination of patient co-morbidity and the degree of exposure to both antibiotics and *C. difficile* spores. In elderly hospitalized patients or those with significant co-morbidty, it carries a high mortality. Sigmoidoscopy shows characteristic yellow mucosal plaques (pseudomembranes).

Management: metronidazole 800 mg PO stat, then 400 mg PO tds for 10 days. Oral vancomycin (125 mg qds for 7–10 days) is an expensive alternative.

Prevention: Avoid indiscriminate or unnecessarily prolonged use of antibiotics. Hand washing, barrier nursing, and environmental cleaning to eradicate spores are fundamental to preventing transmission in hospitals.

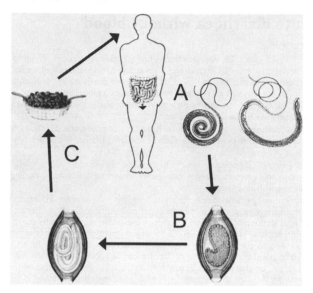

Fig. 6.3 Life cycle of *Trichuris trichiura*: The adult worms are ~5 cm long (the male, shown on the left, is more tightly curled) and live mainly in the large bowel. The eggs are shed in large numbers and become embryonated (infectious form) after ~2 weeks to ~6 months in the environment. They are then ingested e.g. on food or on fingertips, to become new adult worms. (Adapted from G. Piekarski, *Medical parasitology in plates*, 1962 and reproduced with kind permission of Bayer pharmaceuticals.)

Acute diarrhoea without blood

Rotavirus

In developed countries, viral infections (mainly rotavirus) account for up to 60% of all gastroenteritis in children <5 yrs and occur in seasonal outbreaks. In contrast, rotavirus causes <5% of all episodes of diarrhoea in developing countries, but 40–50% of episodes require hospitalization. It is responsible for >600,000 childhood deaths each year. Nearly all children in the tropics have been infected by the age of 2 years.

Clinical features: Vomiting occurs early; fever is common; the diarrhoea is usually watery and large volume. Colicky abdominal pains, ill-defined tenderness, and exaggerated bowel sounds are common.

Management: Supportive, aiming to prevent dehydration. The WHO diarrhoea management scheme (see later) should be followed, including treatment with zinc salts.

Dietary management: Since rotavirus infection is common in infants, dietary management is important to avoid malnutrition. Continue breast-feeding. Lactose malabsorption is common but intolerance is usually only a clinical problem in severe cases. Children with mild diarrhoea should be encouraged to continue eating a normal diet in order to limit weight loss. If diarrhoea continues or is severe, lactose can be reduced by mixing milk with cereals or changing to a lactose-free diet, but calorie intake should be maintained. As with all diarrhoeal episodes, once the child improves or is hungry, extra food should be given to make up for weight loss. Beware confusion with surgical causes of diarrhoea in the neonate such as Hirschsprung's disease, intussusception, and necrotizing enterocolitis.

Prevention: Rotavirus infection is highly contagious, difficult to prevent, and causes outbreaks in hospitals. Two rotavirus vaccines are available which prevent severe illness and hospitalizations (chapter 22).

Other viral causes of diarrhoea

- *Astroviruses:* are single-stranded RNA viruses that occur worldwide and cause diarrhoea, mainly in children and the elderly. The diarrhoea is similar to rotavirus, although generally milder. *Diagnosis*: PCR; ELISA may be useful for diagnosis of outbreaks.
- *Enteric adenovirus*: serotypes 40 and 41 cause diarrhoea, possibly more in developed countries. Clinical features similar to other viral diarrhoeas. *Diagnosis*: electron microscopy or ELISA.
- *Noroviruses (small, round structured viruses e.g. Norwalk virus):* are human enteric caliciviruses and the most important viral cause of water and food-borne diarrhoeal outbreaks in both developing and developed countries. Shell fish have been implicated in some outbreaks. They are the most common viral cause of epidemic diarrhoea and vomiting in adults ('winter vomiting disease'). *Transmission*: faeco-oral ± airborne; nosocomial transmission is common. *Clinical features*: vomiting common at onset and may be severe; watery diarrhoea rarely severe and usually lasts 12–24 h. *Diagnosis*: radioimmunoassay or PCR may be used in an epidemic.

Management of viral diarrhoea: Rehydration. Follow WHO diarrhoea treatment guidelines for management of diarrhoea in children (see later).

Causes of acute diarrhoea without blood

Systemic infections
- Malaria, especially *P. falciparum*.
- Sepsis.

Viruses
- Rotavirus.
- Astrovirus.
- Enteric adenovirus.
- Noroviruses.

Bacteria
- Early or mild shigellosis; *Salmonella* or *Campylobacter* infections.
- Enterotoxigenic *E. coli* (ETEC) (e.g. traveller's diarrhoea).
- Enteropathogenic *E. coli* (EPEC).
- Enteroaggregative *E. coli* (EAEC).
- Enterotoxin-producing strains of *Staphylococcus aureus*.
- *Cholera*.
- *Clostridia spp.*

Protozoa
- Giardiasis.
- Cryptosporidiosis.
- *Cyclospora cayetenesis*.

Strongyloidiasis

Food toxins

Enterotoxigenic *E. coli* (ETEC)

ETEC accounts for 20% of diarrhoeal cases, second only to rotavirus as a cause of inpatient gastroenteritis in developing countries. Transmission is by the faeco-oral route mainly via contaminated food, less commonly water. It accounts for ~80% of travellers' diarrhoea.

Clinical features: toxins stimulate Cl⁻, Na⁺, and water efflux into the intestinal lumen, resulting in voluminous, watery diarrhoea after an incubation period of 1–2 days. Vomiting and abdominal cramps are frequently a feature and up to 10 motions per day may be passed.

Diagnosis: depends on identification of the LT or ST toxins from *E. coli* cultured from faeces, but these tests are usually only available in specialized laboratories. Simple culture of *E. coli* in stools is not helpful.

Management: Supportive. Children should be managed according to WHO guidelines. See box for travellers' diarrhoea.

Prevention: General methods to prevent food contamination. Specific ETEC vaccines are under development but are not yet widely available.

Enteropathogenic *E. coli* (EPEC)

EPEC are strains of *E. coli* that include the classic pathogens O111 and O55 and other serotypes which adhere to Hep-2 cells in culture and human intestinal mucosal cells. In severe infections, the mucosal brush border is lost by a process of vesiculation resulting in malabsorption and osmotic diarrhoea. EPEC are a major cause of infantile diarrhoea that can be devastating. Transmission is by the faeco-oral route. Epidemics of hospital-acquired infection occur and recent hospitalization is a risk factor for infection. It is also a cause of traveller's diarrhoea.

Clinical features: range from acute watery diarrhoea to severe, prolonged, or relapsing diarrhoea, usually with mucus but no blood. Initially, there may be vomiting and fever. Epidemics can occur affecting mainly infants, with an untreated fatality reaching 50%.

Diagnosis: depends on either serotyping of *E.coli* in stools, adherence pattern to Hep 2 cells in culture, or DNA probes for the virulence plasmid. Serotyping is not very reliable or specific, and cell culture techniques and DNA probes are usually only available in specialist centres.

Management: rehydration. Give antibiotics to vulnerable individuals such as infants (e.g. co-trimoxazole 15 mg/kg qds for 5 days for infants >1 month old), depending on local resistance patterns.

Prevention: avoid routinely placing newborns in nurseries (encourage mothers and babies to stay together and avoid shared equipment). Enforce strict handwashing in neonatal nurseries and special care units.

Enteroinvasive *E. coli* (**EIEC**)

EIEC are endemic in developing countries and cause 1–5% of episodes of diarrhoea presenting to health services. Like Shigella, EIC can invade and multiply in epithelial cells. Clinically resembles shigellosis but dysentery is less common. Specific diagnosis is only available in reference laboratories. Management is supportive; treat as for *Shigella*.

Enteroaggregative *E. coli* (**EAEC**) and diffuse-adherent *E. coli* (**DAEC**)

These bacteria have a characteristic adherence pattern to Hep-2 cells. They are an important cause of diarrhoea — EAEC mainly in infants and travellers' diarrhoea and DAEC in preschool children. Clinical features vary from asymptomatic infection to watery diarrhoea, often persistent. Definitive diagnosis by Hep-2 cell assay is only available in specialist centres. Management is supportive. Antibiotics may be indicated for severe episodes; ciprofloxacin is most effective.

Cholera

Vibrio cholerae is the main cause of dehydrating diarrhoea in adults. Clinical episodes range from asymptomatic infection to acute fulminant watery diarrhoea which, if untreated, may be fatal.

Microbiology: Vibrios are Gram-negative, aerobic, comma-shaped bacteria. Several serovars of *V. cholerae* are recognized. Serovar 01 is responsible for the vast majority of cholera epidemics (see box). It is killed by heating at 55°C for 15 mins and by most disinfectants, yet it can survive in seawater for up to 2 weeks. In most cases, the bacteria survive for only limited periods on foodstuffs, with the notable exception of chitinous shellfish upon which they may survive for 14 days if refrigerated.

Transmission: Natural reservoirs of *V. cholerae* have been reported in brackish water, estuaries, and sea water in association with copepods and other zooplankton but the most important reservoir is thought to be humans. Infection usually requires a large infective dose and occurs via contaminated food or water. The incubation period ranges from a few hours to 5 days. Only a minority of infected people develop symptoms; studies suggest that there are ~40 asymptomatic carriers of the El Tor biotype for every symptomatic case (~5:1 for classical biotype). This is true both in endemic areas and during outbreaks, hence the need for meticulous hygiene.

Clinical features: If symptomatic, varies from mild, self-limiting diarrhoea to severe, watery 'rice water' diarrhoea of up to 30 litres per day. Diarrhoea leads to electrolyte imbalances, metabolic acidosis, prostration, and can cause death from dehydration within hours. Vomiting starts shortly after the onset of diarrhoea in 80% of cases. Shock typically follows ~12 h later, with impaired consciousness due to hypovolaemia and hypoglycaemia. This is particularly serious in children who, unlike adults, may have a mild fever. Renal failure, ileus, and cardiac arrhythmias may precede death; the elderly or those with low gastric acid, such as alcoholics, are especially vulnerable. Muscular and abdominal cramps are common due to loss of Ca^{2+} and Cl^- ions.

Diagnosis: In epidemics, the diagnosis may be made on clinical grounds alone. In non-epidemic situations, acute watery diarrhoea resulting in severe dehydration or the death of a patient over 5 yrs suggests cholera. Dark-field microscopy of faecal material shows comma-shaped bacteria darting about; this is quickly halted upon addition of diluted 01 antisera. Transportation of samples should be in alkaline peptone water; samples should be kept cool. Culture requires selective media such as TCBS agar. If possible, specimens should be sent to a reference laboratory for bio- and serotyping.

Management: Treatment consists mainly of meticulous rehydration, usually with oral fluids. This will reduce mortality to <1% (see below for rehydration regimens). The most common error is underestimation of the volume of ORS or IV fluid required. In emergencies where ORS is not available, sucrose and rice-water-based solutions can be given with success.

Antibiotics should be given to severe cases, where they have been shown to reduce both the volume and duration of diarrhoea.

- *Adults*: Azithromycin 1 g PO given as a single dose is drug of choice. Doxycycline 300 mg PO is an alternative (except pregnant women). If resistance reported, alternative antibiotic regimes are furazolidine 100 mg PO qds, or erythromycin 250 mg PO qds, or co-trimoxazole 960 mg PO bd, all for 3 days; or ciprofloxacin 1 g as a single oral dose.
- *Children*: give azithromycin 20 mg/kg (max 1 g) PO stat; or erythromycin 12.5 mg/kg PO qds, furazolidine 1.25 mg/kg PO qds, or co-trimoxazole 5–25 mg/kg PO bd, all for 3 days.
- **In pregnancy**, use erythromycin 250 mg PO qds for 3 days; furazolidine 100 mg PO qds for 3 days is an alternative.

Epidemiology of *V. cholerae*

V. cholerae serovar 01 is the causative agent of cholera. There are two biotypes of the 01 serovar: **classical** and **El Tor**. Each of these biotypes is further divided into three serotypes: Ogawa, Inaba, and Hikojima. The classical biotype caused the first 6 cholera pandemics in south Asia during the 19th and early 20th centuries. The El Tor biotype was first recognized in 1906 but until 1963 was restricted to Sulawesi in Indonesia. During the 1960s, the 7th pandemic started with spread of the El Tor biotype, Inaba serotype, out of Indonesia into South Asia, Africa, and, since 1991, Latin America. This biotype has now replaced the classical biotype throughout much of the world, except Bangladesh.

Other *V. cholerae* serovars cause a cholera-like illness. The 0139 serotype first appeared in southern India in 1992. Unlike other non-01 strains, it causes cholera with similar epidemiological and clinical pictures to 01. In Bangladesh, it is reported to affect mainly adults. Previous exposure to the 01 serovar does not confer protection.

Prevention: Public health measures aimed at improving food and water hygiene and sanitation are the most important factors. Currently, two oral cholera vaccines are available (chapter 22) and are recommended for travellers to areas known to have a cholera epidemic. The use of vaccines in epidemics has not been fully evaluated and should not deflect resources from treatment facilities and prevention of spread.

Health education: Is essential in preventing outbreaks and limiting the spread of infection during an outbreak. Advice should include food and water hygiene, as well as other measures such as disinfecting patients' clothing by boiling for 5 mins, drying out bedding in the sun, burying stools, etc. In larger health centres, patient excreta may be mixed with disinfectant (e.g. cresol) or acid before disposal in pit latrines. Semi-solid waste should be incinerated. Funerals have been a source of spread and preventative measures should be instigated to minimize the risk of mourners arriving from uninfected areas and potential contamination from ritual washing of the dead and funeral feasts.

The cholera outbreak

It is obligatory to notify the WHO of all cholera cases. Suspected cases should be reported immediately by health authorities and laboratory confirmation sent as soon as it is obtained. This should be followed by weekly reports containing the number of new cases and deaths since the last report, the cumulative totals for the year, and, if possible, the age distribution and number of patients admitted to hospital, recorded by region or other geographical division. This data should be sent to WHO headquarters as well as to the appropriate regional office.

Usually, there is a national coordinating committee to implement and regulate control and prevention measures, though often it is up to the front-line doctors to initiate the process and maintain close collaboration. Mobile control teams may be needed in inaccessible areas or in countries with no national coordination and these are responsible for establishing and operating temporary treatment centres, training local staff, educating the public, carrying out epidemiological studies, collecting stool, food, and water samples for laboratory analysis, and providing emergency logistical support to health posts and laboratories. Emergency treatment centres may be needed if appropriate facilities do not exist or are swamped with patients. Strict isolation or quarantine measures are not needed. The most crucial factor affecting survival is access to treatment centres with trained staff and intravenous and oral rehydration capability.

Estimated minimum supplies   **PUBLIC HEALTH NOTE**
needed to treat 100 patients
during a cholera outbreak[1]

- 50 packets of ORS solution (1 litre).
- 20 bags of 1 litre Ringer's lactate solution[2], with giving sets.
- 10 scalp vein sets.
- 3 adult NG tubes, 5.3 mm outside diameter (16 French), 50 cm long.
- 3 paediatric NG tubes, 2.7 mm diameter (8 French), 38 cm long.

For severely dehydrated adults
- 60 doxycycline 100 mg capsules (3 capsules per patient) or.
- 40 azithromycin 500 mg tablets (2 tablets per patient).

For children
- 120 erythromycin 250 mg tablets (6 tablets per patient broken into half).

For pregnant women
- 240 furazolidine 100 mg tablets (12 tablets per person).

If selective chemoprophylaxis is planned
The additional requirements for 4 close contacts per severely dehydrated patient (~80 people) are:
- 240 capsules of doxycycline 100 mg (3 capsules per person).

Other necessary supplies
- 2 large water dispensers with tap for bulk ORS manufacture.
- 20 1-litre bottles, 20 half-litre bottles for ORS dispensing.
- 40 200 ml cups.
- 20 teaspoons.
- 5 kg cotton wool to sterilize skin (e.g. with 70% alcohol) for IV access prior to insertion of cannulae.
- 3 reels of adhesive tape to secure IV cannulae and NG tubes.

1. The supplies listed are sufficient for IV fluid followed by oral rehydration salts for 20 severely dehydrated patients and for ORS alone for 80 patients.

2. If Ringer's lactate solution or equivalent unavailable, physiological saline may be substituted.

Giardiasis

Giardia intestinalis (also known as *G. lamblia, G. duodenalis*) is the most common human protozoan GI pathogen, having a worldwide distribution. Its prevalence can reach ~30% in the tropics, with infection being highest in infants and children. It causes ~3% of traveller's diarrhoea.

Transmission: The cysts can survive for long periods outside the host in suitable environments (e.g. surface water). Importantly they are NOT killed by chlorination. Infection follows ingestion of cysts in faecally contaminated water (rarely food) or through direct person to person contact. Partial immunity may be acquired through repeated infections.

Clinical features: In endemic areas, asymptomatic carriers are common. Symptoms usually begin within 3–20 days of infection; most patients recover within 2–4 weeks, although in 25% of travellers, symptoms persist for up to 7 weeks. Diarrhoea is the major symptom; it is watery initially, becoming steatorrhoeic and often associated with nausea, abdominal discomfort, bloating, weight loss, and sometimes sulfurous, offensive burps. Giardiasis can be the cause of abdominal pain without diarrhoea in children. Some patients develop a chronic diarrhoea associated with weight loss of up to 20% of ideal body weight, fat malabsorption, deficiencies (particularly of vitamins A and B12), and, in some cases, 2° hypolactasia.

Complications: In hyperendemic settings, infections are universal and usually asymptomatic but some studies have documented retardation of growth and development in severely affected infants and children, in whom malabsorption exacerbates malnutrition. Chronic giardiasis is associated with allergic and inflammatory conditions such as lymphoid nodular hyperplasia. Protein-losing enteropathy, lactose intolerance, and irritable bowel syndrome can also occur.

Diagnosis: detection of cysts (and occasionally trophozoites) in faecal samples by light microscopy. Examine 3 separate samples, since cysts are excreted only intermittently and diagnostic sensitivity is low. Trophozoites may be detected in biopsies of small intestine mucosa. ELISA tests can detect faecal *Giardia* antigens. Since mixed enteric infections and asymptomatic carriage of *Giardia* is so common, identification of the parasite does not guarantee that it is the causative agent of the diarrhoea. Serology is not useful because of cross-reactivity in non-infected individuals in endemic areas.

Management
1. Rehydration and symptomatic relief are usually sufficient.
2. If symptoms persist, an anti-giardial drug will decrease the severity and duration of symptoms. Drug failure due to resistance is increasing. Recommended drugs include metronidazole 2 g od PO for 3 days, or tinidazole 2 g as a single oral dose.

Prevention: Attention to personal hygiene, appropriate treatment of water supplies, encouraging breastfeeding (shown to partially protect against infection).

Cryptosporidiosis

The protozoon *Cryptosporidium parvum* is a common opportunistic infection in HIV +ve patients. It is also a common cause of childhood diarrhoea in the immunocompetent. Transmission is mainly through contaminated water. It accounts for 2–20% of childhood diarrhoea in the developing world, and infections contribute to growth faltering during the first year of life. Although usually mild, severe or persistent diarrhoea may occur.

Clinical features: acute diarrhoea is indistinguishable from diarrhoea due to other causes. Abdominal cramping pain is often a feature. Cryptosporidium should be sought in persistent (chronic) diarrhoea; in AIDS patients it may be severe, mimicking cholera, and/or be very prolonged.

Diagnosis: faecal detection of the oocysts (4–6 μm diameter red spheres on modified ZN stain). Oocysts can also be seen in sputum on occasions. ELISA detection kits are available.

Management: Rehydration with symptomatic relief; as yet, no drug has been shown to be effective against this organism. Wider use of highly active antiretroviral therapy (HAART) in people with AIDS has reduced the prevalence of severe cryptosporidiosis.

Cyclospora

Cyclospora cayetanensis is a protozoan coccidian parasite now recognized to be a frequent cause of diarrhoea in developing and developed countries. Transmission is via contaminated water or food; raspberries, basil, and lettuce have been incriminated.

Diagnosis: is by finding typical oocysts in faeces which are 7–10 μm diameter and contain a 'morula' of 8 spherical bodies. The oocysts are also irregularly acid-fast when stained with modified Zn stain.

Clinical features: watery diarrhoea which is most severe in non-immune travellers. Mild fever, fatigue, anorexia, and weight loss may occur. The illness can last for weeks.

Management: co-trimoxazole 960 mg PO bd for 7–10 days.

Strongyloidiasis

The nematode *Strongyloides stercoralis* commonly infects humans world-wide, particularly in parts of S. America and S.E. Asia. It is a serious condition in the immunosuppressed and may cause acute, relapsing, or persistent diarrhoea. There are two adult forms of the worm and two larval forms, one of which is infective.

Life cycle: Complex (see Fig. 6.4) since reproduction can take place in either of two cycles: an external cycle involving free-living worms or an internal cycle. Contamination of skin or buccal mucosa with larvae-containing soil permits initial penetration of larvae and infection. The larvae travel to the lungs and enter the bronchi, eventually passing into the small intestine, where they mature into adults. Eggs produced by the female pass out in the faeces and continue the external cycle.

Autoinfection occurs by either bronchial larvae producing progeny or filariform larvae not passing out in the stool but reinvading bowel or perianal skin. This can produce indefinite (>40 years) multiplication within the host, not requiring further infection. The pre-patent period from infection to the appearance of larvae in the stools is ~1 month.

Clinical features: Infection is usually asymptomatic, except for autoinfection through perianal skin. The immune response limits the infection to the small bowel and also the number of adult worms.

Larval penetration causes petechial haemorrhages and pruritis at the site of entry, frequently with a linear, red eruption (larva currens) as the larvae migrate under the skin. This is normally transient, but may be followed by congestion and oedema. A creeping urticarial rash may occur in pre-sensitized individuals following re-infection. Symptoms similar to bronchopneumonia with consolidation may result from larval invasion of the lungs; it is accompanied by eosinophilia and resembles TPE. Watery diarrhoea with mucus is a frequent symptom; its intensity depends on worm burden. It often alternates with constipation. In severe cases, chronic diarrhoea with malabsorption may ensue.

In the immunosuppressed, those co-infected with HTLV-1, malnourished, or debilitated, massive tissue invasion may occur with severe diarrhoea, ileus, hepatomegaly, and multi-system disease due to blood/lymphatic spread ('hyperinfection syndrome'). Granulomas and/or abscesses occur in liver, kidneys, and lungs, and there may be serous effusions; CNS involvement produces pyogenic meningitis and encephalopathy. Eosinophilia may or may not be a feature. Death usually results from Gram-negative septicaemia.

Diagnosis: Adult or rhabditiform larvae may be detected in the stool, although simple stool microscopy is an insensitive test. Other methods include the modified Baermann technique, agar plate culture, ELISA, serology, and stool culture using charcoal. Look for infection in those who are, or are about to be, immunosuppressed (e.g. on steroids).

Management: Treat all infected patients, not just the symptomatic.
1. Albendazole 400 mg PO bd for 7 days.
   (Alternatives: ivermectin 200 mcg/kg PO od for 2 days; or thiabendazole 25 mg/kg PO bd for 2 days, or 5 days in disseminated infection.)

Prevention: Requires improving hygiene, encouraging footware, and education on a community level, as well as monitoring and evaluation.

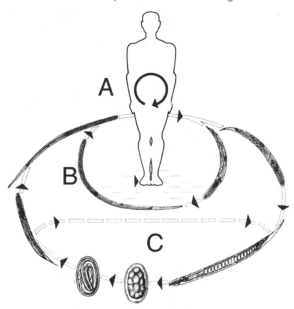

Fig. 6.4 Life cycle of *Strongyloides stercoralis*: The female worms are ~2 mm in length and live in the small intestine; they produce eggs parthenogenetically. In the auto-infectious life cycle (A), these hatch within the bowel and larvae penetrate the intestinal wall to produce more adult worms. Alternatively (B), the larvae may be passed in faeces into environmental surface water, and infect new hosts through intact skin (when walking barefoot in puddles). In a third life cycle (C), free-living adult worms give rise to eggs and then larvae, which infect new hosts. Infective larvae are called 'filariform', and those freshly passed in stool are 'rhabtidiform' larvae. (Adapted from G. Piekarski, *Medical parasitology in plates*, 1962 and reproduced with kind permission of Bayer Pharmaceuticals.)

Food poisoning

Food Poisoning is a general term referring to gastrointestinal symptoms which occur after eating specific foods. When symptoms occur within a few hours of eating the food, this is usually due to a toxin present in the food. Microbial infections usually have a longer incubation period as the pathogen proliferates in the intestine.

Table 6.1 Food poisoning from bacteria or their toxins

Organism/toxin	Principal foods	Time after food	Clinical features
Staph. aureus	Meat, poultry, dairy produce, prepared foods	1–6 h	D, V, AP
Bacillus cereus	Fried rice, sauces, vegetables	1–5 h 6–16 h	V D, AP
Red bean toxin		1–6 h	D, V
Scombrotoxin	Fish	1–6 h	D, flushing, sweating, mouth pain
Mushroom toxin		1–6 h	D, V, AP
Ciguatera	Fish	1–6 h	Fits, coma, renal/liver failure
Salmonella spp.	Meat, poultry, eggs, dairy produce	8–72 h (mean 12–36 h)	D, V, AP, fever
Campylobacter spp	Poultry, raw milk, eggs	1–10 days (mean 2–5 days)	D, AP
Clostridium perfringens	Cooked meat	8–24 h (mean 8–15 h)	D, AP, V
Vibrio parahaemolyticus	Seafood	4–96 h (mean 12 h)	D, V, AP, cramp, headache
Shigella spp.	Faecal contamination	1–7 days (mean 1–3 days)	D(bloody), V, fever
Clostridium botulinum	Poorly canned food, smoked meats	2 h–8 days (mean 12–36 h)	Diplopia, paralysis
Listeria monocytogenes	Dairy produce, meat, vegetables, seafood	1–7 weeks	Septicaemia, septic abortion
E. coli	Dirty water	8–44 h	D, V, cramps
Yersina enterocolitica	Pork and beef	24–36 h	Fever, AP, D

V = vomiting, D = diarrhoea, AP = abdominal pain

Clostridium perfringens

Clostridium perfringens produces two forms of gastrointestinal disease: simple food poisoning (caused by type A, see box on page 238) and necrotizing enterocolitis (type C).

Necrotizing enterocolitis (pigbel)
This is common in Uganda, South-East Asia, China, and the highlands of Papua New Guinea. It occurs when *C. perfringens* type C is eaten, normally in meat, by people who are malnourished, heavily infected with *Ascaris lumbricoides*, or have a diet rich in sweet potatoes. The latter two are associated with high levels of heat-stable trypsin inhibitors that inhibit the luminal proteases, preventing them inactivating the toxin.

Clinical features: symptoms usually begin 48 h following ingestion but may start up to one week later. It is classified into 4 types:
- **Type I** (acute toxic) presents with fulminant toxaemia and shock. It usually occurs in young children and carries an 85% mortality rate.
- **Type II** (acute surgical) presents as mechanical or paralytic ileus, acute strangulation, perforation, or peritonitis. It has 40% mortality.
- **Type III** (subacute surgical) presents later, with features similar to type II. Mortality is also ~40%.
- **Type IV** is of mild diarrhoea only, though it may progress to type III. In types II and III, a thickened segment of bowel is sometimes palpable. Blood and pus are passed with the stool in severe disease.

Diagnosis: isolation of *C. perfringens* from stool or peritoneal fluid culture. Serological diagnosis is also possible.

Management: type I and II disease require urgent surgery after appropriate resuscitation. Surgery may also be required for type III. Give intravenous chloramphenicol or benzylpenicillin and *C. perfringens* type C antiserum, where available. Milder cases may require glucose and electrolyte infusions, with IV broad-spectrum antibiotics if there are signs of extra-intestinal spread. Give an antihelminthic effective against *Ascaris*. Oral food intake should begin after 24 h.

Prevention: immunization with type C toxoid has greatly reduced the incidence and severity of the disease in Papua New Guinea.

Prevention of food poisoning from bacteria or their toxins PUBLIC HEALTH NOTE

Five key to safe food:
1. Keep food clean
2. Cook thoroughly
3. Separate raw and cooked food
4. Keep food at safe temperatures
5. Use safe water and raw materials

Food handlers should be particularly careful about personal hygiene, especially hand washing after defecation and before touching food. Especial attention should be taken to prevent *S. aureus* contamination from skin, nose, and eye infections of food handlers, who are the most common source of contamination of food (~25% people are carriers). The toxin is not destroyed at boiling temperatures.

Persistent diarrhoea & malabsorption

Persistent diarrhoea (lasting >2 weeks) is the preferred term for episodes starting acutely and associated with gastrointestinal infections. Diarrhoea may be prolonged through several mechanisms (see box opposite). In areas where sanitation and clean water are lacking and diarrhoea incidence is high, most persistent diarrhoea seems to be caused by frequent new infections combined with delayed recovery, often due to nutrient deficiencies. Persistent diarrhoea is accompanied by malnutrition and high mortality in children. Dietary management with continued feeding, correction of micronutrient deficiencies, and antimicrobial treatment of concomitant infections and dysentery (as well as rehydration if necessary) is effective in 80% of children.

Malabsorption

May be due to a range of causes (see box). The key features are:
- Chronic diarrhoea and steatorrhoea: stool is typically loose, bulky, offensive, greasy, light-coloured, and difficult to flush away.
- Abdominal discomfort, distension, flatulence.
- Signs of nutritional deficiency e.g. glossitis, pallor, muscle pain bruising, hyperpigmentation, CNS or PNS signs, skeletal deformity.
- General ill health: anorexia, weight loss, lethargy, dyspnoea, fatigue.
- Features related to underlying cause: surgical scars, systemic disease.

Investigations: FBC, U&Es, ESR, LFTs, stool microscopy and culture. Other tests include faecal fat, INR (deficiency of fat-soluble vitamins), carbohydrate absorption (after glucose or xylose), Schilling test (measure of ileal function), small bowel biopsy via endoscopy, or Crosby capsule.

Hypolactasia and lactose intolerance

- 1° hypolactasia occurs because humans, like most mammals, lose the digestive enzyme lactase as they mature and no longer depend on milk (although a genetic variant in some ethnic groups preserves the enzyme).
- 2° hypolactasia occurs after injury to the intestinal mucosa and is common after GI infections.

In both types a limited capacity to hydrolyse lactose leads to lactose malabsorption. **Lactose intolerance** occurs when incompletely hydrolysed lactose reaches the colon and causes osmotic diarrhoea, abdominal pain, distention, and flatulence. Symptoms depend on the amount of lactose reaching the small intestine at a given time.

Diagnosis: History of worsening symptoms with increased lactose intake (lactose tolerance test), acid stools with positive reducing substances, the hydrogen breath test, or a lactase assay in jejunal biopsy.

Management: Symptomatic intolerance can often be controlled by allowing only small amounts of lactose at a time; slowing gastric emptying e.g. by adding chocolate to milk or mixing milk with cereals; reducing lactose by fermentation as in yogurt; or taking lactase supplements with milk drinks. Total exclusion of milk to avoid lactose is rarely necessary and should be avoided whenever possible in infants because it is often difficult to provide alternative bio-available sources of the many nutrients in milk. Care should be taken to maintain energy and nutrient intakes. If, in severe cases, it is necessary to eliminate lactose-containing products, these may be introduced slowly after 6 weeks depending on symptom recurrence.

Causes of persistent or chronic diarrhoea

Secondary events
- Lactose intolerance due to 1° or 2° hypolactasia.
- Tropical sprue.
- Cow's milk protein intolerance.

Continuing infection
- Strongyloidiasis.
- Cryptosporidiosis.
- Microsporidiosis.
- Enteropathogenic *E. coli*.
- Giardiasis.
- Intestinal flukes.
- Chronic intestinal schistosomiasis.

Delayed recovery
- Malnutrition.
- Zinc deficiency.
- Sequential new infections.

Other causes
- HIV enteropathy.
- Chronic calcific pancreatitis.
- Short bowel disease (e.g. recovered pigbel disease).
- Ileocaecal TB.
- Lymphoma — Burkitt's and Mediterranean.
- Acute and chronic liver disease.
- Inflammatory bowel disease and coeliac disease.
- Irritable bowel syndrome.

Causes of malabsorption

- *Infective*: acute enteritis, intestinal TB, parasitic infections, Whipple's disease, other causes of traveller's diarrhoea.
- *Anatomical/motility*: blind loops, diverticuli, strictures, fistulae, small bowel lymphoma, systemic sclerosis, diabetes mellitus, pseudo-obstruction, radiotherapy, amyloidosis, lymphatic obstruction (TB, lymphoma, cardiac disease).
- *Defective digestion*: chronic pancreatitis, cystic fibrosis, food sensitivity (lactose, gluten), malnutrition, gastric/intestinal surgery, Zollinger–Ellison syndrome, pancreatectomy, biliary obstruction, terminal ileal disease/resection (short bowel syndrome), parenchymal liver disease, bacterial overgrowth.
- *Drugs*: antibiotics, cholestyramine, metformin, methyldopa, alcohol, antacids, purgative misuse, paraaminosalicylic acid.

Post-infective malabsorption (PIM); tropical enteropathy; tropical sprue

This syndrome of malabsorption, haematological abnormality, weight loss and diarrhoea can occur in residents and long-term visitors (>3 months) to the tropics, especially Central America, northern South America, parts of Africa, the Mediterranean coast, Middle East, and Asia. It is by definition a chronic condition; ≥2 months of symptoms are needed to make the diagnosis. Malabsorption significantly reduces energy and nutrient intake quickly leading to malnutrition, especially in children, and to anaemia. For reasons that are not clear, PIM seems to be becoming less common.

Aetiology: PIM is an enigma. It is not clear whether it is a distinct entity which occurs with the persistence of malabsorption after acute infective diarrhoea, or a form of tropical enteropathy (tropical sprue; see below). Both tropical enteropathy and PIM show abnormal jejunal morphology with partial villous atrophy. There is crypt hyperplasia, with T cell infiltration. Changes in gut hormones, disturbed gut motility, and colonic function have been described. Bacterial overgrowth of the small intestine is found but no single organism can be held responsible. An association with certain HLA antigens has been reported suggesting a genetic predisposition.

Clinical features: chronic diarrhoea/steatorrhoea ± flatulence of >2 months duration. Other features include weight loss, glossitis, macrocytic anaemia, fluid retention, depression, lethargy, amenorrhoea, and infertility. Serum folate and vitamin B12 may fall to very low levels. Hypoalbuminaemia and oedema are late signs. Foreign travel or recent GI infection can unmask other chronic GI disorders such as coeliac disease, inflammatory bowel disease, and GI malignancy. Irritable bowel syndrome is reported in 3–10% of people following travellers' diarrhoea episodes.

Investigations: 1-h blood xylose concentration following a 5 g or 25 g loading dose; 72-h faecal fat estimation; Schilling test; serum B12; RBC folate; serum globin; and albumin. Exclude faecal parasites. Barium meal and follow-through will show dilated loops of jejunum with clumping of barium. Endoscopy and jejunal biopsy may show a ridged or convoluted mucosa, depending on the duration of the disease, with T lymphocyte infiltration.

Management

Eliminate bacterial overgrowth with tetracycline 250 mg PO qds for at least 2 weeks.
1. Aid mucosal recovery by providing folate supplements.
2. Provide a suitable diet to promote weight gain.
3. Give symptomatic relief in the acute stages:
• Codeine phosphate 30 mg PO tds *or*
• Loperamide 4 mg PO initially, then 2 mg after each loose stool. Usual dose 6–8 mg od; maximum dose 16 mg od.

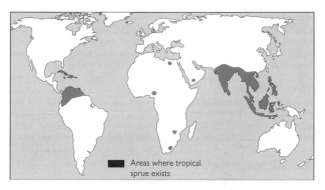

Fig. 6.5 Distribution of post-infective malabsorption (tropical sprue).

Tropical enteropathy and subclinical malabsorption

Individuals living in highly contaminated environments such as commonly found in the tropics fight a constant battle against repeated low-grade viral, bacterial, and parasitic gastrointestinal infections. This is associated with chronic changes in the jejunal mucosa with blunted villi and nutrient malabsorption which recover when the subject leaves the contaminated environment. Tests of nutrient absorption e.g. B12 and xylose absorption tests, are usually abnormal. Tropical enteropathy probably contributes to child growth retardation in developing countries together with energy and micronutrient deficiencies and frequent infectious diseases. Improvement of the condition occurs spontaneously when travellers return to a clean environment. In resident infants, mucosal changes improve with age but persist into adulthood.

Chronic calcific pancreatitis

A syndrome of pancreatic calcification associated with both exocrine and endocrine impairment, commonly encountered in the tropics, especially equatorial Africa, southern India, and Indonesia. Its aetiology is unknown, although childhood kwashiorkor, gastroenteritis, excessive alcohol consumption, dehydration, and ingestion of cassava (*Manhiot esculenta*) have all been implicated.

Clinical features: are of chronic malabsorption with weight loss, often associated with DM (10% of diabetes in E&W Africa) and (sometimes severe) pain. There is an association with pancreatic malignancy.

Management: diabetic control, low-fat diet, and enzyme supplementation (e.g. pancreatin BP 6 g PO with food; dose tailored to individual patient).

Intestinal lymphoma

A wide variety of lymphomas may affect the GI tract, originating in either intestinal lymph nodes (e.g. Hodgkin's lymphoma) or mucosa-associated lymphoid tissue (MALT lymphomas). Small bowel lymphoma is a recognized complication of HIV/AIDS. Weight loss is a common feature and nodal disease may be confused with intestinal TB, as X-ray changes appear similar. Diagnosis requires biopsy.

Whipples disease

Whipples disease is a rare condition caused by the actinomycete bacterium *Tropheryma whippelii*. Classically, there is weight loss, diarrhoea, and malabsorption, but clinical features are protean and often non-specific. Other features include fever, lymphadenopathy, arthralgia (may be transient or migratory), uveitis, culture negative endocarditis, coronary arteritis, myocarditis, and encephalopathy. A histopathological diagnosis is often made incidentally on examination of intestinal biopsy material showing granulomatous inflammation and periodic acid-Schiff (PAS) staining deposits. PCR for the presence of *T. whippelii* in affected tissues confirms the diagnosis. *Treatment*: 2 weeks ceftriaxone 1 g bd IV, then oral co-trimoxazole (alternatives: tetracycline or minocycline) for 1 year.

Other causes of malabsorption

1. Lymphangiectasia: lacteal dilatation (either 1° or 2° to abdominal malignancy) causes a protein-losing enteropathy, hypoproteinaemia, and oedema. Diagnosis requires small bowel biopsy. Treatment: low-fat diet.

2. Abetalipoproteinaemia: a rare AR disorder, usually presenting in childhood due to defective triglyceride transport from the liver and gut. Eventually, neurological dysfunction (peripheral neuropathy, cerebellar ataxia) may follow. Diagnosis is by small bowel biopsy and symptomatic treatment is with low-fat diet and vitamin supplementation.

3. Intestinal parasites: Many GI parasites (e.g. *Giardia, Cryptosporidium, Trichuris, Strongyloides*) can cause diarrhoea. Others (e.g. schistosomiasis, trichinellosis, cysticercosis, clonorchiasis, opisthorchiasis, ecchinococcus) cause hepatic or pancreatic dysfunction. Pancreatic duct obstruction may be caused by ascariasis.

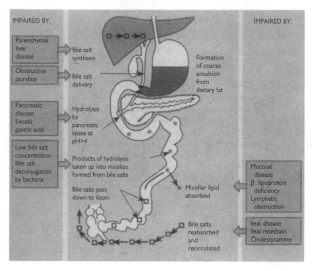

Fig. 6.6 Mechanisms of Steatorrhoea.

Intestinal flukes

These pathogens are common throughout Asia (particularly S.E. Asia), where their prevalence may reach 30% in certain populations. Children are more heavily infected and prone to symptoms.

- *Fasciolopsiasis*: Caused by *Fasciolopsis buski*; infection follows ingestion of metacercaria attached to the seed pods of water plants contaminated by human and pig faeces.
- *Echinostomiasis*: At least 15 *Echinostoma* species infect humans via the consumption of raw or undercooked freshwater snails, clams, fish, and tadpoles. In N.E. Thailand, it is commonly associated with *Opisthorchis* infection.
- *Heterophyasis:* Numerous species of the small (2.5 mm) *Heterophyes* flukes infect humans following consumption of raw aquatic foods and/or insect larvae.

Clinical features: The attachment of parasites to the intestinal mucosa results in inflammation and ulcer formation. Infections are frequently asymptomatic; when symptoms do occur, they are usually mild and non-specific — diarrhoea, flatulence, mild abdominal pains, vomiting, fever, and anorexia. Fasciolopsiasis may produce severe disease with anaemia, malabsorption, oedema, and ascites. Eggs (and sometimes adult worms) of *Heterophyes* spp. may enter the lymphatics after mucosal penetration and be transported to other sites (notably heart, spinal cord, brain, lungs, liver, and spleen) where they cause granulomatous reactions. Myocarditis and neurological deficits may result.

Diagnosis: Faecal examination for eggs, after concentration. Differentiation between *F. hepatica*, *F. buski*, and echinostomes is often difficult. Similarly, heterophydiae eggs closely resemble those of *Clonorchis* and *Opisthorchis*. Recovery of adult worms from post-treatment faeces allows a definitive diagnosis, although in the case of the heterophyids, this is difficult owing to their small size. Extraintestinal cases of heterophyiasis are also difficult to diagnose — they are often only revealed during surgery or autopsy.

Management
1. Praziquantel is the drug of choice, given as 25 mg/kg PO tds for 1 day.
2. Mebendazole or albendazole may be used for echinostomiasis, although praziquantel is recommended in areas where other trematodes are present, due to its broad efficacy.

Prevention: Concentrate on breaking the faeco-oral cycle (e.g. stopping the use of human and pig excreta as fertilizer) possibly combined with community-based praziquantel treatment and education regarding the consumption of raw/undercooked foodstuffs.

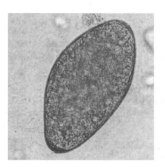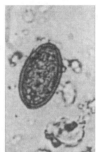

Fig. 6.7 Eggs of *Fasciolopsis buski* (left, 140 × 85 μm) and *Heterophyes heterophyes* (right, 25 × 15 μm).

General management of dehydration

Dehydration due to diarrhoea remains a major cause of childhood death in the developing world. The volume of fluid lost in the stool can vary from 5 ml/kg to >200 ml/kg in 24 h. Electrolyte loss also varies. The total body sodium deficit in young children with severe dehydration owing to secretory diarrhoea is usually about 70–110 mmol per litre of water lost.

The degree of dehydration is graded according to clinical features. In the early stages of dehydration, there are no signs or symptoms. As dehydration increases, thirst, restless, or irritable behaviour develop. Examination reveals decreased skin turgor, dry mucous membranes, sunken eyes, sunken fontanelle (in infants), and absence of tears when crying. In severe dehydration, these effects become more pronounced and the patient may develop signs of hypovolaemic shock, including decreased consciousness, anuria, cool moist extremities, rapid and feeble pulse, low blood pressure, and peripheral cyanosis. Death may follow swiftly without prompt rehydration.

Types of dehydration

1. *Isotonic dehydration*: occurs most frequently and is due to net losses of water and sodium in similar proportion to that in the extracellular fluid (ECF). The serum sodium concentration (130–150 mmol/l) and serum osmolality (275–295 mOsmol/l) are normal. Hypovolaemia occurs due to excess ECF losses. Clinical features are those of hypovolaemic shock (e.g. thirst, reduced skin turgor, dry mucous membranes, sunken eyes, oliguria, and a sunken fontanelle in infants). This progresses to anuria, hypotension, a weak pulse, cool extremities, and eventually coma and death.

2. *Hypertonic (hypernatraemic) dehydration*: reflects a net loss of water in excess of sodium and tends to occur in infants only. It usually results from attempted treatment of diarrhoea with fluids that are hypertonic (e.g. sweetened fruit juices/soft drinks, glucose solution) combined with insufficient intake of water and other hypotonic solutes. Hypertonic solutions cause water to flow from the ECF into the intestine, leading to decreased ECF volume and hypernatraemia. There is a deficit of water, hypernatraemia (Na >150 mmol/l), and raised serum osmolality (>295 mOsmol/l). Clinical features include severe thirst, irritability and convulsions (esp. if Na^+ is >165 mmol/l).

3. *Hypotonic (hyponatraemic) dehydration*: occurs in patients with diarrhoea who drink large amounts of water or other hypotonic fluids containing very low quantities of salt and other solutes. and in patients who receive IV infusions of 5% glucose in water. It occurs because water is absorbed from the gut while the loss of salt continues, producing a net excess of water and hyponatraemia. Serum sodium and osmolality are low (Na^+ <130 mmol/l, Osm <275 mOsmol/l). Clinical features include lethargy and, rarely, convulsions.

All three types of dehydration can be managed with the same oral rehydration fluid and intravenous regimes described on the following pages.

Assessment of dehydration in patients with diarrhoea

1. Look at

Condition	Well, alert	Restless, irritable	Lethargic[1] or unconscious
Eyes[2]	Normal	Sunken	Sunken
Thirst	None	Drinks eagerly, very thirsty	Drinks poorly, unable to drink

2. Pinch the skin to assess skin turgor[3]

	Goes back immediately	Goes back slowly	Goes back very slowly

3. Decide:

	No dehydration	Some dehydration	Severe dehydration

4. Treat:

	Plan A (see p. 252)	Plan B (see p. 254)	Plan C (see p. 256)

Plans B and C require at least two of the four signs to be positive

Notes:

1 A lethargic patient is not simply asleep; the patient's mental state is dull and the patient cannot be fully awakened. The patient may appear to be drifting into unconsciousness.

2 In some infants, the eyes normally appear a little sunken, so ask the mother if the child's eyes appear normal to her.

3 Pinch the abdominal skin in a longitudinal manner with thumb and bent forefinger. 'Goes back slowly' means that it is visible for more than 2 seconds.

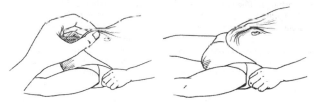

Fig. 6.8 Skin pinch to assess skin turgor. Pinch skin midway between umbilicus and flank, then release skin to observe how quickly it goes back. Skin pinch returns very slowly (≥ 2 seconds) in severe dehydration due to reduced skin turgor. (Reproduced from *Management of the Child with a Serious Infection or Severe Malnutrition* with permission from the WHO.)

Estimation of fluid deficit

A child's fluid deficit may be estimated as follows:

Assessment	Fluid deficit as % body weight	Fluid deficit ml/kg
No signs of dehydration	<5%	<50 ml/kg
Some dehydration	5–10%	50–100 ml/kg
Severe dehydration	>10%	>100 ml/kg

Children with dehydration should be weighed without clothing, as an aid to estimating their fluid requirements. If weighing is not possible, the child's age may be used to estimate the weight. Treatment should never be delayed because scales are not readily available.

Suitable fluids
Many countries have recommended home fluids which should be used in the prevention of dehydration only (i.e. treatment plan A). Whenever possible, these should include at least one fluid that normally contains salt (e.g. oral rehydration solution — ORS; salted drinks such as salted rice water or salted yoghurt; vegetable or chicken soup with salt). Other fluids should be recommended that are frequently given to children in the area, that mothers consider acceptable for children with diarrhoea, and that the mothers would likely give in increased amounts if advised to do so. Such fluids should be safe and easy to prepare.

If there are signs of dehydration, ORS should be used as per treatment plans B and C.
• Teaching mother to add salt (about 3 g/l) to unsalted drinks or soups during diarrhoea is beneficial, but requires education and (initially) supervision. Teach the mother to ALWAYS taste the fluid herself before giving it to the child. It should not taste saltier than tears.
• A home-made solution containing 3 g/l salt and 18 g/l of common sugar (sucrose) is effective, but the recipe is often forgotten, made up incorrectly, and/or the ingredients hard to obtain.

Unsuitable fluids
A few fluids are potentially dangerous and should be avoided during episodes of diarrhoea. Avoid drinks sweetened with sugar that can cause osmotic diarrhoea and hypernatraemia (e.g. soft drinks, Cola, sweetened fruit drinks, sweetened tea).

Oral rehydration solution (ORS)

The formula for ORS recommended by WHO and UNICEF is given in the box opposite. Where bulk preparation is required, multiply the amounts shown by the number of litres required. WHO-ORS is also available in pre-prepared packets for dissolution in water. ORS should be used within 24 h of preparation. When given correctly, ORS provides sufficient water and electrolytes to correct the deficits associated with acute diarrhoea. For children with severe malnutrition, a solution containing 45 mmol sodium (ReSoMal, see formula in box opposite) is preferred.

ORS recipe: to make 1L from bulk ingredients

1. Sodium chloride   3.5 g
2. Glucose   20 g
3. Trisodium citrate, dihydrate   2.9 g
4. Potassium chloride   1.5 g

If glucose and trisodium citrate are not available, use:

Sucrose   27 g

Sodium bicarbonate   2.5 g

- Completely dissolve the sugar and salts in one litre of clean water — boiled or chlorinated water is best.
- ORS solution should be used within 24 h, after which time it should be discarded and fresh solution prepared.
- To make 1 litre of rice-based ORS, boil 50 g of rice powder in 1.1 litres of water. Mix in sugar and salt in the quantities stated above. Use within 12 h.

Dehydration in children with malnutrition

Signs of dehydration are more difficult to assess in children with severe malnutrition, and can be difficult to distinguish from signs of sepsis. As a result, the degree of dehydration is often overestimated.

- Eyes appear sunken because of the absence of orbital fat. Ask the mother if there has been a change.
- Skin turgor is more difficult to assess by skin pinch because of oedema in kwashiorkor and redundant skin in marasmus, but the characteristic dough-like feel of severe dehydration may still be useful.
- Thirst is a useful sign if present. Check by offering water or ORS rather than by asking. Inability to drink also occurs in sepsis.
- Lethargy and coma may be due to sepsis.
- Use ReSoMal (rehydration solution for severely dehydrated children) for oral/NG rehydration if available. This has less Na^+ and more K^+.
- Reserve intravenous fluids for dehydration with shock; give at half the rate for non-malnourished children (15 ml/kg in the first hour). Monitor every 15 min (pulse, respiratory rate, signs of dehydration). If no improvement in hydration status after 1 hour of IV rehydration, reduce fluid replacement rate to 4 ml/kg/hour and assume sepsis.

If in doubt, start parenteral antibiotics.

ReSoMal recipe

Mix the same quantity of electrolytes used to make 1 litre ORS* (see box above) with 2 litres of water, 50 g sucrose, and 45 ml of KCl solution (100 g KCL/1 litre)**

* alternatively use 1 (1 litre) packet of WHO-ORS powder

** or 40 ml WHO-concentrated electrolyte/mineral solution, if available

Treatment plan A: treat diarrhoea without signs of dehydration at home

Use this plan to teach the mother to:
- Continue to treat her child's current episode of diarrhoea at home.
- Give early treatment for future episodes of diarrhoea.

Counsel the mother on the 4 rules of home treatment:

1) GIVE EXTRA FLUID (as much as the child will take)
- Breastfeed frequently and for longer at each feed.
- If exclusively breastfed, give ORS or clean water in addition to breastmilk.
- If not exclusively breastfed, give one or more of the following: ORS solution, food-based fluids (such as soup, rice water, and yoghurt drinks), or clean water.

It is especially important to give ORS at home when:
- The child has been treated with Plan B or Plan C during this visit.
- The child cannot return to a clinic if the diarrhoea gets worse.

▶ *Teach the mother how to mix and give ORS. Give the mother 2 packets of ORS to use at home.*
▶ *Show the mother how much fluid to give in addition to the usual fluid intake.*

Amount of ORS to give according to child's age

Age	After each loose stool	At home
<2 yrs	50–100 ml	500 ml/day
2–10 yrs	100–200 ml	1 litre/day
>10 yrs	As much as tolerated	2 litres/day

Tell the mother to:
- Give a teaspoon every 1–2 minutes for a child <2 yrs.
- Give frequent small sips from a cup for older children.
- Wait 10 minutes if the child vomits, then continue, but more slowly.
- Continue giving extra fluid until the diarrhoea stops.

2) GIVE ZINC SUPPLEMENTS
▶ *Tell the mother how much zinc to give:*
- <6 months → 2 tablets (10 mg total) per day for 14 days.
- ≥6 months → 4 tablets (20 mg total) per day for 14 days.

▶ *Show the mother how to give zinc supplements*
- Infants → dissolve the tablet in a small amount of expressed breastmilk, ORS, or clean water, in a small cup or spoon.
- Older children → tablets can be chewed or dissolved in a small amount of clean water in a cup or spoon.

▶ *Remind the mother to give the zinc supplements for the full 14 days.*

3) CONTINUE FEEDING

- Give the child plenty of food to prevent malnutrition.
- Continue to breastfeed frequently. If the child is not breastfed, give the usual milk.
- If the child is >6 months, or already taking solid foods, also give cereal or another starchy food mixed, if possible, with pulses, vegetables, milk, meat, or fish. Give fresh fruit juice or mashed banana to provide potassium. Give freshly prepared foods. Cook and mash/grind food well.
- Encourage the child to eat; offer food >5 times per day.
- Give the same foods after diarrhoea stops and give an extra meal each day for 2 weeks.

4) WHEN TO RETURN

Take the child to a health worker if the diarrhoea does not improve within 3 days or the child develops any of the following:

- Many watery stools.
- Fever.
- Repeated vomiting.
- Eating/drinking poorly.
- Unable to breastfeed.
- Marked thirst.
- Blood in the stool.

What to do if patient does not improve with ORT

In about 5% of patients the signs of dehydration do not improve or worsen after starting treatment with ORS. The usual causes are:

- Continuing rapid stool loss (>15–20 ml/kg/hr) e.g. in cholera.
- Insufficient ORS intake due to fatigue, lethargy, or lack of supervision.
- Frequent severe vomiting.

Such patients should be admitted to hospital and given ORS by NG tube or Ringer's lactate solution 75 ml/kg IV over 4 h. Consider the possibility of cholera. Close monitoring of patient's progress, hourly at first, is essential.

When not to give ORS

Rarely, ORS should not be given. This is true for children with:

- Abdominal distension due to paralytic ileus (often owing to opiate drugs such as codeine or loperamide, or to hypokalaemia).
- Glucose malabsorption, indicated by a marked increase in stool output as ORS is started. There is no improvement and the stool contains large amounts of glucose.

In these situations, rehydration should be given intravenously until diarrhoea subsides.

Treatment plan B: treat some dehydration with ORS

In clinic, give the recommended amount of ORS over a 4-hour period:
▶ *Determine the amount of ORS to give during the first 4 h:*

Age*	<4 mths	4–11 mths	12–23 mths	2–5 yrs	5–14 yrs	>14 yrs
Weight	<6 kg	6–9.9 kg	10–11.9 kg	12–19 kg	19–30 kg	>30 kg
Volume	200–400 ml	400–700 ml	700–900 ml	900–1400 ml	1.4–2.2 l	2.2–4.0 l

* Use the child's age only when you do not know the weight. The approximate amount of ORS required (in ml) can also be calculated by multiplying the child 's weight (in kg) × 75.

- If the child wants more ORS than shown, give more.
- For infants <6 months who are not breastfed, also give 100–200 ml clean water during this period.

▶ *Show the mother how to give ORS solution*
- Give a teaspoon every 1–2 mins for a child under 2 years.
- Give frequent small sips from a cup for an older child.
- If the child vomits, wait 10 minutes; then continue, but more slowly.
- Continue breastfeeding whenever the child wants.

▶ **After 4 h, reassess the patient using the chart on** 📖 **p 249 and continue plan A, B, or C as appropriate**
- If there are no signs of dehydration, shift to plan A. When dehydration has been corrected, urine will start to be passed and children may become less irritable and fall asleep.
- If signs indicating some dehydration are still present, repeat plan B, but start to offer food, milk, and juice as in plan A.
- If there are signs indicating severe dehydration, treat using plan C.

▶ *If the mother must leave before completing treatment:*
- Show her how to prepare ORS solution at home.
- Show her how much ORS to give to finish 4-hour treatment at home.
- Give her enough ORS packets to complete rehydration. Also give her 2 packets as recommended in plan A.
- Make sure that children receive breast milk or, if >6 months, are given some food before being sent home. Emphasize to the mother the importance of continuing feeding throughout the diarrhoeal episode.
- Explain the 4 rules of home treatment:

(1) **GIVE EXTRA FLUID** (see plan A for recommended fluids)
(2) **GIVE ZINC SUPPLEMENTS**
(3) **CONTINUE FEEDING**
(4) **WHEN TO RETURN**

Monitoring signs during oral rehydration therapy

Check the patient from time to time during rehydration to ensure that ORS is being taken satisfactorily and that signs of dehydration are not worsening. If at any time the patient develops severe dehydration, switch to treatment plan C. After 4 h, reassess the patient following the guidelines in the box on 🕮 p 249. Decide what treatment to give next.

- If signs of severe dehydration have appeared, IV therapy should be started immediately, following plan C. This is very unusual, however. It tends to occur in children who drink ORS poorly and continue to pass large volumes of watery stool during the rehydration period.
- If the patient still has signs of mild dehydration, continue oral rehydration therapy following plan B. At the same time start to offer food, milk, and other fluids as described in treatment plan A. Reassess the patient frequently.
- If there are no signs of dehydration, the patient should be considered fully rehydrated. If this is the case: the skin pinch is normal; the thirst has subsided; urine is passed normally; and the child is no longer irritable and may fall asleep.

Teach the mother to treat her child at home using ORS following plan A. Give her enough ORS sachets for 3 days and teach her the signs that indicate she must bring her child back to the health post.

Meeting normal fluid needs

While treatment to replace the existing water and electrolyte deficit is in progress, the child's normal daily fluid requirements must also be met. This may be done as follows:

- *Breastfed infants*: continue to breastfeed as often and as long as the infant wants to, even during oral rehydration therapy.
- *Non-breastfed infants <6 months of age*: during rehydration with ORS, give 100–200 ml of plain water by mouth. After completing rehydration, resume full-strength milk or formula feeds. Give water and other fluids normally taken by the infant.
- *Older children and adults*: throughout rehydration treatment, offer as much plain water, milk, or juice as is accepted, in addition to ORS.

Treatment plan C: treat severe dehydration quickly

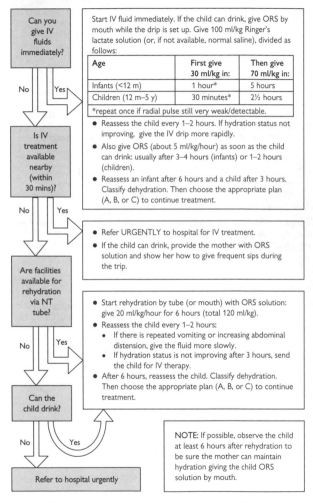

Fig. 6.9 Treatment plan C. (Taken from *Diarrhoea Treatment Guidelines for clinic-based Healthcare* Workers, 2005, with permission of the WHO.)

Monitoring IV rehydration therapy

Patients should be reassessed every 15–20 mins until a strong radial pulse is present. Thereafter, they should be assessed hourly to confirm that hydration is improving. If it is not, the IV fluid may be run at a faster rate.

When the planned amount of IV fluid has been given (6 h for infants, 3 h for older patients), the patient's state of hydration should be reassessed using the chart on 🕮 p 249.

- If the child's eyelids become puffy, liver enlarges, or tachycardia and tachypnoea appear, these may be signs of fluid overload and cardiac failure, especially in malnourished children. Reduce the rate of IV infusion and monitor closely.
- If there are still signs of severe dehydration, repeat plan C. This is unusual, but may occur in cases of cholera and children who pass frequent, watery stools during the rehydration period.
- If the patient shows signs of mild dehydration, discontinue IV fluid replacement and commence oral rehydration with ORS for 4 h according to plan B.
- If there are no signs of dehydration, discontinue IV therapy and commence ORS treatment according to plan A.

Observe the patient for at least 6 h before discharging. For children, ensure that the mother is able to continue giving ORS at home and is aware of the signs that indicate she must bring the child back.

Alternative solutions for IV rehydration

- *Ringer's lactate solution with 5% dextrose* — provides glucose to help prevent hypoglycaemia. If available, it is preferred to Ringer's lactate solution without dextrose.
- *Physiological saline (0.9% NaCl, also called normal saline)* — widely available, it is an acceptable alternative to Ringer's lactate solution but contains neither a base to correct acidosis nor potassium to correct K^+ losses. Sodium bicarbonate or sodium lactate (20–30 mmol/l) and potassium chloride (5–15 mmol/l) may be added.
- *Half-strength Darrow's solution* — is made by diluting full-strength Darrow's solution with an equal volume of glucose solution (50 g/l or 100 g/l). Note that it contains less sodium than is required to replace the sodium lost in diarrhoea.
- *Plain glucose (dextrose) solution should NOT be used* — since it does not contain any sodium, base, or potassium and does not correct hypovolaemia effectively.

Some difficulties encountered in home therapy for diarrhoea

1. The mother is disappointed because the child is not prescribed an antibiotic or given an injection

Explain that diarrhoea will usually stop by itself after a few days. The zinc supplements will help the child get better quicker. In most cases, antibiotics do not help and sometimes can make the diarrhoea go on longer. It is better to see how the child progresses and, if necessary, check to see what germ is causing the diarrhoea so that if antibiotics are needed the doctor can give the right one. Fluid replacement and continued feeding will help shorten the illness and maintain her child's strength and growth.

2. The mother believes that food should not be given during diarrhoea.

Ask her to explain her beliefs about how diarrhoea should be treated. Discuss with her the importance of feeding in order to keep her child strong and growing, even during diarrhoea. There are almost always some foods which are acceptable — find out and encourage these alternatives.

3. The mother does not know what fluids to give her child at home.

Ask her what fluids she can prepare at home and reach an agreement on appropriate fluids for her child.

4. The mother does not have the ingredients to make a recommended fluid.

Ask her if she can obtain the necessary ingredients easily. If she cannot, suggest another home fluid.

5. The child vomits after drinking ORS or other fluids.

Explain that more fluid is usually kept down than is vomited. Tell her to wait 10 mins and then start giving fluid again, but more slowly, just sips at a time from a spoon or cup.

6. The child refuses to drink.

A child who has lost fluid and is dehydrated will usually be thirsty and want to drink, even when there are no signs of dehydration. If the child is not familiar with the taste of ORS, some persuasion and patience may be needed at first. When a child drinks well to begin with but then loses interest, it usually means that sufficient fluid has been given. If the child is not dehydrated, it is not necessary to insist on ORS; other clear fluids can be given as suggested on p 250.

7. The mother is given some ORS packets for use at home but is afraid they will be used up before the diarrhoea stops.

Explain that after the ORS has been used up she should give a recommended home fluid (e.g. rice water) or water or she should return to the health facility for more packets of ORS. In any event, she should continue to give extra fluid until the diarrhoea stops.

Summary of important points in the management of diarrhoea in children

- Infectious diarrhoea very common, esp. ages 6 months — 2 years.
- Always examine the child and follow WHO guidelines for assessing hydration status (📖 p 249).
- Keep in mild the possibility of other non-infectious causes such as intussusception, appendicitis.
- Exclusively breastfed babies may have frequent explosive diarrhoea-like stools but appear well, are not dehydrated, do not lose weight, and usually follow a similar daily pattern of stooling.
- Treat dysentery (visible blood in stools) with antibiotics.
- Avoid antibiotics in non-dysenteric diarrhoea unless severe diarrhoea in a high-risk group (neonates, immune compromised).
- Avoid antimotility drugs (loperamide) in children under 2 yrs.
- Give oral zinc supplements: 20 mg elemental zinc daily for 10–14 days (10 mg daily in children <6 months).
- Continue breastfeeding.
- Continue normal diet, fractioning* diet, and increasing frequency of servings. Reduce lactose if necessary by mixing milk with other foods. Do not dilute formula with water.
- Advise caretaker of signs of alarm in small children:
  - Undue sleepiness.
  - Abdominal distention.
  - Worsening of diarrhoea.
  - Fever.
  - Drinking poorly or unable or unwilling to breastfeed.
  - Visible blood in stools.
- Use all opportunities of contact with carers of young children to advise preventative measures:
  - Exclusive breastfeeding to 6 months.
  - Introduce complementary foods from 6 months.
  - Continue breastfeeding together with other foods to 2 years.
  - Give locally appropriate nutritional advice to ensure sufficient calories and micronutrients.
  - Wash hands frequently with soap.
  - Dispose of infant stools safely, use potties, avoid faecal contamination of play areas.
  - Make up infants' food fresh for each meal.
  - Avoid storing prepared food and bottles at room temperature.
  - Boil water for children if clean water source is not guaranteed.

* Fractioning diet: divide the diet into small frequent amounts. This is especially useful for lactose intolerance as it reduces the amount reaching the duodenum and having to be hydrolysed at any one time.

Management of persistent diarrhoea

This is diarrhoea with or without blood that begins acutely and lasts >14 days. Clinically, these episodes cannot be differentiated from sequential episodes of acute diarrhoea over a prolonged period, but the management is the same. It is usually associated with weight loss and, often, with serious non-intestinal infections. Many children with persistent diarrhoea are malnourished before the diarrhoea starts. Persistent diarrhoea almost never occurs in infants who are exclusively breastfed. Take a careful history and examine the patient well.

The object of treatment is to restore weight gain and normal intestinal function. In most cases, the patient will need to be admitted to hospital for diagnostic tests, treatment, and observation.

Treatment of persistent diarrhoea

1. *Appropriate fluids* to prevent/treat dehydration (See 📖 p 248–257).
2. *Appropriate antimicrobial therapy* to treat diagnosed infections, in particular non-intestinal infections in children (e.g. pneumonia, otitis media, UTI). Look for evidence of *Giardia*, *Shigella*, or *Entamoeba* infection.
3. *A nutritious diet* that does not cause worsening of the diarrhoea. Children will require a minimum of 110 calories/kg per day, which may have to be given via a NG tube if the child is too weak or refuses to eat. For infants <6 months, encourage exclusive breastfeeding but check the baby is gaining weight. If possible help mothers who are not breastfeeding to re-establish lactation (See 📖 Chapter 17).
4. *Where possible, replace animal milk* with yoghurt, a lactose-free formula, or a local diet with reduced lactose (<3.5 g/kg body weight/day). For older infants and young children, use standard diets made from local ingredients. Two diets are given in the box: the first contains reduced lactose, the second is lactose-free for the 30% of children who do not improve with the first diet.
5. *Supplementary vitamins and minerals.* All children with persistent diarrhoea should receive supplementary multivitamins and minerals each day for 2 weeks. Tablets that are crushed and mixed with food are less costly. One should aim to provide at least two recommended daily allowances (RDAs) of folate, vitamin A, iron, zinc, magnesium, and copper. As a guide, the RDAs for a 1-year-old child are:
- Folate 150 mcg.
- Zinc 10 mg.
- Iron 10 mg.
- Vitamin A 400 mcg.
- Copper 1 mg.
- Magnesium 80 mg.

Diet 1 (low lactose)	Diet 2 (lactose-free)
83 calories/100 g	75 calories/100 g
11% of calories as protein	15% of calories as protein
2.7 g lactose in 130 ml/kg body weight/day	
Ingredients	
Full-fat dried milk 11 g (or 85 ml whole milk)	Whole egg (without shell) 36 g
Uncooked rice 15 g	Uncooked rice 10 g
Vegetable oil 3.5 g	Vegetable oil 5 g
Cane sugar 3 g	Glucose 5 g
Water to make up to 200 ml final volume	Water to make up to 200 ml final volume
130 ml/kg provides 110 cal/kg	*145 ml/kg provides 110 cal/kg*
Boil rice to a slurry with some of the water, add other ingredients and rest of water to make up to 200 ml final volume.	Boil rice to a slurry with some of the water, add the whole beaten egg and continue to cook for another minute, stirring well. Add the rest of the ingredients and the water to make up to 200 ml final volume.

Malnutrition and diarrhoea

Diarrhoea is as much a nutritional disease as one of fluid and electrolyte loss. Children who die from diarrhoea, despite good management, are usually malnourished — often severely so.

During diarrhoea, decreased food intake, decreased nutrient absorption, and increased nutrient requirements often combine to cause weight loss and failure to grow. The child's nutritional status declines and any pre-existing malnutrition is made worse. Malnutrition itself makes diarrhoea worse, prolonging it and making it more frequent. This vicious cycle may be broken by continuing to give nutrient-rich foods during diarrhoea and giving a nutritious diet, appropriate for the child's age, when the child is well.

When these steps are followed, malnutrition can be either prevented or corrected and the risk of death from a future episode of diarrhoea is much reduced.

Complications of diarrhoea

Electrolyte disturbances

Knowing the serum electrolyte concentrations rarely changes the management of patients dehydrated due to diarrhoea. In most cases, hypernatraemia, hyponatraemia, and hypokalaemia are all adequately treated by oral rehydration with ORS or IV rehydration with Ringer's lactate. In severe dehydration, however, plasma sodium concentrations may reach extremes and hypokalaemia may produce muscular weakness, dangerous cardiac arrhythmias, and paralytic ileus.

Fever

Fever in a patient with diarrhoea may be due to the organism causing the diarrhoea or, particularly in children, a 2° infection (e.g. pneumonia, otitis media, malaria). The presence of fever should suggest infections, particularly if it persists after the patient is fully hydrated. In areas where *P. falciparum* malaria is prevalent, children with a fever of ≥38°C should be treated with an appropriate antimalarial. High fevers (>39°C) in children should be treated with an antipyretic such as paracetamol. This will reduce irritability and prevent febrile convulsions.

Convulsions

In a child with diarrhoea and convulsions during the illness, the following diagnoses should be considered:

- *Febrile convulsions*: usually occur in children aged 6 months to 6 years (📖 p 15). Treat with paracetamol and tepid water sponging.
- *Meningitis*: needs to be considered in any child or adult following a convulsion. Look for neck rigidity and Kernig's sign. Do a lumbar puncture after checking the retinae for papilloedema (raised ICP) and looking for focal neurological signs.
- *Hypoglycaemia*: occasionally occurs in children with diarrhoea, due to their small hepatic glycogen reserves and insufficient gluconeogenesis. If suspected, give 2–5 ml/kg of 10% glucose solution (or 2.5 ml/kg of a 20% glucose solution) IV over 5 mins. If hypoglycaemia is the cause, recovery will usually be rapid. In such cases, Ringer's lactate with dextrose should be given to the child for IV rehydration. Give carbohydrates as soon as possible to restore liver glycogen.
- *Shigellosis*: Shigella infections can sometimes cause convulsions. Do stool culture for *shigella*.

Vitamin A deficiency

Diarrhoea reduces the absorption of, and increases the need for, vitamin A. In areas where vitamin A deficiency is already prevalent, young children with diarrhoea have an increased risk of developing eye problems. Treat if vitamin A deficiency common locally or suspected clinically.

Doses: 50,000 iu for children <6 months; 100,000 iu for children 6–12 months; 200,000 iu for children >12 months. Give dose on day 1, day 2, and 14 days later or at discharge.

Metabolic acidosis

During episodes of diarrhoea, a large amount of bicarbonate may be lost from the stool. If renal function is normal, this will be replaced. However, renal impairment due to hypovolaemia may result in the rapid development of acidosis. Poor tissue perfusion → excess lactate production. Features of metabolic acidosis are: respiratory compensation (look for deep 'Kussmaul' breathing ± tachypnoea); vomiting; low serum bicarbonate (<10 mmol/l); acidaemia (pH <7.3).

Antidiarrhoeal drugs

These agents, though commonly used, have no practical benefit and are never indicated for the treatment of acute diarrhoea in children. Some of them are dangerous.
* *Adsorbents*: (e.g. kaolin, attapulgite, smectite, activated charcoal, cholestyramine) are of no proven value in the treatment of diarrhoea.
* *Antimotility drugs*: (e.g. loperamide, diphenoxylate with atropine, tincture of opium, paregoric, codeine) reduce the frequency of stool passage in adults, but do not do so appreciably in children. Moreover, they may cause severe paralytic ileus and prolong infection by delaying the elimination of the causative organism/ toxin. Loperamide is useful in traveller's diarrhoea in adults; it should never be used in infants.

Other drugs

* *Antiemetics* (e.g. prochlorperazine, chlorpromazine, metaclopramide) should not be given since they often cause sedation and may interfere with ORS treatment. Vomiting will cease as the patient becomes hydrated.
* *Cardiac stimulants* should never be used to overcome shock and hypotension which may occur in severe dehydration with hypovolaemia. Cardiac output will be restored by fluid resuscitation.
* Blood or plasma is only indicated if there is proven shock.
* Steroids and purgatives are of no benefit and should not be used.

Prevention of diarrhoea

Proper treatment of diarrhoeal diseases is highly effective in preventing death, but has no impact on the incidence of such diseases. Teach family members to adopt preventative measures. Do not overload the mother with technical advice, but emphasize the most important points for each particular mother and child.

1. Measures that interrupt the transmission of pathogens

The infectious agents that cause diarrhoea are usually transmitted by the faeco-oral route. Measures to interrupt transmission should focus on:
• Giving only breast milk for the first 6 months of life.
• Avoiding the use of infant feeding bottles and dummies.
• Improving practices relating to the preparation and storage of weaning foods (to minimize microbial contamination).
• Using only clean water for drinking.
• Washing hands after defecation and disposal of faeces, and before preparing food.
• Disposing of all faeces in a safe manner.

2. Measures that strengthen host defences

• Continuing to breastfeed for the first 2 years of life.
• Improving a child's nutritional status by giving more nutritious food, including foods of animal origin that contain essential minerals such as zinc and other micronutrients. Giving complementary foods more often, from 3 times per day when first introduced at 6 months to 5 times per day at 12 months.
• Immunizing against measles.
• Immunizing against rotavirus.

3. How doctors can help to prevent diarrhoea

• Ensure appropriate in-service training of health facility staff.
• Make sure that all staff are giving consistent messages on diarrhoea prevention and infant feeding.
• Display promotional material on how to treat and prevent diarrhoea.
• Be a good role model (breastfeeding, hand washing, water hygiene, latrine hygiene).
• Take part in community-based activities to promote health.
• Co-ordinate efforts for disease prevention with those of relevant government programmes.

Household strategies for safe drinking water

Provision of safe drinking water requires a safe water source and a safe storage system. Clean water alone is not enough; food hygiene and hand washing are also essential measures to reduce diarrhoea.

- **Boiling**: Bring water to rolling boil for 1 min and allow to cool. Most effective sterilization method: kills most microbes even at high altitude. But it is slow, expensive, requires ~1 kg firewood/litre, contributes to deforestation, danger of scalding, and recontamination is possible.
- **Chlorination**: Add 0.5–1.0 mg/l sodium hypochlorite solution (e.g. liquid laundry bleach, but check no other ingredients), mix well, and leave for 30 mins to kill all bacteria, viruses, and most protozoa; longer exposure in tightly closed container kills *E. hystolytica* and *Giardia spp.* and reduces chlorine taste; not effective against cryptosporidia. Works less well (requires more time) when water is turbid: works best if turbid water filtered or sediment left to settle first. Taste may reduce acceptability. During disinfection, use two containers: while one is in use, the water in the other remains exposed to the chlorine increasing the effectiveness against viruses and protozoa and also reducing the chlorine taste.
- **Iodination**: 8 mg/l iodine sterilizes most microbes within 10–30 mins at 20°C; longer periods for colder water; and up to 8 h to ensure complete sterilization. Taste may reduce acceptability.
- **Sand Filtration** (0.15–0.3 mm particles ≥0.5 m deep, either in a settling tank or a specially designed receptacle): Removes particulate matter and ~50% bacteria, 20% viruses, and 50% protozoa (not cryptosporidia oocysts). Cotton cloth filters remove ~50% bacteria but less effective for viruses and oocysts. Both methods remove the copepod vector of dracunculiasis. Helpful as preliminary stage before boiling or chlorination.
- **Ceramic filters**: Require 1 μm pore size; use a coarser filter first if water turbid to prevent clogging. Relatively expensive. Ideally, boil water first.
- **Sunlight UV-irradiation**: Put 0.5–1 litre water in clean transparent container (e.g. plastic Cola bottle), shake vigorously, and expose to sunlight (e.g. on roof of hut) for 6 h. UV light kills many bacteria and protozoa, but some viruses resistant; more effective if water gets hot. Usually only suitable for small volumes; needs sunlight and preferably hot climate.
- **Flocculation/coagulation**: Not usually used domestically. Reduces turbidity, removes ~30% microbes, enhances action of chlorination or sunlight.
- **Safe carriage and storage of water**: Water is often contaminated by dirt, dust, animals, or bird droppings during collection and storage e.g. by dipping hands or containers into the water store. To minimize contamination use vessels of sufficient size, with the smallest possible opening to prevent hand entry or dipping of utensils, preferably with a cap or lid, and a spout or tap which prevents hand contact. Disinfectant such as sodium chlorite may be added to the water container (as above).

Traveller's diarrhoea

Travellers' diarrhoea affects ~20–50% of the ~12 million travellers to the tropics/subtropics annually, especially those from high-income countries; small children and young adults (perhaps because of higher risk behaviour); backpackers; campers; adventure tourists; and those staying in low-cost accommodation or cruise ships. In addition to upset business or holiday plans, longer-term consequences include chronic or persistent diarrhoea (1–3%), irritable bowel syndrome (3–10%), and Guillain–Barre syndrome (rare). The most common causes are:

Enterotoxigenic E. coli	30–80%	Salmonella spp	3–15%
Campylobacter jejuni	~20%	Giardia intestinalis	0–3%
Shigella spp	5–15%		

Management (see Fig. 6.10):
- Most episodes are self-limiting.
- Increase fluid intake. Eating e.g. broth with noodles or salty crackers with sweetened drinks will provide a balance of carbohydrate and salt.
- Oral rehydration solution (ORS) is preferable if diarrhoea frequent or severe, or if there are signs of dehydration, weakness, or muscle cramps, as it more effectively restores both salts and water deficits.
- Drinks designed for rehydration during sports activities do NOT contain the correct balance of salts for diarrhoea treatment. Sodas and fruit juices are often hyper-osmolar or have high sugar content and can make diarrhoea worse.
- Prompt antibiotic treatment reduces symptom duration (e.g. ciprofloxacin 500 mg bd PO for 3 days).
- Loperamide (4 mg PO once followed by 2 mg after each loose stool) shortens the episode in older children and adults with frequent small volume stools. (**DO NOT USE** loperamide if blood in stools, fever, tenesmus, or other signs of dysentery.)

Prevention: Avoid unpeeled fruit and uncooked vegetables, sauces which are not freshly prepared, and food prepared and handled in unhygienic conditions e.g. by street vendors. Where there is no reliable source of chlorinated water, sterilize water by boiling or with chlorine tablets, or drink bottled water from a reputable source. Avoid bottled water where the bottles are immersed in water or ice to keep them cool. Beware of ice or ice cream, which may be made using contaminated water. When trekking or in isolated places, it is advisable to carry packets of ORS and a course of treatment. Hand sanitizers are useful when handwashing is impossible.

Prophylaxis: Short-term travellers may take prophylactic bismuth subsalicylate (525 mg qds) or antibiotics such as norfloxacillin 400 mg or ciprofloxacin 500 mg daily, but both are associated with some side-effects including a risk of Clostridium difficile associated diarrhoea; early treatment of episodes is therefore preferable.

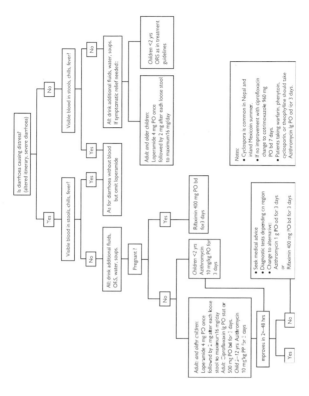

Fig. 6.10 Empirical treatment of travellers' diarrhoea.

Gastroenterology

Section editor   **Marc Mendelson**

Disorders of the mouth and pharynx

Oropharyngeal pathology is a common feature of tropical infections and is most pronounced in HIV disease and those with malnutrition.

Gingivostomatitis and mouth ulcers

Several viruses may cause gingivostomatitis (inflammation of the gums/oral mucosa), including HSV, EBV, and enteroviruses (hand, foot, and mouth disease). If primary HSV gingivostomatitis suspected, particularly in the setting of HIV, give acyclovir (📖 p 562).

Aphthous ulcers are common, and may occur in HIV seroconversion. Oral ulceration also occurs in Behçet's syndrome. Crohn's and coeliac disease, and Stevens–Johnson syndrome. *Treatment*: topical steroid e.g. adcortyl in orabase, hydrocortisone 2.5 mg lozenges, or inhaled steroid (e.g. budesonide or beclomethasone) applied directly to the ulcers; alternatively try tetracycline mouth wash (250 mg in a few ml of water, held in the mouth for 3 mins) tds for 3 days. Severe aphthous ulceration in HIV may require oral prednisolone or thalidomide. If solitary ulcer present for >3 weeks, consider biopsy of ulcer edge to exclude malignancy.

Oral candidiasis

Small, white mucosal flecks with surrounding erythema, common in HIV. Treat with nystatin liquid or amphotericin lozenges qds. In HIV treat with fluconazole 100 mg od for 1 week, especially if oesophageal candidiasis is suspected (dysphagia/odynophagia).

Oral hairy leukoplakia (OHL)

Caused by EBV and associated with advanced HIV disease, OHL appears as poorly demarcated, slightly raised, and corrugated white patches on the side of the tongue or buccal mucosa. Unlike candida, it cannot be scraped off and is painless. OHL does not usually require specific treatment and usually regresses on ARVs.

Gingivitis

Periodontal disease and caries are a major problem in developing countries; prevention focuses on encouraging oral better hygiene. Gingival changes may also occur with anaerobic infection (Vincent's angina), drugs (phenytoin, cyclosporin, or nifedipine), AML, and pregnancy. Haemorrhagic gingivitis may occur in vitamin C deficiency (scurvy). Gingivorrhoea may follow envenoming by certain snake species.

Glossitis

Glossitis is a feature of iron deficiency, vitamin B deficiency, and tropical sprue. Overgrowth of papillae and *Aspergillus niger* result in a black, hairy tongue.

Pharyngitis

Typically due to Streptococci, viruses, or diphtheria. Less commonly may occur in Lassa fever or rabies, and rarely, following ingestion of *Fasciola hepatica*. In developing countries with high incidence of acute rheumatic fever, a single dose benzathine benzylpenicilin 1.2 million units IM decreases the risk of acute rheumatic fever from 2.8 to 0.2%, and should be considered in children with sore throat (esp. children >3 yr old). Necrobacillosis (Lemierre's disease) presents with severe pharyngitis with spread to neck, thrombosis of internal jugular vein, ± embolization of infected thrombus; treatment is with IV penicillin + metronidazole.

Acute necrotizing ulcerative gingivostomatitis

Painful ulceration of the mouth with halitosis and gingivorrhoea. Predisposing factors include malnutrition, HIV, poor oral hygiene, and smoking. Treat with warm saline mouth washes and metronidazole 200 mg PO tds plus penicillin 500 mg PO qds for 5–7 days.

Other benign lesions of the mouth

Salivary gland hypertrophy is common in malnourished children but may also be associated with *Ascaris lumbricoides* infection and as part of diffuse inflammatory lymphocytosis syndrome (DILS) in HIV. Angular stomatitis is commonly a feature of iron-deficiency anaemia, HIV, and riboflavin deficiency.

Malignant lesions of the mouth and pharynx

Buccal squamous cell carcinoma (associated with tobacco, chewing betel nut, ± alcohol) and Burkitt's lymphoma (due to EBV infection) are common, especially in India, S.E. Asia, and tropical Africa. Nasopharyngeal carcinoma (due to EBV infection) is common in the Far East and S. China. Malignant change may be preceded by leukoplakia and epithelial atrophy. Optimum management and outcome rely on early diagnosis. Consider malignancy in chronic (>3 weeks), solitary lesions: examine for cervical lymphadenopathy and biopsy lesion ± lymph nodes. KS causes purple lesions, often on the hard palate. It is usually associated with HIV; treatment is ART therapy.

Cancrum oris (Noma)   PAEDIATRIC NOTE

A serious and often fatal condition in which gangrenous stomatitis rapidly spreads to involve the palate and face following anaerobic infection. It occurs mainly in young, malnourished African children. Management requires wound debridement and antisepsis, antibiotics (IV penicillin plus metronidazole), and nutritional rehabilitation (± surgical reconstruction).

Upper GI tract symptoms

Dysphagia and odynophagia

Dysphagia and odynophagia are difficulty and pain in swallowing, respectively. Dysphagia that has progressed from solids to liquids implies severe narrowing of the oesophagus. Endoscopy ± biopsy is the investigation of choice where available; barium swallow is an alternative. In HIV, a trial of empirical fluconazole 200 mg OD for 2 weeks for oesophageal candidiasis reduces the need for endoscopy.

Dyspepsia

Epigastric or retrosternal discomfort associated with eating. The history often provides a clue to the cause (see box). Causes include peptic ulcer disease, gastro-oesophageal reflux, dysmotility, drugs, and parasitic infections of the GI tract (including hookworm, *Taenia*, *Ascaris*, *Giardia*, and *Entamoeba histolytica*). Suspect malignancy if age >45 y, weight loss, dysphagia, vomiting, haematemesis, or anaemia.

Management

1. Review any drugs that may cause dyspepsia.
2. Trial of antacids, unless malignancy suspected.
3. Endoscopy or barium meal if malignancy or peptic ulcer suspected.
4. Stool microscopy if gastrointestinal parasites suspected. *Note:* presence of parasites does not exclude other causes of dyspepsia.
5. Stop smoking and avoid alcohol.

Helicobacter pylori and peptic ulcer

Helicobacter pylori are motile, Gram-negative rods that live in the mucus layer of the stomach. In developing countries *H. pylori* colonization is almost universal by age 20. Clinical associations include:

- *Peptic ulcer disease* (PUD): Up to 90% patients with duodenal ulcer and >50% patients with gastric ulcer are colonized with *H. pylori*.
- *Gastric cancer*: *H. pylori* causes intestinal metaplasia and atrophic gastritis which are risk factors for adenocarcinoma of the stomach.
- *Mucosa-associated lymphoid tissue (MALT) lymphoma*: Generally, a benign monoclonal proliferation of lymphocytes; tumour histology and clinical features improve with *H. pylori* eradication.
- *Non-ulcer dyspepsia*: The role of *H. pylori* in this condition remains uncertain; trials of *H. pylori* eradication have shown little benefit.

Diagnosis: Options include endoscopy + biopsy, serology, urea breath test and stool antigen test, depending on resources.

Eradication therapy: Proton pump inhibitor or Bismuth-based regimens with 2 antibiotics, e.g. oral omeprazole 20 mg od (or bismuth subsalicylate 2 tabs qds) + amoxycillin 1 g bd (or tetracycline 500 mg bd) + metronidazole 400 mg bd (or clarithromycin 500 mg bd) for 7 days.

Dysphagia: key questions in the history

- Can fluid be drunk normally?
  Yes → suspect stricture (benign or malignant)
  No → possible motility disorder
- Is the dysphagia constant and painful?
  Yes → suspect malignant stricture
- Is it difficult to initiate swallowing?
  Yes → suspect bulbar palsy, especially if swallowing causes cough
- Does the neck bulge or gurgle upon swallowing?
  Yes → suspect pharyngeal pouch
- Is the patient HIV infected?
  Yes → suspect oesophageal candidiasis
- Are there signs of systemic infection or illness?
  Yes → may be manifestation of systemic disease

Causes of dysphagia

- *Malignancy*: carcinoma of the oesophagus, stomach, or pharynx.
- *Extrinsic compression*: mediastinal lymphadenopathy, carcinoma of the lung, retrosternal goitre, left atrial enlargement.
- *HIV-associated*: candidiasis, CMV, HSV, severe aphthous ulceration.
- *Motility disorders*: achalasia, Chagas disease, bulbar/pseudobulbar palsy (incl. bulbar poliomyelitis), diffuse oesophageal spasm, myasthenia gravis, syringobulbia, systemic sclerosis.
- *Benign strictures*: peptic stricture, ingestion of caustics, oesophageal web, iron deficiency anaemia (Plummer–Vinson syndrome).
- *Pharyngeal pouch*.
- *Others*: trauma, foreign body (e.g. bezoar, swallowed fish or animal bone), anxiety (globus hystericus).

Causes of dyspepsia and their typical clinical features*

- *Peptic ulcer disease*: epigastric pain, night waking, and relief by eating food, drinking milk, or taking antacids.
- *Gastro-oesophageal reflux*: retrosternal discomfort, heartburn, and regurgitation/acid brash. Worse lying flat or after large meals.
- *Dysmotility*: early satiety, bloating, and nausea.
- *Drugs*: e.g. NSAIDs, calcium antagonists, nitrates, pyrazinamide.

* Note that although the history often gives a clue to the cause of dyspepsia, it does not replace further investigation of specific causes where indicated.

Disorders of the oesophagus

Gastro-oesophageal reflux disease (GORD)

Heartburn and regurgitation with a bitter, acid taste (acid brash), particularly when lying flat, are the hallmarks of gastro-oesophageal reflux.

Diagnosis: is usually clinical; barium swallow may identify a hiatus hernia.

Management: stop smoking, lose weight if obese, and raise the head of the bed. Advise antacids after meals and at bedtime. Severe cases require H_2 receptor antagonists (e.g. cimetidine 100 mg at night up to 400 mg QID) or proton pump inhibitors (e.g. omeprazole 20–40 mg at night) ± metoclopramide.

Hiatus hernia

Herniation of the stomach through the oesophageal hiatus of the diaphragm. Often asymptomatic; may predispose to GORD or present with acute chest and/or epigastric pain. A fluid level behind the heart on erect CXR, or on Ba meal, is diagnostic. Management is as for GORD.

Columnar-lined (Barrett's) oesophagus

Columnar-lined oesophagus (CLO) represents the severe end of the spectrum of GORD in which there is columnar metaplasia of a segment of the oesophagus. Its importance derives from the risk of progression to oesophageal adenocarcinoma.

Management: adequate treatment of GORD is recommended but often difficult to achieve. Where facilities allow, regular follow-up is advised, with repeated endoscopy + biopsy to detect malignancy early.

Oesophageal cancer

Oesophageal cancer usually affects adults (males: females ~3:1) aged >30 years. Incidence is highest in central/east Africa, Iran, southeast Asia, and northern China. Pre-malignant associations include columnar-lined (Barrett's) oesophagus (for adenocarcinoma), and Plummer–Vinson syndrome and achalasia (linked to squamous cell carcinoma). Other risk factors include smoking, alcohol, and malnutrition.

Clinical features: dysphagia, weight loss, retrosternal pain (± lymphadenopathy). Extensive disease → coughing (due to aspiration or development of oesophago-tracheal fistula), aspiration pneumonia, Horner's syndrome, recurrent laryngeal nerve palsy (hoarse voice).

Management and prognosis: usually rapidly progressive; many patients present late so <5% 5-yr survival. Resection for early stage adenocarcinoma → 5-year survival of >80% if tumour confined to the mucosa, and 50–80% if submucosa involved. Neoadjuvant chemoradiotherapy slightly improves survival in adenocarcinoma. Palliative treatment includes nutrition (oesophageal stenting often required), pain relief, and treatment of complications including aspiration pneumonia.

Gastric cancer

The incidence of gastric cancer varies throughout the tropics; it is especially common in Costa Rica and N.E. Brazil. Risk factors include chronic gastritis, bile reflux, *H. pylori*, pernicious anaemia, ingestion of corrosives, and diet — high salt intake, lack of fresh fruit, and ingestion of toxic nitrosamines from fish.

Clinical features: include dyspepsia, weight loss, malaena, anaemia and abdominal mass. In metastatic disease there may be hepatomegally, deranged liver function tests, lymphadenopathy (left supraclavicular lymphadenopathy = Virchow's node), umbilical deposits (Sister Mary Joseph's nodule), or peritonism.

Diagnosis: requires biopsy for histology and staging.

Management: surgical resection offers the only hope of cure. Palliation aims to relieve pain and obstruction and control haemorrhage.

Upper GI bleeding

Assessment

Haematemesis and/or malaena indicate upper GI bleeding, which may be due to a number of causes (see box). Initial assessment should include a brief history and examination to assess the severity and likely cause. Ask about previous GI bleeds, history of PUD, liver disease, varices, dysphagia, vomiting or weight loss, comorbidity, alcohol, and drugs. Look for signs of liver disease and portal hypotension; do a rectal examination to check for malaena.

- **Mild to moderate bleed**: pulse and BP normal, age <60 y, insignificant co-morbidity, and Hb >10 g/dl (unless chronic anaemia present).
- **Severe bleed**: age >60 y, pulse >100 bpm, systolic BP <100 mmHg, Hb <10 g/dl, significant co-morbidity.

Immediate management

- IV access (two large bore venous cannulae; central venous access to guide fluid resuscitation if severe).
- Take blood for FBC, U&E, LFT, clotting, group and save/cross-match.
- Fluid resuscitate with normal saline or colloid while waiting for blood (if blood required); in dire emergency, use O Rhesus –ve blood.
- Correct clotting abnormalities (vitamin K, FFP, platelets).
- Catheterize if severe and monitor urine output to ensure >0.5 ml/kg/h.
- Monitor vital signs closely.
- Consider urgent endoscopy, and notify surgeons of all serious bleeds on admission; keep patient nil by mouth until stable.

Further management

Further management depends on severity, response to initial treatment, and the underlying diagnosis.

- High-dose IV proton pump inhibitor therapy reduces re-bleeding (but has little effect on mortality).
- Endoscopy helps define cause of bleeding, assess risk of re-bleeding, and plan treatment; repeat endoscopy may be required for rebleeding.
- Endoscopic therapy may be possible for some lesions (e.g. adrenaline injection, sclerotherapy, variceal banding).
- If stable 4–6 h post-endoscopy, allow to eat and drink.
- Treat peptic ulcer disease with proton pump inhibitors and eradicate *H. pylori*. Avoid NSAIDs if possible.
- Repeat endoscopy at 6 weeks for gastric ulcers to ensure response to proton pump inhibitors and exclude gastric cancer.

Oesophageal varices

In portal hypertension, portal-systemic shunts develop in the lower oeso-phagus → dilated oesophageal veins. Variceal bleeding occurs in 20–50% cirrhotic patients, usually within 2 years of diagnosis. Mortality from a first bleed is ~50% and is related to severity of liver disease. Common causes include liver cirrhosis, schistosomiasis, portal vein thrombosis, and Budd–Chiari syndrome (hepatic vein thrombosis).

Management of acute variceal bleed

- Assess and resuscitate as for any upper GI bleed (see opposite page).
- Protect airway: may require intubation and ventilation if uncontrolled bleeding, encephalopathy, hypoxia, or aspiration pneumonia.
- Control bleeding by endoscopic variceal band ligation or sclerotherapy. Balloon tamponade with a Sengstaken–Blakemore tube may be used for emergency short-term control of bleeding; ideally, patient should be intubated and ventilated to reduce risk of aspiration and to aid passage.
- Give octreotide (50 mcg/h IV) for 2–5 days.
- Correct clotting abnormalities (FFP ± vitamin K, platelets).
- Give antibiotics to reduce risk of bacterial sepsis, e.g. ciprofloxacin 500 mg bd for 1 week.

Primary and secondary prevention of variceal bleeding

- Endoscopic variceal band ligation is most effective if available; sclerotherapy also works.
- Reduce portal pressure with propranolol 40–80 mg bd (and/or isosorbide mononitrate 20 mg bd).
- Manage the underlying cause, especially schistosomiasis — periportal fibrosis regresses after treatment. Advise to abstain from alcohol.

Causes of upper GI bleeding

Most common causes
- Peptic ulcer disease.
- Gastritis/gastric erosions.
- Mallory–Weiss tear.
- Oesophageal varices.
- Oesophagitis.
- Duodenitis.
- Malignancy.
- Drugs (NSAIDs, anticoagulants, steroids).

Rarer causes
- Portal hypertensive gastropathy.
- Angiodysplasia.
- Dieulafoy lesion.
- Bleeding disorders.
- Aortoenteric fistula.
- Haemobilia (bleeding from biliary tree).

Acute abdomen

Someone who becomes acutely ill and in whom symptoms and signs are chiefly related to the abdomen has an acute abdomen. Thorough history and examination are essential — abdominal pain may be misinterpreted as body aches and treatment given for malaria, only for peritonitis to be found later. Prompt laparotomy is sometimes essential: *repeated examination is the key to making the decision.*

The most common causes of an acute abdomen are given in Fig. 7.1.

Clinical syndromes that usually require laparotomy

1. **Organ rupture** (e.g. spleen, aorta, ectopic pregnancy). There may be shock and abdominal swelling. Note history of trauma (especially if pre-existing splenomegaly, but note splenic rupture may occur weeks after trauma, and in the absence of trauma).
2. **Peritonitis** (e.g. due to perforated ulcer, diverticulum, appendix, bowel, or gall bladder). The patient lies still and has signs of shock, abdominal tenderness, board-like abdominal rigidity, and absent bowel sounds. Acute pancreatitis may present similarly but does not require laparotomy, so check serum amylase.

Syndromes for which laparotomy may not be indicated

1. **Local peritonitis** e.g. cholecystitis, salpingitis, appendicitis (the latter *will* need surgery). If abscess formation suspected (swelling, swinging fever, ↑WCC) look for sentinel loop on plain AXR; do abdominal USS or CT if available. Drainage may be percutaneous (USS or CT guided) or by laparotomy.
2. **Colic** is pain which regularly waxes and wanes due to muscular spasm of a hollow viscus (e.g. gut, ureter, uterus, or gall bladder), causing the patient to be restless, unlike peritonitis.
3. **Bowel obstruction** causes colicky abdominal pain and distension, vomiting, and (often absolute) constipation, with active 'tinkling' bowel sounds (c.f. reduced bowel sounds in functional ileus). Causes include adhesions (previous surgery), herniae (internal or external), sigmoid/caecal volvulus, tumours, intussusception, TB, and ascariasis. AXR showing dilated loops bowel ± fluid levels helps to distinguish small and large bowel obstruction.

Immediate management

- Fluid resuscitate with normal saline, colloid, or blood as appropriate. Anaesthesia compounds shock, so resuscitate properly before taking to theatre — unless losing blood faster than it can be replaced (e.g. ruptured ectopic pregnancy, leaking abdominal aortic aneurysm).
- Take bloods for FBC, U&E, LFT, Ca^{2+}, amylase, culture, cross-match.
- Insert an NG tube and keep patient nil by mouth; IV maintenance fluids.
- Consider erect CXR, AXR, ± ECG.
- Give broad-spectrum empiric antibiotics initially if infection suspected, and rationalize therapy later in light of investigations and progress.

Non-surgical causes of an acute abdomen

Several non-surgical conditions may present with an acute abdomen. The most common causes are listed in the box below.

Medical causes of acute abdominal symptoms

- Gastroenteritis.
- Typhoid.
- Malaria.
- Myocardial infarction.
- Cholera.
- Porphyria.
- Heroin addiction.

- Pneumonia.
- UTI.
- Sickle cell crisis.
- Polyarteritis nodosa.
- Herpes zoster.
- Thyroid storm.
- Lead colic.

- Diabetic ketoacidosis.
- Abdomino-peritoneal TB.
- *Yersinia enterocolitica.*
- Fitzhugh-Curtis syndrome (*Chlamydia*).
- Pneumococcal peritonitis.
- Henoch–Schonlein purpura.
- Irritable bowel syndrome.

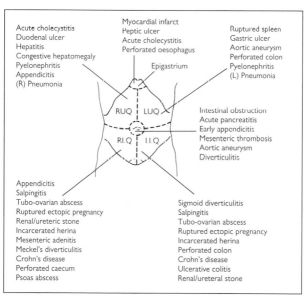

Fig. 7.1 Causes of acute abdominal pain.

Appendicitis

Appendicectomy is the most common emergency abdominal operation. Without surgery, appendicitis may progress to gangrene, perforation, peritonitis, and death. Mortality is highest at the extremes of age, but also in young adults in malaria-endemic areas, where non-specific symptoms may be misinterpreted.

Aetiology Obstruction due to lymphoid hyperplasia or faecolith; super-infection is usually bacterial (rarely, amoebae, *S. mansoni, S. stercoralis, T. trichiura, A. lumbricoides,* or *Taenia* spp. implicated).

Clinical features Increasing central abdominal colic, usually shifting to the right iliac fossa (RIF) depending on the anatomical position of the appendix. Anorexia is common; vomiting or diarrhea may occur. Common signs are flushing with mild fever, tachycardia, RIF tenderness, guarding, rebound tenderness, and Rosving's sign (LIF palpation causes pain in RIF). An appendix mass or abscess may be palpable, due to encasement of the appendix or pus in omentum and bowel loops.

Diagnosis Clinical. Examine the patient repeatedly, since the severity may change. Do a PR (painful on right side), and a PV in women to exclude pelvic disease.

Differential diagnosis See box. USS may differentiate between an appendix mass and an abscess.

Management

1. Prompt appendicectomy is indicated to prevent perforation, unless appendix mass present or surgery otherwise contraindicated. Give metronidazole 500 mg IV or 1 g PR plus cefuroxime 1.5 g IV prior to surgery. Surgery is well tolerated during pregnancy, whereas perforation carries a 30% foetal mortality.

2. If appendix mass present, manage conservatively initially: give metronidazole 1 g PR tds plus either gentamicin 3–5 mg/kg IV daily or chloramphenicol 12.5 mg/kg IV q6 h. Monitor vital signs and size of appendix mass closely. Surgery is indicated if patient's condition deteriorates. Any abscess should be drained. Elective appendicectomy is carried out at ~3 months, once inflammatory adhesions have subsided.

Mesenteric adenitis   PAEDIATRIC NOTE

A viral inflammation of the mesenteric lymph nodes affecting children. Suspect it if there is high fever, vomiting, a history of URTI, and cervical lymphadenopathy. Abdominal signs are usually less severe than in appendicitis and usually subside within 48 h.

Differential diagnosis of RIF pain

Inflammation	Clinical features
Mesenteric adenitis (children)	High fever, vomiting, cervical nodes; improvement with observation.
Meckel's diverticulitis	Usually discovered at appendicectomy; rarely bleeds or causes obstruction.
Caecal diverticulum	May be inflamed, perforate, or bleed; blood PR cannot be attributed to other causes.
Inflammatory masses	?Abdominal mass, weight loss.
TB	Other systemic signs of TB; ascites common.
Crohn's disease/UC	Systemic, eye, joint, and/or anorectal manifestations.
Worm infection	Worms or ova in stool. Chronic history ± weight loss; pruritis ani.
Amoebic colitis	Diarrhoea with blood and mucus; trophozoites in hot stool; patient may be critically ill.
Malignancy	
Lymphoma	Weight loss; lymphoma elsewhere.
Caecal cancer	Anaemia, weight loss, intermittent pain.
Large bowel tumour	Diarrhoea; blood PR; eventually obstruction with caecal distension.
Genital tract pathology	
Salpingitis	Vaginal discharge; pelvic pain; tender on PV.
Ectopic pregnancy	Amenorrhoea, vaginal bleeding, abdominal distension; may be shocked; positive pregnancy test.
Pelvic abscess	Previous salpingitis; ? history of illegal abortion.
Ovarian torsion or bleeding	Severe pain, minimal signs; requires USS. Ovarian cyst/fibroid.
Testicular torsion	Testis is swollen and very tender ± referred pain.
Intra-abdominal testis	Torsion or malignancy (teratoma/seminoma)

Peritonitis

Peritonitis in the tropics is most commonly due to appendicitis, perforated duodenal ulcer, tubo-ovarian infection, typhoid perforation, or amoebic colitis. Consider TB peritonitis if chronic, esp. if HIV positive.

Clinical features: The patient is immobile, anxious, and in obvious pain. There may be fever, sweating, tachycardia, and tachypnoea with use of accessory breathing muscles. Sepsis results in a hyperdynamic circulation initially (warm peripheries, bounding pulse), but shock (cold peripheries, thready pulse) may develop with extravasation of fluid into the peritoneal cavity. Abdominal findings include distended, rigid abdomen which moves poorly with respiration; rebound tenderness, guarding, and absent bowel sounds. In chemical peritonitis (bile, gastric acid, or pancreatic enzymes) pain is intense; the abdomen may be so rigid that distension is minimized. Signs of peritonism may be less in the very young or critically ill (e.g. post-op). Abdominal signs are usually mild in cirrhotic patients with infected ascites (spontaneous bacterial peritonitis).

Diagnosis: is clinical; CXR may show gas under the diaphragm; AXR may show fluid between thickened loops of bowel or distended bowel and fluid levels. USS may show intraperitoneal fluid or collections/abscesses. Free fluid in the abdomen may be aspirated with a fine (21-gauge) needle. Send the fluid for microscopy (pus cells suggest bacterial peritonitis, lymphocytes suggest TB) and protein (to confirm fluid is an exudate). FBC, CRP, U&E, serum amylase, blood cultures are helpful. Diagnostic laparotomy may be required in severe cases.

Treatment
- Immediate management/resuscitation as for acute abdomen (📖 p 278).
- Insert an NG tube and keep patient nil by mouth.
- Give broad-spectrum antibiotics (e.g. IV cefuroxime 750 mg tds or IV ceftriaxone 1 g od, *plus* IV metronidazole 500 mg tds).
- Monitor vital signs and urine output closely.
- Where possible, drain intra-abdominal collections under USS guidance. If USS not available, or if the patient's condition deteriorates, drainage by laparotomy is required.
- In the absence of contraindications, laparotomy is usually indicated for severe, generalized peritonitis.

Female genital tract sepsis

Tubo-ovarian sepsis usually causes local pelvic peritonitis. Many cases may be managed with antibiotics alone — but if patient's condition deteriorates, pelvic mass expands, or perforated uterus suspected (e.g. septic abortion), urgent laparotomy ± hysterectomy is indicated. Rupture of tubo-ovarian abscesses carries a high mortality.

Amoebic colitis

Failure to respond to metronidazole (see 📖 p 222) within 48 h suggests transmural disease ± ischaemic necrosis for which laparotomy indicated.

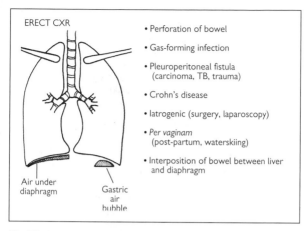

Fig. 7.2 Causes of gas under the diaphragm.

Plain abdominal X-rays (AXR)

These are rarely diagnostic. They are most useful in GI obstruction. Gas patterns are best seen on supine images; erect films may demonstrate fluid levels better. Free intraperitoneal gas (signifying perforation) is best seen as air under the diaphragm on erect CXRs. Small bowel is recognized by its central position and valvulae conniventes, which reach from one wall to the other. Large bowel is more peripheral and the folds (haustrae) go only part of the way across the lumen.

Where to look

1. Gas patterns: look for dilated stomach, small intestine, or colon. Normal diameter of the small intestine is 2.5 cm, colon 5 cm. Dilated small intestine occurs with obstruction and paralytic ileus. Dilated large bowel occurs with obstruction, ileus, and toxic dilatation. Local peritonitis may cause a sentinel loop of intraluminal gas (localized ileus) giving a clue to the site of pathology.

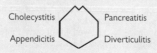

   You must explain any gas outside the stomach, small intestine, and colon. It could be a pneumoperitoneum, or gas in the urinary tract or biliary tree.

2. Biliary tree and urinary tract. The ureters pass near the tips of the lumbar transverse processes, cross the sacro-iliac joints down to the ischial spine, and turn medially to join the bladder. Look for calcification in the gall bladder, kidney, or ureter.

3. Bones: look for scoliosis, degenerative disease, metastatic deposits (osteolytic or osteoblastic), Paget's disease.

4. Soft tissue: look for position of liver, spleen, kidneys, bladder.

Acute pancreatitis

Acute pancreatitis is rare in most tropical countries. Single attacks may occur, or on background of chronic pancreatitis. Progression to haemorrhagic, necrotizing disease may be very rapid with high mortality.

Causes: Gallstones (~50% cases), alcohol abuse (20–25%), other causes of duct obstruction (e.g. *Ascaris*, tumour, hydatid cysts in common bile duct), drugs (e.g. stavudine, sodium stibogluconate and meglumine antimoniate, thiazides, steroids, tetracycline), viruses (mumps, coxsackie, EBV, HAV, HBV), hypercalcaemia, hyperlipidaemia, trauma, scorpion venom, autoimmune diseases (e.g. PAN), hypothermia.

Clinical features: Abdominal pain and vomiting (90% cases) + ↑ amylase/lipase are typical. Peritonism may develop, but as the pancreas is retroperitoneal, abdominal signs are often mild. Jaundice may occur due to oedema around the common bile duct. Severe disease may cause periumbilical (Cullen's sign) or flank (Grey Turner's sign) discoloration.

Investigation: Check serum amylase/lipase (levels peak early and ↓ over 3–4 days), U&Es, Ca^{2+}, glucose, fasting lipids, ABG. Exclude other causes of acute abdomen (📖 p 279). USS for gallstones. If patient deteriorating with severe pancreatitis, CT may show pancreatic necrosis requiring surgery.

Prognosis: assessed using modified Glasgow criteria (see box).

Treatment
- Immediate management/resuscitation as for acute abdomen (📖 p 278).
- Severe pain requires strong analgesia (e.g. morphine 10 mg q4 h plus prochlorperazine 12.5 mg q8 h IM).
- Consider broad-spectrum antibiotic prophylaxis ± surgical necrosectomy in very severe cases (e.g. >30% pancreatic necrosis on CT).
- Following recovery, consider cholecystectomy if gallstones implicated as cause.

Complications
- **Early** = organ failure: acute respiratory distress syndrome, acute renal failure, DIC, hypocalcaemia (may require albumin replacement or 10 ml of 10% calcium gluconate IV slowly), transient hyperglycaemia.
- **Late** (>1 week): pancreatic pseudocyst (may resolve spontaneously or require surgical drainage into bowel; if it becomes infected, it requires drainage). A few patients develop persisting DM.

Chronic pancreatitis
Destruction of the pancreas with atrophy results in some permanent loss of exocrine and endocrine function. This may be characterized by pain, diabetes, and malabsorption with steatorrhoea. 3 main types of chronic pancreatitis are recognized: chronic obstructive, minimal change (often post-acute pancreatitis), and chronic calcific pancreatitis (📖 see Chapter 6, p 244).

Modified Glasgow prognostic score for acute pancreatitis

The following factors are associated with a poor prognosis. The greater the number of factors, the poorer the prognosis.

- Glucose >10 mmol/l.
- Urea >16 mmol/l.
- ALT/AST >200 u/l.
- LDH >600 iu/l.
- pO₂ <8 kpa (60 mmHg).
- Albumin <32 g/l.
- Calcium <2.0 mmol/l.

Severe acute pancreatitis is suggested by the presence of ≥3 factors. Outcome is also influenced by the cause of the inflammation.

These criteria have been validated for pancreatitis caused by gallstones and alcohol (c.f. Ranson's criteria which have only been validated for alcohol-induced pancreatitis).

Right upper quadrant (RUQ) pain

RUQ pain is usually due to liver or gallbladder pathology; other causes include those shown in the box opposite. Important tropical causes include AIDS cholangiopathy, amoebic liver abscess, hydatid liver disease.

Gallstones and biliary colic

Impaction of a gallstone in the gallbladder outlet causing severe, constant pain lasting up to several hours, radiating to the interscapular region, and associated with nausea and vomiting. Complications include:

- Acute cholecystitis: fever ± local peritonism, tender, palpable gallbladder especially on inspiration (positive Murphy's sign), and/or jaundice.
- Ascending cholangitis: RUQ pain, fever, and jaundice (Charcot's triad).

Management: Strong analgesia ± antispasmodics (e.g. hyoscine butylbromide 20 mg IV/IM, repeated after 30 min if necessary). Treat cholecystitis and cholangitis with broad-spectrum antibiotics e.g. cefuroxime 750 mg IV tds + metronidazole 500 mg IV (or 1 g PR) tds, followed by cholecystectomy when the patient's condition allows.

AIDS cholangiopathy

A syndrome of RUQ pain (>90%) and cholestasis ± low-grade fever. Patients occasionally present with asymptomatic cholestasis. Cryptosporidium, cytomegalovirus, and microsporidiosis are the most common causes, but often no organism is identified. 4 types are recognized: papillary stenosis, sclerosing cholangitis-like, combined (>50% cases), and extrahepatic duct strictures (include malignancy). HAART markedly improves prognosis.

Amoebic liver abscess

Amoebic liver abscess (ALA) is the most common form of extra-intestinal amoebiasis (📖 p 223). It may complicate acute amoebic dysentery (~10%) or present months after exposure. ~70% recall no history of diarrhoea.

Clinical presentation: Usually acute (over 2–7 days) with fever, rigors, sweats, and RUQ ± right shoulder tip pain, ± vomiting; left lobe abscesses often → LUQ pain. May also present subacutely with dull RUQ ache, weight loss, fatigue, low-grade pyrexia, and anaemia; antimalarial/ antibiotic treatment may → more subacute presentation. Clinical signs include hepatomegally (often tender); 'punch tenderness' may be elicited if abscess concealed beneath the ribs. Extreme tenderness or oedema of the abdominal wall or intercostal space suggests imminent rupture. There is seldom jaundice or ascites. Right-sided pleural effusion/empyema/lung collapse may occur due to rupture into the pleura. Rupture of a left lobe abscess into the pericardium is usually rapidly fatal.

Diagnosis

- Blood tests characteristically show neutrophilia, ↑ESR, ±↑ALT/ALP.
- CXR may show raised hemi-diaphragm ± pleural reaction and/or basal atelectasis.
- USS characteristically shows a large (usually unilocular) necrotic lesion with some internal debris. During the early 'amoebic hepatitis' stage of the disease, USS may miss the lesion: repeat USS may be required.
- E. histolytica serology is +ve in >95% patients after the first week.
- Stool microscopy is +ve for cysts in 50% (culture = 75%).
- Indications for aspiration are shown in the box. Abscess fluid is odourless and reddish-brown (resembles 'anchovy sauce') rather than yellow pus. Microscopy shows debris (c.f. pus cells in pyogenic liver abscess) and Gram stain does not show organisms; rarely E histolytica trophozoites may be seen.
- Beware misdiagnosing acute ALA as acute cholecystitis or appendicitis.

Management

- Drug therapy is sufficient to cause healing without scarring in most cases. Give metronidazole 800 mg tds (or tinidazole 2 g od) PO for 5 days, followed by diloxanide furoate 500 mg tds (or paromomycin 500 mg tds) PO for 10 days for intraluminal E histolytica eradication.
- Indications for percutaneous drainage are given in the box. Drains may be removed when drainage is minimal (usually after 2–3 days).
- Follow up ALA clinically. (Note: USS may show large liver defects even after successful cure.)

Causes of RUQ pain

Gastrointestinal/hepatobiliary
Acute hepatitis
Amoebic liver abscess
Hydatid liver disease
Liver tumours
AIDS cholangiopathy
Gallstones (biliary colic)
Cholecystitis
Cholangitis
Liver flukes

Other
RLL pneumonia
Right heart failure
Pyelonephritis
Duodenal ulcer
Trichuriasis (whipworm)

Indications for drainage of amoebic liver abscess

- Large left lobe abscess (risk of rupture into pericardium).
- Severely ill patients in whom rupture is considered imminent either clinically or on USS.
- Diagnostic uncertainty — diagnostic aspirate for Gram stain/culture.*
- Lack of response to drug therapy after 3–4 days.

* Adequate drainage is usually indicated for pyogenic liver abscess.

Hydatid disease

Echinococcus granulosus and *E. multilocularis* are responsible for causing cystic hydatid disease and alveolar hydatid disease, respectively.

Cystic hydatid disease

E. granulosus is a small (3–6 mm) cestode (tapeworm) that lives in the small intestine of dogs (also jackals, foxes). Eggs passed in canine faeces are infective to humans. Following ingestion, eggs develop into oncospheres which penetrate the intestinal mucosa and pass in the blood or lymphatics to host viscera including the liver (50–70%), lungs (20–30%), other organs, and peritoneal cavity. Oncospheres encyst in host viscera developing into mature larval cysts. These may be multiple and reach massive proportions.

Clinical features: Liver cysts grow ~1 cm a year, presenting as masses rather than abscesses. Patients may be asymptomatic or present with symptoms related to expansive growth of cysts, including abdominal pain, hepatomegaly, fever, and jaundice. Lung cysts may present when the cyst contents rupture into an airway and are coughed up.

Complications: Cyst rupture may be accompanied by life-threatening anaphylactic shock; conversely, other cysts collapse or disappear spontaneously. Cholangitis may occur due to rupture into the biliary tree. Pyogenic abscesses may form due to bacterial superinfection of cysts.

Diagnosis: The characteristic appearance of cysts on imaging (USS, CT, or MRI) is usually sufficient. Serology may aid diagnosis.

Management

- Most cysts are amenable to percutaneous aspiration-injection-reaspiration (PAIR) treatment (see box). PAIR cure rates are >95%.
- In addition to PAIR, some authorities recommend albendazole 400 mg bd PO for 1–6 months, starting before and continuing after drainage.
- Albendazole treatment alone is not sufficiently reliable, although some individuals with multiple cysts are treated with prolonged courses.
- Surgical removal may be indicated for cysts not amenable to the PAIR approach, especially if at risk of rupture or exerting pressure effects.

Alveolar hydatid disease

Alveolar hydatid disease occurs mainly in the northern hemisphere. *E. multilocularis* causes aggressive local tissue invasion by lateral budding of cysts ± metastasis to other parts of the body (~10% patients to CNS, lungs, bone, and eyes). Liver complications include cholangitis, Budd–Chiari syndrome, and portal hypertension. Due to the aggressive nature of the lesions, many are misdiagnosed clinically/radiologically as malignnancy. Mortality untreated is high (>60% at 10 yrs). Operable cases require wide surgical resection to ensure complete resection of the cyst. Adjuvant albendazole was shown to be of benefit in one case series. In inoperable cases, albendazole provides arrest or cure in some patients.

Percutaneous aspiration-injection-reaspiration (PAIR)

- **Puncture** cyst under USS or CT guidance.
- **Aspirate** ~30% of cyst fluid volume.
- **Inject*** an equal volume of a scolicidal agent such as hypertonic saline (30% saline = 300 g NaCl/litre) or 95% ethanol into the cyst.
- **Reaspirate** cyst contents after 30 minutes.

* **NOTE:** Injection of a scolicidal agent is contraindicated if cyst fluid is bile stained suggesting communication with the biliary tree.

Prevention of hydatid disease   PUBLIC HEALTH NOTE

- Education and hygiene to avoid exposure to/ingestion of dog faeces.
- In hyperendemic populations, periodic treatment of dogs (incl. wild and stray dogs) with praziquantel helps to prevent/control human disease.
- Strict control of livestock slaughtering and disposal of organs helps restrict the access of dogs to potentially contaminated viscera.

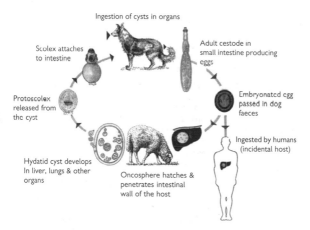

Ingestion of cysts in organs

Scolex attaches to intestine

Adult cestode in small intestine producing eggs

Protoscolex released from the cyst

Embryonated egg passed in dog faeces

Ingested by humans (incidental host)

Hydatid cyst develops in liver, lungs & other organs

Oncosphere hatches & penetrates intestinal wall of the host

Fig. 7.3 Life cycle of *E. granulosus*. (Adapted from G. Piekarski, Medical parasitology in plates, 1962, with kind permission of Bayer pharmaceuticals.)

Liver disease

Jaundice

Bilirubin is formed from the breakdown of haemoglobin. It is conjugated with glucuronic acid by hepatocytes, making it water-soluble. Conjugated bilirubin is secreted into the bile and passes out into the gut. Some of it is taken up again by the liver (enterohepatic circulation) and the rest is converted to urobilinogen by gut bacteria. Urobilinogen is either reabsorbed and excreted by the kidneys, or converted to stercobilin, which colours faeces brown.

Clinical jaundice (icterus) occurs if plasma bilirubin exceeds ~35 mmol/l. Causes may be pre-hepatic, hepatocellular, or post-hepatic/obstructive (see box; for neonatal causes of jaundice, see 📖 p 24). Sclerae and skin appear yellow. Do not confuse normal pale brown sclerae in dark-skinned people with jaundice. Carotinaemia (due to eating excess mangoes, tomatoes, or carrots) also causes yellow skin, especially of the palms and soles, but the sclerae are white.

- *Pre-hepatic jaundice:* excess bilirubin production due to haemolysis, ↓liver uptake, or ↓conjugation leads to ↑ serum *unconjugated* bilirubin.
- *Hepatocellular jaundice:* hepatocyte damage ± some cholestasis.
- *Obstructive (cholestatic) jaundice:* bile excretion impeded by intra- or extrahepatic biliary obstruction → *conjugated* hyperbilirubinaemia; pruritus common (look for excoriations, shiny fingernails); excretion of water-soluble conjugated bilirubin makes urine dark; stools pale as less bilirubin excreted in faeces. Steatorrhoea (fatty, pale, offensive stools that often float) may occur, and malabsorption of fat-soluble vitamins (A, D, E, K) may → osteomalacia and coagulopathy.

Assessment: Ask about alcohol, blood transfusions, sexual activity, tattoos, body piercing, jaundiced contacts, family history, and drugs, including herbal medicines. Examine for hepatomegaly and signs of chronic liver disease. Further investigations depend on clinical features but include FBC, clotting, blood film, Coomb's test, U&Es, LFTs, hepatitis viral serology. Liver USS may show dilatated bile ducts (obstructive jaundice), gallstones, hepatic metastases, or pancreatic mass.

Hepatomegaly

Hepatomegaly is a common finding in the tropics. Palpate liver, noting texture, and percuss to define size (normal liver is <12 cm longitudinally in midclavicular line) — this will differentiate liver ptosis (e.g. due to lung hyperexpansion in COPD). Auscultate for hepatic bruit (e.g. in hepatocellular carcinoma). Look for jaundice and signs of chronic liver disease.

Causes: include viral (e.g. Hep A-E, EBV, CMV, HIV), bacterial (e.g leptospira, syphilis, pyogenic liver abscess, TB), protozoal (amoebic liver abscess), and other parasitic infections (e.g. hydatid, fasciolia, opisthorchis); chronic liver disease (see box); malignancy (metastases, 1° hepatocellular CA); infiltrative conditions (amyloid, sarcoid); Budd-Chiari syndrome; congestive cardiac failure; congenital Riedel's lobe; and polycystic liver.

Causes of jaundice

Pre-hepatic jaundice
- Malaria.
- G6PD deficiency.
- Sickle cell disease.
- Gilbert's syndrome.
- Drugs (📖 p 467).
- Bacterial sepsis.
- Viral haemorrhagic fevers.
- Dyserythropoiesis.
- Crigler–Najjar syndrome (rare).

Hepatocellular jaundice
- Viruses e.g. Hep A-E, EBV, CMV, yellow fever, Lassa fever).
- Other infections e.g. typhoid, leptospira, bartonella, syphilis.
- Alcoholic hepatitis.
- Chronic liver disease/cirrhosis.
- Drugs (📖 p 298).
- Hepatic metastases.
- Hepatocellular carcinoma.
- Liver abscess.
- Hydatid disease (rarely).
- Rotor, Dubin–Johnson syn (rare).

Post-hepatic (cholestatic) jaundice
- Gallstones.
- Pancreatic CA.
- Portahepatic lymph nodes.
- Cholangiocarcinoma.
- Primary biliary cirrhosis.
- Sclerosing cholangitis.
- Viral hepatitis (cholestatic phase).
- AIDS cholangiopathy.
- Ascariasis.
- Fascioliasis.
- Opisthorchiasis/clonorchiasis.
- Choledochal cyst.
- Biliary atresia.
- Hydatid disease (rare).
- Drugs (📖 p 298).

Treatable causes of hepatomegaly without jaundice

Infections
- Amoebic liver abscess.
- Schistosomiasis.
- Plague (*Yersinia pestis*).
- Visceral leishmaniasis.
- Hydatid disease.
- Bartonellosis.
- Trypanosomiasis.
- Fascioliasis/opisthorchiasis.
- Toxocariasis.
- Disseminated TB.
- Malaria.

Cardiac and nutritional causes
- Beri beri.
- Chagas disease.
- Fatty infiltration in Kwashiorkor.

Viral hepatitis

Hepatitis A virus (HAV)

HAV is an non-enveloped RNA picornavirus related to enteroviruses. Transmission is via the faeco-oral route including ingestion of contaminated food or water. It is the most common viral cause of hepatitis worldwide and hyperendemic in many parts of the developing world, especially in areas of poor sanitation, where childhood infection is very common. Serological studies in hyperendemic areas demostrate immunity in most adults (e.g. India ~99%), thus HAV is an uncommon cause of acute hepatitis in adults in these settings. However, infection frequently occurs in non-immunized travellers and secondary cases or outbreaks in developed countries may follow importation of HAV.

Clinical features: Disease severity is proportional to age, ranging from asymptomatic infection (common in children) to fulminant hepatitis (<0.5%). In symptomatic cases, after 1–6 week incubation period, there is a viraemic prodrome including malaise, anorexia, myalgia, headache, arthralgia, nausea, and fever. Symptoms improve as jaundice appears — this is often cholestatic and may last up to several weeks in adults. Hepatosplenomegaly, lymphadenopathy, or a rash may occur. Virus is excreted via the bile in the faeces 1–2 weeks before the onset of jaundice; excretion then declines over the following week. Chronic carriage, relapses, and chronic liver disease do not occur.

Diagnosis: HAV-specific IgM is detectable by symptom onset; HAV-IgG rises 1–2 weeks later and remains elevated for life. ALT/AST rise at the onset and typically settle in 2-6 weeks. ALP may take longer to settle, along with the cholestatic jaundice.

Treatment: is supportive as most infections are self-limiting. Avoid alcohol until LFTs return to normal.

Prevention: Improved sanitation reduces transmission. Faecal shedding of the virus is highest during the incubation and prodromal phase, so by the time of presentation, isolation of patients is of limited value. Immunity following infection is probably lifelong. Non-immune travellers to endemic areas should be vaccinated (see 📖 p 822).

Hepatitis E virus (HEV)

HEV is a non-enveloped, RNA hepevirus endemic in many parts of south, southeast, and central Asia. Transmission and clinical features are similar to HAV, although, unlike HAV, large epidemics affecting mainly young adults have been described. In India, HEV accounts for >50% sporadic hepatitis in adults. Like HAV, most infections are self-limiting. Women in the 3rd trimester of pregnancy are particularly susceptible to fulminant liver failure and death (~20%) for reasons that are poorly understood.

Diagnosis: HEV-specific IgM is detectable at presentation in >90% cases; HEV-IgG rises thereafter. PCR may detect HEV RNA in blood or stool.

Treatment: supportive. No vaccine is yet available. Pooled human immune globulin is not protective.

Hepatitis C (HCV)

HCV is an enveloped, single-stranded RNA flavivirus, with 6 major genotypes and over 50 subtypes. Transmission is predominantly blood borne, and ~2–5 million iatrogenic HCV infections occur annually. The prevalence of HCV infection among Egyptians is >15%, mainly due to mass parenteral anti-schistosomal treatment programmes in the past. Less commonly, sexual and vertical transmission may occur. The risk of infection following needlestick injury from a HCV+ve donor is ~1–3%.

Natural history: Primary infection is usually asymptomatic or accompanied by mild, flu-like symptoms; however, 50–85% go on to develop chronic HCV infection. Non-specific symptoms include malaise, nausea, and abdominal pain. Ongoing cycles of inflammation, necrosis, and apoptosis gradually lead to cirrhosis, which occurs in 2–20% over 20–30 years. Progression is faster in males, those infected at an older age, HIV co-infection (especially if CD4 <200 cells/ml) and/or HBV co-infection, and those with HCV genotype 1. Once cirrhosis present, the risk of HCC is 1–4% per year. Extrahepatic manifestations, which are uncommon, include glomerulonephritis, cryoglobulinaemic vasculitis, and lichen planus.

Diagnosis: HCV antibodies become detectable 6–8 weeks following 1° infection. PCR for HCV RNA is expensive and should only be done if treatment is available, at which point genotyping is also done.

Management: Conservative measures include avoidance of alcohol as this accelerates progression of cirrhosis. Specific therapy is costly. Where available, this is with pegylated interferon and ribavirin combination therapy for 24 weeks. Genotypes 2 & 3 have been shown to have a better chance of treatment success (75–85%). *Contraindications* to therapy include liver failure, ongoing alcohol or substance abuse, pregnancy, and co-existing conditions such as uncontrolled seizures or autoimmune diseases. Response to HCV therapy is less favourable in HIV/HCV co-infection. HAART improves the course of HCV and is the mainstay of therapy for co-infected individuals in resource-poor settings.

Hepatitis B virus (HBV)

HBV is a double-stranded DNA hepadnavirus. It is an important cause of acute and chronic hepatitis and hepatocellular carcinoma. Worldwide ~2 billion people show serological evidence of exposure and ~400 million have active infection. High prevalence areas include sub-Saharan Africa, China, and southeast Asia.

Transmission: The virus is present in the blood and (to a lesser extent) in semen, vaginal secretions, and saliva of actively infected individuals. Transmission occurs via transfusion of infected blood products, use of unsterilized needles, sexually, and among children by close contact through mucosae or minor breaks in the skin. Vertical transmission from mother to child occurs perinatally. High-risk groups include health workers, haemophiliacs, IV drug users, haemodialysis patients, those in institutions, and homosexual men.

Natural history of acute infection: Most 1° infections are asymptomatic, esp. in young children. Symptomatic cases present after an incubation period of 1–4 months with clinical features indistinguishable from other acute viral hepatitides. Death from fulminant hepatitis occurs in ~1%; glomerulonephritis is a rare complication. Following acute infection, there is either complete recovery (with long-term immunity) or persistent infection. The latter occurs in 5–10% infected adults, 30% infected children, and 90% infants infected at birth; it is more common in the immunocompromised.

Serological markers of infection: are shown in Fig. 7.4. Following 1° infection, there is marked viraemia. HBsAg becomes detectable after 4–10 weeks, followed by IgM anti-HBc. As the host immune response targets infected hepatocytes, ALT rises, and HBeAg (which is a marker of active viral replication) becomes detectable. Recovery with viral clearance is accompanied by disappearance of HBsAg and appearance of anti-HBs and anti-Hbe antibodies. During the 'window' period between disappearance of HBsAg and appearance of anti-HBs, acute infection can be confirmed by the presence of anti-HBc.

Persistent infection: is defined as the presence of circulating hepatitis B surface antigen (HBsAg) >6 months post-infection. There may be:
- **Asymptomatic chronic HBV carriage** (sub-clinical persistent viraemia, with normal ALT and normal/near normal liver histology); *or*
- **Chronic hepatitis B** (liver function and histology abnormal). Symptoms are usually non-specific and do not correlate with disease severity. ~20% patients go on to develop cirrhosis, and there is a 100-fold increase in the risk of hepatocellular carcinoma (HCC).

Levels of HBV viraemia are usually lower in persistent infection and decline over time. Persistent HBeAg indicates higher levels of viral replication. Clearance of HBeAg may occur with development of anti-HBe, may be accompanied by a transient rise in ALT ± clinical hepatitis (due to immune-mediated destruction of infected hepatocytes) and usually leads to lower levels of viraemia; a small proportion of patients (~1% per year) will clear the virus permanently and remain immune thereafter.

HBe-negative mutants: Most HBeAg negative patients have low levels of viraemia. However, some have high viraemia levels despite being HBeAg negative, due to a viral mutation in the promoter region of the gene encoding the core antigen which prevents HBeAg expression. Prevalence of these 'pre-core mutants' is higher in certain geographical areas (e.g. Asia 15–20%) and increases with infection chronicity. They appear to be associated with more severe disease and higher risk of cirrhosis.

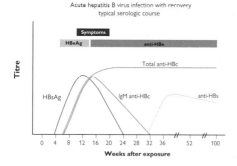

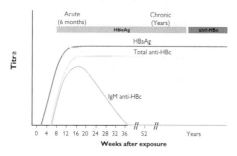

Fig. 7.4 Serological changes in hepatitis B infections. (HBsAg = HBV surface antigen; HBcAg = HBV core antigen; HBeAg = HBV e antigen; anti-HBsAg = antibody to HBsAg; anti-HBcAg = antibody to HBcAg; anti-HBeAg = antibody to HBeAg).

Management of acute HBV infection: Supportive; avoid alcohol. Management of chronic HBV aims to reduce transmission risk and limit/prevent progression to cirrhosis and/or HCC. General measures include avoidance of alcohol (exacerbates liver damage) and drugs which may promote viral replication (e.g. steroids, NSAIDs), and adequate nutrition.

Where available, the goal of medical therapy for chronic HBV is to reduce viraemia and liver damage; complete viral clearance occurs in <5% cases with current regimens. Most studies have concentrated on chronic HBeAg-positive carriers with raised ALT, whose course is easy to follow. Some HBeAg-negative patients with high circulating viraemia may also benefit from treatment. Treatment options currently available:

- **Nucleoside analogues** (e.g. lamivudine) interfere with HBV reverse transcriptase and thereby inhibit viral replication. Lamivudine has been shown to delay clinical progression in patients with chronic HBV and cirrhosis, reducing risk of HCC. However, resistance is seen in >50% patients after 3 years' therapy. The future of HBV treatment is likely to be combination therapy with other nucleoside analogues (e.g. adofevir, tenofovir entecavir, emtricitabine, famciclovir).
- **Interferon alpha** showed modest benefit in clinical trials but is limited by side-effects and has been largely superseded by newer antivirals.

Prevention of hepatitis B infection   PUBLIC HEALTH NOTE

Primary immunization with hepatitis B vaccine is recommended by WHO as part of the expanded programme on immunization (EPI) schedule (see Chapter 22). Studies in Taiwan showed that universal vaccination of children under 5 years reduced the incidence of hepatocellular CA.

Post-exposure immunization should be given to babies born to mothers who are HBV carriers or who had HBV during pregnancy, and to other non-immune individuals exposed to HBV (e.g. following needlestick injury). Passive immunization with hyperimmune hepatitis B immunoglobulin (HBIG)* within 12 h of birth reduces their chances of developing the carrier state by up to 70%; protective efficacy is increased to 90% by combining HBIG with HBV vaccine. Give HBIG* plus HBV vaccine at day 0 and after 1 and 2 months, and a booster at 12 months (accelerated schedule). It is unclear whether the combination of HBIG and HBV vaccination provides significantly better protection than early (<24 h) HBV vaccination alone, and practice varies between countries.

* HBIG doses: adults 500 IU, children 5–9 yrs 300 IU, children <5 yrs and infants 200 IU.

Hepatitis D (HDV, 'delta agent')

HDV is a single-stranded RNA virus that can only replicate in the presence of HBV, and is transmitted by similar routes. ~5% chronic HBV carriers are HDV co-infected, especially in the Mediterranean region, parts of eastern Europe, Africa, the Middle East, and South America. Co-infection leads to more severe acute HBV hepatitis or, in chronic HBV infection, accelerated hepatic failure and cirrhosis. Treatment and prevention is as for HBV (HBV vaccination prevents HDV co-infection).

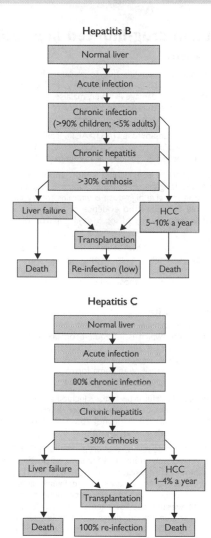

Fig. 7.5 Schematic comparing the natural history of hepatitis B and C infection. (Reprinted from *The Lancet*, 2006, **368**: 896–7, with permission of Elsevier.)

Alcohol and drug-induced hepatitis

Alcoholic hepatitis

Clinical features: Acute hepatitis due to alcohol abuse causes (tender) hepatomegaly and jaundice ± nausea/vomiting, and the systemic inflammatory response to liver damage → fever, malaise, anorexia, and leukocytosis. Depending on the duration and severity of liver damage, signs of chronic liver disease/cirrhosis may be present.

Investigations: ↑liver transaminases (AST>ALT), ↑bilirubin, ↑ALP, ↑WCC, ↑urea. Alcohol excess *per se* may → ↑γGT, ↑MCV, ↓platelets. Reduced hepatic synthetic function in cirrhosis → ↓albumin, ↑PT.

Management: Abstinence from alcohol is most important; manage alcohol withdrawal with reducing course of benzodiazepine (e.g. chlordiazepoxide). Optimize nutrition and give high-dose B vitamins (pabrinex) IV. Consider ascitic tap to rule out SBP. If no evidence of sepsis and severe disease, consider prednisolone 40 mg od for 5 days, tapered off over the next 2–4 weeks.

Prognosis: Scoring systems have been devised to predict outcome (see boxes opposite). Abstinence from alcohol, good nutrition, and steroid therapy (for severe alcoholic hepatitis) have each shown survival benefit: 7-year survival was ~50% in those who continued to drink, compared with ~80% in those who were abstinent.

Drug-induced hepatitis

Drug-associated liver damage is most commonly a result of an idiosyncratic reaction — one which is infrequent, occurs at therapeutic doses with variable latency period, and with a pattern that is consistent for each drug. Injury may result in hepatitis, cholangiohepatitis, or pure cholestasis (see box opposite). Steatosis, granuloma formation, and fibrosis may also occur. Women are at higher risk of drug-induced hepatitis.

Clinical assessment: Careful drug history including use of traditional and complementary medicines or over-the-counter drugs, timing of symptoms in relation to start of drug, and alcohol abuse. Rule out other common causes of liver injury, such as viral hepatitis.

Manangement: Once identified, the drug should either be withdrawn altogether, or very closely monitored for signs of progressive liver damage (e.g. nevirapine hepatotoxicity on instigating HAART). A decision to re-challenge will depend on severity of the liver reaction and on the indication for the drug's use. The risks and benefits of reintroducing a drug should be weighed up. For example, when deciding whether to re-challenge with antituberculous drugs, one should take into account the strength of the initial TB diagnosis and the duration of antituberculous therapy already received.

Glasgow alcoholic hepatitis score (GAHS)

Variable	Score		
	1	2	3
Age (years)	<50	≥50	–
WCC (×10^9/l)	<15	≥50	–
Urea (mmol/l)	<5	≥5	–
PT ratio/INR	<1.5	1.5–2.0	>2.0
Total bilirubin	<125	125–250	>250

GAHS ≥9 associated with 28 day mortality >60%

GAHS ≤5 associated with 28 day mortality <10%

Drugs causing hepatitis

Type of injury	Important drugs
Hepatocellular	Isoniazid, nevirapine, pyrazinamide, Paracetamol
Cholestatic	Erythromycin, rifampicin, chlorpromazine
Allergic	Sulphonamides, sulfones, phenytoin, halothane
Granulomatous	Diltiazem, quinidine
Steatohepatitis	Stavudine, didanosine, tetracycline
Fibrosis	Methotrexate

Chronic liver disease and cirrhosis

Chronic liver disease is common in the tropics due to widespread alcohol consumption and frequent exposure to hepatitis viruses, parasites, bacteria, and toxins. Persistent liver injury causes cirrhosis: irreversible destruction of liver cellular architecture by fibrosis, with nodular regeneration of hepatocytes. Causes are shown in the box opposite.

Clinical features

Variable and depend upon the degree of liver damage and compensation. Symptoms include malaise, pruritus, and reversal of normal sleep patterns (if encephalopathic). Ask about alcohol, blood transfusions, sexual activity, tattoos, body piercing, jaundiced contacts, family history, and drugs, including herbal medicines. There may be hepatomegaly in early cirrhosis, although fibrotic contraction typically causes the liver to shrink as the disease progresses. Examine for Dupuytren's contracture (associated with alcohol excess), jaundice, and extra-hepatic signs of chronic liver disease including portal hypertension (PHT) and hepatic encephalopathy:

- *Face and skin*: jaundice, hepatic fetor, excoriations.
- *Hands*: leuconychia, clubbing, palmar erythema, bruising, asterixis.
- *Chest*: gynaecomastia, loss of body hair, spider naevi, bruising.
- *Abdomen*: splenomegaly, ascites, testicular atrophy.
- *Legs*: oedema (due to hypoalbuminaemia), muscle wasting.

Hyponatraemia occurs due to 2° hyperaldosteronism, and osteomalacia may occur due to altered vitamin D metabolism.

Diagnosis

Abnormal LFTs reflect hepatocellular damage (pattern often dependent on aetiology); ↓albumin and prolonged prothrombin time reflect reduced liver synthetic function. USS (which shows characteristic cirrhotic liver architecture) and liver biopsy (check PT, platelet count, and Hb before biopsy) are the mainstay of diagnosis.

Management and prognosis

Depend on the severity and underlying cause. Cirrhosis is an irreversible condition, so the aim is to limit further damage, treat complications, and support the patient.

- Avoid alcohol and hepatotoxic drugs (e.g. paracetamol).
- Treat dehydration and intercurrent infections.
- Ensure adequate nutrition.
- Treat ascites (📖 p 304).
- Management and prevention of PHT (📖 p 304) and variceal bleeds (📖 p 277).
- Colestyramine 4–8 g od PO for pruritis.
- If possible, treat underlying cause —e.g. peri-portal fibrosis in hepatic schistosomiasis is partially reversible with praziquantel treatment.

Causes of chronic liver disease/cirrhosis

- Alcoholic liver disease.
- Viral hepatitis (hep B, C).
- Haemochromatosis.
- Autoimmune hepatitis.
- Cryptogenic.
- Primary biliary cirrhosis.
- Wilson's disease.
- Alpha-1-antitrypsin deficiency.
- Drugs.

Hereditary haemochromatosis

An inherited disorder of iron metabolism in which intestinal iron absorption is increased leading to iron deposition in multiple organs including liver, heart, pancreas, pituitary, adrenals, skin, and joints. Inheritance is autosomal recessive in the majority of cases.

Clinical features

The classic triad is of hyperpigmentation, hepatomegaly, and diabetes (30–50%). Fatigue and arthralgia are early symptoms. Cardiac involvement with heart failure and dysrrhythmias is common, as is arthropathy; hypogonadism may occur 2° to pituitary involvement and/or cirrhosis. Presentation is usually in the 4th–6th decade, due to slow accumulation of body iron. Men are more frequently and severely affected, probably due to female menstrual iron loss. Complications include cirrhosis (9 times more likely in patients drinking >60 g alcohol/day) and hepatocellular carcinoma, which occurs in 30% of cirrhotic patients with haemochromatosis.

Diagnosis

↑ferritin, ↑transferrin saturation >80%, ↑serum iron, ↓TIBC. LFTs, blood glucose, ECG ± echo. Joint X-rays may show chondrocalcinosis. Liver biopsy to assess severity of liver disease. Where available, genotype for mutations. Differential diagnosis includes haemosiderosis (see below) and other causes of 2° iron overload (e.g. thalassaemia and sideroblastic anaemia); other causes of chronic liver disease (📖 p 301); and porphyria cutanea tarda.

Management

Venesection is the mainstay of treatment and has been shown to reduce morbidity and mortality: remove 1 unit blood (~500 ml, 250 g iron) weekly initially, until mildly iron deficient; then maintenance venesection of 1 unit every 2–3 months. Aim to maintain serum ferritin <50 ng/ml and transferrin saturation <50%. Avoid vitamin C supplementation which accelerates iron mobilization, increasing pro-oxidant and free-radical activity. Assess and manage end-organ dysfunction such as cardiomyopathy and diabetes. Screening of all first-degree relatives is advised: check serum ferritin ± genotyping where available.

Haemosiderosis ('Bantu siderosis')

Haemosiderosis (a focal or general increase in tissue iron stores) affects the liver in populations in some regions of southern Africa (and to a lesser extent in some other tropical areas) and is linked to chronic ingestion of beer brewed in iron containers. Co-factors for chronic liver disease such as high alcohol intake are also commonly present.

Clinical features: Hyperpigmentation, hepatomegaly (portal fibrosis/cirrhosis), and cardiac failure occur. Ascorbic acid deficiency is often present. Associated osteoporosis may → vertebral collapse.

Management: similar to hereditary haemochromatosis, with regular venesection. Use of alternative containers for brewing and storage of beer helps prevent disease progression/occurrence.

Primary biliary cirrhosis (PBC)

A chronic granulomatous cholangiohepatitis causing destruction of inter-lobular bile ducts. The aetiology is thought to be autoimmune. 90% of patients are women. Associations include thyroid and pancreatic disease, Sjogren's syndrome, and localized cutaneous scleroderma.

Clinical features: Vary widely but include fatigue, hepatosplenomegaly, clubbing, xanthomata, xanthelasma, arthralgia, and features of cholestasis (📕 p 290), cirrhosis (📕 p 300), and portal hypertension (📕 p 304).

Diagnosis: Often diagnosed incidentally following discovery of abnormal LFTs. ↑ALP, ↑γGT, slightly ↑AST/ALT; ↑bilirubin in late disease. Liver USS to exclude extrahepatic biliary obstruction. Antimitochondrial antibodies highly specific. Liver biopsy and/or ERCP confirm diagnosis.

Management: symptomatic: colestyramine for pruritis, low-fat diet, and vitamin supplementation. Monitor for signs of portal hypertension. Death commonly occurs within 5 years in severe disease.

Wilson's disease

A rare, autosomal recessive disorder of copper excretion leading to toxic accumulation of copper in liver and brain (hepatolenticular degeneration). Clinical features reflect chronic liver disease and basal ganglia damage (tremor, dysarthria, dyskinesias, parkinsonism, and eventually dementia). When present, Kayser–Fleisher rings (greenish-brown pigment at the cor-neoscleral junction) are pathognomonic, but may only be seen with slit lamp and often absent in young children.

Diagnosis: ↓serum caeruloplasmin levels, ↑24 h urinary copper excretion. Liver biopsy shows ↑copper (but also raised in chronic cholestasis). MRI may show typical changes in basal ganglia.

Management: Lifelong chelation therapy with penicillamine. Screen children and siblings and treat asymptomatic homozygotes.

Indian childhood cirrhosis

A disease presenting in children aged 1–3 years in the Indian subconti-nent. It may follow a subacute, acute, or fulminant course, ranging from a viral type acute hepatitis to florid cirrhosis. There is fibrosis with micro- and macronodular degeneration and, although progression to hepatocel-lular CA is rare, mortality is high. The cause is unknown, although a high copper intake (e.g. from milk stored in copper vessels), possibly coupled with an inherited defect of copper absorption/metabolism has been implicated. There is no specific treatment.

Portal hypertension (PHT)

PHT may be a sequel to any chronic liver disease, although cirrhosis and schistosomiasis are the most common causes in the tropics. It is useful to split causes according to the level of obstruction (see box).

Clinical features: ↑portal pressure → splenomegally and ascites; development of porto-systemic venous collaterals → oesophageal/gastric varices (the most serious complication, see ▢ p 277), caput medusae (distended collateral abdominal veins radiating from the umbilicus), and haemorrhoids. Look for signs of chronic liver disease.

Management
- Treat underlying cause where possible.
- Manage and prevent oesophageal variceal bleeds (▢ p 277).
- Prompt treatment of SBP (below) and hepatorenal syndrome (▢ p 306).
- TIPS (transjugular intrahepatic portosystemic shunting) is an option where available, but expensive and shunt stenosis is common.

Ascites

Ascites occurs in PHT due to a combination of sodium and water retention (due to splanchnic arterial vasodilation and ↓splanchnic arterial pressure → release of vasoconstrictors and antinatriuretic factors), ↑portal hydrostatic pressure, and ↓plasma oncotic pressure (↓albumin).

Management: includes general measures to ameliorate cirrhosis and PHT, and specific treatment to reduce ascites:
- *Moderate ascites* Give low-dose diuretics (spironolactone 50–200 mg od or amiloride 5–10 mg od); if response poor or peripheral oedema present, add furosemide 20–40 mg od for the 1st few days. Aim for 300–500 g weight loss/day (800–1000 g if peripheral oedema).
- *Massive ascites* (rapid accumulation with abdominal discomfort): Drain ascites with plasma expander cover (e.g. 20% albumin 100 ml IV per litre drained); remove drain within 24 h to minimize infection risk. High-dose diuretics are a less effective alternative (spironolactone 400 mg od plus furosemide 160 mg od). Irrespective of which method used, diuretics should be used to prevent re-accumulation.
- *Refractory ascites* Repeated ascitic drainage 2–4 weekly; consider TIPS.

Spontaneous bacterial peritonitis (SBP)

Spontaneous infection of ascitic fluid, usually with intestinal pathogens (e.g. *E. coli*), which occurs in 10–30% of patients with ascites. There may be abdominal tenderness or signs of sepsis, but often asymptomatic/non-specific presentation, therefore consider in any patient with ascites who deteriorates. Hepatorenal syndrome complicates in up to 30% episodes.

Diagnosis: Microscopy and culture of ascitic fluid: SBP defined as ≥ 250 polymorphonuclear cells/mm^3.

Treatment: Broad-spectrum antibiotics e.g. ceftriaxone, pending culture results. Consider 2° prophylaxis (e.g. norfloxacin 400 mg od) as recurrent episodes common (70% at 1 year). Albumin (1.5 g/kg initially and 1 g/kg at 48 h) reduces the incidence of hepatorenal syndrome.

Veno-occlusive disease

Thrombosis of smaller hepatic veins due to toxins such as pyrrolizidine alkaloids contained in certain herbal teas (e.g. *Helotropium*, *Crotalaria*, and *Senecio*). It is an important cause of PHT in Jamaica, South Africa, central Asia, and south west USA.

Causes of portal hypertension

Pre-hepatic
- Hyper-reactive malarial splenomegaly (increased portal blood flow).
- Portal vein occlusion (e.g. lymphoma, pancreatic CA).
- Portal vein thrombosis (e.g. severe dehydration).
- Splenic vein occlusion (following neonatal umbilical sepsis).

Hepatic (sinusoidal)
- Cirrhosis.
- Schistosomiasis (*S. mansoni* or *S. japonicum*).
- Hepatocellular carcinoma (HCC).
- Veno-occlusive disease.
- Congenital hepatic fibrosis.
- Drugs (e.g. dapsone).

Post-hepatic
- Congestive cardiac failure (e.g. rheumatic fever, TB pericarditis).
- Endomyocardial fibrosis.
- Inferior vena cava obstruction.
- Hepatic vein thrombosis (Budd–Chiari syndrome e.g. in pregnancy).

Causes of ascites

- Portal hypertension (see box above for causes).
- Abdomino-peritoneal TB.
- Hypoproteinaemia (e.g. nephrotic syndrome).
- Right heart failure.
- Chylous ascites.

Liver failure

In the tropics, liver failure usually results from viral hepatitis or alcohol. Less common but significant causes include drug-induced hepatitis (TB treatment or paracetamol overdose), other infections (e.g. leptospirosis), and acute fatty liver of pregnancy. Onset may be acute with no preceding illness or jaundice (fulminant hepatic necrosis). However, liver failure occurs more commonly in patients with pre-existing cirrhosis. These patients have a chronic deterioration with infection, lethargy, GI bleeds, diuretic usage, and/or electrolyte disturbances.

Clinical features

Include jaundice, fetor hepaticus (breath smells like pear drops), hypoglycaemia, sepsis (which may be overwhelming), ascites ± SBP, coagulopathy, hepatic encephalopathy, and hepatorenal syndrome.

Hepatic encephalopathy: Liver failure leads to build up of ammonia which enters the brain where astrocytes clear it, producing glutamine in the process. ↑ osmotic pressure due to excess glutamine causes fluid to enter cells → cerebral oedema and hepatic encephalopathy. Early signs include lethargy, asterixis (liver flap), constructional apraxia (e.g. inability to copy a 5-pointed star), and reversed sleep pattern with diurnal somnolence, which may progress to confusion, drowsiness, incontinence, ataxia, ± ophthalmoplegia, extra-pyramidal signs, and eventually coma.

Hepatorenal syndrome (HRS) occurs in ~10% patients with advanced cirrhosis and ascites and is thought to be due to severe intravascular hypovolaemia causing renal vasoconstriction. Two types are recognized: type 1 is characterized by progressive oliguria and rapid rise creatinine, often precipitated by SBP; type 2 is commonly seen in patients with refractory ascites, who have gradual increase in creatinine. Prognosis is poor: median survival without treatment is <1 month for type 1. Where available, vasopressin analogues (e.g. terlipressin 0.5–2 mg bd IV) plus albumin may be effective in up to two thirds of patients with type 1 HRS.

Management

- Monitor vital signs, neuro obs, blood glucose, and urine output closely.
- Treat hypothermia and hypoglycaemia.
- Monitor FBC, U&Es, LFTs, and clotting.
- Control active bleeding with FFP/platelets; give Vitamin K 10 mg od IV for 3 days to correct PT (less effective in established cirrhosis).
- Insert NG tube (unless oesophageal varices). Consider NG feeding.
- Avoid sedatives, hepatotoxic drugs, drugs metabolized by the liver, and NSAIDs (risk of GI bleed).
- Give lactulose (and/or neomycin) to ↓ammonia absorption from GIT.
- Manage coma in hepatic encephalopathy (Chapter 10) and monitor for signs of ↑ICP (consider mannitol).
- Ensure careful control of fluid balance.
- Investigate and treat suspected infection promptly (e.g. SBP).
- Liver transplant, where available, sometimes offers the only hope of survival or cure.

Hepatocellular carcinoma (HCC)

HCC is common, particularly in men aged 20–40 years, and causes an estimated 1 million deaths per year worldwide. It is the most common 1° cancer of men in sub-Saharan Africa, with a male incidence as high as 100/100,000 in Mozambique. It is also common in parts of Asia and the western Pacific.

Aetiology and risk factors

- Chronic hepatitis B and, to a lesser extent, hepatitis C are thought to cause ~80% of HCC cases worldwide.
- Aflatoxin B ingestion: the toxin is produced by the plant mould *Aspergillus flavus*, which commonly grows on groundnuts (peanuts) but is also found on maize, millet, peas, and sorghum. Levels of food contamination in Mozambique are the highest in the world.
- Cigarette smoking.
- Alcohol: HCC is 5× more common in males who drink >80 g alcohol per day than in non-drinkers.

Clinical features

RUQ pain, weakness, and weight loss. Hepatomegaly occurs in 90%, cachexia and ascites in 50%, abdominal venous collaterals in 30%, jaundice in 25%. A hepatic bruit is audible in half of cases. Bone metastases may cause pathological fractures and there may be signs and sequelae of portal hypertension (e.g. bleeding from oesophageal varices).

Diagnosis

Clinical. CXR may show a raised R hemidiaphragm. ALP and α-fetoprotein usually ↑. Other Ix: USS, CT scan, biopsy.

Management

HCC is a rapidly growing tumour and treatment is usually palliative. In the tropics, presentation may be fulminant, with death occurring within weeks of diagnosis. Aim to relieve pain and reduce symptoms (e.g. anti-pruritic agents, drain ascites, transfusions for anaemia). Chemotherapy, radiotherapy, and transplantation are disappointing. Surgical resection provides the only prospect for cure, although this is only possible in ~2% of cases at presentation.

Prevention: HBV vaccination and avoidance of risk factors (above).

Hepatic neoplasia

Liver metastases are less common in the tropics than in the developed world. Clinical features may relate to the underlying primary cancer or may be non-specific (e.g. malaise, lethargy, weight loss). The liver may have a characteristic knobbly feel on palpation. Jaundice is relatively uncommon as a presenting feature. *Investigations*: USS and biopsy are the best means of determining the cause of focal liver lesions.

Differential diagnosis of the irregular liver

Cystic lesions: amoebic (or pyogenic) abscess — both usually very tender in a febrile, toxic patient; congenital liver cysts, polycystic liver, or hydatid cyst — all non-tender, no fever unless secondarily infected.

Solid lesions: are likely to be malignant. Surgical resection of small, solitary lesions may be attempted. If the patient is terminally ill, omit all investigations and concentrate on palliation.

Primary cancers which cause liver metastases

Male
- Stomach.
- Lung.
- Colon.
- Uterus.

Female
- Breast.
- Colon.
- Stomach.
- Carcinoid.

Rarer malignancies
- Pancreas.
- Leukaemia.
- Lymphoma.

Liver flukes

Liver trematodes (or flukes) are an important cause of human disease and prevalence rates may exceed 50% in some endemic areas. All are transmitted by food contaminated with infective metacercariae.

Opisthorchiasis and clonorchiasis

Approx. 17 million people are infected by the 3 closely related species of human liver flukes *Clonorchis sinensis* (E. Asia), *Opisthorchis felineus* (E. Europe, N. Asia), *O. viverrini* (Thailand, Laos), and *O. guayaquilensis* (Ecuador). In N.E. Thailand, where the prevalence of *O. viverrini* infection reaches up to 25%, it is believed to contribute to the high incidence of cholangiocarcinoma.

Life cycle and transmission: Humans are infected following ingestion of raw or undercooked fish containing metacercariae (see Fig. 7.6). Adults can live in the biliary tree for years. Pathology results from bile duct inflammation caused by large numbers of adult flukes.

Clinical features: Asymptomatic hepatomegaly is common, although USS may reveal gallbladder enlargement, sludge, gallstones, and poor function. RUQ pain, anorexia, dyspepsia, diarrhoea, and fullness are common symptoms; fever, eosinophilia, obstructive jaundice, weight loss, ascites, and oedema occur in more severe cases. Some patients have a sensation of something moving within the liver.

Complications: Gallstones and intrahepatic stones are common complications. Risk of cholangiocarcinoma due to *O. viverrini* infection is related to worm burden (5-fold increased risk for mild infection, 15-fold for heavy infection). Acute opisthorchiasis (*O. felineus*) presents with fever, tender hepatomegaly ± splenomegaly, and eosinophilia (up to 40% of WCC) soon after exposure to a large dose of metacercariae.

Diagnosis: is usually by detection of eggs in stool (may not be present in complete biliary obstruction or low worm burden). Adult worms may also be identified by ERCP or during surgery. Percutaneous bile aspiration is not recommended due to the high risk of biliary peritonitis and haemorrhage. Serology (± stool antigen detection assays) are available in some endemic areas.

Management: Praziquantel 40 mg/kg PO stat is often effective. Heavy Clonorchis infection may require up to 75 mg/kg tds for 2 days.

Prevention of clonorchiasis/ opisthorchiasis	PUBLIC HEALTH NOTE

- Improved sanitation and prohibition of the use of night soil in fishponds.
- Cook freshwater fish thoroughly; discourage consumption of raw fish.
- Saturated salt solution recommended for fish storage (but unproven).
- In non-endemic areas, suspect import of dried or pickled fish.
- Molluscicidal control of snail vectors is not feasible.

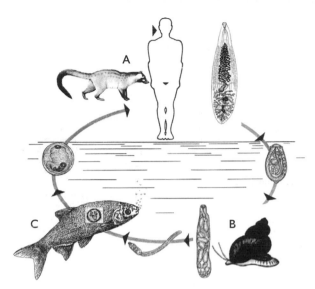

Fig. 7.6 Life cycle of *Opisthorchis* or *Clonorchis*: (A) the adult flukes living in the biliary tree of the carnivorous host (e.g. man or palm civet) shed ova into the bowel. Sewage contaminates fish ponds in which freshwater snails (B) live. In the snails, the parasites develop into miracidia, redia, and then cercariae which infect freshwater fish (C). The carnivore completes the cycle when ingesting metacercariae in the flesh of uncooked fish. (Adapted from G. Piekarski, *Medical parasitology in plates*, 1962, with kind permission of Bayer Pharmaceuticals.)

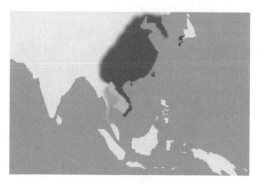

Fig. 7.7 Geographic distribution of *Clonorchis* and *Opisthorchis* (*C. sinensis* — black; *O. viverrini* — dark grey; *C. sinensis* and *O. viverrini* — light grey).

Fascioliasis

Fascioliasis is primarily an infection of animals, with man as an 'accidental' host. Nevertheless >2 million people worldwide are estimated to be infected with *Fasciola hepatica* or *F. gigantica*. Adult flukes live in the biliary tree of the primary hosts (usually sheep for *F. hepatica* and cattle for *F. gigantica*), passing eggs which are excreted in faeces. In water, ciliated miracidia hatch and infect an intermediate snail host. Free-living cercariae leave the snail, attaching to aquatic plants such as watercress where they become metacercaria. Following ingestion, the metacercariae excyst in the duodenum and migrate through the small intestinal wall into the liver and peritoneum. Larvae migrate to the common and hepatic ducts maturing into adult flukes.

Clinical features

Although many infections are asymptomatic, the pre-patent larval stage lasting 3–4 months may be accompanied by abdominal pain, weight loss, fever, and eosinophilia. During chronic or biliary stage fascioliasis, a small number of the adult flukes live in the bile ducts and shed eggs into the faeces. Patients are frequently asymptomatic, but may have symptoms and signs of biliary pain or obstruction.

Diagnosis

Eggs can be seen in the faeces within 2–4 months of infection, but identification may require repeated samples. Serology is useful for diagnosis, but cross-reaction has been reported with other worms. There may be an eosinophilia, and USS ± further imaging may be useful. Dietary history is important, particularly in outbreaks and in returning travellers.

Management

Single-dose triclabendazole 10–20 mg/kg PO is the treatment of choice, with low incidence of side-effects. The 2nd line drug is bithionol which requires 10–15 days' treatment and causes side-effects in up to 50%. Praziquantel is NOT active against *F. hepatica*.

Prevention of fascioliasis   PUBLIC HEALTH NOTE

- Avoid eating raw watercress/other aquatic plants, especially from grazing areas.
- Exclude animals from commercial watercress beds.
- Avoid the use of livestock faeces to fertilize water plants.
- If practicable, treat livestock.
- Consider molluscicides to eliminate mollusks (not considered feasible in most settings).

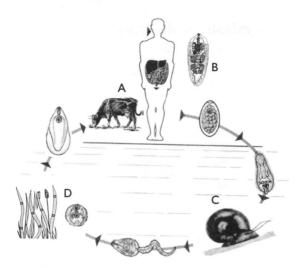

Fig. 7.8 Life cycle of *Fasciola hepatica*. The mammalian hosts (A), usually cattle, sheep, or man, become infected when ingesting aquatic plants (e.g. watercress) or grasses at the edges of fresh water. The ingested metacercariae excyst to form young flukes which migrate through the wall of the intestine and through the capsule of the liver and liver parenchyma until they reach a large bile duct. There the adult fluke (B), which is 2–4 cm long, lives for many years, passing its large (140 m) operculated eggs via the bile duct into the faeces. The eggs hatch in fresh water and undergo development in pond snails (C) into cercariae. These attach themselves to aquatic plants (D) which are ingested to complete the life cycle. (Adapted from G. Piekarski, *Medical Parasitology in Plates*, 1962, with kind permission of Bayer Pharmaceuticals.)

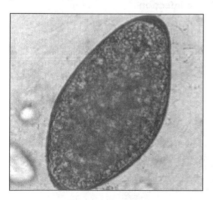

Fig. 7.9 *F. hepatica* egg in a faecal smear (~140×50 μm).

Schistosomiasis (Bilharzia)

A common, chronically debilitating, and potentially lethal disease affecting ~200 million people worldwide (with ~600 million people at risk), second only to malaria in socio-economic importance. It is caused by infection with the blood trematodes (flukes) *Schistosoma mansoni*, *S. japonicum*, *S. haematobium*, and, occasionally, *S. mekongi* or *S. intercalatum*. In most cases, infections are light or moderate. It is usually a slow, insidious disease but may give rise to renal failure, colitis, periportal fibrosis, and bladder carcinoma.

Life cycle and disease burden

Transmission occurs when humans are exposed to water infested with the intermediate snail host while swimming, washing, or collecting water (Fig. 7.10). Schistosome cercariae released from the snails penetrate human skin and enter blood vessels, passing via the lungs to the liver, where they mature into adults. Adult worms may migrate to vesical plexus (*S. haematobium*) or mesenteric veins (other species). The adults mate and may produce eggs for several years. Some of the eggs pass into the urinary tract (*S. haematobium*) or into the bowel (other species) before being excreted in urine or faeces. Other eggs lodge in the bladder or bowel mucosa, or are carried in the blood to ectopic sites (e.g. lungs, liver, CNS). Disease is caused by the granulomas around the eggs.

Adult worms do not multiply, so the level of infection and disease is proportional to the degree of exposure. Usually, there is a slow accumulation of egg granulomas; clinical illness occurs after several years. Infection peaks in early adult life with both sexes equally affected. Infections may be very severe in those with regular exposure e.g fishermen on African rivers/lakes, rice farmers in Philippines. Prevalence and intensity of infection decrease in older age groups due to less water contact and acquired immunity.

Clinical features — Acute infection

- **Early reaction (swimmers' itch)** occurs hours after infection. It is a pruritic papular rash with oedema, erythema, and eosinophilia caused by reaction to cercariae upon skin penetration. It resolves spontaneously within 10 days and is rare in people living in endemic areas.
- **Katayama fever** (acute toxaemic schistosomiasis) is a rare, but often severe, immune complex mediated seroconversion illness which occurs 1–3 months after 1° infection. It is most severe with *S. japonicum* and *S. mansoni*. *Clinical features* include fever, rash, chills, sweating, anorexia, headache, diarrhoea, cough, hepatosplenomegaly, lymphadenopathy, and giant urticaria. There is usually marked eosinophilia and raised immunoglobulins, and serial serology shows rising titres of anti-schistosomal antibodies. Usually no ova, or only scanty ova, are found in specimens as egg output is only beginning at this stage. It only occurs in non-immunes on first exposure to schistosomiasis (e.g. travellers from non-endemic areas), and usually subsides after several weeks (although egg output may remain high).

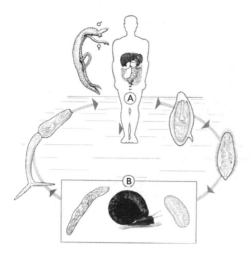

Fig. 7.10 Life cycle of schistosomiasis. The adult worms live in venous plexuses in the pelvis; the male wraps around the female and encloses it in its gynaecophoral canal. The human host (A) sheds ova in stool or urine; these hatch, releasing miracidia which infect the freshwater snail host (B). After further development, cercariae are released into the water, which penetrate the skin of humans during water contact. (Adapted from G. Piekarski, *Medical Parasitology in Plates*, 1962, with kind permission of Bayer Pharmaceuticals.)

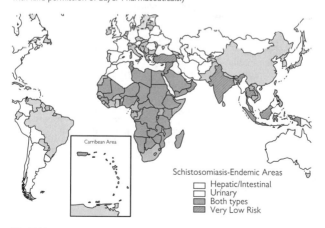

Fig. 7.11 Global distribution of schistosomiasis. (Reproduced from *Health Information for International Travel 2005–2006*, Centre for Disease Control and Prevention, 2005, with permission from Elsevier.)

Clinical features — Chronic disease

In chronic disease, eggs induce granulomatous inflammation and fibrosis which may affect many organs:

- *Hepato-splenic disease (hepatic periportal fibrosis):* may cause hepatosplenomegaly (often massive) and portal hypertension with porto-systemic collateral circulation, ascites, and oesophageal/gastric varices. Liver enzymes and albumin are usually normal, with few stigmata of liver failure until very late stages. Hypersplenism may result in pancytopaenia. The USS appearance is characteristic. Even if other causes of liver cirrhosis may co-exist, it is wise to treat for schistosomiasis because even established periportal fibrosis may improve substantially with treatment.

- *Intestinal disease:* eggs may reach both the superior and inferior mesenteric venous plexuses (and superior haemorrhoidal veins in S. japonicum disease) and pass through to the intestinal mucosa to involve both small and large bowel. Chronic inflammation of the large bowel may cause intermittent, bloody diarrhoea with tenesmus, pseudopolyp formation, hypoalbuminaemia, and anaemia, giving a clinical picture similar to that of ulcerative colitis or proctitis.
  A 'bilharzioma' is a mass of schistosomal eggs, which may be found in the omentum and/or mesenteric lymph nodes. Other features include protein-losing enteropathy, intussusception, and rectal prolapse.

- *Genitourinary disease:* chronic sequelae of S. haematobium infection include bladder fibrosis and calcification with reduced volume, and blockage of vesicoureteric orifice resulting in ureteric obstruction, hydroureter, hydronephrosis, reflux, and secondary infection. Patients may present with terminal haematuria or haemospermia. There is an increased risk of squamous cell carcinoma of the bladder at a relatively young age. Other pelvic structures, including fallopian tubes, may be affected.

- *CNS disease:* is a rare but serious complication of ectopic egg deposition. Eggs of S. japonicum may embolize to the brain to cause meningoencephalitis or focal epilepsy. S. mansoni or S. haematobium eggs occasionally embolize to the spinal cord, causing cauda equina syndrome, a transverse myelitis-like syndrome, paraplegia, or bladder dysfunction.

- *Pulmonary disease:* embolizing eggs (esp. S haematobium) occasionally occlude the pulmonary capillary bed, leading to pulmonary hypertension. There may be fatigue, syncope, chest pain, and signs of RV failure (raised JVP, tricuspid incompetence, peripheral oedema).

- *Other sites:* very rarely, there may be placental, genital, arthropathic, or cutaneous schistosomiasis.

- *Bacterial superinfection:* bacteria (e.g. Salmonella spp) may colonize adult worms, providing a source for bacteraemic episodes.

Diagnosis

Rests upon a history of exposure and clinical signs ± demonstration of eggs in the urine (*S. haematobium*) or faeces/rectal biopsy specimen (other species) or serology. Urine dipstick for blood is a sensitive screening method for urinary schistosomiasis. Filtration or sedimentation of urine prior to microscopy increases yield. Thick faecal smears (Kato–Katz preparation) are examined under relatively low power. Collected eggs may be hatched in fresh water to demonstrate miracidia. Depending on the presentation and site of infection, other methods include liver biopsy and further radiological imaging.

Management

Permanent cure is achievable in non-endemic areas but not usually feasible in endemic areas due to the high rate of re-infection. In cases where treatment does not achieve a full cure, egg production is nevertheless decreased by > 90%.

Katayama fever: Drugs are poorly active against the early migratory phase parasites (schistosomules). Give oral prednisolone to suppress the acute reaction, then praziquantel 40 mg/kg PO as a single dose. Repeat praziquantel after ~1 month.

Chronic disease

- Praziquantel is the drug of choice. It is effective against all schistosome species (plus cestodes and other snail-borne trematodes). For most species, give 2 doses of 20 mg/kg PO 4–6 h apart (3 doses 4 h apart for *S. japonicum*). If possible, take after food. *S. mekongi* may require repeated doses. For CNS disease, give 75 mg/kg as 3 divided doses 4 h apart. Paediatric dosage is the same. Cure rate is ~70%.
- Oxamniquine is an alternative for *S. mansoni* only. It is contraindicated in pregnancy; drug resistance is reported; and availability is limited.
- Metrifonate is an alternative for *S. haematobium* only. 3 doses are required, 2 weeks apart. Drug availability is limited.

Surgical treatment is not recommended — even chronic/fibrotic lesions will improve, especially in the young, and CNS disease may show resolution even after treatment.

Control of schistosomiasis   PUBLIC HEALTH NOTE

- Education and improved sanitation.
- Mass treatment of high-risk groups in high endemic areas (school-aged children, women of childbearing age, certain occupational groups).
- Personal protection e.g. rubber boots for rice farmers.
- Avoid recreational swimming in at-risk areas.
- Rapid, vigorous drying following contact may kill any cercariae which have not fully penetrated skin.
- Molluscicides (costly and have environmental consequences).

Ascariasis

Ascaris lumbricoides is a soil-transmitted roundworm accounting for ~60,000 deaths annually. ~25% of the world's population are infected, with prevalence approaching 95% in parts of the tropics.

Life cycle

Eggs containing larvae are ingested and hatch in the small intestine. Larvae penetrate the intestinal wall and migrate via the bloodstream through liver and heart to the lungs, where they penetrate alveoli and ascend the tracheobronchial tree to be swallowed. Returning to the intestine they develop into mature worms, beginning egg production ~2 months after initial ingestion. Adult worms live ~10–24 months and female worms lay ~200,000 eggs/day. Eggs passed in faeces persist in warm humid soil for up to 6 years and are resistant to cold and normal detergents. Children in rural areas have the highest burden of infection, as do communities which use human faeces as fertilizer.

Clinical features

Most infections are asymptomatic. Heavy infection produces symptoms proportional to worm burden, especially in children:
- Larval migration: 1–7 days after infection, larvae may invoke a hypersensitivity response with cough, wheeze, eosinophilia, and patchy infiltrates on CXR (Löffler's syndrome). Ectopic migration to the CNS occasionally causes convulsions, meningism, and insomnia. Ocular granulomas, similar to those of *Toxocara canis*, may occur.
- Adult worms: mild infections usually asymptomatic, but may cause appetite suppression, abdominal discomfort, and dyspepsia. Heavier infections (particularly in children) may cause anaemia and malabsorption of vitamins A & C, proteins, fats, lactose, and iodine. Growth retardation and cognitive impairment are frequently seen.
- A bolus of adult worms may cause bowel obstruction (usually near the ileocaecal valve), intussusception, volvulus, or perforation, which may be fatal. One study in Nigeria reported intestinal obstruction in 1:1000 infected children.
- Individual worms may enter the common bile duct, pancreatic duct, or appendix, leading to obstructive symptoms and 2° bacterial infections.
- Eggs released into the peritoneum may cause granulomas and chronic peritonitis resembling TB peritonitis.
- High fever or exposure to anaesthetics can cause adult worms to migrate (e.g. to stomach). Worms are often vomited up by febrile patients; rarely they migrate to ectopic sites (e.g. Eustachian tubes).

Diagnosis

Marked eosinophilia occurs during larval migration; differential diagnosis of this stage includes toxocariasis, hookworm, strongyloidiasis, schistosomiasis, and TPE. Intestinal infection is diagnosed by identifying worms or eggs in faeces (colour plate 5). Worms may be seen on AXR or Ba studies as string-like or tramline shadows.

Management

- Albendazole 400 mg PO stat (½ dose if <3 yrs) kills adult worms. Alternatives in adults/children >1 y: mebendazole 500 mg PO stat or 100 mg bd for 3 days; or pyrantel pamoate 11 mg/kg PO stat (max 1 g).
- Treat Loeffler's syndrome with prednisolone, followed by albendazole 2–3 weeks later to kill adult worms.
- Intestinal or biliary obstruction is best managed conservatively (analgesia, NG tube, antispasmodics, IV fluids, liquid paraffin) followed by antihelminthic treatment once the acute phase is over.
- Laparotomy may be necessary for worsening/persistent obstruction, appendicitis, or intestinal perforation. Sometimes the bolus of worms can be 'milked' into the colon by the surgeon.

Prevention of ascariasis   PUBLIC HEALTH NOTE

Education: improve hygiene and protect food from dirt.
Sanitation: prevent soil contamination by faeces disposal (e.g. latrines).
Mass treatment: is indicated when prevalence of infection >50% or frequency of heavy infection (>50,000 eggs/g faeces) ≥10% in pre-school children. Give single-dose albendazole or mebendazole to women (annually) and pre-school children (2–3 × per year).

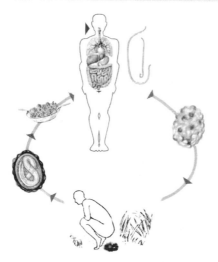

Fig. 7.12 Life cycle of *A. lumbricoides*. Vegetable gardens are faecally contaminated by eggs, which become embryonated (infectious) after 1–7 weeks in the soil. The ingested eggs hatch in the intestine, larvae migrate through lungs (see text), then are swallowed to become adult worms (females up to 40 cm, males smaller). (Adapted from G. Piekarski, *Medical parasitology in plates*, 1962, with kind permission of Bayer Pharmaceuticals.)

Toxocariasis

The canine and feline roundworms *Toxocara canis* and *T. catis* have a worldwide distribution. Humans are an accidental host: adult worms do not develop in humans, yet larvae migrate around the body and may persist for >10 years, causing visceral larva migrans and ocular disease.

Life cycle

Eggs excreted in dog or cat faeces (particularly from puppies) become embryonated in the soil and are later ingested by humans. Larvae hatch in the stomach, penetrate the intestinal mucosa and enter the circulation via mesenteric blood vessels, from where they may migrate to the brain, eye, and other organs.

Clinical features

Depend upon the density of infection:

- **Visceral larva migrans**, which occurs predominantly in children <5 years old, is characterized by heavy infection. Although asymptomatic infection may occur, typically there is fever, hepatomegaly ± splenomegaly, bronchospasm, and eosinophilia. CNS involvement (with seizures, encephalopathy, and/or neuropsychiatric symptoms), myocarditis, and nephritis are described. In most cases, the disease resolves spontaneously within 2 years, although it can be fatal, particularly if there is CNS involvement.
- **Ocular toxocariasis** usually manifests in slightly older children (5–10 years) and is an important cause of decreased visual acuity in the tropics. It usually presents with unilateral visual impairment. Peripheral involvement of the retina by subretinal granulomata and choroiditis closely resembles retinoblastoma in the early stages. Diffuse endophthalmitis or papillitis and secondary glaucoma can occur.
- **Co-infection** with *Ascaris* and *Trichuris* may also occur. 2° infection with gut bacteria carried by the larvae is common.

Diagnosis

Clinical suspicion; history of exposure, particularly to puppies; eosinophilia, fever ± organ involvement, hypergammaglobulinaemia, and elevated isohaemogglutinin titre.

ELISA using recombinant antigens to 2nd stage larvae has ~92% specificity and reasonable sensitivity (~78% for titre 1:32). CXR may show mottling in lung disease. Demonstration of larvae is very difficult, though they are sometimes present at the centre of granulomatous lesions at biopsy or post mortem.

Management

Albendazole 400 mg PO bd for 5 days; alternatively, thiabendazole 50 mg/kg PO daily in 3 divided doses for 7–28 days; or diethylcarbamazine 3 mg/kg PO bd for 21 days. Steroids may be required for ocular disease.

Prevention of toxocariasis Public health note

- Educate pet owners; avoid contamination of soil by dog and cat faeces in areas immediately adjacent to houses and child play areas.
- Control stray dogs and cats.
- Regular deworming of cats and dogs beginning at 3 weeks of age.

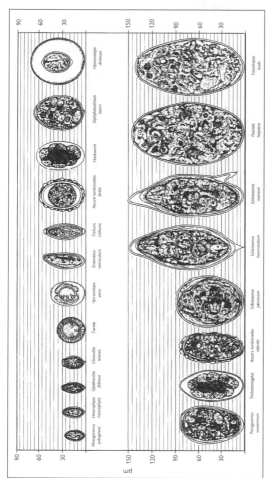

Fig. 7.13 Relative size and appearance of helminth eggs. (Reproduced with permission by the WHO from *WHO Bench Aids for the Diagnosis of Faecal Parasites*.)

* *Schistosoma mekongi* and *Schistosoma intercalatum* have been omitted. Eggs of *S.mekongi* measure 51–78 μm; eggs of *S.intercalatum* measure 120–240 μm long.

Lower GI bleeding

Lower GI bleeding occurs less frequently than upper GI bleeding and presents with passage of red blood per rectum. (Rarely, very brisk upper GI bleeds may result in passage of red blood PR rather than malaena.)

Causes: In the absence of diarrhoea, the most frequent cause is haemorrhoids. Other causes include lower GI malignancy, diverticular disease, angiodysplasia, inflammatory bowel disease, typhoid fever, and amoebic or bacterial dysentery (📖 see Chapter 6). Other causes in the setting of HIV/AIDS include TB, disseminated fungal infection (e.g. histoplasmosis), and intestinal KS.

Diagnosis and immediate management
1. Resuscitate as for upper GI haemorrhage (📖 p 276).
2. Detailed history and examination, including rectal examination. Stool colour gives an indication of the level of pathology in the GI tract (in general, the darker the stool, the higher the cause). Be alert for symptoms and signs of typhoid fever and constitutional symptoms of TB.
3. Proctoscopy and rigid sigmoidoscopy ± biopsy where appropriate.

Further management: depends on the cause. In many cases, bleeding will cease spontaneously with bed rest. Prolonged bleeding will necessitate further investigation (e.g. colonoscopy). Consider keeping patient nil by mouth (give IV fluids) initially or if there is a risk surgery may be required. For large bleeds, involve a surgical team at an early stage.

Diverticular disease

A diverticulum is an out-pouching of the gut wall which may be congenital, but is more commonly acquired due to raised intra-luminal pressure (e.g. 2° to straining at stool due to constipation) which forces the mucosa to herniate through the muscular layers of the gut wall. The condition is less common in many parts of the tropics, probably due to a diet high in fibre. Patients typically present with altered bowel habit, LIF colic (relieved by defecation), and painless rectal bleeding. Diverticula may become infected (diverticulitis), causing fever, leukocytosis, raised ESR. Treat with bed rest, high-fibre diet, and (if infected) antibiotics. Monitor for signs of perforation (>40% mortality).

Colorectal carcinoma

Lower GI malignancy remains relatively uncommon in the tropics. *Risk factors* include a high-fat, low-fibre diet; prolonged colonic transit time; polyposis coli; and ulcerative colitis. Tumours may be annular, polypoid, or ulcerous. *Clinical features* include altered bowel habit, blood/mucus PR, tenesmus, and non-specific features of malignancy (weight loss, lethargy, anorexia, etc). Anaemia and/or faecal occult blood may suggest lower GI bleeding. Abdominal or rectal examination may reveal a palpable mass. *Late presentation* may be with bowel obstruction or perforation. Perform lower GI endoscopy + biopsy where available (proctoscopy/sigmoidoscopy/colonoscopy, depending on the site). The Duke's classification is used for tumour staging. With complete surgical resection, the prognosis of Duke's A carcinoma is good.

Inflammatory bowel disease (IBD)

Both Crohn's disease and ulcerative colitis are rare in the tropics, although cases are reported from more developed areas. The usual presentation is with weight loss and diarrhoea with blood and mucus. Severe disease may present with intestinal obstruction or toxic dilatation of the colon. Anorectal fissures/fistulae and oral or perineal ulceration may also complicate Crohn's disease. Associated extra-intestinal manifestations include erythema nodosum, pyoderma gangrenosum, anterior uveitis, arthritis, sacroiliitis, primary sclerosing cholangitis, renal stones, malnutrition, and amyloidosis. *Diagnosis* requires sigmoidoscopy/colonoscopy and biopsy. *Management* of the acute case is with systemic steroids (or topical prednisolone enemas if disease is localized to the rectum). Exclude infective aetiology (e.g. amoebic dysentery) as best as possible first. 5-ASA drugs such as sulfasalazine and mesalazine form the backbone of maintenance therapy. Severe cases may require surgery.

Haemorrhoids (piles)

Haemorrhoids are prolapsing anal cushions, normally associated with constipation and/or childbirth; varicosities of the anal canal may also occur in severe portal hypertension. Presentation is with bright red PR bleeding, prolapse, and/or discomfort (pain may be severe if thrombosis occurs). They are classified and treated as follows:

- *First degree*: prolapse down the anal canal but not out of it; therefore only recognized at proctoscopy. Treatment is sclerotherapy by injecting 2 ml of 5% phenol in oil.
- *Second degree*: prolapse through the anus but reduce spontaneously. Treatment is with sclerotherapy or rubber band ligation.
- *Third degree*: as above but require digital reduction.
- *Fourth degree*: remain permanently prolapsed. Treatment is with rubber band ligation or haemorrhoidectomy.
- *Thrombosed piles* are treated with analgesia and bed rest. The clot may be expressed under local anaesthetic, usually relieving the pain.

Prevention: high-fibre diet; avoid straining during defecation.

Childhood causes of rectal bleeding	PAEDIATRIC NOTE
Newborn	**Characteristics**
Swallowed maternal blood	Tarry red blood, spontaneous resolution
Haemorrhagic disease	Coagulopathy, haemorrhage elsewhere
Stress ulcer; haemorrhagic gastritis	Difficult labour/delivery; CNS injury, sepsis
Necrotizing enterocolitis (NEC)	Associated with prematurity
Neonate/infant	
Milk allergy	Occult bleeds, colic, diarrhoea, atopy
Mid-gut volvulus	Bile-stained vomitus, pain, obstruction
Intussusception	Usually <2 y old (see 📖 p 17)
Bleeding Meckel's diverticulum	Congenital; often painless; anaemia
Any age	
Henoch–Schonlein purpura	Pain, arthralgia, haemolytic anaemia (📖 p 219)
Haemangioma/telangiectasia	Congenital; may be cutaneous lesions
Other (IBD, peptic ulcer, varices, etc)	As for adults

Around the anus

Pruritus ani

Peri-anal itching/discomfort may be caused by:

- Skin infection or damage e.g. due to enterobiasis, tinea cruris, psoriasis, contact dermatitis, lichen planus, lichen sclerosis, leukoplakia, *Corynebacterium minutissimum* (the causative agent of erythrasma).
- Surgical conditions e.g. haemorrhoids, fissure-in-ano, fistulae, skin-tags, polyps, malignancy.

Enterobiasis (threadworm, pinworm)

The soil-transmitted helminth *Enterobius vermicularis* is a common infection of young children worldwide.

Life cycle: Transmission is usually faeco-oral (pruritus ani → scratching → eggs transferred on fingers or under fingernails from anus to mouth; eggs may also be carried on contaminated bed linen or fomites) or by retro-infection in which larvae hatching at the anus migrate back upwards into the bowel. Ingested ova hatch in the stomach and larvae migrate to the appendix and caecum where they invade the crypts and mature into adult worms (9–12 mm long by 2–4 mm wide). The female migrates through the anus (usually at night) and lays eggs on the perianal skin and perineum, which are then carried on the faeces or picked up under the fingernails during scratching. There is no multiplication inside the body. The cycle takes about 2–4 weeks.

Clinical features: In the majority of cases, infected individuals are asymptomatic until the female deposits her eggs perianally. This induces intense pruritus. General symptoms include insomnia, restlessness, loss of appetite and weight; children are often irritable and frequently have enuresis. Worms can enter the vulva and cause vulvitis with a mucoid discharge and pruritus. Worms may also occasionally be found in the ears and nose. Very rarely, the worms gain access to the abdominal cavity and cause chronic peritonitis and granulomata. 2° bacterial infection of skin damaged by scratching is a common problem.

Diagnosis: Requires detection of eggs on swabs from either the perianal region (use sellotape), under the fingernails, or (less commonly) in the faeces. Occasionally, adult worms may be seen around the anus (usually with an 'element of surprise' at night!).

Management: Really only beneficial in symptomatic individuals since reinfection is virtually inevitable in most cases, unless there is change in behaviour. Where possible, treat the whole family and school members. A single dose of albendazole 400 mg PO (children 12–24 months 200 mg) or mebendazole 100 mg repeated after 2–3 weeks.

Prevention of recurrent   PUBLIC HEALTH NOTE
threadworm infection

- Education to improve personal hygiene.
- Scrub children's hands before meals and after defecation.
- Keep fingernails short.
- Wash bedclothes, underwear, and nightclothes regularly at ≥55°C for several days after treatment.

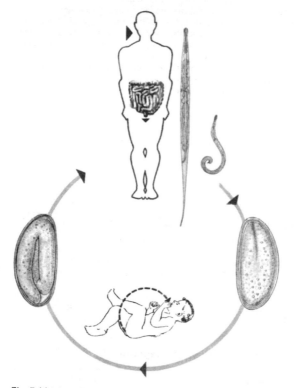

Fig. 7.14 Life cycle of threadworm (*Enterobius vermicularis*). Eggs are ingested (e.g. from fingers which have scratched itchy perianal skin). Larvae hatch in the intestine, develop, and penetrate the mucosa. The male and female worms mate in the intestine and the smaller males die; the gravid females (about 12 mm long) migrate through the anus and deposit up to 10,000 eggs on the perianal skin. (Adapted from G. Piekarski, *Medical parasitology in plates*, 1962, with kind permission of Bayer Pharmaceuticals.)

Visible 'worms' in stool

Some helmith infections may present following direct observation of worms in the stool. These include *Ascaris lumbricoides* (📖 p 318), *Taenia saginata* and *Taenia solium* (the beef and pork tapeworms), and *Hymenolepsis nana* (the dwarf tapeworm).

Taenia saginata (the beef tapeworm)

This is common wherever raw beef is eaten (e.g. Ethiopia). Mature proglottids of the bovine tapeworm *Taenia saginata* are highly motile and conspicuous in the faeces of infected individuals. Occasionally, proglottids (white, 16×8 mm, flat, motile) may be felt emerging independently from the anus, causing embarrassment. The adult worm is typically 3–5 m long (though some reach 10 m) and attaches, via suckers, to the upper small intestine wall. Humans are the only definitive host and usually acquire infection from eating raw or undercooked beef containing a larva-filled cysticercus. Adult worms may shed up to 50,000 eggs per day for 10 years or more. Patients may complain of vague abdominal pain, distension, anorexia, and nausea, although infection is often asymptomatic.

Diagnosis: Eosinophilia is not usually a feature. Eggs may be seen on faecal microscopy but are often absent because they are contained within proglottids — if the stool is negative, ask the patient to collect proglottids to show you. Intact proglottids can be speciated according to the number of uterine branches.

Management: Give praziquantel 10 mg/kg PO as a single dose.

Prevention: Avoid eating undercooked beef (cysts are destroyed by temperatures >48°C). Improve sanitation. Avoid cattle grazing in areas used for open-field defecation.

Taenia solium (the pork tapeworm)

Cysts are eaten in poorly cooked pork (the intermediate host) and mature in the small intestine. The adult worm measures 2–3 m (up to 8 m) and attaches to the mucosal surface by two encircling rows of hooklets. Unlike *T. saginata*, humans are also readily infected by the larval form of the tapeworm after ingesting eggs excreted by a human carrier (often auto-infection from faecal-oral contamination), causing human cysticercosis (see 📖 p 440). Symptoms of adult worm infection are as for *T. saginata*. The proglottids are smaller (~12×6 mm) and less motile.

Management: Give praziquantel 10 mg/kg PO as a single dose.

Hymenolepsis nana (the dwarf tapeworm)

Measuring 3–4 cm, *H. nana* is seldom seen in the stool but may give rise to abdominal symptoms like other tapeworms. However, unlike the other tapeworms, *H. nana* has both larval and adult stages in humans and does not require intermediate hosts. Infection with several hundred worms is common. Since encystation occurs within small intestinal villi, there is immune stimulation, resulting in eosinophilia. Characteristic eggs are seen on faecal microscopy.

Management: Give praziquantel 20 mg/kg PO as a single dose.

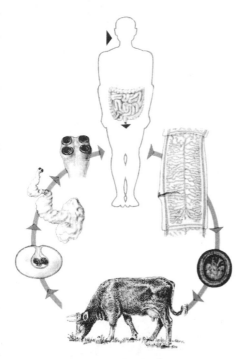

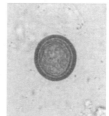

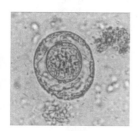

Fig. 7.15 Life cycle of *T. saginata*. Man ingests the cysticercus in beef, which evaginates, and the scolex attaches to wall of the intestine. The adult worm grows to several metres length in the intestine, releasing gravid segments (proglottids) and some free eggs. Cattle become infected when grazing on grass contaminated with faeces. (Adapted from G. Piekarski, *Medical parasitology in plates*, 1962, with kind permission of Bayer Pharmaceuticals.)

Fig. 7.16 Egg of *H. nana* (30 × 45 mcm) and of *T. solium* (30 × 45 mcm diameter).

Cardiology

Section editor   **Bongani Mayosi**

Cardiology in developing countries

The pattern of cardiovascular disease is changing in developing countries. Although infectious diseases still dominate clinical medicine in many countries (especially in Africa), increasing urbanization with its attendant risk factors of smoking, hypertension, and obesity are producing a new pattern of disease which includes stroke, diabetes mellitus, and ischaemic heart disease. While ischaemic heart disease is increasing in Latin America, India, and China, the disease is still rare in rural parts of sub-Saharan Africa, India, and South America. Rheumatic heart disease, tuberculous pericarditis, and infectious (Chagas' disease) and other cardiomyopathies remain major contributors to circulatory disease in many developing countries.

Acute rheumatic fever and rheumatic heart disease still disable young patients and are the most common causes of heart failure in children and young adults. Facilities for medical and surgical treatment are often lacking. HIV co-infection has led to a large increase in cases of tuberculous pericarditis, carrying a mortality of 40% in HIV+ patients. The cardiomyopathies are endemic in many developing countries. Peripartum cardiomyopathy is highly prevalent in parts of Africa; endomyocardial fibrosis occurs in the peri-equatorial tropical regions of Africa, America, and India.

Chagas' disease is the major cause of disability secondary to tropical diseases in young adults in Latin American countries. Congestive heart failure caused by Chagas' cardiomyopathy is the most frequent and severe clinical manifestation of *Trypanosoma cruzi* infection, and is associated with a poor prognosis and a high mortality when compared to heart failure due to other causes.

Chest pain

Central chest pain

Nature
- A constricting pain suggests angina, oesophagitis, or anxiety.
- A sharp pain may be from the pleura or pericardium (both may be exacerbated by deep inspiration, movements or positions, postures).
- Prolonged, crushing, tight ('like an elephant on my chest'), intense pain unrelated to position or breathing suggests myocardial infarction (MI).
- The pain of aortic dissection is often felt in the back.

Pains that are unlikely to be cardiac in origin include:
- Short, sharp, stabbing or pricking pains.
- Pains lasting <30 seconds, however intense.
- Well-localized left submammary pain ('in my heart, doctor').
- Pains of continually varying location.

Ask about
- Radiation (to shoulders, neck, jaw, or arms — especially left: suggests lesion of the heart, aorta or oesophagus).

- Precipitating and exacerbating factors (exercise, emotion, or palpitations suggest ischaemia; food, lying flat, hot drinks, or alcohol suggest oesophagitis. However, a meal may also precipitate angina).
- Alleviating factors (N.B. glyceryl trinitrate relieves both cardiac pain and oesophageal pain, but acts much more rapidly in the former). Pericardial pain classically improves on leaning forward.
- Associations (e.g. dyspnoea and/or palpitations, pallor, sweating, feeling of impending doom, nausea and vomiting — can be present with both an inferior MI and GI pathology).
- Risk factors for ischaemic heart disease (age >55 years, previous angina/MI, smoking, diabetes, hypertension, hyperlipidaemia).

Non-central chest pain

May still be cardiac in origin, but other conditions enter the differential diagnosis (see box). The more common conditions include:

- Pleuritic pain.
- Musculoskeletal pain.
- Gall bladder disease.
- *Varicella zoster* (shingles).
- Pancreatitic disease.

Causes of chest pain

Cardiovascular
Myocardial ischaemia
Myocardial infarction
Aortic dissection
Aortic aneurysm
Large pulmonary embolus
Tumours (primary)

Airway
Intubation
Central bronchial carcinoma
Inhaled foreign body
Tracheitis

Mediastinal
Oesophageal spasm
Oesophagitis
Mediastinitis
Sarcoid lymphadenopathy
Lymphoma

Pleuro-pericardial
Pericarditis
Infective pleurisy
Pneumothorax
Pneumonia
Autoimmune disease

Chest wall
Rib fracture
Rib tumour
Muscular strain
Thoracic nerve compression
Costochondritis
Thoracic varicella zoster
Coxsackie B infection

Other
Anxiety, hyperventilation
Panic attacks, tabes dorsalis
Gall bladder disease
Pancreatic disease

Angina

Classically, this is central, crushing chest pain that may radiate to the jaw, neck, or one or both arms. It may be felt only in the jaw or arm, or be felt as tightness across the chest. It represents myocardial ischaemia and may be precipitated by exertion, anxiety, cold, or a heavy meal and be associated with dyspnoea, pallor, and faintness. It is relieved by rest and nitrates. In most cases, it is caused by coronary artery disease, but may be due to valvular heart disease (aortic stenosis, aortic regurgitation, mitral stenosis), hypertrophic cardiomyopathy, and hypoperfusion from dysrrhythmias, arteritis, or anaemia. Indigestion is the most common differential diagnosis. Ischaemic heart disease is particularly common in people of Asian, Melanesian, Polynesian origin (who also have high incidence of NIDDM). The incidence is also higher in black than in white Americans. Angina is graded clinically using the Canadian Cardiovascular Society (CCS) grading system—see box.

Diagnosis

On the ECG look for ST depression, flattened (or inverted) T waves, and evidence of old infarcts (Q waves). If available, do an exercise ECG 48 h after the angina settles. Take blood for FBC and ESR to exclude non-atheromatous causes (see above), and cardiac enzymes, as available, to exclude myocardial infarction.

Management

Risk factor modification: Stop smoking, prudent diet (↓ lipids and ↑ fruit and vegetable intake), ↓ weight, exercise more. Look for hypertension, diabetes, and hyperlipidaemia and treat as appropriate. Start:
- *Aspirin:* 75–150 mg od.

Anti-anginal therapy: Start with glyceryl trinitrate (GTN) 300 to 600 mcg either sublingually or as a spray at 0.4 mg per dose prn up to every hour. If inadequate, switch to triple therapy:
1. *Beta-blockers:* e.g. atenolol 50–100 mg PO od. (contra-indicated in asthma).
2. *Slow-release calcium antagonists:* e.g. nifedipine MR 30 mg–90 mg PO od; felodipine 5–10 mg/day, diltiazem 60 mg PO 2–3 times od, increasing to max 360 mg od. (contra-indicated in fertile women). Short-acting Ca^{2+} blockers ↑ cardiac events.
3. *Isosorbide mononitrate or dinitrate* (as available): mononitrate 10–60 mg/d (od or bd); dinitrate 10-60 mg tds. NB: need nitrate-free interval of 7 h in every 24. When drugs fail to control angina (CCS Class II to IV, see box), coronary angiography is indicated to consider revascularization either by percutaneous coronary intervention (PCI) or by coronary artery bypass grafting (CABG) for the relief of symptom.

Unstable angina

Unstable angina is new onset angina of at least CCS III severity (see box), or angina that is rapidly worsening and present on minimal exertion or at rest or within 30 days of MI.

Management: aspirin, clopidogrel, beta-blocker, and bed rest. Give unfractionated heparin 7500–10,000 IU IV q4 h to keep APTT twice control, if monitoring is available. (If available, low molecular weight heparin does not require monitoring.) If pain persists or recurs or high TIMI risk score ≥5 (see below) refer for specialist assessment/angiography/revascularization.

Grading of angina pectoris by the Canadian Cardiovascular Society (CCS)

Class I	Angina occurs only with strenuous, rapid, or prolonged exertion.
Class II	Slight limitation of ordinary activity: angina occurs on walking or climbing stairs rapidly, walking uphill, walking or stair climbing after meals, or in cold, or in wind, or under emotional stress, or only during the few hours after awakening.
Class III	Marked limitation of ordinary physical activity: angina occurs on walking 1 or 2 blocks on the level and climbing one flight of stairs in normal conditions and at a normal pace.
Class IV	Inability to carry on any physical activity without discomfort — anginal symptoms may be present at rest.

Risk of myocardial infarction or death

(thrombolysis in myocardial infarction (TIMI) IIB trial risk score*)

Prognostic variable	Point
>2 angina events within 24 h	1
Use of aspirin within 7 days	1
Age ≥65 years	1
>3 coronary risk factors	1
Known coronary obstruction	1
ECG: ST-segment deviation	1
Elevated cardiac enzymes	1
Total	7

* Risk of adverse outcome (death, repeat MI) ranges from 5% (score 0 or 1) to 41% (score 6 or 7)

Preventing ischaemic heart disease (IHD)

The prevention of IHD applies to three groups:
1 Cardiovascular health promotion in children and adolescents — promote healthy diet, no smoking, and high physical activity.
2 1° prevention of adults without overt features of cardiovascular disease.
3 2° prevention in adults with established cardiovascular disease (i.e. MI, peripheral vascular disease, or stroke).

Interventions

- *Diet*: advocate consumption of a variety of fruits, vegetables, whole grains, dairy products, fish, legumes, poultry, and lean meat. Fat intake is unrestricted prior to 2 years of age. After age 2, limit foods high in saturated fats (<10% of calories per day), cholesterol (<300 mg per day), and *trans*-fatty acids. Limit salt intake to <6 g per day.
- *Smoking*: avoid beginning cigarette smoking and exposure to environmental tobacco smoke, and complete cessation for those who smoke.
- *Physical activity*: >60 minutes/day of moderate to vigorous physical activity, and sedentary time must be limited (e.g. limit TV time to <2 h/day).

The following 1° prevention interventions are of proven cost effectiveness in adults who do not have overt cardiovascular disease:
- Prudent diet, smoking cessation, and physical activity.
- Identification and treatment of hypertension, diabetes, and familial hyperlipidaemia.
- Statins in patients with diabetes and hypertension with multiple risk factors.

The following 2° prevention interventions are of proven value and cost effectiveness in adults with overt cardiovascular disease:
- Prudent diet, smoking cessation, and physical activity.
- Statins in patients with IHD, stroke, and peripheral vascular disease.
- Angiotensin-converting enzyme inhibitors for all patients with MI, PVD, stroke.
- Cardiac rehabilitation following MI.

Myocardial infarction (MI)

This is the irreversible necrosis of part of the heart muscle, almost always due to coronary artery atherosclerosis.

Clinical features: the pain is usually of greater severity and duration (>30 minutes) than angina, though similar in nature and usually associated with nausea and vomiting, sweating, pallor, and distress. In the elderly and diabetics, small MIs may be painless. There may be tachycardia, tachypnoea, cyanosis, mild pyrexia (<38.5°C). The BP may be ↑, normal, or ↓. There may also be features of the complications (e.g. dyspnoea, basal lung crepitations, pericardial rub, or the pan-systolic murmur of mitral incompetence or VSD).

Diagnosis: ECG and cardiac enzymes. Diagnosis is based on (i) history (ii) ECG changes, and (iii) cardiac enzymes in order to allow the classification into ST-elevation MI (STEMI) or non-ST-elevation MI (NSTEMI). Troponins, where available, are the investigations of choice.

Other tests: CXR — look for features of heart failure, change in cardiac size (ventricular aneurysm), or aortic dissection. Measure haemoglobin, white cell count, and platelet count; urea, creatinine, sodium, potassium, and glucose.

ECG changes in MI

An initially normal ECG progresses to tall T waves and ST elevation (>2 mm in two chest or >1 mm in two adjacent limb leads for a diagnosis of STEMI). Alternatively, patient may develop new onset LBBB. Within 24 h, the T wave inverts as ST elevation begins to resolve. Pathological Q waves (>1 small square in width and >2 mm in length) form within a few days. These may persist or completely resolve in 10%. T-wave inversion may or may not persist. If ST elevation persists, suspect ventricular aneurysm.

Site of infarct

- *Anterior*: changes occur in V2–5.
- *Septal*: changes in V1–3.
- *Inferior*: changes in II, III, and aVF.
- *Lateral*: changes in I, aVL, and V6.
- *Posterior*: look for the reciprocal (i.e. inverted) changes in the anterior leads V1–3; dominant R wave (= inverted Q wave); and ST depression (= inverted ST elevation) with the clinical features of an infarct. May be associated RV infarct — ask for V4R ECG lead (lead V4 placed in mirror image position over right chest) which will show ST elevation.

Non-Q-wave infarcts: (formerly called 'subendocardial infarcts') do not involve the whole thickness of the myocardium and thus have the ST changes but not the Q waves.

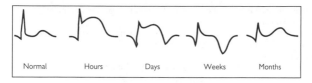

Fig. 8.1 ECG changes following MI.

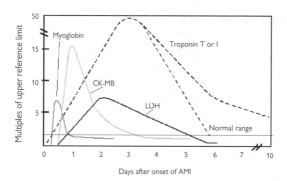

Fig. 8.2 Release patterns of cardiac markers (Wu, A.H., *Journal of Clinical Immunoassay* 1994, 17, 45–8.)

Immediate management of MI

The greatest risk of death is in the 1st hour — prompt action can and does save lives.

- Relax and reassure the patient.
- Give oxygen by face mask if hypoxic or left heart failure/pulmonary oedema suspected. Finger pulse oximetry is then recommended to monitor arterial O_2 saturation.
- Insert an IV line and give pain relief (morphine 10 mg by slow IV injection, followed by further 5–10 mg doses as necessary; half the dose in elderly or frail patients.)
- Give GTN 0.3–0.6 mg sublingual tablet or spray.
- Give aspirin 300 mg PO stat, then 75 mg od thereafter.
- Give clopidogrel, initially 300 mg, then 75 mg PO daily on admission, in conjunction with aspirin.
- If STEMI, refer to a centre where streptokinase (see box opposite) or 1° percutaneous coronary intervention may be given within 12 h.
- Give a beta-blocker (e.g. atenolol 5 mg IV over 5 min, 50 mg PO 15 mins later, then 50 mg bd) unless the patient has heart failure or asthma. It will ↓ cardiac O_2 demand, infarct size, and risk of dysrrhythmias and septal rupture.
- Start the patient on an oral ACE inhibitor 24 h after the infarction. Titrate dose against BP.

- Start statin therapy in hospital in all patients regardless of initial cholesterol level.
- Tight glycaemic control with insulin in patients with type 2 diabetes is required in the peri-infarction period.
- Prohibit smoking.
- At least 24 h bed rest with continuous ECG monitoring and q6 h temp, pulse, RR, BP. Perform frequent clinical examination for complications (📖 p 339).
- Daily ECG, cardiac enzymes, U&Es (and CXR if there is worsening lung function) for the subsequent 2–3 days.

Post-infarct management

If the post-MI period is uncomplicated, the patient may be mobilized by day 2 or 3. If there are no complications, the patient can usually be discharged by day 3 and gradually ↑the amount of exercise done over 1 month. The patient should not drive during this period. Strongly discourage smoking and give dietary advice.

Prognosis: depends upon the degree of LV dysfunction, presence of significant dysrrhythmias, heart size on CXR, presence of post-MI angina, and the presence of pulmonary oedema. In the UK, mortality rates for the first year after discharge are 6–8% with over half these deaths occurring in the first 3 months.

Long-term treatment: patients with no complications and good prognostic indices should be discharged and followed by the general practitioner. All patients should be advised to modify their risk factors.

All patients should ideally take aspirin (indefinitely), clopidogrel (for at least 9–12 months), beta blocker (for >18 months), an ACE inhibitor (indefinitely), and a statin (indefinitely).

Thrombolysis

Streptokinase is the most widely available thrombolytic agent. Give 1.5 million units streptokinase in 100 ml 0.9% saline IV over 1 h. Carries ~1% risk of stroke. Other side effects include hypotension (usu responds to slowing down or stopping infusion), nausea, vomiting, haemorrhage, anaphylaxis (rare). tPA, rPA, and tNK are more expensive thrombolytics than streptokinase, but slightly more effective and cause less hypotension.

Contraindications to thrombolytic therapy

A thrombolytic agent should not be given if the patient:
- Has had a stroke or active bleeding (e.g. peptic ulcer) within the last 2 months
- Has systolic BP>200 mmHg
- Has had surgery or trauma in the past 10 days
- Has a bleeding disorder or uses anticoagulants
- Is pregnant
- Is menstruating
- Has had previous streptokinase treatment between 4 days and 1 year previously (in the case of streptokinase).

Complications of MI

1. Post-infarct angina: (within 30 days of MI): is associated with ↑mortality and occurs in up to 30%. Treat vigorously with nitrates, beta-blockers, Ca^{2+} channel blockers, heparin, and aspirin. Angiography is indicated.

2. Arrhythmias: see ALS protocols below.

- *Sinus bradycardia* — may be due to infarct or medication (beta-blocker). Usually no action is required if the patient is haemodynamically stable.
- *Supraventricular tachycardia* — a sinus tachycardia is common post-MI. Atrial fibrillation (AF) occurs in 10% and should be rapidly controlled to avoid the onset of ventricular tachycardia (VT) and infarct spread. Use beta blockade. AF is usually transient, but, if necessary (in presence of heart failure or hypotension, or refractory to other treatments), conversion back to sinus rhythm can be achieved by DC cardioversion or IV amiodarone (see 🕮 p 344).
- *Ventricular arrhythmias* are most common in the first few hours post MI and may be heralded by ventricular premature beats. VT>120 bpm may progress to ventricular fibrillation (VF). Treat with an IV beta-blocker. Correct low serum potassium level. Amiodarone (300 mg IV over 20–60 min; then 900 mg over 24 h) may be added if VT recurs. VF may occur in the first few hours or days and needs emergency treatment. It carries a poor prognosis in the presence of cardiogenic shock or failure. Accelerated idioventricular rhythm can occur after any MI with reperfusion (following thrombolysis) — it is usually benign, not affecting cardiac output, and needs no treatment.
- *Nodal rhythms*: have a narrow QRS complex, normal axis usually, but have no associated P wave (or it may come after the QRS). They are usually intermittent and self-limiting, but in a large MI may ↓ both cardiac output and BP. Treat with atropine or a temporary pacemaker.
- *Conduction disturbances*: all degrees of AV block may occur, most commonly in inferior MIs (20%). 1st-degree block needs no treatment. 2nd-degree block is usually Wenckebach and only requires treatment if there is symptomatic bradycardia. 3rd-degree block often follows second-degree block and is usually temporary. Again, treat with atropine or isoprenaline if symptomatic. In extensive anterior MIs, damage to the conducting system will cause complete and progressive AV block that will require pacing, possibly permanently. Heart block in inferior MIs is usually temporary, lasting <5 days.

3. Myocardial dysfunction

- *Left ventricular failure* (see below).
- *Cardiogenic shock*: severe failure causing hypotension, tachycardia, oliguria, distress, and peripheral shutdown. It may be due to: acute MR, severe LV dysfunction, cardiac rupture, VSD, arrhythmias, RV infarct. Treatment is with face mask O_2, IV diuretics (if LVF), fluids (if RV infarct), inotropes. Evidence from clinical trials supports invasive intervention in cardiogenic shock post-MI.

4. Right ventricular infarct: occurs in one-third of inferior infarcts but is clinically significant in less. There is ↓BP and ↑JVP with clear lung fields on auscultation. Lead V4R (see 🕮 p 336) on the ECG may show ST elevation. Treatment is with IV fluids to ↑LV filling. Inotropes may be useful.

5. Mechanical defects

- *Papillary or septal rupture* occurs in <1% of all MIs and may occur 1–7 days after an anterior or inferior MI (MR most commonly after infero-lateral MIs, VSD after septal MIs). Listen for new murmurs and basal crepitations, and watch for clinical deterioration. Urgent surgery is indicated for papillary muscle rupture with acute MR; early closure of VSD is advised.

- *Left ventricular aneurysm*: occurs in 10–20% of anterior MIs. The apex beat is diffuse and there may be atypical/stabbing chest pain, accompanied by ST elevation lasting 4–8 weeks. They rarely rupture but are associated with emboli, arrhythmias, and CCF. Patients may require lifelong anticoagulation. Surgical removal of aneurysm is indicated in intractable heart failure, recurrent ventricular tachycardia, and frequent embolism in spite of anticoagulation.

- *Cardiac rupture*: usually results in rapid death 2–7 days post-MI. It occurs in <1% of MIs. A small or incomplete rupture may be sealed by the pericardium, forming a pseudoaneurysm that needs prompt surgical repair.

6. Pericarditis: 20% of patients have a pericardial rub after 24 h. There is chest pain, relieved by sitting up and varying with respiration. It is usually self-limiting but a single-dose NSAID (e.g. indomethacin 100 mg PR) may be very effective, avoiding the need for long-term therapy.

- *Dressler's syndrome*: is an autoimmune pericarditis occurring 1–10 weeks post-MI in 5% of patients. There is fever, leucocytosis, and, occasionally, pericardial or pleural effusion. Treatment is with NSAIDs ± corticosteroids.

7. Mural thrombus: is common in large MIs and may cause arterial emboli, leading to strokes, gut/limb/renal infarcts. Usually diagnosed by echocardiography; needs warfarin for ≥3 months.

Advanced life support (ALS) protocols

Most sudden deaths result from dysrrhythmias associated with acute MI or chronic IHD. Successful resuscitation following a cardiopulmonary arrest is most likely if:
- The arrest is witnessed.
- Basic life support is started promptly and
- Defibrillation (if appropriate) is carried out as early as possible.

Basic life support (BLS)

The purpose of BLS is to maintain adequate ventilation and circulation until a means can be obtained to reverse the underlying cause of the cardiac arrest.
- Remember **A**, **B**, and **C** — **A**irway, **B**reathing, and **C**irculation.
- Ensure that it is safe to approach the patient.

Airway: Remove foreign bodies from the airway (including false teeth); use suction if necessary. Tilt the head back (unless a neck injury is suspected) or do jaw thrust.

Breathing: Is the patient breathing? If not, assist via a mask (with 100% O_2) and bag ventilation if available, or mouth-to-mouth resuscitation until intubation is possible. If there is upper airway obstruction, a cricothyrotomy may be needed. If there is a tension pneumothorax, relieve it before proceeding further.

Circulation: Is there a pulse in the carotid arteries? If not, begin external cardiac massage until defibrillation (under the guidelines below) is possible.

If you are alone and the patient is unconscious, assess whether going/calling for help would be of more benefit than attempting resuscitation alone. It is hard to leave an injured/unconscious person, but their only realistic hope of survival may be if you go straight for help.

ALS treatment algorithms for cardiopulmonary arrest

The algorithm shown opposite is a summary of the methods used in the ALS training scheme. The methods involve skilled procedures which should only be attempted by qualified staff, since improper use of defibrillators could result in more harm being done to the patient, as well as harm to those carrying out the resuscitation. It is strongly recommended that all medical staff read the ALS (or equivalent) course book and practise arrest protocols in 'mock' arrest scenarios.

Note: If at any stage a spontaneous pulse is felt, defibrillation should stop and the patient be ventilated. Watch for peri-arrest dysrrhythmias (see below). Intubation and IV access should take <30 seconds. If difficult, they should be delayed until the next loop of the cycle. If defibrillation remains unsuccessful, consider changing the paddle positions or the defibrillator.

ALS protocols are presented with the kind permission of the Resuscitation Council (UK) Ltd., and are also given on the inside back cover of the book for easy reference in emergency.

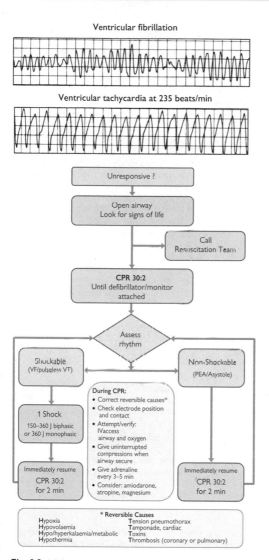

Fig. 8.3 Adult cardiac arrest algoithm. (Reproduced with kind permission of Resuscitation council (UK) Ltd).

Cardiac dysrrhythmias

These most commonly occur in the setting of an acute MI, but may also occur during chronic ischaemia.

Clinical features: are usually of 'funny turns', collapse, and palpitations. Distinguish from epilepsy — a witness may help in this.

Investigations: FBC, U&E, Ca^{2+}, glucose, TFTs, CXR, ECG. Arrange echocardiography if cardiomyopathy or valvular disease is suspected.

Atrial fibrillation (AF)

AF is an ineffective, irregular atrial tachycardia, which results in irregular ventricular contraction. Common causes are MI, ischaemia, MV disease, hyperthyroidism, hypertension, and excess alcohol intake. Also: cardiomyopathy, pericarditis, sick sinus syndrome, CA bronchus, endocarditis, atrial myxoma, and haemochromatosis. It is a significant risk factor for stroke.

Clinical features: an irregularly irregular pulse with a first heart sound of varying intensity and the apex rate greater than the radial rate. The patient may be breathless and complain of palpitations. ECG shows a chaotic baseline with no P waves and irregularly irregular QRS complexes.

Therapeutic strategy

The therapeutic goals in patients with AF are:
- To identify and treat the underlying cause or risk factor for AF.
- A choice of restoration and maintenance of sinus rhythm (rhythm control) versus acceptance of the arrhythmia and control of ventricular rate (rate control).
- Assessment of thrombo-embolic risk and antithrombotic treatment for patients at risk. Anticoagulation with warfarin is superior to antiplatelet therapy.

Identification of the underlying cause

This is the first step in the management of all patients with AF. The underlying cause (listed above), if any, must be addressed prior to or at the same time as initiating specific treatment for AF.

Rhythm control

Using electrical cardioversion, drugs, ablation, or surgery may be particularly useful in younger patients with structurally normal hearts and paroxysmal AF, or persistent AF of recent onset. Both electrical and chemical cardioversion carry risk of embolization of atrial thrombus, so should only be attempted within 48 h of new AF onset, or in patient adequately anticoagulated for >6 wks, or if pre-cardioversion transoesophageal echo shows no thrombus.

Rate control

- Appropriate in elderly patients with hypertension or structural heart disease and persistent or permanent arrhythmia, especially if this can be tolerated symptomatically.
- Use drugs (usually β or calcium channel blockers with or without digoxin) or, occasionally, atrioventricular node ablation and implantation of a permanent pacemaker.

Antithrombotic treatment

Anticoagulation with warfarin is indicated in patients with AF (paroxysmal or persistent) with:
- Previous stroke or transient ischaemic attack.
- Valvular or other structural heart disease.
- Hypertension.
- Diabetes.
- Age >65years.
- Left ventricular dysfunction and/or left atrial enlargement on echo.
- Warfarin carries a risk of bleeding which should be balanced against its likely benefits and discussed with the patient in each case.

Bradycardia

If the bradycardia is acute and symptomatic (usually post-MI):
- Treat or remove the underlying cause (e.g. beta-blockers, NB eye drops).
- Give atropine 0.3–0.6 mg slowly IV, repeating to a max. of 3 mg in 24 h.
- Alternatively, try isoprenaline 1–4 mcg/min IV (increasing to 8 mcg/min if necessary for Stokes–Adams attacks).
- Temporary pacing may be needed for unresponsive bradycardia. Chronic bradycardia necessitates permanent pacing.

Other causes of arrhythmias and conduction disturbances

- Drugs (mostly those used to treat arrhythmias).
- Cardiomyopathy.
- Myocarditis.
- Thyroid disease.
- Electrolyte disturbances.

Heart failure

Heart failure is a clinical syndrome of effort intolerance which is due to a cardiac abnormality and is usually associated with neurohumoral adaptations leading to salt and water retention. Thus, heart failure is a syndrome and not a diagnosis — i.e. the patient may have features consistent with heart failure, but always ask what is the cause?

Causes of heart failure

- Hypertension.
- Ischaemic heart disease.
- Heart muscle disease — cardiomyopathy, myocarditis, infiltrative diseases (haemochromatosis, sarcoid, amyloid), Chagas' disease, Beri–Beri.
- Valvular heart disease — aortic stenosis/regurgitation, mitral stenosis/ regurgitation.
- Pericardial disease — effusive/effusive-constrictive/constrictive pericarditis.
- Congenital heart disease.
- Other causes — prolonged tachycardia, thyrotoxicosis, alcohol and other toxins (e.g. chemotherapy, cocaine), pregnancy, severe anaemia, Paget's disease, arteriovenous fistula, phaeochromocytoma.

Fluid overload involves pushing the myocardium too far over the Starling length–tension relationship (initially, stretching results in ↑ contractile force, but beyond the apex of the curve, further stretch results in ↓ force), resulting in ↓ cardiac output. The neurohumoral activation of the renin-angiotensin-aldosterone system leads to salt and water retention.

Based on clinical manifestations, heart failure may be classified as left, right, or biventricular failure.

Left ventricular failure (LVF)

Dominated by pulmonary oedema, resulting in exertional dyspnoea, orthopnoea, paroxysmal nocturnal dyspnoea, wheeze, cough, and fatigue.
- *Signs:* tachypnoea, tachycardia, basal lung crackles, third heart sound, pulsus alternans, cardiomegaly, peripheral cyanosis, pleural effusion, ↓ peak expiratory flow.
- *CXR signs* — see box.
- *ECG* changes will depend on the specific cause.
- *Echocardiography* may differentiate between valvular and pericardial lesions.

Right ventricular failure (RVF)

RVF causes dependent oedema (i.e. in the legs if standing, in the sacrum if supine), abdominal discomfort, nausea, fatigue, and wasting. Usually 2° to chronic lung disease or LVF.
- *Signs:* raised JVP, hepatomegaly (may be pulsatile if tricuspid regurgitation is present), and pitting oedema.

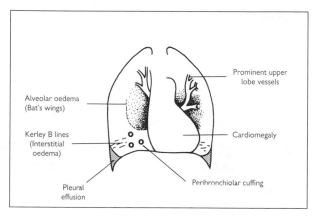

Fig. 8.4 CXR changes in heart failure.

Management of heart failure
- Identify and treat the cause if possible.
- Treat reversible exacerbating factors (e.g. anaemia, arrhythmia, electrolyte disturbance, infection, non-adherence to treatment).
- Restrict salt and alcohol intake.
- Avoid NSAIDs as they cause fluid retention. They may also interact with diuretics and ACE inhibitors to cause renal failure.
- Drug treatment:
  - Start with a diuretic (usually loop sealing) — monitor weight daily. Adjust the dose of diuretic to achieve 'dry weight' with optimal symptoms.
  - Once stabilized, begin an ACE inhibitor (see box).
  - Consider low-dose spironolactone (25–50 mg od) if available and the patient is not hyperkalaemic, and/or adding an inotrope such as digoxin.
  - Beta blockers: introduce cautiously once patient is clinically stable (not in acute severe heart failure), starting at a low dose and titrating up the dose slowly ('start low, and go slow').
  - Angiotensin receptor blockers: indicated in patients who do not tolerate ACE inhibitors (e.g. cough, angioedema).
  - A combination of isosorbide dinitrate and hydralazine has been shown to be effective add-on treatment in African-American patients.

Treatment of resistant heart failure Search for other causes and check patient compliance with drug regimes and daily weighing.
- Admit to hospital for bed rest, anti-thromboembolic stockings, heparin 5000 units SC tds, furosemide IV up to 4 mg/min, and training in the use of the weight scale in fluid and symptom management.
- Increase the ACE inhibitor or venodilator dose to the maximum tolerated; consider metolazone where available. Often adding in a thiazide to a loop diuretic will cause synergistic diuresis.
- In extreme circumstances, consider using IV inotropes for a short time only (e.g. dobutamine, starting at 2.5–10 mcg/kg/min, or dopamine starting at 2–5 mcg/kg/min; increasing both according to response up to a maximum of 40 mcg/kg/min (dobutamine) or 20–50 mcg/kg/min (dopamine)).
- Sometimes a degree of peripheral oedema and exercise limitation must be accepted in order to avoid unacceptable symptoms of low output.

Starting an ACE inhibitor

- Watch for hypotension after the 1st and 2nd doses.
- Check the BP. If <100 mmHg systolic, give the first doses in hospital if possible.
- Ensure the patient is not salt or volume depleted (e.g. due to D&V).
- Check for aortic stenosis or mitral stenosis (relative contraindication), and renal artery stenosis.
- If there is symptomatic hypotension, give 0.9% sodium chloride infusion (plus atropine if the patient is bradycardic).
- **Contraindications:** significant hypotension, angioedema, renal artery stenosis, pregnancy, porphyria.

Other precautions

- Check U&Es and creatinine routinely and stop the ACE inhibitor if there is significantly worsening renal function. However, urea and Cr will often rise when ACE inhibitors or diuretics are first used. This is not necessarily a reason to stop — levels will usually plateau and drop later. Monitor closely; stop if Cr/urea increase >20% or continue to rise.
- Weigh the patient regularly to monitor the response and train the patient to maintain ideal 'dry weight' by adjusting the diuretic dose as needed.
- Monitor WCC and urine protein if there is co-existent connective tissue disease.
- Beware of other interactions: Li^+ (levels ↑), digoxin (levels may ↑), NSAIDs (urea and K^+ ↑), anaesthetics (BP ↓).
- Watch for K^+ derangement (usually ↓) through diuretic action. Mild hypokalaemia is well tolerated without the need for K^+-sparing diuretics as long as: (i) the K^+ is >3.5 mmol/l, (ii) there is no predisposition to dysrrhythmias, and (iii) there are no other K^+-losing conditions (e.g. cirrhosis, chronic diarrhoea).

However, do not be put off trying a patient on an ACE inhibitor by these cautions. Most patients tolerate them very well and gain a significant benefit from them.

Shock

Shock is inadequate perfusion of vital organs due to hypotension.

Clinical features: tachycardia (unless on beta blockers or in spinal shock), hypotension (although in fit adults there may be >10% blood loss before any BP change, which is often an initial rise in diastolic pressure — i.e. a narrowing of the pulse pressure), pallor, faintness, sweating, and cold peripheries with poor capillary refill.

Causes of shock

Cardiogenic shock

Failure of the heart to pump sufficient blood around the circulation. It may occur rapidly or after progressive heart failure. It carries a high mortality and may be due to dysrrhythmias, tamponade, pneumothorax, MI, myocarditis, endocarditis, PE, aortic dissection, drugs, hypoxia, sepsis, and acidosis.

Management: Treat the cause, if known. Give O_2 mask if hypoxaemic. Monitor ECG, urine output, ABGs, U&Es, CVP. Consider inotropic agents (see previous page) adjusted to keep the systolic BP >80 mmHg. Refer to a specialist if possible.

Anaphylactic shock — see box.

Endocrine failure — see Addison's disease (📖 p 518) and hypothyroidism (📖 p 514).

Septic shock — see 📖 p 670.

Hypovolaemic shock

Due, for example, to trauma, ruptured aneurysm, or ectopic pregnancy.

Management prevent further blood loss and aim to restore circulatory volume as quickly as possible until the pulse rate falls and the BP starts to rise. Give whole blood where possible (crossmatched if there is time, otherwise use Rh -ve blood). Whilst waiting for blood to arrive, give warmed crystalloids such as Hartmann's solution or a synthetic colloid.

For the last two causes of shock, the immediate need is rapid IV fluid replacement.

Points on fluid resuscitation

- Use the largest vein and largest cannula possible.
- Add pressure to the fluid bag to speed the infusion.
- If access is difficult, it may be necessary to cut down to a vein (e.g. 2 cm above and anterior to the medial malleolus).
- If this fails, intraosseous infusion is possible using specific cannulae below and medial to the tibial tuberosity; especially useful in children.
- Give extra fluid if there are fractures: ribs 150 ml, tibia 650 ml, femur 1500 ml, pelvis 2000 ml.
- Double these estimates if there are open fractures.
- Remember to splint fractures and apply traction to ↓ blood loss.

Anaphylaxis

Anaphylactic shock requires prompt energetic treatment of laryngeal oedema, bronchospasm, and hypotension. It may be caused by exposure to insect venom (bee stings), food (eggs, peanuts), drugs (antibiotics, aspirin; especially if given IV) and other medicinal products (e.g. vaccines, antivenom).

Management

1. Stop infusion if this has caused the anaphylaxis.
2. Secure the airway, give O_2.
3. Give adrenaline 0.5 mg (0.5 ml of a 1:1000 solution) IM.
4. Repeat every 5 mins until BP and pulse both ↑. (Patients on non-cardioselective beta-blockers may not respond to epinephrine in usual doses; they may need salbutamol IV for 48 h.)
5. Give an antihistamine (e.g. chlorphenamine 10–20 mg by slow IV injection). Continue this PO for 48 h.
6. Continuing deterioration requires additional treatment with IV fluids and IV aminophylline or nebulized salbutamol. Assisted ventilation and emergency tracheostomy (for laryngeal oedema) may be required.
7. Give hydrocortisone 100–300 mg IV slowly; may need oral steroids tapered for a few days depending on the antigen.

If there is doubt about the adequacy of the patient's circulation, it may be necessary to give the epinephrine/adrenalin IV as a dilute solution.

Anaphylactic reactions require prior exposure to the antigen. Anaphylactoid reactions appear clinically similar but occur when large quantities of allergen are infused IV (e.g. antivenoms rich in Fc antibody portions). Prior skin testing does not exclude the possibility of a subsequent anaphylactoid reaction since the reaction is dependent on the quantity of antigen injected. Always have adrenaline already drawn up when injecting antivenoms.

Hypertension

Hypertension (HT) is an increasing problem in the tropics, particularly in urban areas, where lifestyles are becoming similar to those in the West. Environmental factors are chiefly involved in this process, since in these same countries, HT is virtually unheard of in rural populations, living traditional lifestyles. It is a major risk factor for MI, stroke, renal and heart failure, and peripheral vascular disease. Treatment aims to ↓ incidence/progress of complications.

Clinical features: people are usually asymptomatic until irreversible damage has occurred.

Symptoms: dizziness, fatigue, headache, palpitations. *Signs:* raised BP (although BP may be normal with heart failure); if 2° HT, there may be signs of the 1° disease; end-organ damage (e.g. LV hypertrophy, heart failure, retinopathy, proteinuria, uraemia). **BP should be checked** with the correct sized cuff, sitting (erect and supine in the elderly/suspected postural drop) after at least 5 and preferably 15 mins relaxing, and checked twice.

Who to treat?

All patients should be advised to lose weight, exercise, ↓ Na intake/↑ K intake, and address co-risk factors (e.g. smoking).

1. Where BP is >180 mmHg systolic or >95 mmHg diastolic, confirmed on 3 separate occasions over 1-2 days, treatment should be started. If severe or in the presence of associated conditions (e.g. heart failure), treat immediately — see box.
2. Where the initial BP is >140/90 over several weeks:
   • If no vascular or end organ complications and no diabetes, advise non drug Rx and reassess in 3 months. If still high, start drug therapy.
   • If any of the above are present, start drug therapy.
3. Isolated systolic hypertension (systolic >160 mmHg, diastolic <90 mmHg) in persons >60 yrs should be monitored over 3 months and treated if it persists, preferably with a low-dose thiazide diuretic ± low-dose beta-blocker.
4. Hypertension during pregnancy can be treated with methyldopa; beta-blockers and Ca^{2+} channel blockers can be used during the third trimester.
5. In diabetics and patients with vascular risk factors, aim should be BP<125/85.

Investigations: recheck the BP on at least 3 separate occasions. Search for a cause (particularly in the young). U&E, Cr, glucose, plasma lipids, MSU (twice), renal USS, 24 h urinary catecholamines/urinary VMA, ECG, CXR, fundoscopy.

Specific indications/agents and contraindications

• *Carotid atherosclerosis* — calcium channel blockers.
• *CHF* — ACE inhibitor, beta-blocker, and spironolactone.
• *Chronic kidney disease* — ACE inhibitor or ARB.
• *Diabetes* — ACE inhibitor or ARB.
• *ECG left ventricular hypertrophy* — ARB or ACE inhibitor.
• *IHD* — beta-blockers, Ca channel blockers (not short-acting ones).

- *Resistant hypertension* — spironolactone.
- *Secondary prevention of stroke* — ACE inhibitor plus diuretic or ARB.
- *Reserpine* — still used; cheap, effective, keep dose <0.5 mg/day.
- *PVD* — beta-blockers exacerbate.
- *Gout* — diuretics exacerbate/trigger.

Accelerated HT

Rapidly increasing BP with end-organ damage. It is heralded by sudden onset heart failure, renal failure, encephalopathy (convulsions/coma), or a diastolic BP >140 mmHg. Untreated, mortality is 90%; treated, it carries a 5-yr survival of only 60%. See box for managment.

Management of HT

Aim to ↓ incidence of stroke, heart and renal failure, and MI.
- *Non-drug therapy.*
Stop smoking (not itself a risk factor for HT; only for MI/stroke)
↓ sodium, alcohol intake, weight if obese
↑ intake of potassium, fresh vegetables, and fruit
↑ exercise
- *Drug therapy:* explain that the patient may need to be on tablets for life, even though had no symptoms, and may even feel worse. Encourage patient to return to a doctor if there are unacceptable side-effects and not simply to stop taking the medication.

Suggested approach
- Start with a thiazide diuretic (e.g. bendroflumethiazide 2.5 mg od PO) as first-line therapy. Use lowest possible dose; check plasma K^+ 4 wks after starting therapy).
- If not controlled, start either an ACE inhibitor (e.g. captopril 6.25 mg tds), or angiotensin receptor blocker (ARB) if ACE inhibitor intolerant, and/or a Ca^{2+} channel blocker (e.g. modified-release nifedipine 10–40 mg PO bd) as 2nd- or 3rd-line therapy.
- If still uncontrolled, add a beta-blocker (e.g. atenolol 25–50 mg PO od) as 4th-line treatment.
- If the HT is still not resolved (<10% will not respond to one or a combination of these drugs), seek expert help before starting centrally acting antihypertensives (e.g. moxonidine, clonidine) or vasodilator agents (e.g. hydralazine).
Always try to stop ineffective drugs.

Management of accelerated HT
- Bed rest, use of IV furosemide 40–80 mg, IV glyceryl nitrate 5–10 mcg/min, nifedipine 5 mg.
- Drugs noted above for Rx of HT should be used.
- Patients need close monitoring; may need specialist evaluation/ opinion. Dihydralazine should be used with caution.
- Drop in BP over hrs or days, not mins (increased risk of stroke).
- Do not lower BP in acute stroke unless >220/120. If so, lower slowly by 15–20% every 24 h.

Rheumatic fever

Rheumatic fever (RF) is an important cause of cardiovascular morbidity and mortality throughout the developing world. Group A beta-haemolytic streptococcal (*Streptococcus pyogenes*) pharyngitis leads, in 3–6% of cases, to rheumatic fever, due to an immune cross-reactivity between the bacteria and connective tissue.

It is a disease of the poor, the overcrowded, and the poorly housed, with children being chiefly affected. The disease is often more severe in the developing world than in the West. This severity reflects a failure of health services to prevent recurrences of acute rheumatic fever. If these recurrences can be prevented, many patients who have carditis in their 1st attack will eventually lose their murmurs and have normal or near normal hearts.

Clinical features

- *Arthritis*: occurs in 80% of cases. Typically an asymmetrical and migratory 'flitting polyarthritis' affecting large joints; the pain is severe while swelling is often modest. Onset is acute and subsides over a week; as one joint improves, a second gets worse. This process may continue for 3–6 weeks. There is a dramatic response to aspirin.
- *Carditis*: occurs in 40–50%. It is the most serious manifestation of acute RF, causing death acutely in <1% of cases. It may affect only the endocardium (valvulitis, often MR ± AR, 'mild carditis'), or the myocardium and pericardium may also be involved ('severe carditis').
- *Chorea*: occurs in 10% after a longer incubation period. Sydenham's chorea is emotional lability and involuntary movements (face, limbs, esp. hands). More common in girls; one-third have no cardiac involvement. Seldom affects those with arthritis.
- *Erythema marginatum*: <5% cases.
- *Subcutaneous nodules*: now rare.

Diagnosis: Based upon the revised Jones criteria (see box) and requires (i) evidence of recent streptococcal infection plus (ii) either two major criteria, or one major and two minor criteria.

Management

- Bed rest until the child feels better.
- Anti-inflammatory drugs to suppress the inflammatory process:
  - Aspirin 20–25 mg/kg PO qds. Continue for 3–6 weeks if heart is not involved; 3 months in mild carditis; 4–6 months in severe carditis.
  - In severe carditis, prednisolone 0.5 mg/kg qds may be given for 2 weeks.
- Treat as for heart failure from other causes.
- Sodium valproate 7.5–10 mg/kg PO bd for 3 months for chorea (alternative haloperidol 0.05 mg/kg od).

Primary prevention of rheumatic fever

There is good trial evidence to show that the treatment of suspected streptococcal pharyngitis in children with one dose of IM benzathine penicillin ↓ the risk of developing rheumatic fever by 80%. Sixty children need to be treated to prevent 1 episode of rheumatic fever.

Secondary prophylaxis is essential for all patients

Give benzathine benzylpenicillin 1.2 million units (children <30 kg, 600,000 units) IM every 2–4 weeks, duration as follows:
- >5 yrs or until age 21, whichever is the longer, for patients with carditis but no residual heart disease.
- 5 yrs or until age 21 yrs, whichever is the longer, for patients who did not have carditis.
- Lifelong prophylaxis is recommended for patients with carditis and residual heart (valvular) disease (WHO, 2004).

(Alternative for penicillin-allergic patients is erythromycin 250 mg bd PO.)

Revised Jones criteria

A. Evidence of recent group A streptococcal infection
- Positive throat culture or rapid streptococcal antigen test.
- Elevated or rising streptococcal antibody titre.

B. Major manifestations
- Carditis.
- Polyarthritis.
- Chorea.
- Erythema marginatum.
- Subcutaneous nodules.

C. Minor manifestations
Clinical findings
- Arthralgia.
- Fever.

Laboratory findings
- Elevated acute-phase reactants (ESR or C-reactive protein).
- Prolonged PR interval.

Any effort that will make the IM injection less painful, and therefore less frightening for the child, will make 2° prophylaxis more successful. Painful monthly IM injections for a young child can be a very frightening prospect that could make the child unwilling to take this life-saving treatment.

Infective endocarditis

Fever + regurgitant murmur = endocarditis until proven otherwise.

50% of endocarditis is on normal valves. When it is caused by highly pathogenic bacteria like staphylococci, pneumococci, and β-haemolytic streptococci, endocarditis follows an acute course, often with serious emboli, heart failure, and death. The course is subacute if *Streptococcus viridans* affects valves previously damaged by RF or other causes. Endocarditis often occurs on prosthetic valves (2%), in which case the involved valves often need replacing.

Pathogenesis

Any bacteraemia, especially following dental procedures, GU manipulation, or surgery may expose the valves to colonization. In the UK, *Streptococci viridans*, *Enterococcus faecalis*, and *Staphylococcus aureus* are common. Rarely fungi, *Coxiella*, or *Chlamydia* species infect valves; Gram-negative bacteria (e.g. *E. coli*) almost never cause infective endocarditis. Rare non-infective causes include SLE and malignancy. Right-sided disease is more common in IV drug users, leading to pulmonary abscesses.

Clinical features

Include evidence of:

- *Infection*: fever, malaise, night sweats, finger clubbing, splenomegaly, anaemia.
- *Heart murmurs*: especially regurgitation of aortic or mitral valves; sometimes murmurs change from day to day — not because the vegetation is changing rapidly, but because fever accentuates the murmur and because valve regurgitation may suddenly develop. Usually, the murmurs deteriorate until treatment is effective.
- *Embolic events*: vegetations on valves may cause embolic events (e.g. strokes or acute limb ischaemia). Occasionally, embolic abscesses or mycotic aneurysms form.
- *Vasculitis*: microscopic haematuria, splinter haemorrhages, Osler nodes (painful lesions on finger pulps), Janeway lesions (painful red patches on the palms), Roth spots (on fundoscopy), and renal failure.

Diagnosis

Take 3 blood cultures from different sites at different times — it is not necessary to time the cultures with fever spikes, as the bacteraemia is relatively constant. Always take blood cultures before starting antibiotics — a delay of a few hours is seldom critical. At least one culture will be positive in 99% of cases. ESR, FBC, U&E, Cr, echocardiography may show the vegetations on valves. Perform urinalysis for haematuria.

Management

For fully sensitive streptococcal infection, give benzylpenicillin 1.2 g IV q4 h plus synergistic doses of gentamicin 60–80 mg IV bd for 2 weeks. Then, if there is a good clinical response, switch to amoxicillin 1 g PO tds for 2 weeks. Less sensitive streptococcal isolates require 4 weeks of penicillin plus gentamicin. For *S. aureus* infections, give flucloxacillin 2 g IV q4–6 h and gentamicin as above for 2 weeks, then IV flucloxacillin for 2 weeks.

Use vancomycin or teicoplanin if MRSA suspected. For *S. epidermidis* infections, use vancomycin and rifampicin for ≥4 weeks.

If 'blind' empirical therapy is required, give benzylpenicillin and gentamicin and add in flucloxacillin if the endocarditis is acute in onset. Wait for blood culture results. This recommendation is based on streptococcal infections being the most common cause of endocarditis. Alter these recommendations according to the local circumstances.

Prognosis

30% mortality in the UK from staphylococcal endocarditis, 14% with anaerobic infection, and 6% with sensitive streptococci.

Prevention

Prophylaxis required

- Previous history of endocarditis.
- Prosthetic valves.
- Congenital heart disease (except secundum ASD).
- All acquired valvular heart disease.
- Hypertrophic cardiomyopathy with mitral regurgitation.
- Mitral valve prolapse with regurgitation.
- Surgically corrected shunts/conduits.

Prophylaxis not required

- Previous CABG.
- Pacemakers/implated cardio-defibrillators.
- Mitral valve disease without regurgitation.
- Previous rheumatic fever without valve defects.
- 'Innocent' murmurs.

Procedures requiring prophylaxis

- Any dental procedure that causes bleeding from gingiva, mucosa, or bone.
- Tonsillectomy.
- Rigid bronchoscopy.
- Incision of abscess.
- Vaginal delivery with chorioaminonitis.
- 'Dirty' surgery/procedure.

Procedures not requiring prophylaxis

- Natural shedding of teeth.
- Caesarian section.
- Vaginal delivery without infection.
- 'Clean' procedures.

Antibiotics

- Amoxicillin 3 g PO 1 h before procedure under local anesthetic.
- If allergic to penicillin or >1 course of penicillin in last month, give clindamycin 600 mg PO 1 h before procedure.
- For procedures under general anaesthetic, give amoxicillin 3 g PO 4 h before the procedure and again as soon as possible after the procedure.
- For procedures under general anaesthetic in patients at high risk (antibiotics in the previous month, prosthetic valve, or allergic to penicillin), refer all procedures to hospital. Amoxicillin plus gentamicin (or vancomycin in penicillin-allergic patients) can be used for such patients.

Cardiomyopathies

Disease of the myocardium → cardiac dysfunction, resulting in heart failure, arrhythmia, and sudden death.

1. Dilated (congestive) cardiomyopathy

Cause may not be identifiable, but recognised causes include alcohol, unrecognized HT, pregnancy, HIV, or previous myocarditis.

Clinical features: are of heart failure. Apex diffuse and displaced, often functional valvular incompetence and murmurs. May be AF (especially in alcoholics) and associated emboli. Typically, the patient is male 40–50 years old. HIV cardiomyopathy occurs in younger patients.

Diagnosis and management: echocardiography shows a dilated hypokinetic heart with involvement of all cardiac chambers. However, in HIV-associated cardiomyopathy the left ventricle may be of normal size but severely hypokinetic. Evaluation is in three stages:

1. *Non-invasive clinical evaluation* — reversible causes including HT, alcoholism, thyrotoxicosis, infiltration (iron, amyloid, sarcoid) tachycardia-induced cardiomyopathy, DM, myocarditis, and phaeochromocytoma must be excluded.
2. *Invasive evaluation* — coronary angiography and endomyocardial biopsy in patients with risk factors for IHD or ECG suggestive of MI or when infiltrative disorders or myocarditis are suspected.
3. *Family evaluation* — if no cause found, screen 1st degree relatives by ECG and echo to exclude familial dilated cardiomyopathy. Full evaluation yields a cause in 50–75% cases. Cause linked to prognosis; investigation important when possible. Mortality of idiopathic dilated cardiomyopathy high — 40% by 3 yrs.

2. Peripartum cardiomyopathy

Dilated cardiomyopathy beginning in last month of pregnancy or <5 months postpartum, with no other history of heart failure and with no discernible cause for the heart failure.

Risk factors: high parity, age, low socio-economic status. Myocarditis found in 50% in some series, but mechanism unclear. Cultural practices such as eating Na^+-rich foods in hot climates during pregnancy may have a role. The combination of increased circulatory demand (± anaemia), heat (→ peripheral vasodilatation), and high salt load might lead to a high output dilated cardiac failure.

Investigation and management: as for heart failure. In about 50% cases there is irreversible cardiac dysfunction. Dysrrhythmias, persistently dilated heart, and systemic or pulmonary emboli mark poor prognosis. Consider *sterilization* in patients with irreversible cardiac dysfunction beyond 6 months follow-up.

3. Restrictive cardiomyopathy

Due to endomyocardial stiffening, resembling constrictive pericarditis. Often due to endomyocardial fibrosis in which hypereosinophilia (possibly triggered by helminthic infection, especially filariasis) damages the myocardium. Mural thrombus formation produces a fibrotic mass. Rare causes are amyloid or carcinoid.

Clinical features: may begin with a febrile illness, facial oedema, and dyspnoea that may progress to death within months. Most patients are seen in chronic stage with heart failure. Clinical features may be either LV or RV, or a combination. LV disease consists of MR (never MS or AR cf. RF) with an S₃, and progressive pulmonary hypertension. RV disease (usually TR) results in gross ascites and markedly elevated JVP but often minimal peripheral oedema. May be exophthalmos, central cyanosis, delayed puberty, ↓ pulse pressure, and AF. Murmurs may be heard (cf. pericardial disease). Pericardial effusion common in endomyocardial fibrosis.

Diagnosis: CXR varies from massive cardiac shadow (aneurysm of R atrium, or pericardial effusion) to almost normal. Echo and Doppler studies show fibrosis of inflow tracts with involvement of ventricles and regurgitation of mitral and tricuspid valves. Pericardial effusion and thrombi in the atria or ventricles also seen.

Management: Acute treatment is supportive. If there is hyper-eosinophilia, look for and treat cause. In established disease, resist the temptation to drain the ascites, since it may cause the patient to lose protein. Digoxin may control ventricular rate if there is AF.

4. Hypertrophic cardiomyopathy

Hypertrophic cardiomyopathy is unexplained ventricular hypertrophy (i.e. hypertrophy in absence of hypertension, aortic stenosis, DM, obesity, or other cause) leading to obstruction of the LV outflow tract in 20% cases (i.e. hypertrophic obstructive cardiomyopathy, HOCM). Over 90% of cases show autosomal dominant inheritance. Genetic counselling and screening of 1st degree relatives essential.

Clinical features: Dyspnoea, angina, syncope, palpitations. May be a double impulse at apex, jerky pulse, S₄, late systolic murmur. ECG almost always abnormal, showing LVH, Q waves, and deep T-wave inversion. ECG abnormalities precede the echocardiographic onset of cardiac hypertrophy which manifests from adolescence onwards.

Management: Beta-blockers for angina and treat dysrrhythmias. Uncontrolled AF needs anticoagulation. Consider high-risk patients (i.e. family history of sudden death, syncope, abnormal BP response to exercise) for implantable cardioverter defibrillator.

5. Acute myocarditis

Inflammation of myocardium, may present like an MI. *Causes:* viral (coxsackie virus), diphtheria, RF, drugs, other infections; Angina, dyspnoea, arrhythmia, tachycardia, and heart failure. Exclude MI, pericardial effusion. Management is supportive.

6. Left atrial myxoma

Rare benign tumour, developing from atrial septum causing left atrial obstruction (as in MS), emboli, AF, fever, weight loss, and raised ESR. May be a family history. Rarely, a tumour 'plop' on auscultation. 2:1 female excess. Differentiate from MS by occurrence of emboli without AF or on echo. *Treatment:* excision. May recur.

Pericardial disease

Pericarditis

In the tropics, this is commonly due to TB or pyogenic infection.

- *Tuberculous pericarditis* is especially important in the areas of high HIV prevalence. Spread is probably from the adjacent lymph nodes and pleura. The effusion may be massive in HIV; echocardiogram may show strands of fibrin floating in the effusion.
- *Acute pyogenic pericarditis* results from generalized bacteraemia derived from, or associated with, a 1° focus elsewhere.
- *Other causes:* any infection (especially coxsackie virus), malignancy (such as KS in HIV +ve people), uraemia, MI, Dressler syndrome, trauma, radiotherapy, connective tissue diseases, and hypothyroidism.

Clinical features

Pericarditis: a sharp constant sternal pain, which may radiate to the left shoulder, down the left arm, or to the abdomen. It is relieved by sitting forward, and worse by lying on the left, coughing, inspiring, or swallowing. Auscultation may reveal a scratchy superficial pericardial rub, loudest at the left sternal edge. In a large effusion, the rub is generally lost, and heart sounds are heard faintly.

Pericardial effusion: depends on the speed at which it is formed. If formed quickly, the pericardium cannot stretch and so pressure rises and the heart is compressed to produce cardiac tamponade. There is a fall of cardiac output (↓ BP), ↑ JVP, Kussmaul sign (JVP rises with inspiration), tachycardia, impalpable apex, pulsus paradoxus, peripheral shut down, and quiet heart sounds. In more chronic effusions, signs of heart failure predominate with severe ascites and hepatomegaly. Percussion reveals an increased area of cardiac dullness in the retrosternal and right parasternal areas, and the apex beat is impalpable or felt within the area of dullness. Impending tamponade or restriction is first indicated by elevated JVP; however, the JVP may be so high that the patient must be examined sitting or standing upright. Patients with pyogenic pericarditis are extremely unwell with signs of severe sepsis.

Diagnosis: ECG classically shows upwardly concave (saddle shaped) ST segments in all leads except lead AVR, with no reciprocal changes. In pericardial effusions, CXR shows a large globular heart (and may show pleural effusions). ECG has low voltages and changing QRS complexes (electrical alternans = a changing axis beat to beat). Echocardiography is diagnostic with an echo-free zone showing the heart surrounded by effusion. In exudative effusions, fibrinous strands are clearly seen within the fluid. Differentiate from an MI and PE.

Constrictive pericarditis

Encasement of the heart in a non-expansive pericardium, usually following TB infection. Features are as for chronic effusion; however, the heart is small on CXR and may show calcification, especially on the lateral CXR. The onset is usually insidious, with ascites, oedema, hepatomegaly, proteinuria being found. The patient may or may not be breathless. Often the JVP is so far elevated that it is missed on routine inspection of the neck.

Management

Pericarditis: find and treat the cause.
- Give analgesia with NSAIDs if pericardial pain is present.
- For TB pericarditis, commence anti-TB treatment for 6 months and perform an HIV test. It is uncertain whether adjunctive steroids prevent death or constriction.
- *Pericardial effusion*: find and treat the cause (e.g. antibiotics for bacterial infections; anti-TB drugs for TB).
- *Tamponade* requires urgent drainage. Aspirate with a 50 ml syringe, fitted with a long needle and two-way tap, inserting upwards and to the left of the xiphisternum. Watch the ECG monitor to know if the myocardium is touched. Patient should be propped up 45°. Watch the ECG monitor to know if the myocardium is touched. Adjunctive steroids are effective in reducing the re-accumulation of pericardial fluid.
- *Recurrent pericardial effusion*, especially of pyogenic origin, requires surgery draining through a pericardial window or pericardiotomy.
- *Constrictive pericarditis*: requires surgical excision of the pericardium.

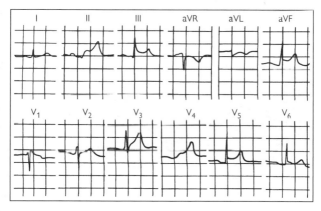

Fig. 8.5 ECG changes in pericarditis.

Renal medicine

Section editors   **Sally Hamour**
                      Dwomoa Adu

Assessing renal function

The kidneys regulate fluid, electrolyte, and acid base balance; eliminate potentially toxic substances; and produce renin and erythropoietin. The renal tubular synthesis of 1,25-dihydroxycholecalciferol from the major circulating form of vitamin D, 25-hydroxycholecalciferol, is catalyzed by the enzyme 1α-hydroxylase.

Serum creatinine: is simple to measure and widely available. However, the serum creatinine concentration remains in the normal range until the GFR has fallen by around 40%. It is therefore not a useful measure of *early* renal impairment.

Glomerular filtration rate (GFR): The normal range for the GFR is 88–174 ml/min in men and 87–147 ml/min in women. GFR is estimated by calculating the creatinine clearance (CCr). This requires a 24-hour urine collection; for this reason, equations have been devised to estimate either the creatinine clearance or GFR and these are widely used.

Calculated creatinine clearance (Cockroft Gault formula)

This formula is widely used for the calculation of creatinine clearance from the serum creatinine but suffers from the limitations inherent to the inaccuracies of measuring serum creatinine.

$$\text{Calculated creatinine clearance (ml/min)} = \frac{1.2 \times [140 - \text{age (yrs)} \times \text{weight (kg)}]}{\text{plasma creatinine (µmol/L)}}$$

In females, the result is factored by 0.85 to account for lower creatinine production.

Modification of Diet in Renal Disease (MDRD) estimation of GFR.

This is calculated as follows:

GFR (ml/min/1.73 m^2) = 186 × (Creatinine (µmol/l × 0.0113)$^{-1.154}$ × age$^{-0.203}$.

In females multiply result × 0.742; in Afro-Caribbeans multiply × 1.21. A useful table and online calculator for estimating the MDRD GFR can be downloaded from *http://www.renal.org/eGFR/about.html*

Urine analysis

- **Colour**: see box opposite.
- **Transparency**: cloudiness may be due to infection, blood, pus, chyle, or crystals of phosphate (white) or urate (yellow).
- **Smell**: an unpleasant smell is commonly due to a UTI (bacteria split urea to release ammonia). Antibiotics or vitamins may also cause a smell.
- **Specific gravity (SG)**: normally 1.002–1.025. A low SG suggests diabetes insipidus; a high SG suggests dehydration or diabetes mellitus (large amounts of dissolved glucose).

Chemical analysis

Dipsticks can be used to detect pH, protein, glucose, ketones, blood, urobilinogen, bilirubin, and nitrites in the urine. If dipsticks are not available, simple lab tests can be used to detect urine abnormalities (e.g. heat coagulation test for protein and Benedict's test for reducing substances).

- **pH**: the urine is normally acidic (range 4.5–8.0).
- **Protein**: see proteinuria (📖 p 366).
- **Glucose**: modern dipsticks are specific for glucose. The Benedict's test detects reducing substances in the urine (glycosuria, salicylates, ascorbic acid, and galactose). Renal glycosuria is an impaired ability of the kidney tubules to reabsorb glucose, and may be due to normal variant or be part of renal tubular disease (e.g. Faconi's syndrome).
- **Ketones:** are found in diabetic ketoacidosis and starving patients.
- **Nitrites:** their presence suggests a UTI, but their absence does not exclude it. False positives may be seen after a protein-rich meal or vitamin C ingestion.
- **Blood:** dipsticks rely on the peroxidase activity of Hb. Intact red cells give a punctate staining, while free Hb or myoglobin give a homogeneous colour. Confirm by urine microscopy — intact red cells will be seen in haematuria, but not haemoglobinuria or myoglobinuria.

Urine analysis by colour

Pale/colourless	Yellow/orange	Red	Brown	Black
Overhydration Diabetes insipidus	Dehydration Bilirubin	Haematuria Haemoglobin	Bilirubin Haemoglobin	Severe haemoglo- binuria
Post- obstructive diuresis	Rifampicin Tetracycline	Myoglobin Porphyrins	Myoglobin Nitrofurantoin	Methyldopa Melanoma
Excessive beer consumption	Sulfasalazine Riboflavine Clofazimine	Beetroot	Metronidazole Phenothiazines	Ochronosis

Abnormal urinary sediment

The urine is centrifuged, supernatant poured off, and the sediment then microscoped.

Cells

- *Red cells*: see haematuria (📖 p 368).
- *Leukocytes*: usually indicates a UTI. May also occur in glomeru- lonephritis and interstitial nephritis. If a sterile pyuria persists, consider TB of the urinary tract.

Casts

- *Hyaline casts or fine granular casts*: consist of mucoprotein and are a non-specific finding. Found in normal urine, febrile illnesses, after exercise, in concentrated urine, and in renal disease.
- *Coarse granular casts*: granules derive from degeneration of embedded cells. They are more usually pathological and are seen in glomerulonephritis.
- *Red cell casts*: indicate glomerular bleeding and are a sign of glomerulonephritis.
- *White cell casts*: indicate an acute pyelonephritis.

Proteinuria

Normal protein excretion is <150 mg/day and includes albumin (<30 mg/day), Tamm–Horsfall protein, and other small proteins.

- Microalbuminuria: is daily excretion of between 30–300 mg albumin/ 24 h. It is not detected by dipsticks — special methods are needed for detection. It is abnormal and an early feature of diabetic nephropathy.
- Dipsticks become positive for protein when albuminuria is >300 mg/ 24 h (macroalbuminuria).
- Dipsticks are very sensitive to albumin but are insensitive to Bence–Jones protein and light chains found in urine in myeloma.

If persistent proteinuria is present, the next step should be to quantify this. Most centres now use a urine albumin/creatinine ratio or a urine protein/creatinine ratio rather than a 24-h urine protein excretion.

Causes of persistent proteinuria

- **Postural (orthostatic) proteinuria**: absent proteinuria after overnight rest, but mild proteinuria after 2 h of standing and quiet walking. Patients are asymptomatic and have no haematuria; other investigations are normal. Renal Bx is not indicated and long-term prognosis excellent.
- Renal disease.
- Other causes: exercise induced, CCF.

Chyluria

Chyle in the urine makes it resemble milk or rice water. It results from rupture of lymphatic varices, producing a fistula between the lymphatic system and urinary tract. It is relatively common in the tropics, especially where filariasis is prevalent. It must be differentiated from pyuria, phosphaturia, and lipuria. A rose/pink colouration to the urine may mean that there is also haematuria.

- Commonly caused by parasites blocking lymphatics, often *W. bancrofti*.
- Non-parasitic chyluria is rare and usually involves stenosis or obstruction of the thoracic duct (eg. neoplastic infiltration, trauma, TB).

Clinical features: usually relapse and remit over a long period. Main symptom is passage of milky white urine; there may be loin pain, ureteric colic, passage of clots (may cause retention), and fever.

Diagnosis: urine microscopy reveals chylomicrons and fat globules. IVU, cystoscopy (2 h after a fatty meal) to detect site of lesion; lymphography may be required. Look for a cause. Measure 24-h urine, protein excretion, and serum proteins (to assess albumin loss).

Management: treat filariasis, although lesions may be irreversible; >50% resolve spontaneously. A low-fat diet and a high fluid intake reduces the risk of urinary stasis and clot formation. If the chyluria is severe and/or accompanied by episodes of dysuria, colic, retention, and/or weight loss, surgical repair should be considered.

Haematuria

Blood in the urine always requires investigation. It may be:
- Microscopic: with ≥5 red blood cells per high-powered field, or
- Macroscopic: (i.e. seen with the naked eye) if >0.5 ml of blood is present per litre of urine.

While almost half of patients presenting with haematuria in the West have neoplastic lesions, in the developing world, a large number of other diseases present with bleeding from the urinary tract.

Causes

- *Surgical*: renal stone disease; transitional cell or squamous carcinoma of the bladder, ureter, or pelvis; renal cell carcinoma; trauma; benign prostatic hyperplasia; AV malformations.
- *Medical*: UTI, schistosomiasis, TB, glomerular disease (IgA nephropathy, glomerular nephritis, SLE), polycystic kidneys (PCK), infarction, bleeding diatheses.

Investigating haematuria

Focus on stones, urological malignancy, UTIs and schistosomiasis (in endemic areas) before considering the rarer medical causes. Ask the following questions:

- **Is it true haematuria?** Check other causes of red urine (see 📖 p 365).
- **What is its timing in relation to micturition?** Early haematuria suggests a low (urethral/genital) bleeding site, while late haematuria (i.e. at the end of voiding) suggests a bladder site; red colouration throughout micturition implies a ureteric or renal lesion.
- **Is the haematuria painful?** Carcinoma and schistosomiasis tend to be painless, whilst cystitis, obstruction (e.g. stones), and infection are commonly painful.
- **Is there?** dysuria and fever (UTI), poor stream (urethral/bladder neck lesion), loin pain (ureteric obstruction due to tumour, stone, or clot), family history (PCK), or a history of trauma.

Diagnosis: urine microscopy (red cell casts and dysmorphic red cells suggest glomerular bleeding), culture, and cytology of a midstream urine sample; renal USS; IVU; cystoscopy, FBC, blood urea.

Haemoglobinuria: is caused by intravascular haemolysis due to toxins/venoms, falciparum malaria, incompatible blood transfusions, G6PD deficiency, paroxysmal nocturnal haemoglobinuria, chronic cold agglutinin disease, microangiopathic haemolytic anaemia, march haemoglobinuria.

Myoglobinuria: is caused by rhabdomyolysis (muscle destruction) after muscle injury, excessive contraction (convulsions, hyperthermia, very heavy exercise), viral myositis (influenza, legionnaires' disease), and drugs/toxins (alcohol, snake venoms). Myoglobinuria may be idiopathic.

Urinary schistosomiasis

Schistosoma haematobium causes urinary schistosomiasis in Africa and parts of the Middle East. *S. intercalatum* and hybrid species between *S. haematobium* and other species can produce atypical clinical pictures, with ectopic localization of worms. For distribution and life cycle, see 📖 p 315. Worm eggs stimulate a T-cell-mediated immune response, producing eosinophilic granulomata in the bladder, uterus, and genitals. Eggs may also affect the GI tract, lungs, liver, skin, and CNS.

Transmission

Depends on
• Human (definitive host) availability and water-contact activities.
• *Bulinus* snails (intermediate host).
• *S. haematobium* strain.
• The host–parasite relationship.
• The host's immune response.

Prevalence increases to a peak at 15 yrs, after which there is a plateau until 30 yrs, at which point it begins to decline (due to age-related changes in water-contact, increased immunity, and death of adult worms).

Clinical features

• *Egg deposition*: begins 3 months after infection, often accompanied by painless haematuria which may persist for months–yrs, together with dysuria, pain, malaise, and mild fever.
• *Established infection*: haematuria often decreases in the chronic stage, unless there is 2° infection, ulceration, or malignancy. Fibrosis and calcification of the bladder reduce its volume, producing frequency and dribbling. Other complications include perineal fistulae and 2° bacterial infection. In severe cases, there may be urinary retention, stasis, stone formation, and renal failure. In men, involvement of the seminal vesicles causes eggs to shed in semen ('lumpy' semen); prostate, epididymis, and penis are uncommonly affected. In women, ulcerating, polypoid, or nodular lesions may be seen in the vulva, vagina, and cervix. The ovaries, fallopian tubes, and uterus are rarely affected. *S. haematobium* infection may be associated with ectopic pregnancies and infertility.

Diagnosis

Visualization of parasite eggs in the urinary sediment, bladder biopsies, or rectal mucosal snips. Schistosome antigens may also be detected immunologically. Antibodies to Schistosoma develop 6–12 weeks post exposure and serology can be performed at this time (ELISA). Look for bladder calcification on AXR ('foetal head' sign); IVU may be useful, and USS can show bladder wall thickening or hydronephrosis.

Treatment

See 📖 p 317. Praziquantel is effective against all species of schistosomes; a single dose of 40–60 mg/kg usually being curative. The patient should be followed up at 2 and 6 months for urinalysis and clinical assessment of improvement.

S. haematobium and bladder cancer

The association between bladder cancer and chronic heavy S haematobium infection is well-recognized. There is a lag period of at least 20 yrs between infection and the development of cancer. 75% of patients (with squamous carcinoma) in Egypt are <50 yrs old; by contrast, in non-schistosome areas, most patients (with adenocarcinoma) are >65 yrs. It is more common in males, smokers, and those working with aromatic amines (e.g. in the rubber industry).

Clinical features: haematuria, cystitis, and obstruction. Spread is local to pelvic structures, via the lymphatics to the iliac and paraaortic nodes, and via the blood to liver and lungs.

Investigation: urinalysis, FBC. AXR may show a calcified bladder wall. IVU, cystoscopy, and biopsy. Staging is as follows:
T1 — tumour in mucosa or submucosa. Not felt at examination under anaesthesia (EUA).
T2 — superficial muscle involved. Rubbery thickening at EUA.
T3 — deep muscle involved. Mobile mass at EUA.
T4 — invasion beyond bladder. Fixed mass at EUA.

Management: T1 and T2 — cystoscopic diathermy. Consider intravesicular chemotherapy or BCG administration. T3 — radical surgery and radiotherapy. T4 — palliation (long-term catheterization).

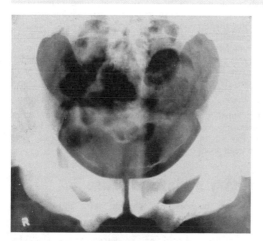

Fig. 9.1 Bladder calcification in urinary schistosomiasis — the 'foetal head' sign. Such patients commonly have well-preserved bladder function.

Kidney lumps

Enlarged kidneys tend to bulge forwards, whilst perinephric abscesses or collections tend to bulge backwards. A tender loin mass may suggest an obstructed kidney but, if there is evidence of psoas muscle spasm, a perinephric abscess is more likely. With acute obstruction, or development of pyonephrosis, guarding is common and the mass difficult to define. With chronic obstructed states and tumours, the mass is usually better defined and less tender. Bilateral, irregular kidneys suggest polycystic renal disease. A horseshoe kidney may present as a central abdominal mass, whilst ectopic kidneys may be felt lower in the loins, in the iliac fossae, or even suprapubically.

Kidney tumours

There are three main types of renal tumours:
1. **Nephroblastoma:** (Wilm's tumour): is an undifferentiated mesodermal tumour of children which may be sporadic or familial; 95% are unilateral.
2. **Urothelial tumours:** may arise in the renal pelvis, ureters, urethra, or bladder. In the West, transitional cell carcinoma accounts for 90% of urothelial malignancies, whilst in Africa squamous CA predominates due to a high incidence of urinary schistosomiasis. Tumours may lead to chronic urethral strictures, obstruction, and recurrent infection.
3. **Renal carcinoma (hypernephroma):** the majority of renal cell carcinomas are clear cell carcinomas. Classic symptoms are of loin pain, a mass, and frank haematuria. Anaemia and hepatic dysfunction are commonly present, sometimes with polycythaemia due to increased erythropoietin secretion. These tumours are often discovered as an incidental finding on ultrasound.

Diagnosis: by imaging with USS or CT scan and CXR (for metastases).

Management: Standard treatment of localized tumours is by radical unilateral nephrectomy. Five-year survival in patients with localized disease is 90% but this falls to 9% in patients with metastatic disease. Drug treatments have been disappointing so far.

Genitourinary hydatid disease

After passage through the portal system, right heart, and pulmonary circulation, eggs of *Echinococcus granulosus* and *E multilocularis* may come to rest in the genitourinary system. Cysts form in the kidney, bladder, prostate, seminal vesicles, and epididymis, in descending frequency. For details, see 🕮 p 288.

Renal masses

Unilaterally palpable	*Bilaterally palpable*

Unilaterally palpable
- Renal cell carcinoma.
- Hydro/pyonephrosis.
- Acute pyelonephritis.
- Polycystic kidneys (asymmetrical enlargement).
- Hydatid disease.

Bilaterally palpable
- Polycystic kidneys.
- Bilateral hydro/pyonephrosis.
- Bilateral renal cell carcinoma.
- Amyloid, lymphoma, acromegaly.

Polycystic kidney disease

Autosomal dominant polycystic kidney disease (APKD) is a single gene disease occurring in ~1 in 500 live births and a major cause of chronic kidney disease. 85–90% of cases are due to a germ line mutation in the PKD1 gene and 10–15% due to a mutation in the PKD2 gene that encode the proteins polycystin1 and 2, respectively.

Clinical features: The main symptoms are renal pain, gross haematuria, and urinary infections but the diagnosis can be made with an incidental finding of an abdominal mass. Hypertension is common; its treatment slows progression of renal failure. Cysts are commonly found in the liver and pancreas. Some families have intracerebral aneurysms that may lead to intracerebral or subarachnoid haemorrhage.

Over 50% of patients develop end-stage renal failure. End-stage renal failure or death develops earlier in patients with PKD1 (53 years) than in those with PKD2 (69.1 years).

Diagnosis: USS shows enlarged kidneys with characteristic multiple cysts. Look for a family history.

Management: Supportive. Treat hypertension and UTIs. For infected cysts, co-trimoxazole, and ciprofloxacin have good penetration. Manage bleeding conservatively. CRF is the usual cause of death unless there is access to dialysis or transplantation. Consider screening family members for asymptomatic disease. Most affected individuals have cysts by age 20 years.

Autosomal recessive polycystic disease

This is less common than the autosomal dominant variety and is found in 1 in 20,000 live births. Often causes death in *utero* or in the neonatal period from pulmonary atresia. Renal failure and fibrosis develop in those children who survive.

Urinary tract infection (UTI)

UTIs may progress rapidly in the tropics and complications are common, especially in the malnourished. Infection is commonly due to gram-negative gut organisms, most frequently *E. coli* (70%). UTIs are common in women.

Clinical features

- *Cystitis*: abrupt onset of frequency, dysuria, urgency, supra pubic pain, and tenderness; occasionally haematuria, incontinence, retention.
- *Acute pyelonephritis*: features of cystitis, plus high fever ± rigors, loin pain, nausea and vomiting, D&V (in children).

Ask about: previous infections including STD, recent urinary instrumentation, diabetes, childhood UTI, known urinary tract abnormalities, renal colic, stone disease, obstructive uropathy.

Examine for: loin tenderness, renal mass, large prostate, meatal ulcers, vaginal discharge, pelvic mass on vaginal examination, hypertension, signs of CRF.

Is it a complicated UTI?

UTI in a male is usually caused by prostatic hypertrophy, sometimes with prostatitis. UTIs in pregnant women should be treated with care, as premature labour may follow. Complicated UTIs often complicate urinary tract abnormality (congenital, obstruction, calculi); reflux; neurogenic bladder; recent urinary instrumentation; female genital mutilation. UTI in a child is often a sign of vesico-ureteric reflux, urethral stricture, or other abnormalities. Diabetes and immunosuppression predispose to UTIs.

Diagnosis

Ask for a clean-catch midstream urine specimen. Sterile bags are useful in infants and children. Visually inspect the urine for turbidity and haematuria. Test the urine for leukocytes and nitrites (blood and protein alone have low specificity/sensitivity). Send specimens for microscopy (pyuria, bacteria, epithelial cells) and culture. Pyuria with a growth >10^5 colony forming units per mL of urine, of a single recognized urinary pathogen, confirms UTI. However, genuine mixed growth may occur in complicated UTI and lower counts may be significant, particularly in men and with slow-growing organisms.

Perform further investigations: if recurrent UTI, first UTI in men, UTI in children, overt or persistent haematuria, sterile pyuria. Recurrent UTIs in infants, particularly with reflux, may be a cause of progressive renal failure.

Further investigations: include USS, IVU, micturating cystourethrogram and DMSA scan for scars in children.

Sterile pyuria

Consider partially treated UTI, TB or other atypical organisms, chlamydia, candida, calculi, bladder tumour, prostatitis, papillary necrosis (the elderly, over-use of NSAIDs), polycystic kidneys, appendicitis.

Management of a UTI

- Advise increasing fluid intake, frequent voiding, double micturition, and post-coital voiding.
- Antibiotic treatment should be started empirically. Be guided by local sensitivities. Except for pregnant women, asymptomatic bacteriuria does not usually require antibiotics.

Lower tract infection (cystitis): 3–5 days of any of the following: trimethoprim 200 mg BD; ciprofloxacin 500 mg BD; cefalexin 500 mg BD.

Upper tract infection (pyelonephritis) or complicated UTI: 2 weeks of antibiotics. Start with IV 3rd generation cephalosporin (e.g. ceftriaxone 2 g OD) or ampicillin 1 g 6-hrly plus ciprofloxacin; with clinical improvement, change to one of the oral agents used for lower tract UTI (ideally guided by microbiology results) but continue for 2 weeks total.

If the urinary tract is obstructed (urethral valves/stricture, prostate, stones), urgent decompression is required (urinary catheter; suprapubic catheter; nephrostomy — guided by USS).

Recurrent UTIs: emphasize frequent voiding and double micturition. Short-term prophylactic antibiotics (e.g trimethoprim 100 mg at night) may break the cycle of infections. Cefalexin 500 mg after sexual intercourse may be helpful. Investigate children under 5 years for reflux nephropathy and tract abnormalities.

Renal calculi and renal colic

Renal and ureteric calculi are less common in agricultural economies than in the West, and are seen less frequently in Africa than Asia and the Middle-East. M:F ratio is 2.5:1. Epidemiological factors such as diet, affluence, climate, and metabolic factors are significant. Congenital renal abnormalities (e.g. polycystic disease, horseshoe kidney) with urinary stasis, GU schistosomiasis, and TB predispose to stone disease. Overall, 80% of stones are calcium oxalate; triple phosphate stones (staghorn calculi) are associated with UTI, usually *Proteus* spp; uric acid and cysteine stones are uncommon.

Clinical features: can occur at any point in the urinary tract. Stones in the ureter cause renal colic with sudden onset of agonising paroxysms of pain. The pain radiates from the loin to groin and the patient often cannot lie still. Kidney stones may cause loin pain with abdominal/loin tenderness with haematuria. Bladder stones cause strangury — urgent desire to pass something which will not pass. Common sites of obstruction are vesico-ureteric and pelvi-ureteric junctions.

Diagnosis: Kidney-Ureters-Bladder (KUB) AXR for calculi (90% of urinary stones are radio opaque). Dipstick for blood. Screen for UTI. USS or IVU to look for stone and obstruction. Blood tests: U&E, uric acid, Ca^{2+}, bicarbonate.

Management

1. Increase fluid intake. Treat infection.
2. Give pain relief: NSAIDs (beware renal impairment) or opiates for severe colic.
3. Most stones will pass spontaneously: >70% of ureteric stones <4 mm wide will pass spontaneously in one year while <10% of stones > 8 mm wide will pass. Stones that are likely to pass without complications can be managed conservatively.
4. If there is obstruction, infection, or bilateral involvement, seek urgent urological advice. Decompress the renal tract before renal failure occurs. Stones can sometimes be removed by extracorporeal shock wave lithotripsy or surgery.

Prevention: avoid oxalate-rich foods (spinach, beetroot, green peppers, almonds, cashew nuts, cocoa, grapefruit juice, orange juice, black tea, cola drinks) and excessive dietary protein. There is a high risk of recurrence without preventative management regarding fluid intake and diet. Ideally, a dietary history, metabolic screen, and stone analysis are performed if facilities allow.

Glomerular disease

Glomerulonephritis (GN) is more common in the tropics than temperate regions and the frequency of infection-associated GN is higher.

Clinical features

GN may present with:
1. asymptomatic microscopic haematuria or frank haematuria.
2. proteinuria.
3. nephrotic syndrome.
4. acute nephritis (haematuria, proteinuria, oliguria).
5. acute renal failure (rapidly progressive glomerulonephritis).
6. chronic renal failure (CRF).
7. hypertension.

The glomerular response to injury is fairly restricted. Glomerular appearances seen on microscopy may be idiopathic or secondary to infection or auto-immune disease (see table opposite). >70% of all glomerulonephritis is idiopathic. A careful search for possible infections is important.

Diagnosis

- **Urine**: proteinuria; dysmorphic RBCs (and RBC casts in proliferative GN) on microscopy; albumin/creatinine or protein/creatinine ratios.
- **Blood**: serum creatinine, albumin, lipid profile, U&E, FBC, ESR.
- **Serology**: (to help determine the cause) ANA, dsDNA, complement C3 & C4 (immune disease); HBsAg, anti-DNAase B, ASOT, Hep C and HIV antibody (infections); ANCA (vasculitis); anti-GBM Ab (Goodpasture's disease).
- **Radiology**: renal USS.
- **Renal biopsy**: where available.

Management of GN

In many cases, GN resolves after treating the infection. In other cases, depending on the aetiology, histology, and chronicity, GN may be amenable to treatment. In a resource-poor setting, where histological classification is unavailable, management is usually based on the clinical syndrome.

General principles

- salt restriction.
- ACE inhibitors or angiotensin receptor blockers (check creatinine and potassium 2/52 after starting and after each dose increase).
- careful use of diuretics.
- aim for a BP of <130/80 mmHg.
- avoid further renal insults e.g. nephrotoxins, NSAIDS.

Specific treatment

Primary GN is usually treated with steroids and immunosuppression. However, these carry significant risks, particularly in the tropics, and require experienced supervision. In addition, effort must be made to ensure that the patient does not have chronic infection (with e.g. strongyloides, amoebiasis, viral hepatitis, or HIV) that might be exacerbated by such treatment.

Table 9.1 Glomerular pathology

Glomerular histology	Idiopathic	Secondary
Minimal change nephropathy	+	Lymphoma (rare)
Focal segmental glomerulosclerosis	+	Reduced renal mass, *Schistosoma mansoni*, HIV-associated nephropathy, sickle cell anaemia
Membranous nephropathy	+	Hepatitis B infection, lupus, carcinoma, *Schistosoma mansoni*, syphilis, leprosy, filariasis
Proliferative glomerulonephritis	+	Streptococci, *Schistosoma mansoni*, leprosy, lupus, *Wuchereria bancrofti*, onchocerciasis
Mesangiocapillary glomerulonephritis (Membranoproliferative glomerulonephritis)	+	Lupus, sickle cell anaemia, *Schistosoma mansoni*, onchocerciasis, hepatitis C

Nephrotic syndrome

The nephrotic syndrome is characterized by proteinuria (>3 g/24 h or albumin/creatinine ratio >300), hypoalbuminaemia, oedema, and hypercholesterolaemia. Most cases of the nephrotic syndrome in the tropics are idiopathic; some are secondary to:

- infections, including HIV, hepatitis B, hepatitis C.
- diabetic nephropathy.
- autoimmune diseases e.g. SLE, Henoch–Schönlein purpura.
- neoplasia (especially lymphoma and carcinoma).
- amyloid (leprosy, tuberculosis), sickle cell disease.

Clinical features

Facial and peripheral oedema with ascites and pleural effusions if severe. Urine is frothy. Complications include:

- **Venous thromboembolism** — renal vein thrombosis is a recognized complication. Suspect it if there is sudden loss of renal function with haematuria, esp. with back pain. Treat with anticoagulants.
- **Infection** — especially pneumococcal peritonitis. Consider prophylaxis with penicillin V 500 mg BD while oedematous; treat infections.
- **Hypercholesterolaemia** — treat in chronic cases.
- **Hypovolaemia and ARF** — check postural BP, monitor urine output.

Management

- Give an adequate protein diet.
- Restrict salt intake.
- Give diuretics to relieve oedema. Use cautiously since volume depletion may be present (postural drop in BP, low urine output).
- Monitor U&E and creatinine twice weekly and weigh daily.
- Use ACE inhibitors to reduce proteinuria.
- Treat hypercholesterolaemia with statins if chronic.
- Consider prophylaxis with penicillin V during oedematous state (risk of pneumococcal peritonitis).
- Treat the cause in secondary GN. Use immunosuppression with steroids ± 2nd line agents in primary GN depending on histology, with cautions described above.

Minimal Change GN

Presents with nephrotic syndrome and is less common in children in tropical areas. Treatment is with high dose steroids and the long-term prognosis is excellent although time to remission is slower in adults and the rate of remission is lower.

Membranous GN

Common in children and adults in tropical areas. Up to 60% may respond to six months treatment with steroids.

HIV-related Nephropathy

In tropical areas, this ranges from HIV associated nephropathy with proteinuria to the nephrotic syndrome. The typical histological lesion is a collapsing focal semental glomerulosclerosis. Other lesions include HIV immune complex disease, membranous nephropathy, mesangial hyper-cellularity, post infectious glomerulonephritis and IgA nephropathy. Management comprises generic treatment of GN (as for other causes of GN, in particular ACE inhibitors) and commencement of HAART.

Hepatitis B associated glomerulonephritis

Occurs mainly in children who are carriers for hepatitis B. The majority of affected patients are male and the age of onset is between 2 and 12 years. The histological lesion is of a membranous nephropathy. Most children go into spontaneous remission but adults often progress to renal failure. The management is with conservative measures in children but anti-viral treatment in adults.

'Quartan Malarial Nephropathy'

The previously suggested association between chronic *P malariae* infection and nephrotic syndrome remains unsubstantiated.

Acute nephritis

Most often due to post-streptococcal glomerulonephritis in the tropics; occurring 2–3 weeks after a beta haemolytic streptococcal throat, ear, or skin infection (impetigo, infected scabies, or infected eczema).

Clinical features: haematuria, oliguria, fluid retention (with mild oedema, elevated JVP), hypertension, and variable uraemia. *Complications* include hypertensive encephalopathy, pulmonary oedema, acute renal failure; rarely, rapidly progressive glomerulonephritis and CRF.

Diagnosis: haematuria, ± red cell casts, proteinuria, elevated blood urea and creatinine, reduced creatinine clearance, and elevated anti-DNAase B, ASOT. Culture throat and skin for streptococcus. CXR may show pulmonary oedema.

Renal oedema

Oedema is often the presenting feature in both nephrotic syndrome and acute nephritis. It can occur in ARF and CRF.

- *Nephrotic syndrome*: the mechanism of oedema in the nephrotic syndrome is unclear. It is due in part to glomerular damage → large protein loss in urine → hypoalbuminaemia → reduction of colloid osmotic pressure → oedema due to transudation of fluid from capillaries to the extracellular fluid compartment → reduced intravascular volume → activation of the renin-angiotensin-aldosterone system → 2° hyperaldosteronism with retention of salt and water → increase in oedema. However, only 1/3 of patients are hypovolaemic and the others are normovolaemic or hypervolaemic.
- *Acute nephritis*: glomerular inflammation → reduction in glomerular filtration → retention of sodium and water → increased intravascular volume → increased hydrostatic pressure within capillaries → oedema due to transudation of fluid into extra cellular fluid compartment.
- *Renal failure*: oedema occurs in acute or chronic renal failure due to volume overload: Na^+ and water intake exceeds the kidney's capacity to excrete them due to the loss of glomerular filtration.
- *Other causes of generalized oedema*: CCF, cirrhosis of the liver, malnutrition, hypothyroidism, drugs (NSAIDs, calcium channel blockers, oestrogens, and steroids), pregnancy, and idiopathic oedema.

Management of acute nephritis

1. Restrict fluid intake, if oliguric, to 500 ml plus urine output over past 24 h.
2. Restrict salt and potassium in diet.
3. Give diuretics (e.g. furosemide) IV or PO and antihypertensive treatment (not β blockers which may precipitate pulmonary oedema).
4. To eradicate residual streptococcal infection, give oral penicillin V 500 mg qds for 10 days; or single dose of benzathine penicillin 900 mg IM; or if allergic to penicillin, erythromycin 250–500 mg QDS.

Acute renal failure with pulmonary oedema requires specialist treatment and/or dialysis. The prognosis is usually good. Proteinuria and abnormal urinary sediment may persist for up to 2 years — if it persists for longer, consider biopsy.

Acute renal failure (ARF)

ARF complicates many diseases in the tropics. Causes are roughly 60% medical, 25% surgical, and 15% obstetric. If ARF is part of multiple-organ dysfunction, it carries a poor prognosis. The prognosis is better when the ARF is isolated e.g. following snake bite or malaria.

- *Pre-renal ARF*: ARF is 2° to hypoperfusion (dehydration, shock, blood loss, hypotension, or septicaemia). Patient will be volume-deplete and urine is concentrated. Requires careful fluid resuscitation.
- *Intrinsic renal disease*: e.g. leptospirosis, falciparum malaria, massive intravascular haemolysis from G6PD deficiency and drugs/infections, snake bite, post streptococcal GN, rhabdomyolysis, history of drugs, toxins, IV contrast.
- *Post-renal ARF (obstruction)*: distended bladder, palpable kidneys (hydronephrosis), pelvic mass, large prostate. USS is diagnostic. A urinary catheter will relieve lower tract obstruction.

Clinical features

- Raised blood urea, creatinine, and potassium.
- Oliguria (<500 ml/day) or anuria (occasionally non-oliguric). Patient may be dehydrated or fluid overloaded depending on the underlying cause.
- Anorexia, nausea and vomiting, confusion, pericardial rub.
- Acidosis — Kussmaul breathing or 'air hunger' (deep, sighing breathing).
- Bruising, GI bleeding due to uraemic platelet dysfunction.

Diagnosis

- *Examine urine*: absence of a urinary sediment suggests a pre-renal cause; proteinuria, red cells, and red cell casts suggest glomerulonephritis.
- *Blood*: urea, creatinine, electrolytes, ABG, FBC.
- *Radiology*: US scan of kidneys to exclude obstruction; CXR for pulmonary oedema.
- *Renal biopsy*: if expertise available and cause unclear.

Course and progress: most patients with ARF have acute tubular necrosis (ATN). The oliguria lasts up to 6 weeks with rising urea and creatinine, followed by a polyuric recovery phase. Careful management is required.

ARF in pregnancy: common causes are post-abortion septicaemia, pre-eclampsia and eclampsia, antepartum and postpartum haemorrhage, *abruptio placentae*, and puerperal sepsis.

Management of acute renal failure

1. Examine the patient and assess volume status (JVP, skin turgor, peripheral perfusion, mucous membranes, pulmonary crepitations, peripheral oedema, heart rate, postural BP).
2. Optimize fluid balance. Give fluids if dry; if overloaded, see if there is a response to diuretics.
3. Catheterize to exclude lower tract obstruction and monitor urine output. Remove after 12 h if anuric. Arrange renal tract USS.
4. Consider urgent dialysis for pulmonary oedema, hyperkalaemia, and acidosis.
5. Prevent GI bleeding e.g. with ranitidine 150 mg bd or PPI.
6. Record fluid input and output, daily weight, daily U&E.
7. Once fluid replete, limit fluids to 500 ml + previous days' losses.
8. Treat sepsis.
9. Avoid nephrotoxic or K^+-sparing drugs; adjust doses of other drugs.
10. Start a low-potassium diet.
11. During the polyuric recovery phase, avoid dehydration and hypokalaemia.

Management of complications of ARF

Pulmonary oedema: sit upright, lower legs, give oxygen. Offload with nitrate infusion and IV furosemide. If no response, urgent dialysis is needed for removal of fluid. Consider removing 500 ml of blood as emergency measure before dialysis, if very severe.

Hyperkalaemia: serum K^+ can rise rapidly in patients who are hypercatabolic and/or acidotic. See opposite for management.

Metabolic acidosis: if pH <7.1, cautiously give slow IV bicarbonate. Optimize hydration and attempt to establish a urine output.

Management of hyperkalaemia

- If ECG changes are present or potassium >6.5, protect the heart with 10–20 ml of 10% calcium gluconate by slow IV injection with ECG monitoring (this will not alter serum potassium). Repeat if ECG changes persist.
- Give soluble insulin 5–10 units with 50 ml of 50% glucose by IV infusion over 15 minutes.
- Give nebulized salbutamol 2.5 mg (salbutamol shifts K^+ intracelluarly).
- In refractory hyperkalaemia, particularly in the anuric patient, dialysis is required.
- Cation exchange resins (calcium resonium, polystyrene sulphate) 15 g qds PO or as enema increase faecal K^+ excretion and are used to prevent hyperkalaemia. Give with lactulose to prevent constipation. Furosemide will increase potassium loss if the patient is well-filled and passing urine.
- Remember to stop medications that increase potassium and consider dietary potassium intake.

Dialysis

Many countries are unable to offer chronic dialysis programmes. However, short-term renal replacement therapy with either peritoneal dialysis or haemodialysis can be life-saving in acute renal failure. There is evidence to suggest that haemodialysis improves outcome in renal failure due to malaria or sepsis. However, this requires specialist equipment and expertise and may be unavailable outside large regional centres. Peritoneal dialysis may be more affordable and requires less training.

Intermittent peritoneal dialysis (PD)

Instil 1–2 litres of dialysate over ~10 mins into the peritoneal cavity via a peritoneal dialysis catheter. Keep the dialysate within the peritoneal cavity for 30 mins before allowing it to drain out by gravity over ~30 mins. Dialysate may be pre-prepared or formulated locally.

Complications of dialysis

Infection, including access-related sepsis (line sepsis, PD peritonitis, exit site infection), remains the most significant complication and may be life-threatening. Additional complications include bleeding, thrombosis, or air embolism in haemodialysis and catheter blockage and fluid leaks in peritoneal dialysis.

Chronic kidney disease (CKD)

CKD results from progressive and irreversible loss of renal function. Remarkably, kidneys have sufficient reserve to support life with as little as 8% of their original nephrons functioning. Below this level, patients develop uraemic symptoms — dialysis and/or transplantation is then required for survival. The prevalence of CKD in tropical countries is unknown but is likely to be higher than in temperate countries. There is evidence of an increasing burden of CKD in tropical countries.

Causes: in tropical countries, glomerulonephritis, hypertension, and diabetic nephropathy are major causes of chronic renal failure, as is obstructive uropathy (e.g. chronic urinary schistosomiasis affecting lower ends of ureters).

Clinical features

There are few symptoms of chronic renal failure until the GFR is reduced to <20% when tiredness due to anaemia develops. There may be fluid overload and hypertension. Uraemia may cause anorexia, vomiting, hiccups, peripheral neuropathy, confusion, and drowsiness.

Biochemical features: hyperkalaemia and acidosis are not marked until the GFR falls <20 ml/min. Exceptions to this are patients with tubulointerstitial disorders. In most patients, salt and water balance is maintained until the GFR falls <15% of normal, although this may occur earlier in diabetes. Patients with glomerular disease and hypertension, especially those with hypertensive heart disease, may retain salt and water and develop heart failure.

Bone features: increased blood levels of parathyroid hormone occur in very early renal failure as the GFR falls <50–60 ml/min. This is probably due to inappropriately low levels of 1,25-dihydroxycholecalciferol and not to hyperphosphataemia with consequent hypocalcaemia, as previously thought. With advanced renal failure, there is impaired renal synthesis of 1,25-dihydroxycholecalciferol from its precursor 25-hydroxycholecalciferol. The consequences of this are renal osteodystrophy. Vitamin D deficiency leads to osteomalacia, and hyperparathyroidism to the development of bone erosions and osteitis fibrosa.

Anaemia: Hb concentrations tend to be maintained until the GFR falls <30 ml/min, at which time anaemia occurs. There are many reasons for CKD anaemia, especially the failing kidney's inability to produce sufficient erythropoietin to drive bone marrow production of red blood cells.

Diagnosis

- *Blood*: urea & creatinine, electrolytes, Hb, FBC, Ca2+, PO4, urate, glucose, ESR, serum proteins & electrophoresis (if myeloma suspected).
- *Urine*: analysis, microscopy, culture, 24-h collection for proteinuria and creatinine clearance.
- *Imaging*: AXR or USS (for renal size, obstruction).
- *Renal biopsy*: especially in patients with normal-sized kidneys and mild to moderate CRF, when the cause of CRF is unknown.

Pathophysiology of CKD

- Glomerular hypertrophy resulting from nephron loss is accompanied by glomerular hyperperfusion, hyperfiltration, and hypertension. These in turn produce progressive glomerular sclerosis, tubulointerstitial atrophy, and scarring.
- Reducing intraglomerular pressures by good blood pressure control, in particular with angiotensin blockade, slows down progression of renal failure.

KDOQI classification of CKD

The estimated GFR using the MDRD equation is a much better reflection of renal impairment then serum creatinine (see 🕮 p 364).

The KDOQI (Kidney Disease Outcomes Quality Initiative) committee has used the eGFR, in mL/min/1.73 m^2 and derived from the MDRD equation, to classify the stages of chronic kidney disease as follows.

Stage	Description	GFR	Diagnosis
1	Kidney damage with normal or increased GFR	>90	Proteinuria, haematuria
2	Kidney damage with mild decrease in GFR	60–89	Proteinuria, haematuria
3	Moderate decrease in GFR	30–59	Early chronic kidney disease
4	Severe decrease in GFR	15–29	Late chronic kidney disease
5	Kidney failure (ESRD*)	<15 or dialysis	Renal failure

* ESRD = end stage renal failure.

Management of CKD

Treat the cause and reversible contributing factors
- Relieve obstruction.
- Avoid nephrotoxic drugs; discontinue NSAIDs in patients with CKD.
- Treat infections.

Prevent progression
- Maintain good glycaemic control in diabetes mellitus.
- Maintain blood pressure less than 130/80 mmHg. Aim for 125/75 mmHg in patients with a urine albumin/creatinine ratio >100 or proteinuria >1 g/24 h.
- ACE inhibitors and Angiotensin II receptor blockers (ARBs) are effective in slowing progression of renal failure and should be used especially when there is proteinuria (see opposite).
- Low-salt diet if oedematous/hypertensive; Low-potassium diet if hyperkalaemia.

Referrals
- Patients with microscopic haematuria as well as proteinuria and renal impairment require urgent nephrology referral.
- Patients with a rising creatinine over days or weeks should be assumed to have ARF and referred urgently.
- Arrange urgent ultrasound kidneys and bladder in patients with urological symptoms.

Management of anaemia
- Consider erythropoietin when Hb falls to <10.5. However, first, exclude other causes of anaemia (e.g. deficiency of Fe, folate, B12); investigate as appropriate. Fe supplements are frequently required.
- A major side-effect of erythropoietin is hypertension; therefore, regular monitoring of blood pressure is essential.

Management of bone disease
- Start a calcium-containing phosphate binder when serum phosphate is >1.6 mmol/L. To be taken with meals 2–3 times a day.
- If serum parathyroid hormone (PTH) is greater than 2 times the upper limit of normal, start alfacalcidol 0.25 mcg per day and increase. Maintain PTH level between normal to 2 times normal.
- Once a patient is on calcium supplements or alfacalcidol, monitor calcium and phosphate 3-monthly and parathyroid hormone 6-monthly.

Management of cardiovascular risk
- Chronic kidney disease at least doubles the risk of cardiovascular disease. Management of risk factors such as smoking, exercise, blood pressure, and lipids should be strongly reinforced.
- For cholesterol treatment, statins are generally safe but fibrates should be avoided.

Starting angiotensin blockade

- Check creatinine and potassium two weeks after starting an ACE inhibitor or angiotensin II receptor blocker and after any increase in dose. There is usually a slight decline in GFR. Discontinue drugs only if GFR drops by more than 20% and consider referral to nephrology to exclude renal artery stenosis.
- In patients with impairment of renal function who are on an ACE inhibitor or ARB, do not use potassium-sparing diuretics (spironolactone/amiloride) or NSAIDS because of the risk of hyperkalaemia.
- Treat hyperkalaemia (K^+ 5.5–6.0) with furosemide and recheck in 2 weeks. Discontinue angiotensin blockade if K^+ >=6.0 mmol/L.

Neurology

Section editors **Jeremy Farrar**
Diana Lockwood (leprosy)

Acute confusional state (ACS)

Clinical features: clouding of consciousness is the most important sign. Patients also have a short attention span and are easily distractable. They may be disorientated in time and place. They often appear bewildered and have impaired immediate recall and recent memory.

Check carefully for signs of reduced consciousness, particularly drowsiness. This may be a warning of impending coma (see 📖 p 396). Psychiatric causes of confusion (e.g. schizophrenia, paranoid state) and early dementia do not present with drowsiness.

Delirium

This is more florid than ACS. It also manifests typically with disorientation, confusion, and reduced attention but, in addition, the patient is often frightened, irritable, and more profoundly disorientated. The patient may have frightening hallucinations and/or delusions, and exhibit aggressive behaviour.

Causes: see box. Most common causes will vary with age.
- *Systemic infection*: check chest, urinary tract, surgical wounds, IV cannula sites, CSF.
- *Chronic subdural haematoma:* may present with ACS.

Management
Treat cause if one can be recognized.
1. At night, turn the lights on to improve the patient's orientation.
2. Give 50 ml of 20% dextrose IV if hypoglycaemia is suspected.
3. Treat disturbed behaviour with chlorpromazine 25–50 mg IM/PO q6 h or haloperidol 1.5–3 mg PO tds initially or 2–10 mg IM, repeated as necessary q 4–8 h to a maximum daily dose of 18 mg.
4. Avoid benzodiazepines.

Nursing is very important in ACS — if possible, use a well-lit room with familiar staff. Attempt to reassure the patient.

Dementia

Unlike confusional states and delirium, there is no disturbance of consciousness in dementia. It is a chronic or progressive condition characterized by impaired higher mental function (e.g. memory, reasoning, comprehension) and emotional and behavioural changes. Common causes are Alzheimer's disease and multiple strokes (vascular dementia). Uncommon but treatable causes include communicating hydrocephalus; vitamin B12 or B1 deficiency; hypothyroidism; syphilis; cysticercosis; brain tumour; chronic subdural haematoma. HIV can cause a dementia that is responsive to antiretroviral therapy.

Management: Identify the few patients with treatable causes. Aim to supply others with general support so that they may have the highest quality of life possible. Remember that the family will also need support. Information useful to Alzheimer's disease patients and their carers is available on the web at *www.alz.org*

Common causes of acute confusion/delirium at presentation (they may all progress to coma)

- CNS infection (malaria; meningitis — including TB meningitis; encephalitis; HIV-related infections).
- Systemic infections.
- Hypoxia.
- Metabolic causes (e.g. hypoglycaemia, hyerglycaemia).
- Alcohol — excess or withdrawal.
- Drugs.
- Head injury/concussion.
- Stroke.
- Mental illness such as schizophrenia.
- Raised intracranial pressure.
- Epilepsy (post-ictal).

Coma

A persistent pathological state of unconsciousness. In the comatose patient, immediately ensure a clear airway, check that they are breathing, establish haemodynamic stability, and check for life-threatening injuries.

Take a history: from relatives or bystanders — did anyone see how the patient became unconscious? Is there any past medical history such as diabetes, alcohol abuse, or drug overdose that might explain the coma?

Examine: the patient in an attempt to distinguish metabolic causes of coma from brainstem causes — see below. It is particularly important to identify coma due to brainstem compression since surgical relief of the enlarging mass may be urgently required. Use the Glasgow coma score (GCS) — see below.

Useful clinical features

• Fever	Meningitis or encephalitis
	Cerebral malaria
	Metabolic coma of infection
• Hypothermia	Hypothyroidism; hypothermic coma
• Hypertension	Coma may be due to stroke
• Hypotension	Shock
• Pallor, cyanosis	Metabolic disease
• Bleeding, bruising	Head trauma

Progressive deterioration: suggests brainstem compression. Look for focal CNS signs. Search for asymmetry (e.g. in response to pain or in the face during expiration). If the response to pain is different, the side with lower response in the GCS is the side with hemiparesis.

Diagnosis
There are three broad categories.

1. *Metabolic*
• Normal pupil responses.
• Normal or absent eye movements depending on the depth of coma.
• Suppressed, Cheyne–Stokes, or ketotic respiration.
• Symmetrical limb signs, usually hypotonic.

2. *Intrinsic brainstem disease*
   From the outset there may be:
• Abnormal pupil responses and eye movements.
• Abnormal respiratory pattern.
• Bilateral long tract and cranial nerve signs.

3. *Extrinsic brainstem disease due to compression*
   Papilloedema and hemiparesis **with progressive**
• Loss of pupillary responses.
• Loss of eye movements.
• Abnormal respiratory pattern.
• Long tract signs.

Management of an unconscious patient

1. *ABC*: ensure adequate airway, oxygenation, and circulation.
2. *Obtain a reliable history*: check for signs of injury or trauma especially to the head. Record the vital signs — temperature, pulse, BP, respiratory rate, O_2 saturations. Check capillary or venous blood glucose.
3. *Assess the level of coma*: use the Glasgow coma score (see box). Check for meningism, pupillary light reflex, corneal reflexes, fundi, and focal neurological signs in the limbs. Do brainstem reflexes, Doll's eye movements, and caloric tests if brain death is suspected.
4. *Investigate*: do the following — Hb, WCC, urea, electrolytes, glucose, calcium, liver enzymes, and arterial gases. Also do blood cultures if the patient is febrile, a malarial film if the patient is from an area endemic for malaria, a toxicology screen if it is an overdose or poisoning case, or a CSF examination if there is meningism (beware rising intracranial pressure). Do ECG, EEG; X-ray the skull and chest; CT/MRI the head if indicated and available.

5. *Determine the cause and treat:*
- *Coma with focal signs* — e.g. subdural or extradural haematoma or SOL may require definitive neurosurgical drainage and steroids, mannitol, etc., to lower intracranial pressure.
- *Coma without focal signs* — e.g. hypoglycaemia (give 50 ml of 20% glucose IV); opiate poisoning (give IV naloxone); cerebral malaria (give artemisinin derivatives if available or quinine); overdose (give gastric lavage and/or appropriate antidote).
- *Coma and meningism* — e.g. meningitis or subarachnoid haemorrhage, treat with antibiotics.

6. *Care: nurse in the ITU or high-dependency ward:*
- Monitor the level of consciousness using the GCS.
- Determine pupillary size, equality, and response to light.
- Check vital signs.

These should all be done at regular fixed intervals varying from every 15 mins to every 4 h depending on the clinical situation. Pay special attention to respiration, circulation, skin, bladder, and bowels.

Prognosis: depends mainly on the cause, depth, and duration of the coma. The combination of the absence of the pupillary light reflex and corneal and brainstem reflexes at 24 h indicates a grave prognosis. The persistence of deep coma for greater than 72 h also has a poor prognosis.

Glasgow coma score (GCS)

Assess on admission and then at regular intervals to follow progress and predict prognosis.

Best motor response

6   Carries out request (obeys a command)
5   Localizes pain
4   Withdraws limb in response to pain
3   Flexes limb in response to pain
2   Extends limb in response to pain
1   Does not respond to pain

Best verbal response

5   Orientated in time and place
4   Responds with confused but understandable speech
3   Spontaneous speech but inappropriate and not responsive
2   Speech but incomprehensible
1   No speech

Eye opening

4   Opens eyes spontaneously
3   Opens eyes in response to speech
2   Opens eyes in response to pain
1   Does not open eyes

Add together the best response in each group. Roughly:
GCS 1–8 = serious injury
GCS 9–12 = moderate injury
GCS 13–15 = minor injury

The simpler AVPU scoring system can also be useful

A Alert
V Responds to vocal stimulo
P Responds to pain
U Unresponsive

Headache

The brain parenchyma is insensitive to pain. Headaches result from distension, traction, or inflammation of the cerebral blood vessels and dura mater. Pain is referred from the anterior and middle cranial fossae to the forehead and eye via the trigeminal nerve, and from the posterior fossa and upper cervical spine to the occiput and neck via the upper three cervical nerves. Both infratentorial and supratentorial masses can lead to frontal headaches by causing hydrocephalus.

Causes of a headache

- *Acute meningeal irritation*: due to subarachnoid haemorrhage or meningitis caused by bacteria, viruses, fungi, or metastases.
- *Rising intracranial pressure*: see 📖 p 402.
- *Many infectious diseases*: cause a headache during the acute phase. Locally important infections need to be determined (e.g. malaria; meningitis — including TB; trypanosomiasis; typhoid, arboviral and typhus fevers; fungal infections).
- *Giant-cell arteritis*: may rapidly result in blindness. Occurs in elderly. There may be a tender engorged occipital or temporal artery; ESR markedly raised. Temporal artery biopsy may confirm the diagnosis, but do not delay giving steroids while awaiting biopsy.
- *Migraine*: headaches which occur at intervals (not daily) associated with N&V, anorexia, photophobia, phonophobia, and in 20% of cases, visual, mood, sensory, or motor disturbances. Most first attacks occur while young. Identify and avoid precipitating factors; give analgesia (paracetamol, NSAIDs, or codeine) plus metoclopramide 10 mg (not in children). Ergotamine useful in 50% of patients. Chemoprophylaxis may work for regular migraines.
- *Tension headache*: most common cause of headache. Normally a benign symptom due to an identifiable cause (e.g. overwork, family stress, lack of sleep, emotional crisis). It is often a daily occurrence unlike migraine headache, getting worse as the day goes on. Visual disturbances, vomiting, and photophobia do not occur. Management involves thorough examination and reassurance of its benign course, analgesia (usually paracetamol 1 g qds), and rest. Ask about drugs, caffeine, and alcohol. Amitriptyline starting at 10 mg at night, increasing by 10 mg each week up to 75 mg, is also often of benefit. Tension headaches may be part of a depressive illness. Check for other signs or symptoms such as mood change, loss of appetite, weight, or libido, or a disturbed sleep pattern.
- *Analgesia-induced headache*: follows long-term inappropriate use of analgesia. History reveals increasing and frequent use of multiple analgesics. *Management*: reassurance followed by stopping all forms of analgesia. The headache initially worsens before improving.
- *Others*:
  - Trauma.
  - Drugs.
  - Hypertension.
  - Cluster headaches.
  - Indomethacin-sensitive headaches.

Pain may be referred: to the forehead and temple from the orbits, paranasal sinuses, teeth, skull, or spine pathology, and venous sinuses.

The major responsibility of a physician faced with a patient with a headache is to exclude a treatable, structural, or dynamic cause. Specifically, exclude either a SOL or meningitis. Check for:
- Localizing signs.
- Papilloedema.
- Neck stiffness.
- Rash.

Raised intracranial pressure (↑ICP)

Clinical features
Include
- *Headache:* often worse in the morning due to CO_2 retention during sleep → cerebrovascular dilatation, possibly waking the patient from sleep; made worse by coughing, straining, standing up; relieved by paracetamol in the early stages.
- *Alteration:* in the level of consciousness (drowsiness).
- *Vomiting:* (may relieve the headache; sometimes the 1st sign of raised ICP).
- *Hypertension, bradycardia.*

Failing vision and decreasing consciousness are ominous signs. Papilloedema is frequently not present.

Pathophysiology
Initially, mechanisms such as reducing CSF volume allow the CNS to compensate for rising ICP as may occur with a slow-growing tumour. However, if the ICP continues to rise or if the increase is acute and the compensatory mechanisms overwhelmed, the brain often becomes laterally displaced and pushed towards the foramen magnum at the base of the skull. The medial temporal lobe (or uncus) is then forced down through the tentorial hiatus, or a cerebellar tonsil is forced through the foramen magnum, causing the brainstem to become compressed (coning). This produces the following progressive changes:
- Level of consciousness decreases, drowsiness → coma.
- Pupils become dilated and unresponsive, initially on the side of the mass, then bilaterally.
- Posture becomes decorticate, then decerebrate.
- Slow deep breaths → Cheyne–Stokes breathing → apnoea.
- *Beware* of ipsilateral hemiparesis and VI cranial nerve palsy as false localizing signs (they may occur 2° ↑ ICP in the absence of focal intra-cranial pathology).

Causes
SOL; cerebral oedema; hydrocephalus. The cerebral oedema may surround a tumour or result from infection (cerebral malaria, encephalitis), trauma, or hypoxic cell death.

Management
If possible, establish the cause with a CT/MRI scan.
1. Sit the patient up at ~30–40° to increase venous drainage from the brain.
2. Ensure adequate oxygenation — ventilate if necessary.
3. Give mannitol 5 ml/kg of a 20% solution IV over 30–60 mins to reduce cerebral oedema.
- In severe oedema, dexamethasone 12–16 mg IV stat by slow IV injection may also be used.
- If less severe oedema, give dexamethasone 4 mg IM q6 h.
4. If the patient has a positive malaria blood film, see management of cerebral malaria (📖 p 40).
5. Control seizures if present.
6. If a SOL is believed to be responsible, refer to a neurosurgeon. If the ICP progresses rapidly, urgent decompression with burr holes may be life-saving —see 📖 p 430.

Acute pyogenic (bacterial) meningitis

A multitude of microbes — bacteria, viruses, parasites, and fungi — can cause meningitis. However, bacterial meningitis is the most important since it has a high fatality rate and is readily treatable. All febrile patients with a history of headache should be examined for signs of meningism.

Aetiology

In children and adults, bacterial meningitis is frequently due to:

- *Neisseria meningitidis* (Gram −ve intracellular diplococci).
- *Haemophilus influenzae* B (Hib) (Gram −ve rods).
- *Streptococcus pneumoniae* (Gram +ve capsulated diplococci).

Meningococcus causes epidemics (see 🕮 p 406), while previous head injury, sinusitis, otitis media, or pneumonia predispose to pneumococcal meningitis. Hib meningitis is most common in children <5 yrs. Other bacteria are less common (e.g. *S. aureus*, *Pseudomonas* spp) or occur in particular groups or regions (e.g. *Streptococcus suis* in S.E. Asia; Group B streptococci and *E. coli* in neonates; Listeria in pregnant women, immunosuppressed, and neonates).

TB meningitis is also an important cause of meningitis — see 🕮 p 146 and 408.

Clinical features

Headache, fever, N&V, photophobia, and stiff neck. Cardinal signs of meningism are:

- Neck stiffness — passively flex the head (chin towards chest); this results in pain and resistance in a patient with meningism.
- Kernig's sign — passively straighten the leg with hip flexed (>90°); this causes pain and resistance by stretching inflamed nerve roots.

Neurological signs are not normally focal in pyogenic meningitis and include: lethargy, delirium, coma, convulsions. Lower cranial nerve palsies and retention of urine are common in TB meningitis. Acute complications include raised ICP, seizures, sepsis, paralysis, SIADH.

Check the skin (particularly on the back, buttocks, and soles of the feet) and conjunctivae carefully for any abnormal skin colour and purpura. Cold hands and feet and leg pains are also very early markers of meningococcal septicaemia and should be recognized early as this can be rapidly fatal. If present or if unsure treat for meningococcal infection immediately.

Diagnosis

Take blood for culture, FBC, U&E, (and malarial parasites); lumbar puncture (if no evidence of SOL or ↑ ICP) for CSF examination.

Prognosis

Mortality varies with age and organism. Perinatal, neonatal, and childhood mortality varies from 50–80%. Similarly, mortality is increased in old age. In adults, mortality with pneumococcus is 30–40%, Haemophilus 20–30%, meningococcus 10–15% (much higher with septicaemia). The main long-term complications include paralysis, deafness, visual loss, epilepsy, and mental retardation.

Management

1. On suspicion, give immediate antibiotics — see below.
2. Give supportive measures: fluids, oxygen, maintain normal electrolytes, generous pain relief, and tepid sponging to reduce temperature.
3. IV dexamethasone 0.4 mg/kg 12-hrly × 2 days is recommended for adults and children with acute bacterial meningitis in developed countries. However, two large studies from Malawi demonstrated no benefit from steroids in the treatment of bacterial meningitis in childhood or in adults. In Vietnam, in a similar study in adults, there was a dramatic reduction in mortality with steroids. The difference may lie in the rates of HIV, later presentation, and choice of antibiotic. In HIV-coinfected patients not on anti-retroviral drugs, there may be no benefit of steroids.

Initial empiric antibiotic regimens for presumed bacterial meningitis in adults — choose one of:

- Benzylpenicillin 2.4 g (4 mega units) IV q4 h for 10–14 days *and/or* chloramphenicol 12.5–25 mg/kg or 1 g IV q6 h for 10 days.
- Ceftriaxone 2–4 g IV daily in 1–2 divided doses.
- Ampicillin 2 g IV every 4-6 h for 10 days.

Paediatric IV doses — PAEDIATRIC NOTE

- *Benzylpenicillin*: neonate — 50 mg/kg bd (<7 days old) or tds (7–28 days old); children >1 month old — 50 mg/kg every 4–6 h (max 2.4 g q4 h).
- *Chloramphenicol*: neonate <14 days old —12.5 mg/kg; children >14 days old — 12.5 mg 12.5–25 mg/kg qds.
- *Ceftriaxone*: neonates — 20–50 mg/kg (avoid in neonatal jaundice); children <50 kg — 50 mg/kg; children >50 kg — adult dose.
- *Ampicillin*: neonates 50 mg/kg bd (<7 days old) or tds (7–21 days old), or qds (21–28 days old); children >1 month old — 50 mg/kg 4-6 hourly (max 2 g q4 h).

Local recommendations based on antibiotic sensitivity:
1.
2.
3.

Chloramphenicol

The WHO reaffirms the value of chloramphenicol in infections such as meningitis and severe bacterial infections due to bacteria resistance to other antibiotics.

Chloramphenicol has one serious toxicity — aplastic anaemia. Estimates of frequency are 1 in 10,000 to 1 in 70,000 courses of therapy (which are similar to estimates of death due to penicillin anaphylaxis: 1 in 40,000 courses). The WHO's Expert Committee on the Use of Essential Drugs, after due consideration of the risks and benefits of chloramphenicol, concluded that it is essential for modern medical practice in all countries.

Epidemic meningococcal disease

There are at least 9 different serogroups of *Neisseria meningitidis* (meningococci), of which three — groups A, B, and C — cause outbreaks of meningitis. Serogroup A meningococcus is the most important. It is responsible for the explosive epidemics that continue to devastate sub-Saharan Africa on an almost annual basis. It is also the main cause of endemic meningitis in this area of Africa with rates that are higher than the epidemic rates in other parts of the world. Types A and C have both been responsible for large outbreaks in the rest of the world.

Some strains of meningococci appear to be more virulent than others. Large epidemics occur when such strains encounter populations of nonimmune individuals in areas of poverty during particular climatic conditions (e.g. dry season, dust storm). In between epidemics, the bacteria survive in the community in the nasopharynx of carriers.

Vaccination: is essential for stopping an epidemic once it has begun. Kits for such campaigns are available from the WHO. Advice on organizing a campaign is also given in a WHO book — see below.

Chemoprophylaxis: only for household contacts of cases: rifampicin 600 mg (10 mg/kg for a child, 5 mg/kg for children <1 yr) PO bd for 2 days. (Alternative: ciprofloxacin 500 mg PO as a single dose; child 2–5 years 125 mg; child 5–12 year 250 mg.)

Viral meningitis

Enteroviruses, such as ECHO and coxsackie viruses, are important causes of epidemic viral meningitis worldwide, while arboviruses cause sporadic disease in endemic regions. Other causes of sporadic viral meningitis include polio, mumps virus, EB virus, HIV, varicella-zoster virus, CMV, and HSV.

Clinical features are similar to bacterial meningitis but the headache is less severe and the neck less stiff. It is diagnosed by examination of CSF. The identity of the causative virus during epidemics may already be clear. In sporadic cases, peripheral signs may suggest the aetiology such as genital or rectal lesions (HSV), skin blisters (herpes zoster), orchitis (mumps, lymphocytic choriomeningitis virus), rashes (enterovirus), parotid swelling (mumps). The prognosis is usually good, with complete resolution.

Other causes of meningitis

- Mycobacteria — *M. tuberculosis* (📖 p 146 and 408).
- Fungi — *Cryptococcus neoformans*, *Candida albicans*.
- Parasites — *Naegleria fowleri*.

For details on setting up a surveillance system and organizing the logistics of a mass vaccination campaign, see the following book: *Control of epidemic meningococcal disease: WHO practical guidelines* (Edition Fondation Marcel Merieux, 1995). Available from the WHO.

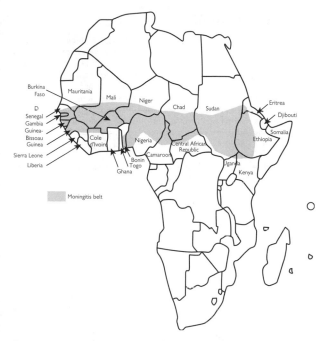

Fig. 10.1 The meningitis belt of Africa. (Reproduced with permission from *Control of Epidemic Meningococcal disease: WHO practical guidelines* (2nd edition)).

Chronic meningitis

TB meningitis or *Cryptococcus neoformans* (also: disseminated fungal infections; cysticercosis in children) typically present with a longer history (>7 days), headache, and low-grade fever. Confusion and drowsiness are common and may be due to hydrocephalus. Papilloedema, visual symptoms, and specific nerve lesions (particularly VI, VII, and urinary retention) may occur. Signs of infection at other sites (e.g. lungs) may also be found. In patients who are co-infected with HIV, the CSF cellular response in TB meningitis may be neutrophilic and this can be confused with pyogenic meningitis. Although often called chronic meningitis, these patients still represent a medical emergency and delayed therapy can lead to a significantly worse prognosis.

Diagnosis: the cause can be determined by examination of CSF; subsequently treat for the relevant infection. Both cryptococcal and TB meningitis occur commonly in immunosuppressed patients, particularly AIDS, but they also occur in previously healthy individuals.

Eosinophilic meningoencephalitis

Follows CNS infection with the nematodes *Angiostrongylus cantonensis*, *Gnathostoma spinigerum*, or *T solium* (causing cysticercosis, see 📖 p 440).

Angiostrongyliasis — results from the ingestion of *Angiostrongylus cantonensis* larvae in infected snails or contaminated shrimps, fish, and vegetables that are eaten raw or inadequately cooked. The larvae migrate to the brain, where they induce an immune response to dead parasites, and then to the eyes and lungs. Initial presentation is of acute, intermittent intense headache without fever; malaise; N&V; cranial nerve palsies; ± meningism. If severe, there may be fever, ↓ GCS, and spinal cord involvement. The eyes are commonly involved. The role of antihelminthics and steroids remains controversial. Dying parasites can elicit a strong immune reaction that can be fatal. It is normally a self-resolving condition — give sedatives, analgesia; the headache responds well to LP every 3–7 days. Treat with antihelminths (albendazole) and steroids. Eye involvement requires surgery to remove the nematode.

Spinocerebral gnathostomiasis is usually acquired by eating inadequately cooked, infected fish, or shrimps, following which *Gnathostoma spinigerum* larvae migrate to the CNS. It frequently presents with intensely painful radiculitis followed by rapidly advancing myelitis → paraplegia with urinary retention or quadriplegia, or as a cerebral haemorrhage in a previously healthy person. Treatment is as for angiostrongyliasis with antihelminthics (albendazole) and steroids.

Primary amoebic meningoencephalitis (PAM)

PAM is a rare but frequently fatal infection that follows intranasal infection with *Naegleria fowleri* while swimming in warm fresh water. The amoebae invade the CNS through the cribiform plate and cause extensive tissue necrosis. Headache occurs first, then fever, meningism, coma, convulsions. The patients are seriously ill. The CSF shows neutrophils, red cells, and amoebae on wet microscopy. The prognosis is poor. *Acanthamoeba* cause a similar syndrome, granulomatous amoebic encephalitis (GAE), in immunosuppressed individuals.

Management: amphotericin B 1 mg/kg IV (it is usual to give a smaller test dose first). Also, give amphotericin intrathecally (via a reservoir) — start with 0.025 mg, then increase to 0.25–1 mg (TOTAL, NOT per kg) on alternate days.

Table 10.1 CSF indices in cerebral infections of different aetiology

Cause	Normal CSF	Pyogenic bacteria	TB	PAM	Virus	Cryptococcus
Appearance	Clear and colourless	Cloudy or purulent	Clear, yellowish, slightly cloudy	Clear or slightly cloudy	Clear	Clear or slightly cloudy
White cells (majority)	$<5/mm^3$	$>200/mm^3$ (neutrophils)	$>10/mm^3$ (mononuclear)	$>200/mm^3$ (neutrophils)	$>10/mm^3$ (mononuclear)	$>10/mm^3$ (mononuclear)
Glucose	2.5–4 mmol/l (45–72 mg%)	Markedly ↓ or absent	Low	Normal or slightly ↓	Normal	Low
Total protein	0.15–0.4 g/l	Raised	Raised	Normal or slightly ↓	Raised	Raised
Microscopy	None	Gram: pus	Ziehl–Neelsen: AFB present	Wet: motile amoebae	None	India ink +ve

Encephalitis

Virus infection of the brain parenchyma is termed encephalitis. It is characterized by impairment of cerebral function, in contrast to meningeal infection that does not involve actual brain tissue.

Epidemics of encephalitis occur seasonally in many parts of the world and are important causes of death and disability in the young and elderly. The equine encephalitides have recently caused widespread epidemics in South America. Herpes simplex virus encephalitis (HSV) is the most important cause of sporadic encephalitis worldwide since it is treatable and, therefore, should be considered in all cases. However, Japanese encephalitis far outstrips HSV in actual numbers.

Clinical features: high fever, headache, N&V, followed by convulsions, confusion, and changes in level of consciousness. Some patients also present with meningism, focal neurological signs, abnormal behaviour, and/or raised ICP. Severe cases result in prolonged coma, hemiparesis, dystonia, decorticate or decerebrate posturing, and respiratory failure. Neurological sequelae such as mental retardation, hemiparesis, and behavioural abnormalities are particularly common after Japanese encephalitis, untreated HSV encephalitis, and post-infectious/vaccination encephalomyelitis.

Diagnosis: is via lumbar puncture. LP is contraindicated if there is evidence of raised ICP or focal signs.

Management: except for HSV encephalitis (see below), management is supportive with careful control of seizures (using phenytoin) and pyrexia. Beware respiratory failure and raised ICP (📖 p 402). The effectiveness of corticosteroids in preventing cerebral oedema is unclear.

Post-infectious or post-vaccination encephalomyelitis

On rare occasions, infection or vaccination elicits an antiviral immune response that results in CNS immunopathology and an encephalitic picture. It usually occurs after infection with measles, rubella, herpes zoster, mumps, and influenza and after vaccination with the Semple form of the rabies vaccine (but the relative risk is very small compared with the benefits of vaccination).

Herpes simplex virus (HSV) encephalitis

HSV encephalitis should be considered in the differential diagnosis of any patient presenting with an encephalitic picture. Focal signs relate to the frontal and temporal cortices and limbic system. It is particularly important since it is the only encephalitis for which there is effective treatment.

Management: aciclovir 10 mg/kg q8 h by slow IV infusion for 10–14 days. Untreated HSV encephalitis has a mortality rate of 40–70% and many survivors have neurological sequelae. Aciclovir markedly decreases mortality and the incidence of sequelae.

Japanese encephalitis

A common arboviral encephalitis of E., S., and S.E. Asia. Historically, it has been an infection of young children in wet season epidemics and more common in rural areas. However, this is changing as the vector adapts to an urban lifestyle. Widespread childhood vaccination campaigns in some countries have reduced the incidence of clinical disease. West Nile virus is a very closely related virus that causes encephalitis in parts of Africa and Central Europe and has recently spread to the USA.

Transmission: is via the bite of Culex mosquitos (e.g. *Culex tritaeniorhynchus*). The virus's primary hosts are birds such as herons, from which it is passed to domestic pigs by mosquitoes. It is amplified in these pigs before transmission to humans (a dead-end host). Most infections are subclinical — ~1 in 300 infections results in encephalitis.

Clinical features: after an incubation period of 6–16 days and a non-specific prodrome illness lasting a couple of days, the sudden onset of fever is accompanied by severe headache, meningism, N&V, and hyper-excitability, or decreased consciousness. Seizures are common in children. Neurological signs such as cranial nerve palsies, tremor and ataxia, parkinsonism, and upper limb paralysis develop. Together with a lowered consciousness level, they follow a variable course. Around 25% of patients die; many survivors have serious long-term neuropsychiatric disabilities (e.g. parkinsonism, paralysis, mental retardation). Spontaneous abortion and foetal death may occur in pregnant women. Japanese encephalitis virus is now a recognized cause of acute flaccid paralysis. Dengue (a related flavivirus) can also cause an encephalopathic illness.

Equine encephalitides

Three alphaviruses — Western, Eastern, and Venezuelan equine encephalitis viruses (EEVs) — cause widespread epizootics of encephalitis in horses in the USA, Central America, and the northern regions of S. America. The EEVs are not common causes of human encephalitis, but VEEV has recently caused large epidemics in both horses and humans in Colombia and Venezuela. The virus is amplified during horse infections and may subsequently cause human encephalitis.

Transmission: rodents and birds are the primary hosts of these viruses; transmission to humans is via Culex, Culiseta, and Aedes mosquitoes.

Clinical features: most infections are subclinical. There may be a short febrile illness with rigors (in VEEV also: sore throat, features of URTI, and diarrhoea). In a few cases, the illness is biphasic: recovery from the febrile illness is followed by encephalitis. Adults do not usually have sequelae; in contrast, many young children and infants are left with permanent neurological effects after encephalitis. Mortality is high (~10%) in this group.

Nipah virus encephalitis

Nipah virus has caused an outbreak of encephalitis in Malaysia and Singapore and appears to be endemic now in South Asia (Bangladesh). The causative agent was a new paramyxovirus named Nipah, closely related to the Hendra virus described in Australia, and potentially a new genus. The Nipah virus is a zoonosis infecting pigs and fruit bats. There is no specific treatment.

Rabies

A uniformly fatal illness, still common in many parts of the tropics, that is caused by the rabies virus (or, very rarely, a related lyssavirus). Once clinical symptoms have appeared, the patient will die. However, if the infection is caught soon after transmission and before the onset of clinical symptoms, rabies can be prevented by post-exposure vaccination. Increasing availability and affordability of vaccines and increasing their uptake by rural populations is pivotal in controlling rabies.

Transmission: is by the bite of an infected mammal, most commonly stray dogs (but also wild dogs, wolves, foxes, cats, and skunks) in endemic regions. The virus does not pass though intact skin; however, infected saliva can infect already damaged skin (e.g. by dogs' claws) and mucosae. Bites by vampire bats and inhalation of virus in bat-filled caves are methods of transmission in central and south America.

Clinical features: after an incubation period that normally lasts 20–90 days, prodromal symptoms develop: itching, pain, or paraesthesia at the site of the bite; followed by fever, chills, malaise, weakness, headache, and neuropsychiatric symptoms. Furious or paralytic rabies develops depending on the major locus of infection.

- *Furious (brain) rabies*: the pathognomic feature is hydrophobia — inspiratory muscle spasm (arched, extended back with arms thrown up) ± laryngeal spasm, associated with terror. While initially stimulated by attempts to drink water or wash, it soon becomes provoked by many stimuli. It may end in convulsions with cardiorespiratory arrest. Other features include: hyperaesthesia; generalized arousal (lucid periods alternating with wild, hallucinating, or aggressive periods); cranial nerve defects; meningism; involuntary movements; autonomic nervous system/hypothalamic changes — hypersalivation, lachrymation, ↑ or ↓ BP and temperature, SIADH, diabetes insipidus.
- *Paralytic (spine) rabies*: prodromal symptoms are followed by flaccid paralysis that ascends symmetrically or asymmetrically from the bitten area, pain, fasciculation, sensory disturbances; paraplegia and loss of sphincter control; ultimately, paralysis of muscles of respiration and swallowing.

Complications include: aspiration and bronchopneumonia; pneumonitis and myocarditis; pneumothorax after inspiratory spasms; cardiac arrhythmias; haematemesis; rarely ↑ ICP.

Diagnosis: history of dog or bat bite plus neurological features; immunofluorescence of viral antigen in base of hair roots in skin biopsy; isolation of virus from body fluids during 1st week.

Prevention: controlling the mammalian reservoir through vaccination; decreasing human exposure to infected mammals; vaccination of persons at high risk and those bitten by mammals (post-exposure vaccination, 📖 p 416).

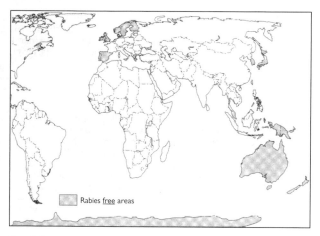

Fig. 10.2 Worldwide distribution of rabies.

Management of rabies infection

There is currently no effective treatment for an individual with signs and symptoms of rabies infection. In this situation, management is symptomatic with sufficient analgesia and sedation to relieve pain and terror. ITU care will prolong life by preventing or controlling complications.

Post-exposure prophylaxis

Vaccination within days of exposure is 100% effective in preventing the progression of the infection to encephalitis. However, the cheap Semple vaccine that is used most widely in the developing world is itself capable of initiating encephalitis. It is made by isolating virus from infected sheep's brains. Unfortunately, an immune response to sheep CNS components left in the vaccine can produce severe CNS disease with a 3% mortality.

Recent efforts to make the safer, tissue culture-grown, human diploid cell vaccine more affordable have involved using small doses intradermally (ID). Studies with such regimens have shown that they induce an immune response extremely quickly and that patients require fewer clinic visits. The regimens have been found to be 100% effective and without major side-effects.

Procedure: see box
- **Clean** *the wound* — this kills virus in superficial wounds. Scrub wound with soap/detergent and wash under running water for >5 mins. Liberally apply virucidal agent: 40–70% alcohol, or aqueous iodine. Debride as required.
- **Give anti-tetanus toxoid.**
- **Consider prophylactic antibiotics.**
- **Give vaccine.** The various regimens are below.
- **Give rabies immunoglobulin** if possible, either human RIG 20IU/kg or equine RIG 40IU/kg (in the latter case, have drugs already drawn up to treat an anaphylactic reaction). Give half the dose IM and infiltrate the remaining half around the wound.

Vaccine regimens for post-exposure prophylaxis

Sheep brain vaccine (Semple) Give 2–5 ml vaccine SC into the abdominal wall daily for 14–21 days. Boosters should be given after the course is finished.
Tissue culture vaccines
- 2-site intradermal method (2–2–2–0–1–1)
  Days 0, 3, and 7: 0.1 or 0.2 ml ID at each of 2 sites (deltoids)
  Days 28 and 90: 0.1 or 0.2 ml ID at 1 site (deltoid)
- 8-site intradermal method (8–0–4–0–1–1)
  Day 0: 0.1 ml ID into 8 sites (2× deltoids, suprascapulum, lower quadrant abdominal wall, thighs)
  Day 7: 0.1 ml ID into 4 sites (2× deltoids, thighs)
  Day 28: 0.1 ml ID into 1 site
  Day 91: 0.1 ml ID into 1 site

ID regimens require the use of Mantoux-like syringes and must cause a raised macule to appear immediately (like BCG vaccination).

Minor exposure

(including licks of broken skin, scratches, or abrasions without bleeding)
- Start vaccine immediately.
- Stop treatment if the dog/mammal remains healthy for 10 days.
- Stop treatment if dog's/mammal's brain proves negative for rabies by appropriate investigation.

Major exposure

(including licks of mucosa and minor or major bites)
- Immediate rabies immunoglobulin and vaccine.
- Stop treatment if dog/mammal remains healthy for 10 days.
- Stop treatment if dog's/mammal's brain proves negative for rabies by appropriate investigation.

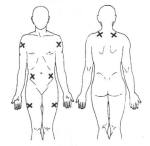

Fig. 10.3 Sites for the 8-site intradermal method of post-exposure vaccination. The use of multiple sites ensures that as many groups of lymph nodes are activated as possible, enhancing the immune response.

Tetanus

Contamination of a wound with the bacterium *Clostridium tetani* can result in severe neurological sequelae due to endotoxin production. The toxin tracks back up the nerves innervating local muscles, entering the CNS; it also enters the blood and passes to other muscles where it is again transported back up peripheral nerves to the CNS. There it blocks the release of inhibitory neurotransmitters, resulting in widespread activation of both motor and autonomic nervous systems. Muscles of the jaw, face, and head are involved first because of the shorter axonal paths, but all muscle groups become involved in most cases. Activation of opposing groups results in rigidity. Protracted uncontrolled muscular spasms of the chest result in ineffective breathing and hypoxia. Death is due to respiratory complications, circulatory failure, or cardiac arrest.

Tetanus is easily prevented by vaccination: its incidence worldwide is directly related to the prevalence of immunization — where immunization rates are high, tetanus is a rare disease; where immunization rates are low, it is a common condition, particularly of neonates who become infected at birth. Immunization of pregnant women prevents neonatal tetanus. Currently ~800,000 people die each year.

Transmission
C. tetani spores are ubiquitous in the environment and can infect even the most trivial cuts, typically on feet, legs, hands, and feet. Neonatal infection occurs via the cut umbilicus from the use of a dirty knife or the practice of applying dung to the stump.

Clinical features
There is an incubation period of 7–10 days, but this is variable and many patients cannot recall the injury. The *period of onset* (between the first symptom and the onset of spasms) varies between 1 to 7 days and is a good prognostic indicator: the shorter the interval, the more severe the disease.

The first symptom is often trismus (due to stiffness of masseters producing difficulty in opening the mouth). As the condition progresses, other muscle groups become rigid, including muscles of the face (producing characteristic look: risus sardonicus), skeleton (→ difficulty in breathing; opisthotonos; rigid limbs), and swallowing (→ aspiration).

Spasms are an exaggeration of the underlying rigidity and occur in more severe disease either as a reflex response to stimuli (touch, sounds, sights, emotions) or spontaneously. They may be mild and brief, or prolonged and very painful. Prolonged thoracic spasms may result in respiratory failure; laryngeal spasms in death from anoxia. In severe disease, the patient has a fever, tachycardia, and an unstable CVS, mostly due to involvement of the autonomic nervous system — see box.

Neonatal cases present with inability to suckle; they go on to develop characteristic opisthotonos (see 📖 p 28).

Diagnosis: is be made on clinical features alone.

Prevention: by active vaccination of children and pregnant women (📖 see also Chapter 22); good wound toilet and passive vaccination following injuries; and provision of clean facilities for childbirth.

Grading of tetanus severity

- *Grade I (mild):* mild to moderate trismus; general spasticity; no respiratory problems; no spasms; little or no dysphagia.
- *Grade II (moderate):* moderate trismus; well-marked rigidity; mild to moderate but short-lasting spasms; moderate respiratory failure with tachypnoea >30–35/min; mild dysphagia.
- *Grade III (severe):* severe trismus; generalized spasticity; reflex and often spontaneous prolonged spasms; respiratory failure with tachypnoea >40/min; apnoeic spells; severe dysphagia; tachycardia >120/min.
- *Grade IV (very severe):* features of grade III plus violent autonomic disturbances involving the CVS. These include: episodes of severe hypertension and tachycardia alternating with relative hypotension and bradycardia; severe persistent hypertension (diastolic >110 mmHg); severe persistent hypotension (systolic <90).

Complications

- *Respiratory:* collapse; aspiration, lobar, or bronchopneumonia (often due to Gram −ve organisms); anoxia due to prolonged laryngeal spasm; severe hypoxia and respiratory failure in severe tetanus if patient is not paralysed and ventilated; unexplained tachypnoea and respiratory distress; ARDS. Complications also include those of tracheostomy and prolonged ventilation.
- *CVS:* (mostly mediated by ANS): persistent tachycardia, hypotension or hypertension; labile hypertension; severe peripheral vasoconstriction → shock-like state. Autonomic storms are characterized by sudden sinus tachycardia + severe hypertension followed by sudden bradycardia and hypotension; they may precede cardiac arrest. Increased vagal tone is shown by sudden bradycardia — sucking out of the trachea may lead to an arrest. Dysrhythmias include: SVT; junctional rhythms; atrial and ventricular ectopics; short bursts of self-resolving VT. Hyperthermia (hypothermia is very rare).
- *Sudden death:* caused by many of the above complications, massive PE, or unidentified event.
- *Sepsis:* most commonly nosocomial.
- *Renal insufficiency.*
- *Mid-thoracic vertebral fracture:* occurs during severe spasms; there are usually few sequelae and healing occurs without incident.

Management of tetanus

Management of severe tetanus can be extremely difficult, particularly in the open ward where conservative management has an appalling mortality rate. Ideally, ALL patients should be treated in an ITU setting.

However, careful management of the patient with particular attention to critical care and ventilatory support can markedly improve the prognosis where an ITU is not available.

If ventilators are limited, they should be kept for patients with:
• Grade IV disease.
• Grade III disease uncontrolled by sedatives.
• Serious respiratory complications.

Give immediate care on admission (see box). Subsequent management depends on the severity of the condition.

Grade I — beware complications of septic wound. Observe carefully since grade I tetanus can progress to more severe disease. For sedation/ muscle relaxation, give diazepam 5 mg PO tds (neonatal dose 2 mg PO tds). Alternative: chlorpromazine 50 mg (adult), 25 mg (child), or 12.5 mg (neonate) IM qds (phenobarbital can be added if essential).

Grade II — as for grade I but increase sedation/muscle relaxation. Increase dose of diazepam up to 4-fold in adults (do not exceed 80–100 mg/day because of risk of respiratory depression). Give by slow IV infusion over 24 h.

The ideal sedative/muscle-relaxant schedule ensures continuous sedation such that the patient can sleep but can be woken up to obey commands. An objective guide is relaxation of abdominal muscles.

Perform a tracheostomy (may prevent death due to prolonged laryngeal spasm and anoxia). If laryngeal spasm occurs, promptly give chlorpromazine 50 mg IV (alternative: diazepam 10–20 mg IV).

Grade III — treat as for grade II but also paralyse and ventilate. Reduce diazepam dose to 30–40 mg over 24 h. Give pancuronium 2–4 mg (poorer alternative: gallamine 20–40 mg) IV, titrated for each patient to give sufficient neuromuscular blockade for efficient ventilation. Initially, give every 1–1.5 h (1st 1–2 wks), then extend interval as the patient improves. Check with periodic arterial blood analysis, if available. Spasms still occur under paralysis but they need not affect ventilation; pancuronium can be stopped when spasms cease. Continue ventilation until patient can be weaned off.

Grade IV — as above, with addition of drugs that act on the CVS if deemed *essential* for grossly deranged haemodynamics.
• Hypotension — give volume load; if ineffective or contraindicated, use dopamine to keep systolic BP >100 mmHg.
• Hypertension (systolic >200, diastolic >100 mmHg) — propranolol 5–10 mg PO or nifedipine 5 mg sublingual.
• Bradyarrhythmia or persistent tachyarrhythmias.

Overall aims of care

- Maintain adequate arterial PaO_2 and O_2 saturation.
- Maintain fluid, electrolyte, and acid-base balance.
- Maintain circulatory support in grade IV hypotensive patient.
- A central venous line is very useful if available.

Management on admission

All patients should receive:

- *Antiserum (antitoxin)* — preferably human tetanus immunoglobulin 150 units/kg IM in multiple sites; otherwise equine antiserum 10,000 units by slow IV injection, but *be prepared for an anaphylactic reaction* in all patients receiving equine antiserum and have treatment ready.
- *Antibiotics* — metronidazole 500 mg IV q8 h for 7–10 days (poorer alternative: benzylpenicillin 1.2 g IM or IV q8 h for 8 days).
- *Local infiltration of antiserum* — is of uncertain efficacy but is recommended in some parts of the world.
- *Magnesium* — can help reduce the need for muscle relaxants and sedatives and may be helpful in reducing autonomic dysfunction and is safe at an intravenous loading dose of 40 mg/kg over 30 minutes, followed by intravenous infusion of 2 g/hour for patients >45 kg and 1.5 g/hour for patients ≤45 kg.
- *Wound toilet* — performed after other steps, to remove necrotic tissue. Delay suturing.
- *Vaccination* — before discharge.
- Prevent, detect, and promptly treat any infection.
- Detect early hyperpyrexia — treat with paracetamol and wet cloths.

Critical care and nursing is essential

- Reduce external stimuli — physical examination must be gentle.
- Keep airway patent — use *gentle* suction to remove saliva and secretions at the back of the throat.
- Take exquisite care of the tracheostomy.
- Gently and frequently change the patient's posture.
- Use physiotherapy to keep lungs patent — give a small IV bolus of diazepam before physiotherapy. In the paralysed patient, perform physiotherapy when the action of pancuronium (gallamine) is at its maximum.
- Keep up patient's nutrition: 3500–4000 calories (including >100 g protein) by NG tube is required each day.

Stroke

A rapidly developing focal loss of cerebral function which lasts more than 24 h in a person with no history of recent head injury. In the industrialized world, mostly due to cerebral infarction after a thrombotic or embolic event (~80%). The situation may differ in the developing world — see box. Around 20% of stroke patients die within the first month; intracranial haemorrhages have a higher fatality rate than those following cerebral infarction. The history of a sudden event is crucial in establishing a diagnosis.

Transient ischaemic attacks (TIAs) — are defined as an acute loss of focal cerebral or monocular function that lasts less than 24 h. They indicate that the person is at increased risk of a stroke (~5%/yr) and death due to thromboembolic events such as stroke or MI (~10%/yr).

Risk factors

Include hypertension (HT), ischaemic heart disease, atrial fibrillation, TIAs, peripheral vascular disease, DM, smoking.

Clinical features

The neurological deficits are varied but commonly come on rapidly. It may be possible to relate the clinical features to the known anatomy of particular cerebral blood vessels but collateral blood supply makes this difficult. Infarcts affecting the cerebral hemisphere may cause contralateral hemiparesis (→ upper motor neurone paralysis after initial spinal shock), sensory loss, homonymous hemianopia, and/or dysphasia. Infarcts affecting subcortical structures such as thalamus and basal ganglia can cause mixed or isolated motor and/or sensory defects or ataxia. Brainstem infarcts can have profound affects: quadriplegia, visual and/or respiratory problems, locked-in syndrome. There is often a transient hypertension that settles.

Management

It is essential to *think about rehabilitation* early in the patient's illness. Do not ignore this issue until the patient has developed joint contractures that will prevent physical recovery.

- Give aspirin 150 mg daily if cerebral haemorrhage excluded.
- Take great care of the airway in the unconscious patient. Turn the patient often to avoid bedsores.
- Ensure adequate nutrition and hydration.
- Slowly and carefully lower BP if very high (>130 diastolic; >240 systolic).
- If there is an identified source of thromboemboli (other than endocarditis), anticoagulate as for a DVT.
- Check for treatable causes such as giant-cell arteritis.
- Watch out for causes of neurological deterioration — see box.
- If there is evidence of cerebral oedema, consider giving mannitol.

Prevention

Recovery for most patients is rarely complete and primary prevention is important. Reduce the risk of strokes by controlling risk factors, particularly HT and smoking, in individuals and populations. In patients who have had

TIAs or previous strokes, it is important to control HT and reduce the chance of further thrombotic events by giving aspirin 75 mg PO od. Assuming no contraindications, anticoagulation is required for patients with AF, clotting disorders, or recurrent DVT.

Main causes of stroke in sub-Saharan Africa

- Hypertension (haemorrhagic stroke).
- Atherosclerosis (thrombotic stroke).
- Rheumatic heart disease (embolic),
- Others: Haemoglobinopathies (including sickle cell disease)
  HIV
  Subarachnoid haemorrhage
  Unexplained (mainly young persons).

Causes of neurological deterioration after stroke

- *Local* — extension of thrombus; recurrent embolism or haemorrhage; haemorrhagic transformation of the infarct; post haemorrhage vasoconstriction; further ischaemia; cerebral oedema; brain shift and herniation; hydrocephalus; epileptic seizures.
- *General* — hypoxia (pneumonia, PE, cardiac failure); hypotension; infection; dehydration; hyponatraemia; hypoglycaemia or hyperglycaemia; drugs; depression.

Stroke rehabilitation

Without rehabilitation and physiotherapy, the patient risks spending the rest of her/his days in a wheelchair or bedbound. It is essential to start physiotherapy as soon as the patient is medically stable, to give the best chance of regaining hand and arm function and of walking. Aim to regain independence.

- Rehabilitation is 24-h process. Good work during the day can be ruined by a night in a bad position. It may be useful to teach the patient's relatives the basics of physiotherapy so that they can both look out for bad positioning and help the patient perform exercises.
- Initially, encourage the patient to participate in therapy for about 20 mins, 3 times a day. This can be increased with time.
- The patient needs regular turning to prevent bed sores (q4 h).
- Physiotherapy should **NEVER** be painful. The expression 'no pain, no gain' has no place in rehabilitation.

General guidelines

- The stroke patient initially has decreased tone. At onset, rehabilitation attempts to increase power in the limbs. However, over time tone may increase so much that the limbs become spastic with fixed deformities. A hand left bunched up and curled under the arm is useless. Gentle repetitive exercises should be able to reduce the tone. Work on the opposite movements to those that cause the hand to bunch up: extension at the shoulder, elbow, wrist, and fingers.
- Normal movement is easier if the person is completely relaxed. This is accomplished by supporting the whole body as in Fig. 10.4.
- The aim of stroke rehabilitation is for normal movement. Some patients will neglect one side — ensure that the patient is able to see both arms and hands at all times. Reinforce the message that they are symmetrical. The patient can practise doing actions with weak limbs (e.g. picking up a cup, stepping from one foot to the other while sitting) by carefully noting the action with the normal limb, and then copying this with the weak limb.

Repetition of a movement over a period reinforces plastic adaptation. After a stroke, the brain has to relearn how to do things. It needs to practise. However, repetition can strengthen both bad and good habits, so it is essential to get the practised movements right.

Early stage

- It is important to support and position the patient carefully, paying particular attention to the hemiplegic shoulder to reduce the risk of injury. Nos. 1–3 in Fig. 10.4 show how to cushion the patient.
- Relatives or nurses should roll the patient carefully (no. 4). As patient becomes stronger, teach rolling from side to side, and then to get up from lying (nos. 5 and 6). The patient will often need help.
- Frequent changes in position are good.

Aim to maintain muscle length (prevent contractures) with *gentle* passive/active movements into extension, taking particular care over the Achilles tendon, and the flexors of elbow, wrist, and fingers.

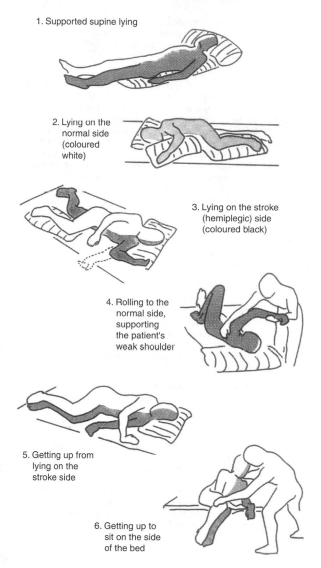

1. Supported supine lying

2. Lying on the normal side (coloured white)

3. Lying on the stroke (hemiplegic) side (coloured black)

4. Rolling to the normal side, supporting the patient's weak shoulder

5. Getting up from lying on the stroke side

6. Getting up to sit on the side of the bed

Fig. 10.4 Patient support and positioning in stroke rehabilitation (continued p 427).

- Encourage selective and controlled movements. It is better to work slowly to get good control of arm and hand movements than to be able rapidly to regain function with gross abnormal limb movements.

Basic principles for this early stage
- *Aim for symmetry* — sit the patient in a good position with adequate support. Set the arms forward. Sit the patient out for short periods if trunk control is poor. This is important; practise transferring weight from side to side — this will make it easier for him/her to shift weight from one leg to the other while learning to walk again.
- *Aim for good control of movement* — in particular, the patient needs to be able to control the transference of body weight in sitting and in standing. The patient needs to lean forward to get up. This is best learned with a high seat initially (and something in front to help build confidence). With progress, the seat can be lowered and the front support shifted to the side, before trying a chair.
- *Aim for trunk control* — in sitting, before trying to stand and, in particular, during the act of moving from sitting to standing.
- *Aim for balance* — in standing and stepping before walking.

Walking stage
- Aim for normal gait — equal stride length and equal time on both sides.
- The patient may require support on one or both sides.
- Start walking with the *unaffected* leg. This means that the patient must have already learned to shift weight from leg to leg.
- Walking aids — use a wheeled frame/rollator or a normal walking stick (a quadruped stick should be a last resort).
- The patient may require help with a 'drop foot'.
- Use mime, gestures, repeating and rephrasing movements, and physical prompts to help the patient. Allow time for slow synapsing.
- Little and often is a better way to build stamina and sustain carry-over from one session to another.

Some 'don'ts' for stroke rehabilitation
- *Do not ask the patient to try harder* — *avoid* effort as it increases tone and gross patterns of movement.
- *Do not ask the patient to squeeze a ball* — this encourages the arm flexors that are already too strong.
- *Avoid a painful shoulder* — do not make any arm movements unless the whole shoulder, including the scapula, is relaxed and supple. *Support for a weak arm* may be useful temporarily (e.g. while concentrating on walking).
- *Never lift under the stroke arm or pull it* — the muscles that hold the shoulder are weak and the joint easily dislocated.
- *Prevent dislocation* — support the forearm and hand forwards with natural weight through the elbow.

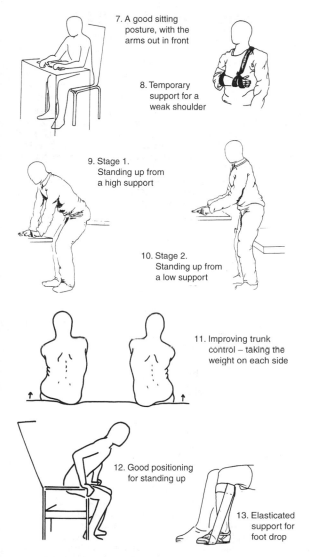

7. A good sitting posture, with the arms out in front

8. Temporary support for a weak shoulder

9. Stage 1. Standing up from a high support

10. Stage 2. Standing up from a low support

11. Improving trunk control – taking the weight on each side

12. Good positioning for standing up

13. Elasticated support for foot drop

Fig. 10.4 Patient support and positioning in stroke rehabilitation (continued from p 425).

Subarachnoid haemorrhage (SAH)

An acute bleed into the subarachnoid space that produces a sudden intense headache, sometimes accompanied by nausea and vomiting. This is classically described as 'like being hit on the back of the head'. Most cases are caused by ruptured aneurysms. Other causes are rare mycotic aneurysms (due to endocarditis) and arteriovenous malformations (more frequent in young patients). 15% have no identified cause.

Clinical features: the conscious level may be impaired. The more severe the bleed, the lower the conscious level, and the worse the prognosis. Other features include: headache with meningism; vomiting; fits. Focal signs are rare. The patient is often irritable and drowsy; the headache may last for weeks. Complications include vascular spasm that contributes to cerebral ischaemia.

Beware: worsening conscious level, the appearance or worsening of a neurological deficit (e.g. development of hemiparesis, dilatation of a pupil), or systemic changes such as ↑BP that may indicate ↑ ICP.

Diagnosis: is by clinical findings with LP (and early CT scan if available). The CSF is uniformly blood-stained in the first few days. Xanthochromia (straw-coloured supernatant) may be present if at least 6 h have elapsed since the onset of the bleed. It may be present for up to 14 days. However, if meningitis forms part of the differential diagnosis, the LP should not be delayed.

Management: involves neurosurgery in many cases to evacuate an intracerebral haematoma or clip the aneurysm. Medical treatment involves extended bed rest, analgesia, sedation (beware masking of deterioration in conscious level), and cautious control of hypertension. IV hydration (3L/day) is strongly advised. Nimodipine (60 mg PO q4 h for 2–3 weeks, starting within 4 days of haemorrhage) decreases the incidence of vascular spasm.

Some SAH are preceded by minor herald bleeds that also elicit an intense headache ± meningism or back pain. If suspected, refer for evaluation since surgical treatment at this time may prevent a later severe bleed. Rebleeding occurs in ~30% of cases; it is a common cause of death.

Subdural haemorrhage

A slow venous bleed that follows damage to veins crossing from the cortex to venous sinuses. May even occur after minor trauma in those predisposed: elderly, alcoholics, people with clotting disorders, epileptics. Presentation can occur months after the forgotten accident as chronic bleeding slowly increases the size of the haematoma.

Clinical features: typically there is a lucid interval between the injury and the onset of neurological symptoms. Common acute symptoms include headache, vomiting, fluctuating levels of consciousness; less often, mood changes, irritability, incontinence, drowsiness. Signs may include changes in pupil size, distal limb weakness, and increased reflexes; less commonly, fits and dysphasia.

Management
This requires a neurosurgical opinion and, if possible, a CT scan — evacuation through burr holes is recommended for most cases (Fig. 10.5). It is possible that minor haematomas will resolve spontaneously. With appropriate management the outcome is good in all ages — ~90% return to normal. It is therefore important to consider the diagnosis in a confused elderly person.

Extradural haematoma

An arterial bleed that normally results from a skull fracture after head injury (e.g. assault, road traffic accident). The haematoma enlarges rapidly and, unless evacuated equally rapidly, there is a high risk of brain herniation and the patient's death. Suspect when the conscious level declines in a patient with head injury. Unilateral dilation of a pupil, which is sluggish or unresponsive to light, is ipsilateral to the side of the haemorrhage.

Management: do a CT scan, if possible, to localize the expanding lesion. Further management depends on the distance to a neurosurgeon. If close, give mannitol before transferring the patient. If the neurosurgeon is remote, a burr hole will be required to prevent brain herniation.

In this situation, unless a burr hole is done rapidly, the patient will die or suffer brain damage. You and the patient have nothing to lose and everything to gain. An inelegant burr hole now will do much more good than an elegant operation one hour or more later.

How to do a burr hole

1. *Incision*
- Shave the scalp if there is time.
- Local anaesthetic is not usually necessary.
- Make a 4 cm incision over the site of fracture or injury: this is usually in the temporal region (just above the zygomatic arch), where a curved incision is made (see Fig. 10.5 – 1, opposite) so that it can be enlarged.
2. *Incise right down to the bone.* Do not stop to control bleeding.
3. *Scrape back the pericranium* (periosteum) using a periosteal elevator (or similar instrument) to expose the skull.
- Insert a mastoid retractor (Fig. 10.5 – 2) — this will stop all the bleeding.
- Leave the retractor in.
4. *Perforate the bone using a perforator* (Fig. 10.5 – 3)
- Dark blood will ooze out.
- The dura will not be seen as it is stripped away by the blood clot.
- Do no more than *JUST* perforate the skull.
- This will create a conical hole.
5. *Enlarge the perforation using a burr* (Fig. 10.5 – 4)
The burr will enlarge the hole so that it is nearly cylindrical.
6. *The blood clot will immediately ooze out.*
- Suck the blood away by applying a sucker to the burr hole but
  **DO NOT INSERT SUCKER INTO THE CAVITY This will cause
more bleeding and might damage the brain.**
- It is now safe to transfer the patient to a neurosurgical unit.
- Leave the scalp retractor in; organize for its return.
- Leave in the endotracheal tube and leave a drip up.

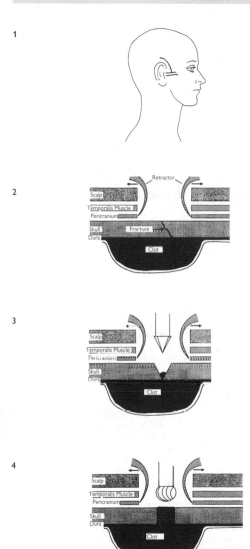

Fig. 10.5 How to do a burr hole.

Blackouts

The most common causes of blackouts are epilepsy and syncope (see box). A reliable eyewitness account is helpful.

Syncope is the brief loss of consciousness due to an acute reduction in cerebral blood flow. It is the most common cause of recurrent episodes of disturbed consciousness and may be precipitated by anxiety or pain. It is due to ↓ venous return to the heart leading to ↓ cardiac output, or an inadequate response of the heart when ↑demand requires ↑cardiac output. Causes include hypotension, vagal slowing of the heart, neuropathy, dysrhythmias, aortic stenosis, vertebrobasilar ischaemia (TIAs), carotid-sinus syndrome.

Space-occupying lesions (SOL)

Classically present with focal neurological signs, ↑ ICP, or seizures. Focal neurological signs can be used to localize the mass but beware false localizing signs due to ↑ ICP rather than direct pressure from the lesion (unilateral or bilateral sixth cranial nerve palsy most common; also third and fourth cranial nerve palsies; uncal herniation may rarely cause an ipsilateral hemiparesis and/or contralateral homonymous hemianopia).

Causes
- Infection — tuberculoma, cysticercosis, echinococcosis, bacterial or amoebic brain abscess, paragonimiasis, schistosomiasis, toxoplasmosis, fungal granulomata.
- Tumour — glioma, meningioma, metastases, lymphoma, pituitary adenoma, cysts.
- Others — aneurysm, haematoma.

Hydrocephalus

In older children and adults, the skull will not expand if the intracranial pressure rises. Blockage of CSF flow through the ventricles or a failure to reabsorb CSF results in a build up of pressure or hydrocephalus. While producing an increasing head circumference in young children, it results in rising intracranial pressure in older persons that will need urgent management. It exists in two forms:
- *Non-communicating hydrocephalus* — due to blockage of CSF flow through the ventricles, normally at foramina or aqueduct between ventricles and/or basal cistern. Caused by any SOL, such as tumour or cyst, or stenosis of the aqueduct. The location of the blockage must be identified and the blockage removed surgically, or a shunt placed.
- *Communicating hydrocephalus* — due to CSF obstruction in basal cisterns or subarachnoid space (the CSF still flows out of the ventricular system but it cannot be reabsorbed in the arachnoid villi). It may result from intracranial haemorrhage or meningitis (acute pyogenic or chronic); the cause is often unknown. Presents with a triad of

dementia, incontinence, and gait disturbance. (This condition is also called normal pressure hydrocephalus). Repeated lumbar taps with treatment of any underlying cause may be sufficient.

Causes of blackouts

- Vasovagal syncope.
- Postural hypotension.
- Hyperventilation.
- Cardiac arrhythmia.
- Hypoglycaemia.
- Vertebro-basilar TIAs.
- Epilepsy.
- Hypoxia.
- Hysteria.

It is important to measure blood levels of:
- Glucose.
- Na^+.
- K^+.
- Ca^{2+}.
- Mg^{2+}.

Epilepsy

Epilepsy is the continuing tendency to have seizures — spontaneous paroxysmal discharges of neurons that result in clinical symptoms.

It is common, with around 40 million people affected worldwide. Its incidence is higher in the developing world than the industrialized world: approximately 1% of the population has epilepsy due to higher incidence of infection and head injury. Unfortunately, at present only ~15% of cases are treated adequately and many people suffer unnecessarily. There is a great need to both reduce its incidence in the developing world (by decreasing the number of head injuries and infections) and find ways of providing adequate supplies of affordable effective antiepileptic drugs to poorer countries.

Causes
70% unknown, 30% known.
- Infection — cysticercosis, tuberculoma, schistosomiasis, paragonimiasis, sparganosis, hydatid disease, toxoplasmosis, toxocariasis, cerebral malaria, cerebral amoebiasis, syphilitic gumma, and HIV.
- Epilepsy can also be a late consequence of almost any meningeal or brain parenchyma infection.
- Brain injury — due to either head injury (such as assault or RTA) or antenatal head injury (may also be due to post-natal injury but this is now believed to be less important).
- Unknown — many may actually be due to very small areas of focal dysgenesis (hamartomas).
- Eclampsia — urgent delivery is required.
- Inherited diseases.
- Alcohol.
- Brain tumour or metastasis.
- Metabolic causes.
- Degenerative disorders (in elderly).
- Vascular disease.
- Drugs.

Clinical features
Will depend on the class of seizure — see below.
- There may be an aura or warning before the attack.
- In grand mal attacks, the person has generalized convulsions usually with tonic-clonic movements of all four limbs. The patient loses consciousness and may bite his/her tongue and be incontinent of urine or, rarely, faeces.
- Post-ictally, there may be a period of confusion, drowsiness, a failure to remember the onset, and a headache with a tendency to sleep.

Seizure classification
Important for choice of drug therapy. Origin and spread of the seizure:
- A seizure that remains localized to its area of origin is a *partial seizure.*
- A seizure that subsequently spreads from this region to involve the whole brain is termed a *secondarily generalized seizure.*
- A seizure that originates in centrally positioned cells and activates all parts of the brain simultaneously is a *generalized seizure.*

Principles of antiepileptic drug therapy

- Establish a clear clinical diagnosis.
- Get EEG supporting evidence if possible.
- Choose a drug, considering the:
  - Seizure type(s).
  - Patient's age.
  - Price.
  - Interaction with other drugs.
  - Possibility of pregnancy.
- Give one drug only.
- Begin with modest dosage, building up slowly over 2–3 months.
- Give full information to the patient concerning:
  - Names and alternative names of the drug supplied.
  - The main side-effects of the drug.
  - The need for compliance with instructions.
  - Possible interactions with other medications.
- Monitor progress, seizure frequency, and side-effects.
- Ensure adequate supplies.

Clinical features of the seizure

1. *Partial seizures:* have signs and symptoms referable to a part of one hemisphere.

- *Simple* (consciousness is not impaired, e.g. in focal motor seizures which may start in a toe, finger, or the angle of mouth).
- *Complex* (consciousness is impaired with signs of temporal lobe activity, e.g. olfactory aura followed by automatism of facial expression, behaviour, hallucinations).
- *Secondarily generalized.*

2. **Generalized seizures:** do not have any features that are referable to only one hemisphere.

- *Absences* (petit mal) brief ~10 sec pauses (e.g. stops talking mid-sentence, carries on where left off). Classically, has pathognomic 3Hz activity on EEG.
- *Tonic-clonic* (grand mal) sudden onset with loss of consciousness, body stiffens for up to 1 min. before jerking, post-ictal drowsiness.
- *Myoclonic* and *akinetic* seizures.

Management

If the seizure appears to have a focal onset, look for a treatable underlying cause, particularly infectious (if available, use CT or, better, MRI). Patients should be warned not to drive.

First-line drugs: see a formulary for details of use and side-effects.

- *Phenobarbital* — start at 1 mg/kg PO od, building up to 3.0 mg/kg (max 180 mg) od. First choice for partial and generalized tonic-clonic seizures. Should not be used to treat the seizures associated with cerebral malaria. Its side-effects in children appear to be acceptable.
- *Carbamazepine* — start at 100 mg PO bd, building up to 600 mg bd if tolerated. First choice for tonic-clonic seizures in association with partial seizures; reserve drug for partial seizures alone.
- *Sodium valproate* — start at 300 mg PO bd, building up to 750 mg bd (max = 2.5 g/day). First choice for typical absences, myoclonic and akinetic seizures, and tonic-clonic seizures in association with typical absences.
- *Phenytoin* — start at 2.5 mg/kg PO od, building up to 5.0(max ~8.0)mg/kg PO od. Reserve drug for tonic-clonic and partial seizures (not for absences). It is a toxic drug and plasma levels should ideally be monitored.
- *Other drugs* — include clonazepam, ethosuximide, and the newer expensive drugs (vigabatrin, lamotrigine, gabapentin).

Changing drugs: Persist with an old drug until it has been used at its maximum dose before considering a change. Introduce the new drug at its starting dose and slowly increase to its mid-range; then start to slowly decrease the dose of the old drug.

Stopping drugs: It is not clear how long any person needs to stay on antiepileptic drugs once the seizures have been controlled. An MRC trial of stopping medication in people who had not had a seizure for 2 yrs showed that 59% of those who stopped medication were seizure-free at 2 yrs compared to 78% who remained on medication. Discuss with the patient what they want: risk of recurrence vs. gravity of the side-effects.

Status epilepticus

Status epilepticus has recently been redefined: 'generalized, convulsive status epilepticus in adults and older children (>5 years old) refers to at least 5 min of (a) continuous seizures or (b) two or more discrete seizures'. This definition reflects the current uncertainty about the relationship between the duration of convulsions and CNS damage. Status epilepticus can result in death, permanent neurological damage, or the onset of chronic epilepsy — risk factors for such sequelae include aetiology, duration of attack, and systemic complications.

Aetiology
~40% occur in known epileptics; other causes include fever or acute CNS infection (particularly in children), head injury, pesticide poisoning, stroke, eclampsia.

Management
- Stop seizures quickly.
- Prevent complications.
- Find and control the underlying causes.
- Remove patient from potential danger.
1. Secure the airway, preferably with Guedal airway, give oxygen.
2. Do not attempt to intubate if the jaw is clenched. Wait for sedation to have its effect.
3. Give 50 ml 20% dextrose as IV bolus unless hypoglycaemia excluded.
4. Give thiamine 250 mg by slow IV infusion over 20 mins if the patient alcoholic: note risk of anaphylaxis.
5. Give diazepam 10–20 mg in 2–4 ml IV or PR at a rate of 5 mg/min. (For children, give 1 mg per year of age.) This should control ~80% of patients. Second (and rarely third) doses may be needed.
6. Beware respiratory depression following bolus diazepam.

If convulsions continue after giving diazepam — manage the patient in ICU if possible
Give phenytoin 10–15 mg/kg as an IV infusion, at <50 mg/min, through a separate giving set. Once seizures are controlled, maintain with phenytoin 100 mg PO or IV q6–8 h. (Alternatively, give phenobarbital 10 mg/kg as an IV infusion, at <100 mg/min. to a maximum of 1 g. Do not give more diazepam. Beware respiratory depression and hypotension. Chlormethiazole is an alternative. Phenobarbital is preferred for fits associated with poisoning.). Check for and treat ↑ ICP.

If convulsions continue after phenytoin
1. Exclude pseudostatus.
2. Check drugs have been given correctly.
3. Then give general anaesthetic and ventilate, whilst treating causative condition. Give thiopental 75–125 mg (3–5 ml of a 2.5% solution) IV over 10–15 secs. Give further doses according to response. Beware hypotension. If large amounts of thiopentone are infused over a long period, it will accumulate and delay recovery.

Cysticercosis

This condition, caused by the pork tapeworm *Taenia solium*, is a common cause of epilepsy worldwide. Humans are the definitive host for this species and normally become infected by eating cysts in undercooked pork meat — see life cycle in Fig. 10.6.

Accidental human ingestion of eggs in faecally contaminated food results in disease with marked morbidity of the CNS, muscles, skin, and eye. The symptoms are caused by the inflammatory reaction to the living and dying parasites (active disease) and long-term effects of the inflammatory reaction to the cysts — fibrosis, calcification, and granulation (inactive disease).

Transmission: by ingestion of food or water contaminated with pig faeces. Poor personal hygiene, particularly amongst food handlers, and faecal pollution of water and irrigated vegetables predispose to infection.

Clinical features: CNS involvement (neurocysticercosis) normally manifests as epilepsy. However, since the number and localization of cysts vary greatly, neurocysticercosis can manifest in a variety of ways including hydrocephalus, dementia (frontal lobe involvement; often in children); infarcts (due to vasculitis); basal meningitis; cranial nerve defects; spinal symptoms.

Subcutaneous and muscular cysts occur in 25% of cases with CNS involvement, but may also occur in isolation — the calcified cysts appear as small, round, painless, firm nodules. The rare involvement of cardiac muscle can result in conduction defects.

Ocular cysticercosis often presents with blurring of vision and the sensation of something moving in the eye. If untreated, it may progress to blindness and eye atrophy.

Diagnosis: active CNS lesions can be identified by CT or MRI; calcified inactive lesions can be seen on CT (and sometimes on X-ray). Serology.

Management

- Patients should be treated with albendazole orally 15 mg/kg/day in two doses for 8–30 days and with oral dexamethasone 0.4 mg/kg/day for 10 days. An alternative is prazaquantel either as a one-day regimen of 25 mg/kg in 3 doses 2 h apart or a 15-day regimen using 50 mg/kg/day orally.
- The one-day regimen should only be used for those with a single or low cyst burden.
- Surgery is usually reserved for subarachnoid and intraventricular cysts causing compression and resulting in hydrocephalus or cord compression.
- Ocular infection should not be treated with drugs. Ocular cysts may need to be treated surgically.

Prevention: health education and public health measures to improve personal hygiene, meat inspection, sanitation on farms, and sewage disposal. Mass treatments in hyperendemic regions and interruption of the parasite's life cycles.

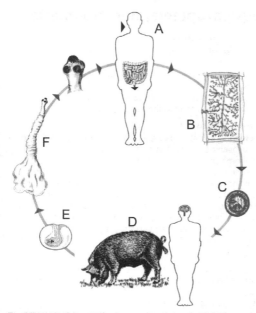

Fig. 10.6 Life cycle of *Taenia solium*. Man (A) is the definitive host, with a tapeworm 3–4 m long in the small intestine. Proglottids (segments, B) of the tapeworm detach and are shed in the faeces, each containing a branching uterus and thousands of eggs (C). When human faecal matter is ingested by man or pig (D) these eggs, which contain an embyo, develop into a larval stage (the cysticercus, E) in muscles, brain, or other tissues. When man ingests uncooked pork containing cysticerci, these evaginate (F) in the human small intestine to form the head of the tapeworm; this elongates and forms new segments, completing the life cycle. (Adapted from G. Piekarski, *Medial parasitology in plates*, 1962, and reproduced with kind permission of Bayer Pharmaceuticals).

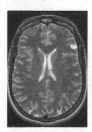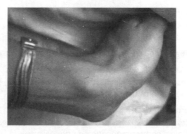

Fig. 10.7 MRI of cysticercus in left fronto-pariental cortex of 35-year-old woman who presented with focal seizures. A cystercus was also visible under the skin of her left wrist. Both lesions disappeared after 4 weeks of albendazole treatment.

Weak legs/paraplegia, non-traumatic

Ask the following questions
- Was the onset gradual or sudden?
- Is the tone spastic or flaccid?
- Is there sensory loss, in particular a sensory level? — a strong clue to spinal cord disease.
- Is there any loss of sphincter control (bowels or bladder)?
- Is there normal sensation around the sacrum and good anal tone?

Sudden weak legs with spasticity
- *Cord compression* — spinal or paraspinal infection or abscess due to TB, Brucella, pyogenic bacteria; tumours (metastases, Hodgkin's or Burkitt's lymphoma, myeloma); disc prolapse; Paget's disease.
- *Cord compression* — is an emergency. It must be considered when there is a rapid progression of leg weakness and/or sphincter failure. Check the perineal area for loss of sensation (saddle anaesthesia).
- *Other causes* — infectious or post-infectious myelitis; cord infarction (due to vasculitis, thrombosis of anterior spinal artery, trauma or compression, dissection of aortic aneurysm, surgery); tetanus; carcinomatous meningitis.

Sudden weak legs with flaccidity/acute flaccid paralysis
- *Cauda equina compression* — a neurosurgical emergency. Causes: tumour; prolapsed disc; canal stenosis; TB; cysticercosis; schistosomiasis.
- *Poliomyelitis* — see 🕮 p 444.
- *Other causes* — acute cord trauma/infarction; myelitis (in early stages with back pain, fever, double incontinence, sensory loss at defined level surmounted by a zone of hyperaesthesia); Guillain–Barré syndrome; rabies; lumbosacral nerve lesion; hypokalaemic periodic paralysis.

Chronic spastic paraparesis
- *Causes* — cord compression (e.g. cervical spondylosis); syringomyelia; tropical spastic paraparesis (TSP, due to HTLV-1); MND; subacute combined degeneration of the cord (vitamin B_{12} deficiency); konzo; and lathyrism.

Chronic flaccid paraparesis
- *Causes* — peripheral neuropathies; myopathies; nerve trauma; and tabes dorsalis.

Weak legs + no sensory loss: motor neurone disease (MND)

Absent knee jerks with extensor plantar responses
- *Causes* — Friederich's ataxia; taboparesis; MND; subacute combined degeneration of the cord; DM.

Unilateral foot drop
- *Causes* — DM; stroke; prolapsed disc; MND; organophosphorous poisoning; common peroneal nerve palsy.

Principles of management of paraplegia

- Prevention of pressure sores by turning every 2 h.
- Attention to bladder and bowels (urinary catheter if incontinent).
- Adequate hydration and nutrition.
- Prevent complications: aspiration and pneumonia (ensure adequate swallowing), DVT (support stockings/heparin), contractures (physiotherapy), malaria (mosquito net).
- Treat the underlying cause.

Poliomyelitis

This disease, usually of young children, is caused by the poliovirus, an enterovirus. The virus selectively infects and destroys anterior horn cells in the spinal cord, resulting in the cardinal sign of polio — acute flaccid paralysis (AFP). The clinical disease is relatively uncommon, however (~99% of infected people show no paralytic manifestations).

A worldwide vaccination effort is under way to eradicate it. Whilst polio has been a major cause of disability worldwide, it may soon be just a memory.

Transmission: via ingestion of faecally contaminated food or water, or via droplet spread from the respiratory tract.

Clinical features: the prodromal symptoms are common to many infections and practically indistinguishable: fever, malaise, headache, drowsiness, sore throat.

In a minority, CNS disease (preparalytic disease) follows with abrupt onset of fever, headache, body pains, sensory disturbances, and neck stiffness — due to poliovirus meningitis. Flaccid paralysis then occurs in ~65%, developing asymmetrically over a variable time, particularly affecting the lower limbs. The paralysis rarely progresses after 3 days or after the temperature falls. There is some recovery of function over the following weeks or months, as some damaged anterior horn cells recover. Death is relatively uncommon but results from aspiration or airway obstruction (bulbar paralysis) or respiratory failure (respiratory paralysis). A rare complication is slow deterioration of limb or bulbar function after many years — the post-polio syndrome.

Diagnosis: is clinical, with retrospective serological analysis.

Management: is supportive. Bed rest is essential; give analgesia, sedation. Avoid injections (see box).

Prevention: vaccination and improved public health.

Guillain–Barré syndrome (GBS)

A post-infectious demyelinating peripheral polyneuropathy. Some form of infection, mainly respiratory or diarrhoea, precedes the onset of GBS by 1–2 weeks in ~60% of cases. It develops over a few hours (rarely), to several weeks, and is a medical emergency. Respiratory arrest may occur without notice in severe cases; sudden death may also be caused by ANS disturbance of cardiovascular function. These patients need constant observation, in an ITU setting if possible.

Clinical features: include progressive muscle weakness in the limbs of less than 4 wks' duration; distal paraesthesia (less often sensory loss). Back and limb pain may be occasionally present. Also cranial nerve palsies (particularly VII); disturbances; ileus. Monitor respiratory function and heart rhythm; plasma exchange or high-dose immunoglobulin, if available, shortens the hospital stay. Recovery occurs over several weeks or months with remyelination of peripheral nerves.

Warnings

Paralytic poliomyelitis is made worse by IM injections during the preparalytic phase (e.g. injections of antibiotics) or by the muscles becoming fatigued (e.g. after exercise), so a high index of suspicion in endemic regions is important to prevent polio being made worse.

Patients must be carefully observed during the onset of paralysis for signs of life-threatening bulbar and respiratory paralysis. Nurse patients with weak swallowing on their side. Good nursing care, including frequent suction and observations, may delay the need for a tracheostomy — however, perform a tracheostomy early in serious cases.

Polio rehabilitation

Acute stage
- Treatment at this stage is based on: (i) rest (ii) positioning.
- Support the wrist and hands in a functional position with a splint or other support (e.g. pillow).
- Support the ankle — maintain the ankle at 90° and avoid excessive inversion or eversion.

Subacute stage
- Progress from passive movements to active assisted movements, to active movements within the normal range. The movements will depend on the muscle groups affected.
- Progress to standing and walking with assistance — use walking aids if necessary (e.g. stick, crutches). Aim for the best possible function.

Avoid
- Muscle shortening.
- Malformation due to muscle imbalance.

Mono/polyneuropathies

The mononeuropathies are lesions of single nerves; polyneuropathies are lesions of multiple nerves normally due to systemic disease. In some conditions such as leprosy, multiple peripheral nerves may be involved simultaneously — this is termed 'mononeuritis multiplex'.

Polyneuropathies are symmetrical conditions and often affect the peripheries initially, producing a symmetrical glove and stocking distribution. In the tropics, environmental toxins and nutritional deficiencies are important causes of peripheral neuropathies. They may be seen in epidemic form after toxins are released into the environment by industry or in an endemic form in particular regions. Some toxins are used in local forms of medicine or they may contaminate food, liquor, etc. They frequently produce an individually recognizable syndrome. As always, there is no replacement for local clinical experience. In these situations, treatment involves removal of the toxin and/or supplementation with the deficient nutrient. The effects of many neuropathies are permanent.

Causes

Single nerves can be damaged by:
- Trauma.
- Compression.
- Diabetes mellitus.
- Leprosy.

The latter two conditions will often develop into neuropathies affecting multiple nerves, causing a mononeuritis multiplex or widespread peripheral neuropathy.

Polyneuropathies can be caused by

1. *Deficiencies*: vitamin B_1, B_6, and B_{12}; plus a variety of multiple nutrient deficiencies.
2. *Toxins*
- Heavy metals: including lead (motor involvement), thallium (found in rodenticides → alopecia), arsenic (Mee's nail lines, changes in skin pigmentation, skin cancers).
- Drugs: many but particularly isoniazid, ethambutol (affects optic nerve), sulfonamides, chloroquine, clioquinol, metronidazole, phenytoin, didanosine, stavudine.
- Industrial chemicals/solvents (e.g. trio-ortho-cresyl phosphate).
- Pesticides, particularly organophosphorous (OP) compounds.
- Excessive consumption of certain foods (e.g. cassava containing a cyanogenic glycoside) can cause tropical ataxic neuropathy.
3. *Metabolic diseases*: DM, renal or liver failure, alcohol, hypothyroidism.
4. *Infections*: leprosy, HIV.
5. Other causes: genetic diseases, malignancy, connective tissue disease.

Table 10.2 WHO differential diagnosis of acute flaccid paralysis

	Polio	Guillain-Barré syndrome	Traumatic neuritis	Transverse myelitis
Onset of paralysis	24–48 h, from onset to full paralysis	From hrs to 10 days	From hrs to 4 days	From hrs to 4 days
Flaccid paralysis	Usually acute, asymmetrical, principally proximal	Usually acute, symmetrical and distal	Asymmetrical, acute, affecting one limb only	Acute, affecting lower limbs, symmetrical
Muscle tone	Reduced or absent in the affected limb	Global hypotonia	Reduced or absent in the affected limb	Hypotonia in lower limbs
Deep tendon reflexes	Decreased to absent	Globally absent	Decreased to absent	Absent in lower limbs early, increased late
Sensation	Severe myalgia, backache, no sensory changes	Cramps, tingling, hypoanaesthesia of palms/soles	Pain in gluteus muscles, hypothermia	Anaesthesia of lower limbs, sensory level
Cranial nerve	Only when bulbar involvement is present	Often present, affecting nerves VII, IX, X, XI, XII	Absent	Absent
Respiratory insufficiency	Only when bulbar involvement is present	In severe cases; worsened by bacterial pneumonia	Absent	Sometimes
CSF findings	Inflammatory	Albumin-cells dissociation	Normal	Normal or a few cells
Bladder dysfunction	Absent	Transient	Never	Present

Leprosy (Hansen's disease)

Leprosy is a disease that still elicits immense stigma in many communities. It is a chronic inflammatory disease caused by *Mycobacterium leprae* infecting macrophages and peripheral nerve Schwann cells.

Its presentation and progress are determined by the patient's cell-mediated immune response to the mycobacterium. Most people (~95%) develop an effective immune response and clear *M. leprae*. A minority are unable to do so and develop clinical leprosy. The clinical features form a spectrum determined by the immune response (see box). The two poles of the spectrum are tuberculoid (TT; paucibacillary) and lepromatous leprosy (LL; multibacillary). At the TT pole there is a strong (but ineffective) immune response to the bacteria which damages peripheral nerves and skin. At the LL pole, there is cellular anergy towards *M. leprae* with abundant bacillary multiplication. Between these two poles are the borderline patients — borderline tuberculoid (BT), borderline (BB), borderline lepromatous (BL) — with varying immunity and bacterial loads. The polar groups (TT, LL) are stable, but the borderline groups are unstable and experience tissue-damaging reactions.

Transmission: Untreated lepromatous patients discharge bacilli from the nose. Infection occurs when *M. leprae* invades via the nasal mucosa with haematogenous spread to skin and nerve. Leprosy bacilli can survive for several days in the environment. People in close contact with infected people have a greater, but still small, chance of becoming infected. The incubation period is 2–5 yrs for TT cases and 8–12 yrs for LL cases. HIV infection does not appear a risk factor for the development of leprosy.

Clinical features

- *Skin*: the most common lesions are macules or plaques; more rarely papules and nodules or diffuse infiltration. Indeterminate leprosy is an early form of disease often found in screening programmes; lesions can last for months before resolving or progressing to established leprosy.
- *Nerve damage*: occurs in peripheral nerve trunks — great auricular nerve (neck), ulnar nerve (elbow), radial-cutaneous nerve (wrist), median nerve (wrist), lateral popliteal nerve (neck of the fibula), and posterior tibial nerve (medial malleolus) — producing typical patterns of regional sensory and motor loss. Small dermal nerves are also involved producing patches of anaesthesia in TT/BT lesions and glove and stocking sensory loss in LL patients.
- *Other organs*: may be involved: eyes (can → blindness); bones (dactylitis, resorption); testes (orchititis, sterility); nasopharynx (nasal collapse).

Presentation of leprosy

- Patients commonly present with skin lesions, weakness, or numbness due to peripheral nerve lesion or a burn/ulcer in an anaesthetic hand or foot.
- Borderline patients may present in reaction with nerve pain, sudden palsy, multiple new skin lesions, pain in the eye, or systemic febrile illness.
- The ulceration and digit loss seen in leprosy is due to secondary damage in neuropathic hands and feet and is not an intrinsic disease feature.

Table 10.3 Clinical features of leprosy

Classification	Skin lesions	Nerve involvement
Indeterminate	Solitary hypopigmented 2–5 cm lesion. Centre may show sensory loss although both doctor and patient are often uncertain about this loss. May become TT-like.	None clinically detectable
Tuberculoid (TT)	Lesions with well-defined borders and sensory loss. The patch is dry (loss of sweating) and hairless.	May have 1 peripheral nerve affected. Occasionally presents as a mononeuropathy
Borderline tuberculoid(BT)	Irregular plaques with raised edges and sensory loss. Satellite lesions at the edges.	Asymmetrical peripheral nerve involvement
Borderline (BB)	Many lesions with punched out edges. Satellites are common	Widespread nerve enlargement. Sensory and motor loss.
Borderline lepromatous (BL)	Many lesions with diffuse borders and variable anesthesia	As above
Lepromatous (LL)	Numerous nodular skin lesions in a symmetrical distribution. Lesions are not dry or anaesthetic. There are often thickened shiny earlobes, loss of eyebrows, and skin thickening	As above

Diagnosis is based on:
- A typical skin lesion (loss of sensation in TT/BT patients).
- Thickened peripheral nerves.
- Skin smear from lesion edge/ear lobe positive for mycobacteria.
  Test skin lesions for sensation. Palpate peripheral nerves to assess enlargement/tenderness. Assess nerve function by testing the small muscles' power and sensation in hands/feet. Many patients are unaware of their anaesthesia. Eye function should be checked (visual acuity, corneal sensation, and eyelid closure). Serology is not helpful.

Management
1. *Chemotherapy to treat the infection*
   The WHO regimens are given in Table 10.4 below. More than 11 million people have been treated with such multi-drug regimens. Relapse rates are 0.1%/yr. Clinical improvement is rapid and adverse reactions are rare. These drugs are considered safe during pregnancy and breastfeeding. Patients are classified for treatment by the number of skin lesions present, paucibacillary have 2–5; multibacillary >5.

Table 10.4 WHO recommended multi-drug therapy regimes

Leprosy type	Drug treatment		Treatment duration
	Monthly supervised	*Daily self-administered*	
Paucibacillary(2–5 skin lesions)	Rifampicin 600 mg	Dapsone 100 mg	6 mths
Multibacillary(>5 skin lesions)	Rifampicin 600 mg	Clofazimine 50 mg	12 mths
	Clofazimine 300 mg	Dapsone 100 mg	

2. *Educate the patient about leprosy*
   Within 72 h of starting chemotherapy, they are non-infectious. They can lead a normal social life. There are no limitations on touching, sex, sharing utensils. Leprosy is not a curse from God or a punishment. Gross deformities are not the inevitable endpoint of disease. Care and awareness of their limbs are as important as chemotherapy.
3. *Prevent disability*
   Monitor sensation and muscle power in patient's hands, feet, and eyes as part of routine follow-up so that new nerve damage is detected early. Treat any new damage with prednisolone 40 mg daily, reducing by 5 mg/day each month.
   Patient self-awareness is crucial in minimizing damage. Patients with anaesthetic hands or feet need to inspect hands and feet (using a mirror) daily for injuries or infection and dress wounds immediately. Protect hands and feet from trauma ('trainers' are excellent for anaesthetic feet). Identify the cause of any injury so that it can be avoided. Soak dry hands and feet in water and then rub with oil to keep skin moist.
4. *Support the patient socially and psychologically.*

Reactions

Immune-medicated, tissue-damaging phenomena that may occur before, during, or after treatment. They should be treated promptly to prevent serious nerve damage. Do not stop chemotherapy during a reaction.

Reversal reaction (type 1 reaction): is due to delayed type hypersensitivity and occurs in patients with borderline leprosy, affecting up to 30% of BL patients. Skin lesions become erythematous; peripheral nerves become tender and painful. Loss of nerve function can be sudden, with foot-drop occurring overnight. Neuritis may occur without skin lesions or in a clinically silent form without nerve tenderness.

Management: for severe reactions, prednisolone 40–60 mg PO od reduced every 2–4 wks over 20 wks. A few patients may require 15–20 mg prednisolone daily for many months. Response rates vary depending on the severity of initial damage but even promptly treated nerve damage will only improve in 60% cases.

Erythema nodosum leprosum (ENL) (type 2 reaction): due to immune complex deposition and occurs in 20% LL and 5% BL patients. It manifests with malaise, fever, and crops of painful red nodules that become purple and then resolve. If severe, plaques may form with necrosis and ulceration. Iritis common; other signs are bone pain and swollen joints, painful neuritis, lymphadenopathy, iridocyclitis, orchitis, nephritis (rarely).

Management: in moderate and severe cases (systemic features or painful nerves), treat in hospital with one of:
- Prednisolone 60–80 mg PO od, reduced after 2 wks by 5–10 mg every 2 wks (best for short episodes).
- Thalidomide 400 mg nightly for 4 wks. Once a satisfactory response, reduce by 50 mg every 2–4 wks (best drug but contraindicated in women of childbearing age and often not available). Causes drowsiness.
- Clofazimine 300 mg daily, reduced after 3 months (preferred drug for premenopausal women; takes 3–4 wks to have full effect so should be combined with prednisolone initially). Causes brown skin staining.
- Treat iridocyclitis with steroid and homatropine eye drops.

ENL is difficult to treat: some patients develop a chronic relapsing form which may last for up to 5 yrs, but will then resolve.

Ulcers

Ulcers in anaesthetic feet are the most common cause of hospitalization. Ulceration is treated by rest and cleaning. Ulcers should be carefully probed to detect osteomyelitis and sinuses that require surgical debridement. Unlike ulcers in diabetic or ischaemic feet, ulcers in leprosy heal if they are protected from weight-bearing. No weight-bearing is permitted until ulcer heals. Appropriate footwear to prevent recurrence.

Haematology

Section editors   **Sara Ghorashian**
                    Imelda Bates

Anaemia

Anaemia is one of the most common medical conditions; prevalence often reaches 70% in children and pregnant women in developing countries. Anaemia is present when the haemoglobin (Hb) falls below the reference level for the age and sex of the individual (see box). A slight drop in Hb is a physiological response to pregnancy, due to an ↑ in the plasma: red cell ratio. Anaemia in pregnancy is associated with 25–40% of maternal deaths.

Causes of anaemia

Anaemia is due to ↓ red blood cell (RBC) production or ↑ RBC loss/ haemolysis (see Tables 11.1 and 11.2); >1 cause may be present in an individual. The blood film morphology, degree of reticulocytosis, and the size of red blood cells (i.e. mean cell volume — MCV, measured by an automated machine) is helpful in determining the cause (see box p 459).

The MCV is influenced by the cause of the anaemia, age of the patient, and the number of reticulocytes (these have a higher MCV than older erythrocytes).

Reticulocyte count is usually ↑ in RBC loss (unless the patient has insufficient stores of iron and/or folate to mount a reticulocyte response) and is ↓ if rbc production is impaired. An indication of the degree of reticulocytosis is given by the degree of polychromasia seen on blood film examination, as these younger cells appear 'bluer' than older erythrocytes. For an accurate reticulocyte count, special stains are required.

Table 11.1 Causes of anaemia due to ↓ red cell production

Aetiology		Clinical findings	Laboratory tests
Iron, folate, and B12 deficiency	Iron	Koilonychia, angular stomatitis, oesophageal webs	↓ MCV, MCH, MCHC, red cell count, ferritin, serum iron, transferrin saturation ↑ TIBC. Blood film: pencil cells.
	Folate and vitamin B12	Glossitis, ↑ skin pigmentation, sub-acute combined degeneration of the cord (vitamin B12 only)	↓ platelet and white cell count ↑ MCV, MCH; normal MCHC. Blood film: oval macrocytes, hypersegmented neutrophils
↓ erythropoietin	Renal failure		Normocytic anaemia Blood film: 'burr cells'
Anaemia of chronic inflammation		Features specific to the underlying condition	Normocytic anaemia ↓ serum iron, TIBC; ↓/normal transferrin saturation High/normal ferritin
Bone marrow suppression/ dysfunction	Drugs (e.g. cytotoxics), aplastic anaemia, malignant infiltration, alcoholism, hypothyroidism, myelodysplasia	Features specific to underlying condition	↓ platelet and white cell count Normal/↑ MCV

WHO definitions of anaemia*

Age	Hb (g/dl)
6–59 months	<11.0
5–11 yrs	<11.5
12–14 yrs	<12.0
Non-pregnant women	<12.0
Pregnant women	<11.0
Men	<13.0

* Where resources only allow estimation of haematocrit, Hb (g/dl) may be crudely estimated as approximately one third the haematocrit (%). However the accuracy of this estimation varies with age and Hb level, and is least accurate in children under 5 years old.

Table 11.2 Causes of anaemia due to ↑ red cell loss and haemolysis

Aetiology		Clinical findings	Laboratory tests
↑ red cell loss			↑ reticulocyte count, polychromasia (unless very acute)
Haemorrhage	Acute (e.g. post-partum, trauma)	Shock (e.g. tachycardia, hypotension, cold extremities)	MCV normal, Hb and Hct may appear normal initially
	Chronic, (e.g. peptic ulcer, hookworm, schistosomiasis)	Black stools, haematuria	Iron deficiency, ↑ platelets, positive stool/urine examination for parasites
Haemolytic anaemias		Jaundice, dark urine	↑ bilirubin and LDH
Inherited	Haemoglobino pathies (e.g. sickle cell disease, thalassaemia)	Family history, stunting, abnormal growth, hepatosplenomegaly, gallstones, leg ulcers	Blood film, haemoglobin electrophoresis
	Enzymopathies (e.g. G6PD deficiency)	Family history, gallstones, infection or recent drug ingestion	Intravascular haemolysis (e.g. low haptoglobins, haemoglobinuria, haemosiderinuria), enzyme assay
	Membranopathy (e.g. hereditary spherocytosis)	Family history, splenomegaly, gallstones	Extravascular haemolysis (e.g. ↑ conjugated bilirubin, urobilinogen); blood film
Acquired: — immune	Allo-immune (e.g. post-transfusion, haemolytic disease of the newborn)	Transfusion within ~10 days	Blood film (spherocytes), positive direct Coomb's test Red cell antibody
	Auto-immune (e.g. antibody-mediated, drug-induced)	Underlying infection, lymphoma, autoimmune disease, discoloured extremities (cold antibody)	Blood film (spherocytes), positive direct Coomb's test Red cell antibody, red cell agglutination (cold antibodies)

Acquired: — non-Immune	Infections (e.g. malaria, bartonellosis, parvovirus B19, clostridial sepsis)	Underlying infection	Blood film (malaria, bartonella)
	Others (micro-angiopathic haemolysis, burns snake bite)	Splenomegaly	Blood film (red cell fragmentation), thrombocyto-penia, renal failure

Clinical features of anaemia

History

Symptoms of anaemia depend on the rapidity of onset and severity. Chronic anaemia may be asymptomatic because of a compensatory ↑ in cardiac output. Symptoms are usually non-specific: fatigue, headache, dizziness, syncope, dyspnoea, palpitations, reduced work or intellectual capacity. Anaemia may also exacerbate pre-existing intermittent claudication or angina.

The history is important in determining the cause(s) of anaemia: a past and family history of anaemia suggests an inherited disorder, such as haemoglobinopathy or glucose-6-phosphate dehydrogenase (G6PD) deficiency. Haemolysis may be suggested by splenomegaly, jaundice, and dark urine and may be precipitated by infections. Sources of blood loss can be revealed from questions about bowel habit and colour of stools, haematuria, and menstrual history. Ask about recent surgery, childbirth, or trauma. The occupation of the patient may be important e.g. fishermen may be prone to schistosomiasis and farmers to hookworm infection. Poor diet may suggest a nutritional deficiency. Chronic infections such as HIV and TB, renal failure, rheumatoid arthritis, and some drugs used to treat these conditions, may be associated with anaemia.

Examination

Clinical assessment is routinely carried out, but has low sensitivity and specificity for mild — moderate anaemia. Signs include pallor of mucous membranes or nail beds (sensitivity 50–70% for moderate to severe anaemia) and signs of a compensatory hyperdynamic circulation (tachycardia, bounding pulse, cardiomegaly, systolic flow murmur). Severe, decompensated anaemia leads to shock (i.e. thirst, sweating, cold extremities, hypotension, and cardiac failure) — these signs require urgent fluid replacement or, as a last resort, blood transfusion.

Laboratory diagnosis of anaemia

Measure the Hb concentration or packed cell volume (PCV or haematocrit) of venous or capillary blood. For capillary samples from a finger or heel prick, the first few drops of blood should be wiped away to encourage free flow. Avoid squeezing — tissue fluid causes dilution.

Assays

Hb can be measured photometrically (e.g. the haemoglobin-cyanide technique) in which lysed whole blood reacts with a cyanide solution to form haemiglobincyanide. Cyanide is hazardous and the method requires laboratory equipment and skill to produce accurate dilutions.

The HemoCue Hb301 system is portable, battery-operated and designed for accurate measurement of Hb in tropical conditions. No dilution is required — it uses whole blood and is simple and rapid.

The WHO haemoglobin colour scale can be used where no power or equipment is available and an approximate haemoglobin estimation is adequate. The colour of a drop of blood on chromatography paper is matched against a colour scale representing blood of Hb in 2 g/dl increments (range 4–14 g/dl). The test is simple and cheap, but the correct paper must be used and it must be read in good light conditions. Other simple techniques such as the Sahli or Talqvist methods have been shown to be unreliable in field situations.

Measurement of PCV requires a microhaematocrit centrifuge and electricity but can be carried out by non-technical staff. Blood is taken up into capillary tubes directly from a finger prick and centrifuged for 5 min. This separates cells and plasma and the ratio of the length of red cell column to the total length of the blood sample gives the haematocrit.

Causes of anaemia due according to red cell size*

Microcytic (low MCV)	Normocytic (normal MCV)
Iron deficiency	Acute blood loss
Thalassaemia	Anaemia of inflammation
Anaemia of inflammation	Marrow hypoplasia or infiltration
Lead poisoning	Chronic infection
Sideroblastic anaemia	Renal failure

Macrocytic (high MCV)

Megaloblasts in bone marrow	No megaloblasts in bone marrow
Folate deficiency	Myelodysplasia
B12 deficiency	Alcohol
Drugs affecting DNA metabolism	Liver dysfunction
Rare enzyme defects	Hypothyroidism
	Haemolytic anaemia
	Neonate (normal)

* Reference range for mean cell volume (MCV) = 76–96 fL

Iron-deficiency anaemia

This is the most common cause of anaemia worldwide.

Causes of iron deficiency

- ↑ losses: menstrual, gastrointestinal infections (e.g. hookworm, whipworm, amoebiasis), peptic ulceration, carcinoma, oesophageal varices, haemoptysis, haematuria.
- ↑ requirements: lactation, puberty, infancy.
- ↓ intake: ingestion of only milk (human or cow's) beyond 6 mths of age; lack of red meat and/or legumes.
- ↓ absorption: intake of inhibitors of iron absorption with meals (tea, milk, phytates present in grain), achlorhydria, malabsorption.

Women have lower iron stores than men and higher losses due to menstruation, pregnancy, delivery, and lactation. If the mother has sufficient iron stores, a neonate is born with enough stores to last 6 mths. After this, iron requirements must be met from the diet — requirements ↑ with rate of growth. Iron deficiency, therefore, particularly affects children and pregnant or breastfeeding women.

Clinical features: brittle nails, koilonychia, angular stomatitis, glossitis, dysphagia (Plummer–Vinson syndrome).

Laboratory features: (see table 11.1, 📖 p 455). Low serum ferritin (<20 mcg/l) is specific but can be insensitive as it is an acute phase protein. Ferritin >100 mcg/l generally excludes iron deficiency, even in the setting of infection.

Management

1. Ferrous sulphate 200 mg tds. Expect a Hb rise of 1–3 g/dl after 4 weeks of therapy if iron deficiency is the cause of anaemia (this can be used as a diagnostic test). Continue iron therapy for 3 mths after normalization of Hb to replenish stores.
2. Identify and treat the underlying cause and any other haematinic deficiencies (e.g. folate).
3. Severe anaemia with signs of heart failure may require blood transfusion.

Notes

- Severely malnourished children should not receive iron supplements until at least 15 days into a feeding programme because of the ↑ risk of bacterial sepsis and toxicity related to free radicals.
- To improve absorption, oral iron preparations should be taken between meals and with vitamin C (e.g. orange juice, ascorbic acid tablets).
- Oral iron should not be taken with antibiotics or antacids.
- Side-effects include GI upset (try lower dose or take with meals), constipation, green/black stools.

Intravenous iron

Failure to respond to oral iron may be due to malabsorption, poor compliance, ongoing excessive iron loss, concomitant anaemia of chronic disease, or an erroneous diagnosis. The first three may respond to IV iron thereby preventing the need for transfusion. The first dose should be given slowly because of the risk of adverse reactions (e.g. anaphylaxis, local irritation). IM iron injections are not recommended because they are painful, there is a risk of abscess formation, and absorption is unpredictable.

Prevention of iron deficiency

- Nutritional advice: eat meat and legumes with vitamin C (e.g. orange juice) and avoid tea, dairy products, or cereals as these inhibit iron absorption.
- Prophylactic iron supplements: iron supplements have been recommended for children > 6 mths and pregnant women where the prevalence of anaemia exceeds 40% because there is a high probability that iron deficiency contributes to anaemia in these populations. Supervised weekly/twice weekly supplementation schedules are effective for prevention of iron deficiency in school children. However, routine supplementation for children is under review following studies suggesting that where malaria transmission is high, routine iron supplementation may be lead to ↑ malarial and other infections.
- Anti-helminthics: empiric treatment may be helpful in those with anaemia where helminth infections are common.

Anaemia of inflammation

Previously termed 'anaemia of chronic disease', this anaemia is associated with chronic inflammatory or malignant disease in which there is ↓ RBC production, abnormalities of iron utilization, and ↓ erythropoietin levels and/or response. These abnormalities are mediated by cytokines released as a result of the underlying disease and by hepcidin, a molecule released by the liver in response to infection or inflammation that blocks the release of iron from enterocytes and macrophages (as a bacteriostatic measure).

Causes
- Chronic inflammatory disease.
  - *Infectious* (e.g. TB, HIV, lung abscess, osteomyelitis, pneumonia, SBE).
  - *Non-infectious* (e.g. RA, SLE, other connective tissue disorders, sarcoidosis, Crohn's disease).
- Malignancy (e.g. carcinoma, lymphoma, sarcoma).

Clinical features: are of anaemia as well as those relating to the underlying diagnosis

Differential diagnosis: anaemia of chronic renal failure, hypothyroidism, hypopituitarism, other microcytic anaemias (see box, 🕮 p 459).

Laboratory features: mild normocytic (occasionally microcytic), normochromic anaemia. Low reticulocyte count for degree of anaemia. ↓ serum iron and TIBC. Normal or ↑ serum ferritin levels and a low/normal transferrin saturation. ↑ markers of inflammation: ESR, CRP.

Management
1. Treat the underlying cause; recombinant erythropoietin may help anaemia caused by HIV, malignancy, or chemotherapy. Blood transfusions are a last resort.
2. Anaemia of inflammation may be complicated by another form of anaemia (e.g. iron, vitamin B12, or folate deficiency), renal failure, bone marrow failure, hypersplenism, or endocrine abnormality. These must also be addressed.
3. A ferritin <100 mcg/l may suggest concomitant iron deficiency, but there is little response to oral iron because of the block of iron uptake in the small bowel. Intravenous iron may be required.

Sideroblastic anaemia

A rare cause of refractory anaemia caused by deranged heme (haem) biosynthesis in red cell precursors in the bone marrow. This leads to ↓ Hb production and ineffective haemopoiesis. There are two forms:
- *Hereditary*: usually X-linked. Associated with moderate hepatosplenomegaly.
- *Acquired*: either 1° (myelodysplasia) or 2° (myeloproliferative disorders, alcohol, drugs such as isoniazid).

Laboratory findings: Ring sideroblasts in the bone marrow (i.e. erythropoietic cells with iron-containing granules (mitochondria) arranged around the nucleus in a ring)

Hereditary: hypochromia, microcytosis, variation in red cell size and shape, low MCH and MCH(C).

Acquired (myelodysplasia): dysplastic morphology of leukocytes and erythrocytes on blood film, macrocytosis, neutropenia, and/or thrombocytopenia may be present

Management

In severe cases, repeated blood transfusion may be necessary but this risks iron overload. Splenectomy is contraindicated because of an associated thrombotic risk. The hereditary type may respond to high-dose pyridoxine therapy (□ p 652). 1° acquired disease may respond to erythropoietin if available. In 2° disease, treat the underlying cause.

Macrocytic anaemias

Folate deficiency

Folic acid is present in green vegetables and fruits such as bananas. It is absorbed in the duodenum and jejunum. The body's stores of folate are limited and clinical deficiency occurs within 2 months. States of rapid cell division (e.g. growth spurts, pregnancy, haemolytic anaemia) ↑ folate utilization and warrant prophylactic supplementation with 400 mcg folic acid. Reduced dietary intake (e.g. in alcoholics, the malnourished, and elderly) can also lead to clinical deficiency. Mild folate deficiency should prompt testing of, or treatment with, vitamin B12.

Vitamin B12 deficiency

Vitamin B12 is present in meat or dairy animal products. The absorption of vitamin B12 is complex and requires proteases and binding factors released in the stomach and combination with intrinsic factor before uptake in the terminal ileum. Deficiency may result from a block at any of these steps. Stores of vitamin B12 take 2–3 years to deplete even after absorption has ceased. Vitamin B12 is essential for DNA production. The combined metabolic role of vitamin B12 and folate explains the similarity of the clinical and laboratory features in both of their deficiency states. There are unique neurological manifestations of B12 deficiency.

Clinical features

Mild jaundice, glossitis, angular stomatitis, purpura due to thrombocytopenia, sterility, reversible melanin skin pigmentation, and increased susceptibility to infections. Neuropathy due to subacute combined degeneration of the cord (loss of vibration sense, hypertonia, weakness, and sensory ataxia), psychosis, and dementia are specific to a lack of vitamin B12.

Laboratory findings

↑ MCV and MCH, normal MCHC, low reticulocyte count, ↓ WCC and platelets in severe cases. *Blood film*: oval macrocytes and hypersegmented neutrophils, basophilic stippling. Slightly ↑ serum unconjugated bilirubin and LDH because of ineffective erythropoiesis.

Management

Replacement therapy

- Folic acid 5 mg PO daily for 4 months; maintenance requirements depend on underlying disease.
- Hydroxycobalamin (vitamin B12) — 6 injections of 1 mg IM over 1–2 weeks and maintenance with 1 mg every 3 months. Oral vitamin B12 therapy can be given if malabsorption is excluded. Anaemia should resolve over months.

Prophylaxis

Fortification and dietary modification. Consider prophylactic treatment (e.g. folic acid 400 mcg/day) in pregnancy, severe haemolytic anaemia, after partial gastrectomy and ileal resection.

Causes of folate and B12 deficiencies

	Folate	Vitamin B12
↓ Intake	Seasonal shortage Boiling bottle feeds Prolonged storage of food Anorexia Famine Inappropriate weaning Foods Prolonged cooking/reheating Feeding infants with goat's milk Alcoholism	Breastfeeding by B12-deficient mothers Strict veganism Alcoholism
Malabsorption	Diarrhoea in infancy Acute enteric infections *Giardia lamblia* Systemic infections (tb, pneumococcus) Strongyloides Coeliac disease Crohn's disease	Pernicious anaemia Gastrectomy Chronic *G. Lamblia* HIV infection Ileocaecal TB Strongyloides Tropical sprue Crohn's disease Fish tapeworm
↑ *Physiological* *demands*	Growth Pregnancy/lactation	
↑ *Pathological* *demands*	Haemolysis Malignant disease	
Metabolic		Nitrous oxide Chronic cyanide Intoxication (Cassava)

Haemolytic anaemias

Haemolysis is the process by which RBCs are broken down and their components metabolized. This occurs in the reticuloendothelial system (RES) in the hepatic and splenic sinusoids. Under certain circumstances (e.g. sickling crisis, severe oxidative damage), red cells may lyse within the circulation. Red cells normally remain in the circulation for ~120 days but their life span can be shortened due to abnormalities inside the red cells (e.g. haemoglobinopathies, enzymopathies), in/on their membrane (e.g. structural defects, deposition of antibody or complement), or due to mechanisms arising outside the red cell.

The bone marrow is able to compensate up to 5 times the normal turnover rate given adequate haematinics and a healthy marrow (compensated haemolysis); if haemolysis exceeds this or there are haematinic deficiencies or associated disease, anaemia results.

Laboratory findings

- ↑ *Red cell destruction:* unconjugated hyperbilirubinaemia, ↑ LDH, ↑ urinary urobilinogen, ↑ faecal urobilinogen.
- ↑ *Red cell production:* polychromasia, reticulocytosis causing ↑ MCV.
- *Intravascular haemolysis:* ↓/absent haptoglobins, ↓ haemopexin, haem/methaemoglobin, positive Schumm's test (methaemalbumin), haemosiderinuria, haem/methaemoglobinuria.

Genetic abnormalities of RBCs are extremely prevalent in the tropics (and to a lesser extent, in temperate zones). Despite the disadvantage of the homozygous state of some of these abnormalities, they persist within populations because the heterozygous state provides a degree of protection against severe malaria. This is either by altering the environment within the RBC or by conferring resistance to various stages in the parasite's lifecycle. For example, the presence of HbS (📖 p 474) confers a 10-fold reduction in risk of severe malaria. Most of these disorders predispose to a degree of haemolysis.

Acquired haemolytic anaemia

- *Drug-induced immune haemolytic anaemia:* occurs when drugs bind RBCs (e.g. high-dose penicillin), form new RBC antigens (e.g. quinidine), or provoke auto-antibodies (methyldopa, mefenamic acid, L-dopa). A careful drug history (including herbal preparations) is crucial.
- *Autoimmune haemolytic anaemia:* can be caused by cold (IgM) or warm (IgG) antibodies. They may be 1° (idiopathic) or 2° to lymphoproliferative disorders, malignancy, autoimmune diseases, or infections. The direct anti-globulin (Coomb's test) test is positive because the patient's red cells are antibody-coated.
    - *Warm AHA* presents as chronic or acute haemolytic anaemia with splenomegaly. Management includes treating any underlying causes. Specific therapy is with steroids (e.g. prednisolone 1 mg/kg daily) until Hb>10 g/dl, then gradually reduce. Splenectomy is an option if this fails. Blood transfusion may be required in severe cases.
    - *Cold AHA* presents as chronic anaemia made worse by the cold and is associated with Raynaud's phenomenon and acrocyanosis. Management involves treatment of the underlying cause; steroids are not helpful. Advise the patient to keep warm. Chlorambucil can be helpful if there is underlying lymphoma. Splenectomy does not usually help as IgM-coated cells are removed in the liver.
- *Paroxysmal cold haemoglobinuria:* is caused by Donath–Landsteiner antibody (occurs after mumps, measles, chickenpox, syphilis, especially in children). This binds red cells after a cold exposure, causing a complement-mediated lysis which manifests clinically as haemoglobinuria.

Glucose-6-phosphate dehydrogenase (G6PD) deficiency

G6PD deficiency predisposes to oxidative damage of the RBC and therefore haemolysis.

Distribution: G6PD deficiency affects >2 million people with prevalence rates reaching 25%. Fig. 11.1 shows the world distribution of G6PD deficiency. Superimposed are three zones where different G6PD variants reach polymorphic frequencies: zone I (GdMediterranean), zone II (GdMediterranean, GdCanton, GdUnion, GdMahidol), and zone III (GdA). These variants have different clinical severities e.g. GdA causes moderate, intermittent haemolysis whereas GdMediterranean and GdCanton are more severe.

Clinical features: G6PD deficiency has sex-linked inheritance, so is much more common in boys. Most people affected are asymptomatic. The main feature is of episodic haemolysis which may be severe and intravascular in nature, particularly in the non-African mutations. Chronic haemolysis is unusual. In Africa, adults with G6PD deficiency usually only suffer mild haemolysis but neonates may develop severe hyperbilirubinaemia and kernicterus. Haemolytic episodes are precipitated by infection and, to a lesser extent, drugs.

Diagnosis

Between attacks: Tests of enzyme activity rely on NADPH production and its detection by direct fluorescence or by reduction of a coloured dye to its colourless form. These are sensitive, simple, and inexpensive for detecting hemizygous males and heterozygous women.

During a crisis: the blood film may show 'bite' cells and 'blister' cells. Testing for G6PD activity during a crisis is often unhelpful because haemolysis eliminates older erythrocytes which have the lowest G6PD activity, so only the youngest cells (which may have normal G6PD activity) remain. Following a crisis, testing should be delayed for 6 weeks. In more severe variants, a greater proportion of erythrocytes have low G6PD activity so delaying enzyme assays may not be necessary.

Management

- Treat underlying infections avoiding medications known to precipitate haemolysis.
- Withdraw any drug that could have precipitated the crisis.
- Maintain a high urine output (to prevent pre-renal failure).
- Folic acid supplements may be useful if deficiency is possible or if recurrent haemolytic episodes.
- G6PD-deficient babies are prone to neonatal jaundice and, in severe cases, phototherapy and exchange transfusion are necessary.

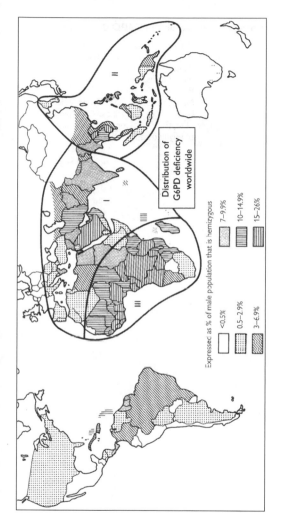

Fig. 11.1 Global distribution of G6PD deficiency.

Examples of drugs to be avoided in G6PD deficiency

Antimalarials	Primaquine, fansidar, maloprim
Sulphonamides/sulphones	Co-trimoxazole, sulphanilamide, dapsone, salazopyrine, sulfamethoxazole
Antibiotics	Nitrofurans, nalidixic acid
Analgesics	Phenacetin
Antihelminths	Naphthol, stibophen, nitrodazole
Miscellaneous	Naphthalene, fava beans, methylene blue, trinitrotoluene, amylnitrates, phenylhydrazine

Pyruvate kinase deficiency

Autosomal recessive inheritance. Mainly affects N. Europeans.
- *Clinical features* are variable. May present with neonatal jaundice or, later, with haemolytic anaemia, splenomegaly, and jaundice.
- *Diagnosis:* blood film shows variable appearances. Definitive diagnosis is by enzyme assay.
- *Management:* is supportive e.g. folic acid supplements, blood transfusion where necessary; splenectomy may improve severe cases.

Red cell membranopathies

These conditions may provide a degree of protection against malaria due to reduced penetration of the erythrocyte by merozoites.

1. Hereditary spherocytosis

Usually autosomal dominant inheritance. Mainly found in N. Europeans.
- *Clinical features are variable:* positive family history, mild anaemia (8–12 g/dl), intermittent jaundice, splenomegaly, pigment cholelithiasis.
- *Diagnosis:* blood film shows spherocytes, ↑ MCH, ↑ reticulocytes, ↑ lysis in osmotic tests, negative direct antiglobulin test.
- *Management:* folic acid 5 mg/day. Splenectomy for those most severely affected (see 📖 p 492).

2. Hereditary elliptocytosis

Autosomal dominant inheritance. Usually asymptomatic; haemolysis may be severe in homozygotes. There may be episodes of jaundice and moderate splenomegaly following intercurrent infections.
- *Diagnosis:* elliptical red cells, parental studies.
- *Management:* is not usually required; folic acid supplements and splenectomy may help if haemolysis is significant.

3. South-east Asian hereditary ovalocytosis

Autosomal dominant inheritance. Common in Malaysia, Indonesia, Philippines, PNG, and Solomon Islands. It is not associated with haemolytic anaemia.

Sickle cell anaemia

The sickle gene is common in equatorial Africa (frequency up to 25%), Saudi Arabia, and S Asia, but less common in the Mediterranean and the mixed populations of the Americas (frequency 5%). It is due to a single point mutation in the Hb β-globin gene chain. When deoxygenated, HbS molecules polymerize into elongated structures causing erythrocytes to deform and haemolyse. Sickled red cells are rigid and block the microcirculation in various organs, causing infarcts.

The inheritance of the disease is autosomal co-dominant (i.e. sickle-cell trait is due to heterozygous inheritance, HbAS). The trait is generally asymptomatic. Sickle cell disease occurs with homozygous inheritance of the gene (HbSS) or co-inheritance of another β-globin chain disorder such as HbC (see below). Sickle cell disease and G6PD deficiency may occur together because of the high prevalence of both conditions in some regions. It provides protection against malaria.

Other sickling syndromes

- *HbSC disease* occurs in west Africa. There is less haemolysis than with HbSS. Some patients are asymptomatic and therefore may present only in adulthood. Splenomegaly is a common clinical finding. Anaemia is less severe than in HbSS but vaso-occlusive complications (e.g. avascular necrosis, proliferative retinopathy) are prominent because of the higher haematocrit and may lead to significant disability in adulthood. Electrophoresis shows two haemoglobin bands, HbS and HbC. The blood film has more target cells than in HbSS as well as irregularly contracted cells.
- *HbSβ⁰thalassaemia* occurs mostly in North Africa, Sicily, and mixed populations of the Americas. Clinically similar to HbSS, there is a lower incidence of stroke. The blood film shows hypochromic microcytic RBCs and target cells. Hb electrophoresis shows HbS, absence of HbA, and elevated HbA2 and HbF. Definitive diagnosis can be made by parental studies or DNA analysis.
- *HbSβ⁺thalassaemia* is the doubly heterozygous condition most commonly seen in west Africa. The clinical course and degree of anaemia is milder than HbSS. However, proliferative retinopathy occurs. Definitive diagnosis with Hb electrophoresis shows HbA 5–30%, HbS 70–95%.
- *HbSD^Punjab and HbSO^Arab* are as severe as HbSS. HbD occurs in Sikh and mixed populations.
- *HbSE, HbSLepore, and HbSHPFH* (hereditary persistence of foetal haemoglobin). All these conditions have a mild clinical course compared to HbSS.

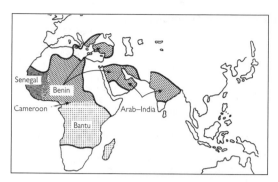

Fig. 11.2 Distribution of haemoglobin S gene and its various haplotypes (Arab-India, Bantu, Benin, Cameroon, Senegal) in the Mediterranean and West Asia.

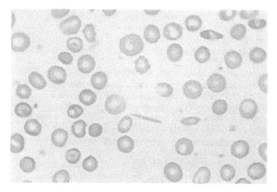

Fig. 11.3 Characteristic sickle-shaped erythrocytes in peripheral blood film in patient with homozygous sickle cell anaemia. (Reproduced with permission from BMJ Publishing Group.)

Clinical features of sickle cell anaemia

Severe haemolytic anaemia punctuated by severe pain crises. Young patients alternate periods of good health with acute crises. Later, chronic ill health supervenes due to organ damage. Symptoms begin after 6 months of age as the HbF level declines. The first signs are often of acute dactylitis due to occlusive necrosis of the small bones of the hands and feet, resulting in digits of varying length. The long bones are affected in older children and adults. Anaemia (Hb 6–8 g/dl; reticulocytes 10–20%) is well–tolerated because of cardiac compensation and a lower affinity of HbS for oxygen.

The severity of complications depends on a number of factors including the proportion of non-sickle Hb molecules (e.g. HbF) and the ratio of α to β chains, which may be modified by concomitant α thalassaemia trait or conditions affecting β-globin chain production (e.g. Bantu haplotype is associated with severe disease, whilst Senegalese and Asian haplotypes are less severe).

Types of crises

- *Painful vascular-occlusive:* frequent and precipitated by infections, acidosis, dehydration, or hypoxia. Infarcts often occur in the axial skeleton, lungs, and spleen. Repeated splenic infarction leads to hyposplenism in adulthood. Crises can involve the CNS (in 7% of patients) and spinal cord.
- *Visceral sequestration:* due to sickling within organs and pooling of blood.
- *Chest:* pulmonary infiltrates on CXR, fever, chest pain, tachypnoea, cough, wheeze. There is often concomitant infection, microvascular occlusion, and bronchoconstriction. Chest crises can arise during a painful crisis; patients should be monitored carefully for this complication, which can be fatal.
- *Haemolytic:* ↑ rate of haemolysis with a fall in Hb. Usually accompanying a painful crisis. Concomitant G6PD deficiency may worsen haemolysis.
- *Aplastic:* arrest of red cell production due to infection with parvovirus and/or folate deficiency. Characterized by a sudden fall in Hb and reticulocytes; emergency blood transfusion can be life-saving.

Complications: pulmonary fibrosis, pulmonary hypertension, stroke, proliferative retinopathy, cardiomegaly, renal concentrating defect, papillary necrosis, osteomyelitis (often due to *Salmonella* spp), skin ulcers, proliferative retinopathy, priapism, hepatic dysfunction, pigmented gallstones. Infectious complications are the most common cause of death. There is a particular risk with encapsulated bacteria (e.g. pneumococcus, meningococcus, haemophilus) because of hyposplenism. Survival is linked to socio-economic conditions.

Laboratory findings

- Hb 6–8 g/dl, ↑ reticulocyte count, normal MCV. If is MCV low, consider concomitant iron deficiency or thalassaemia.
- Sickle cells and target cells in the blood film; features of splenic atrophy (e.g. Howell–Jolly bodies) may also be seen.
- Screening tests such as the sickle solubility test (e.g. with dithionate and Na2HPO4) will be positive in the presence of >20% HbS. These tests are, therefore, also positive in sickle cell trait and compound heterozygotes. They do not require advanced laboratory methods and are widely available. False negative results occur in infants <6 mths old with HbSS because of the predominance of HbF.
- Detection of HbS or other haemoglobin variants, Hb electrophoresis, iso-electric focusing, and high-performance liquid chromatography. Some of these tests provide quantification of the abnormal Hb but are likely to be available only at referral centres. Expect 30–40% HbS with HbAS (≤35% with concomitant α thalassaemia), >90% with HbSS.

Sickle-cell disease and pregnancy

- Sickle-cell disease predisposes to intrauterine growth retardation, pre-eclampsia, pre-term labour, *in utero* foetal death, and ↑ risk of sickle-related complications in the mother. Sickle-cell trait is not a problem, except that pyelonephritis is more common.
- Early access to antenatal care is important to allow monitoring for these complications.
- Folic acid supplements are essential to prevent megaloblastic anaemia and birth defects.
- Delivery should be non-operative where possible. Consider pre-operative exchange transfusion before caesarian section in complicated pregnancies.
- Test neonate for haemoglobinopathy.

Sickle-cell disease and surgery

The incidence of severe complications in sickle-cell patients undergoing surgery is 30–60%, depending on the procedure. Equivalent improved outcomes are shown with either top-up or exchange transfusions. Minor operations can be carried out safely without pre-op transfusion, providing patients are well-hydrated.

Management of painful crises

Acute pain is the most common reason to seek medical attention:

- Exclude other causes of pain.
- Keep hydrated — PO, NG, or IV (if other routes have failed).
- Keep the patient warm.
- O_2 therapy is only necessary if hypoxic.
- Effective pain relief — can reduce time spent in hospital; under-treating can lead to drug-seeking behaviour and a pain-oriented personality.
- Parenteral opiates are often required but IM route can cause abscesses. Monitor the response to analgesia closely; use a pictorial pain scale in children.
- Oral analgesia — NSAIDs are good for bone pain. Give with ulcer-protection (e.g. H2-receptor antagonist or PPI) and monitor renal function. Oral opioids.
- Inhaled NO — risk of subacute combined degeneration of cord with repeated/prolonged use; may be beneficial in acute chest syndrome.

Management of infections

The most common cause of death in sickle-cell disease.

- *Treat bacteraemia rapidly:* start antibiotics empirically if febrile and acutely unwell. Greatest mortality from sepsis with encapsulated organisms; therefore treat empirically to cover S pneumoniae, Hib, N meningitidis (e.g. ceftriaxone 2 g OD). This has the advantage of once-daily dosing. Where microbiological diagnosis is possible, send urine and blood for culture, consider early LP if signs consistent with meningitis, CXR for suspected pneumonia/chest syndrome.
- *Proven/suspected meningitis:* treat with ceftriaxone for 2 weeks.
- *Acute chest syndrome:* usually triggered by infection. Use antibiotic to cover S pneumoniae, Hib, mycoplasma, and C pneumoniae (e.g. cefuroxime and erythromycin). Supportive measures, including bronchodilators. Consider exchange transfusion if severe. Incentive spirometry (use of a spirometer to guide deep respirations at regular intervals) can reduce the risk of acute chest syndrome developing from painful crisis involving the ribs or back.
- *Osteomyelitis:* ideally confirm organism with cultures, or empirically cover S paratyphi, E coli, and S aureus (e.g. cefotaxime and ciprofloxacin). Requires at least 6 weeks of therapy; may require surgery. Monitor closely for recurrence.
- *Malaria:* non-specific cause of fever and associated with mortality in sickle-cell disease.
- *Good supportive care:* is essential to prevent other complications. Monitor fluid balance carefully to prevent overload; treat pain and hypoxia.

Maintenance of health in sickle-cell disease

- *Screening:* greatest mortality <5 years of age so early diagnosis is important to ↓ mortality. Selective screening (e.g. pregnant women, newborn children born to carriers, relatives of those with the disease) may miss a significant proportion of cases so universal screening is being implemented in some wealthy countries.
- *Education:* general health education. Also advise to seek medical attention early (especially if high fever) and to use clean drinking water and insecticide-treated bed nets to prevent malaria. Genetic counselling is important to identify affected relatives and to plan pregnancy.
- *Avoid factors precipitating crisis:* especially dehydration, hypoxia, infections, cold environments.
- *Folic acid supplements:* 1–5 mg/day in adults.
- *Protect against infection:* vaccinate against S *pneumoniae*, Hib, meningococcus, hepatitis B, influenza. Educate parents/patients about reduced mortality with compliance to prophylactic penicillin (125 mg PO bd for children <3 yrs, 250 mg bd thereafter). Advise lifelong anti-malarial prophylaxis.
- *Detection of acute splenic sequestration:* teach parents of young children to palpate the spleen soon after diagnosis and to attend clinic if the child becomes unwell, with an enlarging spleen.
- *Screening for retinopathy:* should be carried out annually from the age of 15 years.

Hydoxycarbamide: ↓ frequency of crises, chest syndrome, hospitalisations, and mortality; should be considered for those with painful crises >2–3 times per year. It is difficult to implement in poorer countries because it requires regular monitoring of FBC to prevent cytopenias and, ideally, of HbF% for maximal effect. It should be avoided in pregnancy.

Indications for transfusion in sickle-cell disease

Transfusions are only indicated in sickle-cell disease in specific circumstances because increasing Hb levels above steady state ↑ the risk of thrombosis. Indications for transfusion include correction of blood loss or ↓ production or sequestration (e.g. post-operatively; during sequestration or aplastic crises; during acute severe illness).

Exchange transfusions: can be performed to ↓ HbS%, and thus the risk of vaso-occlusion. Aim for Hb 10 g/dl, Hct ≤32%, HbS ~30%. Exchange blood transfusions are only beneficial in specific circumstances (e.g. to prevent/↓ risk of stroke, during pregnancy in women with a past history of severe complications).

Thalassaemia

β Thalassaemia

Clinically, β thalassaemia is classified as minor (slight ↓ in β globin chain production, asymptomatic), intermedia (moderate ↓ in β globin chain production, mild symptoms, occasional transfusion requirement), and major (total/almost total reduction in globin chain production, severe symptoms, need for regular transfusion support).

β Thalassaemia minor

Usually heterozygous inheritance. There is palpable splenomegaly and moderate anaemia during pregnancy. This can cause compensatory placental hypertrophy and mild intrauterine growth retardation, but does not significantly affect perinatal mortality.

Diagnosis: mild anaemia (e.g. Hb 9–11 g/dl); blood film shows moderate anisocytosis, microcytosis (MCV<76 fL, MCH<26 pg), hypochromia with a few target and tear drop cells. Basophilic stippling may occur. Hb electrophoresis shows ↑ HbA2(4–6.5%); HbF may also be ↑. *Note:* iron deficiency can mask and co-exist with β thalassaemia minor. Testing for thalassaemia should be delayed until the patient is iron replete.

Management: includes accurate diagnosis to avoid future treatment of the hypochromic anaemia with iron, education about thalassaemic syndromes, and genetic counselling.

β Thalassaemia intermedia

Variable severity from mild haemolytic anaemia to occasional severe anaemia. In general, splenomegaly, bony expansion, and complications of iron overload are present, despite only requiring intermittent transfusion support.

Diagnosis: features are intermediate between those of β thalassaemia major and minor.

General management: As for sickle-cell disease, this involves screening, general health education (active immunization, clean water sources, hygiene measures, use of impregnated bed nets to avoid malaria, early attendance at medical facilities if unwell and especially for febrile illnesses). Specific measures include:

• Folate supplements (5 mg/day for adults).
• Transfusion support — if severe anaemia or failure to thrive, or to suppress erythroid expansion (e.g. in the case of skeletal deformity).
• May need to consider iron chelation if ferritin >1000 mcg/l even if not regularly transfused.
• Splenectomy — hypersplenism can ↑ transfusion requirements. Vaccinations against encapsulated bacteria should be given 2 weeks pre-operatively (see section on splenomegaly).

β Thalassaemia distribution and pathogenesis

β thalassaemia occurs across southern Europe, Africa, the Middle East, India, and south-east Asia, and in immigrants from these areas. It is caused by a variety of mutations of the β globin gene complex. Excess free β globin chains precipitate as inclusion bodies in red cell precursors, leading to their destruction. This causes ineffective erythropoiesis and ↑ splenic uptake of RBCs. There is compensatory ↑ iron uptake and expansion of erythropoiesis within haemopoietic tissues including those in extra-medullary sites. This expansion, together with iron overload and hypersplenism, causes many of the clinical manifestations.

α Thalassaemia

This arises as a result of a defect (usually deletion) of one or more of the four α-globin genes. $α^+$ thalassaemia trait occurs due to deletion or inactivation of a single gene (−α/αα) and is common in Africans. This does not cause anaemia. $α^0$ thalassaemia trait (−/αα) is more common in the Asian and Mediterranean regions; there is mild anaemia and the MCV and MCH are ↓. The blood film shows hypochromic, microcytic red cells and target cells. Screening and genetic counselling programmes in high-prevalence areas ↓ the incidence of compound heterozygotes. Epidemiological studies from Melanesia and Papua New Guinea suggest that $α^+$ thalassaemia protects against malaria.

Unlike β thalassaemia, more severe forms of α thalassaemia affect the foetus and neonate because foetal Hb (α2γ2) requires α chains. Compared to β thalassaemia, α thalassaemia is characterized by haemolysis rather than ineffective erythropoiesis because the tetramers of excess β chains (HbH) are more soluble and less destructive to erythroid cells than α tetramers. HbH inclusions in RBCs can be detected with specific stains, HbH is detected on Hb electrophoresis.

HbH disease

HbH is 5–30% with moderate haemolytic anaemia (Hb 7–10 g/dl). The clinical features often resemble β thalassaemia intermedia. Children may have growth retardation and skeletal abnormalities; there is a variable degree of hepatosplenomegaly. Transfusions are not usually required. Splenectomy may be of benefit.

Hb Bart's hydrops foetalis

The foetus lacks all α genes and is stillborn or dies shortly after delivery.

β **Thalassaemia major**

Often due to inheritance of two different mutations (compound heterozygote) each affecting β globin synthesis. Untreated, most patients die before 5 years of age from cardiac failure or infection.

Clinical features

- *Failure to thrive:* at 3–6 months of age, when the switch from γ to β-chain production should take place; puberty is often delayed and there may be limited development of sexual characteristics.
- *Hepatosplenomegaly:* due to haemolysis, extramedullary haemopoiesis, and later in the disease, iron overload from transfusions. Splenomegaly ↑ blood requirements by ↑ RBC destruction and pooling.
- *Bone expansion:* as a result of intense marrow hyperplasia; leads to skeletal deformity, including the characteristic thalassaemic facies — prominent frontal and parietal bones, maxillary enlargement, and flattening of the nasal bridge. There is osteoporosis (↑ tendency to fracture) and bossing of the skull with 'hair-on-end' appearance on X-ray.
- *Infections:* predisposed to infection for a variety of reasons (e.g. defective splenic function). Severe gastroenteritis caused by *Yersinia enterocolitica* is associated with desferrioxamine treatment. Transmission of viral hepatitis is also increased, probably because of iron overload and transfusion exposure.
- *Iron overload:* due to transfusion therapy (each 500 ml unit of blood contains 250 mg of iron) and ↑ iron absorption. Iron accumulation → liver damage, endocrine damage (failure of growth, delayed or absent puberty, diabetes, hypothyroidism, hypoparathyroidism), and myocardial damage. In the absence of intensive iron chelation, death occurs in the second or third decade, usually from CCF or cardiac arrhythmias. Clinically apparent abnormalities usually appear after ~50 units (12 g of iron) but organ damage and skin pigmentation occur before this.

Diagnosis: severe hypochromic microcytic anaemia with ↑ reticulocyte count. Blood film shows many nucleated red cells, tear drop and target cells, as well as cells of variable morphology and basophilic stippling. Electrophoresis shows absent HbA, ↑ HbF, and variable HbA2 (often ↑).

Management of β thalassaemia major

- *General measures:* as for sickle-cell disease: screening, health education, immunization, clean water sources, hygiene measures, use of impregnated bed nets to avoid malaria, early attendance at medical facilities if unwell (especially with febrile illnesses).
- *Transfusion:* aims to suppress the patient's own (ineffective) erythropoiesis, to prevent bony deformity and to normalize growth. This can be achieved with a regular transfusions of 20 mls/kg packed RBCs every 4–6 weeks to maintain Hb >9.5 g/dl. Start regular transfusions when growth chart monitoring shows failure to thrive (usually around 6–12 months of age). Blood should be matched for ABO, Rh, Kell antigens, and, if possible, filtered to remove WBCs. If blood requirements exceed 300 mls/kg/year then the reason for this should be investigated (e.g. hypersplenism, haemolytic transfusion reactions). Recipients of regular transfusions should receive hepatitis B vaccination and be monitored for transfusion-transmitted infections.
- *Folic acid:* give regularly, especially for dietary insufficiency.
- *Iron chelation:* to prevent/treat overload. Commence in infants after 10–15 units of transfusion. Give desferrioxamine by SC infusion via a syringe pump driver, 20–40 mg/kg over 8–12 h, 3–7 days per week. Desferrioxamine in high doses, especially in children, may lead to neutropenia, high tone deafness, loss of visual acuity, and growth retardation and patients should be monitored for these complications. Other side-effects include joint pain and hepatic dysfunction. The oral chelator, deferiprone, may be considered if parenteral chelation is not possible but it has also been associated with blood dyscrasias. Give vitamin C 100–200 mg daily with chelation to ↑ iron excretion.
- *Splenectomy:* may ↓the amount of blood required. Delay until >6 years because there is ↑ risk of life-threatening infections post-splenectomy before this age. Immunize against encapsulated bacteria two weeks prior to splenectomy (see 📖 p 492).
- *Monitor growth and sexual development:* with weight and height charts as well as clinical examination. Failure to thrive may indicate ↑ transfusion needs or delayed puberty. If secondary sexual characteristics are not adequately developed by 16 years of age, consider testosterone/oestrogen supplements or specialist referral.

Blood transfusion

Blood transfusion can be life-saving in certain circumstances but it should only be a last resort and if indicated by clinical features. Transfusion practice is now very conservative due to increased awareness of risks of transfusion-transmissible infections (TTIs) and better understanding of the role of haemodynamic compensatory mechanisms.

Transfusion-associated risks are high in the developing world because of the high prevalence of TTIs and lack of quality assurance systems. To ↓ the use and need for transfusions, it is important to prescribe according to guidelines and to prevent/treat anaemia effectively e.g. by controlling malaria and improving nutrition.

In countries where supplies of safe blood are scarce, the following may guide the decision to transfuse:
- Signs of severe heart failure.
- Hb <5 g/dl with symptoms.
- Hb <4 g/dl in any situation.
- Acute blood loss resulting in shock or signs of heart failure despite infusion of crystalloid or colloid fluids.
- Need for emergency major surgery with pre-operative Hb<7 g/dl.

Whole blood is used for most transfusions in developing countries. If facilities for refrigerated centrifugation of blood are available, then more efficient use can be made of the blood by splitting it into RBC concentrates and fresh frozen plasma.

Ensuring blood safety and supply

The objective is to make safe blood available:
- Preventing unnecessary transfusions.
- Donor-screening and self-exclusion with a health questionnaire designed to exclude those at high risk of TTIs (e.g. HIV, hepatitis C).
- The use of a panel of voluntary, unpaid donors who have repeatedly tested negative for TTIs and who pass a basic medical test (check pulse, BP, screen for anaemia and other major illnesses).
- Implementation of SOPs for all processes involved in collection, storage, testing, and administration of blood including adequate controls and quality assurance (e.g. two grouping techniques should be used in parallel to prevent fatal ABO-incompatible transfusion reactions).
- Screening all blood for TTIs including HIV, hepatitis B, syphilis, hepatitis C, and, if appropriate, trypanosomiasis and malaria.
- Regular training for those involved in transfusion to ensure competency and safety.
- Use of a closed system allowing collection into blood bags with anticoagulant, testing and, if necessary, division, or fractionation of products.
- Appropriate storage systems in thermostatically controlled fridges with back-up power supplies.
- A labelling system for blood bags, samples, and patient identification as well as a procedure of checks at the bedside to ensure the correct unit is administered to the correct patient.

Administration of blood

Blood should only be removed from the fridge immediately prior to use. When administering a blood transfusion:

- Check the patient details with those of the unit of blood to ensure the unit has been issued to that patient and is compatible with the group of the patient.
- Give IV via a blood-giving set with a filter.
- Keep a record of the volume and units given.
- Check pulse, BP, respiratory rate, temperature at start of transfusion, after 15–30 mins, and every hour during the transfusion. Observe the patient for the first 10 minutes of a transfusion.
- Monitor carefully for signs of fluid overload.

Exchange transfusions

In certain situations, an exchange transfusion is indicated to ↓ the risk of volume overload or to ↓ the concentration of patients' red cells or plasma. For example in:

- Heart failure 2° to anaemia.
- Complications of sickle cell disease.
- Haemolytic disease of the newborn.
- Hyperbilirubinaemia in neonates.

Specialist advice should be sought regarding details of volumes and procedures for exchange transfusion.

Transfusion reactions

1. Severe transfusion reaction: may be due to ABO incompatibility or bacterial contamination of the unit. Heralded by pain at site of cannula, back/chest pain, agitation, dyspnoea, nausea, flushing, or hypotension.

- Stop the transfusion immediately. Do not flush the giving set.
- Ensure IV access, catherize patient, and start fluids to ensure diuresis.
- Monitor renal and liver function, clotting parameters, haemoglobinuria.
- Consider broad-spectrum antibiotic cover after taking blood cultures and send donor unit for culture (if possible).
- Give bronchodilators if wheezing; antihistamine and hydrocortisone as for allergic reaction.
- Laboratory to re-cross match unit, repeat patient's grouping, and monitor for development of red cell antibodies.

2. Simple febrile and allergic reactions: If temperature ↑ by >1°C from baseline or the patient develops urticarial rash or itching, stop the transfusion, check vital signs, give paracetamol, and, if the patient remains well after 15 minutes, restart the transfusion at a slower rate.

3. Delayed transfusion reaction: usually occurs 5–10 days post-transfusion and is due to sensitization to red cells following previous transfusions or pregnancy. Clinical features include fever, hyperbilirubinaemia, and anaemia. Samples should be taken for grouping, direct Coombs' test, repeat cross-matching, and antibody screening and results compared with a pre-transfusion sample.

Acute leukaemias

Characterized by an excessive proliferation of immature haematopoietic cells (blasts) in the peripheral blood. Without treatment, acute leukaemias have a median survival of months. Although they are aggressive disorders, chemotherapy may be curative; this is not the case with indolent haematological malignancies which may not require treatment at diagnosis but are incurable with standard chemotherapy.

Diagnosis: of acute leukaemias relies on analysis of blood and bone marrow samples to establish the origin of the malignant cells and associated genetic abnormalities.

Treatment: is with cycles of chemotherapy. Normal haematopoietic tissue is also affected by chemotherapy, leading to anaemia, neutropenia, and thrombocytopenia, so red cell and platelet transfusions may be required and there is a significant risk of infection.

Acute lymphoblastic leukaemia (ALL) is a common malignancy in children with peaks at 2–5 yrs and >40 yrs. Poor prognostic markers include age <1 or >10 yrs and >30 yrs, presenting white cell count >50 x109/l, and certain cytogenetic abnormalities. Clinical features include bone pain, lymphadenopathy, hepatosplenomegaly, anaemia, haemorrhage, and infections.

Acute myeloblastic leukaemia (AML) has a median age at diagnosis of 70 years. Clinical features are similar to ALL except that in Africa 10–25% of all patients and ~30% of boys may present with a solid tumour (chloroma) e.g. in the orbit or skin. Gum hypertrophy and DIC are features of AML sub-types. Risk factors include exposure to benzene, radiation, and previous cytotoxic therapy. Poor prognosis is associated with age >55 years, poor general state of health, and specific cytogenetic abnormalities.

Causes of lymphadenopathy

Infections	Brucellosis, leptospirosis, typhoid
	Tuberculosis, atypical mycobacteria
	EBV, CMV, HIV, HSV, hepatitis B, measles, mumps, rubella, dengue fever
	Toxoplasmosis, sleeping sickness
	Histoplasmosis, coccidioidomycosis, cryptococcosis
	Lyme disease, syphilis (secondary)
Malignancies	Lymphoma, ALL, CLL, metastatic carcinoma
Autoimmune	Still's disease, SLE, dermatomyositis
Endocrine	Addison's disease, hypothyroidism
Drugs	Atenolol, captopril , cephalosporins, sulphonamides, penicillin

Causes of changes in white cell counts:

↑ *cell count*

Neutrophilia >7.5 x 10^9/l
- Physiological (e.g. Pregnancy).
- Acute bacterial infections (e.g. Pneumonia, UTI, abscess).
- Tissue damage, inflammation, stress (e.g. Burns, dka).
- Malignant disease.
- Drugs (e.g. Steroids).

Basophilia >0.1 x 10^9/l
- Myeloproliferative disorders.
- Allergic reactions.

Lymphocytosis >3.5 x 10^9/l
- Childhood response to infections.
- Certain bacterial infections in adults (e.g. Brucellosis).
- Viral and protozoal infections (e.g. CMV, EBV, toxoplasmosis).
- Lymphoproliferative disorders.

Monocytosis >1.0 x 10^9/l
- Rarely — chronic bacterial infection (e.g. TB).
- Chronic myelomonocytic leukaemia.

Eosinophilia >0.5 x 10^9/l
- Helminth infections (e.g. Hookworm, hydatid disease, schisosomiasis — values >3 x 10^9/l are likely to be due to katayama fever, strongyloidiasis).
- Allergic/skin conditions (e.g. asthma, atopy, drugs, vasculitis, psoriasis) reactive to leukaemia/lymphoma, connective tissue disease.
- Convalescence from viral or other infections, especially in infants.

↓ *cell count*

Neutropenia <2.0 x 10^9/l
- Acute Infection (e.g. Dengue fever, overwhelming bacterial sepsis).
- Certain chronic infections (e.g. visceral leishmaniasis, AIDS).
- Bone marrow failure or drugs (e.g. chloramphenicol).
- Peripheral consumption (e.g. hypersplenism, Felty's syndrome).
- Miscellaneous (ethnic, familial, cyclic, chronic, idiopathic).

Lymphopenia <1.5 x 10^9/l
- Common in many acute infections (e.g. TB, hepatitis, pneumonia).
- Drugs (e.g. corticosteroids).

Lymphoproliferative disorders

Non-Hodgkin's lymphoma (NHL)

A heterogeneous group of tumours of B and T cell origin. Low-grade lymphomas run an indolent course but are incurable, while high-grade lymphomas are more aggressive initially but long-term cure is achievable. High-grade NHLs are more common in Asia and Africa and, in Africa, are associated with malaria. Features include: lymphadenopathy, hepatosplenomegaly, weight loss, night sweats, pruritis, fever, pancytopenia.

Burkitt's lymphoma (BL): is a highly aggressive subtype of NHL. It occurs in malaria-endemic areas, is related to EBV infection, and is the most common childhood cancer in tropical Africa. BL has a male predominance with a peak incidence at 4–7 years but it may also occur in individuals with HIV. It classically involves the jaw but can occur in any extranodal site. Steroids or a single dose of IV cyclophosphamide may provide symptom control and a short-lived remission but intensive chemotherapy is needed to achieve a 70% cure rate.

Hodgkin's Lymphoma (HL)

HL is a malignant proliferation of B lymphocytes. It is more common in males, with two peaks in young adulthood and middle age. There are geographical variations in sub-types; nodular sclerosing HL predominates in published studies, but in developing countries, the mixed cellularity sub-type is more common and has been linked to EBV exposure. HL usually presents as painless lymphoadenopathy and 70–80% of cases are curable with standard radio/chemotherapy.

Chronic lymphocytic leukaemia (CLL)

CLL is characterized by proliferation of mature but dysfunctional lymphocytes and predisposition to infections and, less commonly, autoimmune haemolytic anaemia. The M:F ratio is 2:1 and median age 60. There tends to be a lower incidence in tropical than in temperate regions where it is the most common form of leukaemia. CLL may present with incidental lymphocytosis ($5 - >100 \times 10^9$/l), lymphadenopathy, hepatosplenomegaly, or signs of bone marrow failure. Treatment consists of chemotherapy (e.g. chlorambucil) and transfusions/antibiotics, as required.

Multiple myeloma (MM)

MM is due to infiltration of the bone marrow with malignant plasma cells. The incidence is higher in the islands of the Pacific, the Caribbean, and Africa than in more wealthy countries. Clinical features include bone pain, pathological fractures, osteopenia, hypercalcaemia, renal failure, and bone marrow failure with anaemia, infection, and bleeding. Definitive treatment results in a median survival of 3–5 years. Supportive treatment includes analgesia, transfusions, and bisphosphonates.

Myeloproliferative disorders

A group of disorders characterized by proliferation of haemopoietic stem cells. These cells retain their ability to differentiate, resulting in an excess of mature cells of predominantly one lineage. The disorders share systemic symptoms such as malaise, night sweats, fever, and weight loss. Splenomegaly, gout, and pruritis on contact with water are not uncommon. These disorders are not curable, but may be associated with long survival if treated. Transformation to acute leukaemia or to marrow fibrosis occurs in a minority.

Polycythaemia

Primary polycythaemia (polycythaemia rubra vera) is associated with PCV >56% in females, >60% in males, neutrophilia and/or thrombocytosis, gout, splenomegaly (in 60%), and, less commonly, a thrombotic event. 2° causes should be excluded. Treatment is by venesection to ↓ PCV to <45%, aspirin (75 mg od), and hydroxycarbamide for those at high risk for thrombosis, or with concomitant thrombocytosis. The median survival is ~15 years in non-elderly patients.

Thrombocytosis

Reactive causes of thrombpocytosis include blood loss, iron deficiency, infection, inflammation, hyposplenism, and malignancy. Essential thrombocythaemia is characterized by platelet count persistently $>500 \times 10^9$/l without an underlying reactive cause. Half of patients are asymptomatic, 25% have splenomegaly and 25% have a history of arterial thrombosis at diagnosis. Platelet function may be abnormal in a minority, especially in those with platelets $>1000 \times 10^9$/l. Young patients without risk factors for atherosclerotic disease do not require treatment. Patients at risk of thrombosis should be given low-dose aspirin and some may need hydroxycarbamide to ↓ platelet count.

Chronic myeloid leukaemia (CML)

Due to uncontrolled proliferation of mature myeloid cells; >95% of cases have the Philadelphia chromosome. The median age at diagnosis is 50–60 years, but CML can present in childhood. Most patients present in the chronic phase, which is often asymptomatic. CML inevitably progresses to a blastic phase that is clinically indistinguishable from acute leukaemia and characterized by the proliferation of increasingly abnormal and dysfunctional cells leading to significant morbidity, reduced response to therapy, and death. In chronic phase, hydroxycarbamide 1–2 g should ↓ WCC to normal levels; new treatments may induce remission in the chronic phase. With treatment, the chronic phase may last 2–5 years. The disease is only curable with an allogeneic bone marrow transplant.

Splenomegaly

The spleen is a major site of antigen presentation and platelet reservoir. Splenic macrophages remove damaged or old red cells. The spleen enlarges as a result of over-activity of any of these processes.

The high prevalence of chronic infection/infestation as well as haemolytic anaemias in the tropics means that splenomegaly is a common physical sign. Splenomegaly may produce abdominal distension, discomfort, and early satiety. The spleen is recognized clinically by its movement with respiration, enlargement towards the right iliac fossa, the presence of a notch, and the fact that the upper margin cannot be palpated. Massive splenomegaly may be associated with blood pooling and cytopenias.

Hyperreactive malarial splenomegaly (HMS)

HMS occurs very commonly in areas with high malaria transmission, especially in adults who have taken up residence in the endemic area. HMS is due to polyclonal lymphoid activation because of an abnormal immune response to malaria. HMS is difficult to distinguish from lymphoproliferative disorders, hepato-splenic schistosomiasis, and visceral leishmaniasis, which may co-exist in the same territory. Once other causes have been excluded (see box), HMS is a likely diagnosis. Antimalaria prophylaxis (e.g. proguanil 100 mg/day) for at least 6 months may result in significant regression of the spleen, supporting the diagnosis.

Splenectomy

Indications for splenectomy include trauma, haemolytic anaemia, idiopathic thrombocytopenic purpura, and (infrequently) for the purpose of diagnosis. Post-operatively, especially in the first few years, there is an ↑↑ risk of sepsis (overwhelming post-splenectomy infection — OPSI) from encapsulated bacteria, particularly *Streptococcus pneumoniae*. The risk of OPSI is ~0.5% per year, and even with good resources, mortality is ~50%, so prevention is essential. If possible, elective splenectomy should be delayed until >5 years of age because of increased susceptibility to encapsulated bacteria. Pneumococcal, meningococcal, and *H influenza* b vaccinations should preferably be given at >2 weeks pre-op; if splenectomy is unplanned, they should be given >2 weeks post-op; reimmunization for pneumococcus should be repeated every 5 years. Penicillin V prophylaxis (500 mg bd) should be commenced post-op and continued for life. Patients should be educated about the risk of OPSI and seek immediate attention, or start standby broad-spectrum antibiotics, if they develop a fever with faintness or rigors. There is a greater risk of severe malaria and long-term malaria prophylaxis (or residence outside a malaria area) should be advised. Immediately post-splenectomy, there is a risk of thrombosis because of transient thrombocytosis, or in the case of haemolytic anaemias, a rise in haematocrit.

Common causes of splenomegaly

Infections	SBE, brucellosis, typhoid fever, tuberculosis
	EBV, CMV, HIV, rubella, Hepatitis B
	Toxoplasmosis, malaria (including HMS*), visceral leishmaniasis*, schistosomiasis*, histoplasmosis
Malignancies	Lymphoma*, ALL, CLL*
	Metastatic carcinoma
	Multiple myeloma
	Myeloproliferative disorders* (PRV, myelofibrosis)
Autoimmune	SLE, Rheumatoid arthritis (Felty's syndrome)
Reactive	Auto-immune haemolytic anaemia, haemoglobinopathies*
Congestive	Portal hypertension*, cardiac failure
Other	Sarcoidosis, lipid storage disorders, histiocytosis

* = can give massive splenomegaly ≥10 cm below costal margin

Causes of DIC in tropical countries

Infection	Meningococcal, pneumococcal, staphylococcal
	Ebola, Marburg, Dengue, Lassa fever
	Malaria (rarely)
Malignancy	Disseminated cancer, acute leukaemia
Tissue damage	Burns, fulminant hepatitis, pancreatitis, rhabdomyolysis, fat embolism
Envenoming	Snake bite, Lonomia achelous caterpillars
Obstetric	Septic abortion, abruptio placentae, amniotic fluid embolus, pre eclampsia/eclampsia, retention of dead foetus
Immune	ABO-incompatible blood transfusion
Vascular	Vasculitis, malignant hypertension, atrial myxoma

Disorders of haemostasis

Abnormal bleeding results from disorders of the:
1. vascular endothelium and platelets (primary haemostasis) → bleeding into the skin and mucous membranes, *or*
2. coagulation and fibrinolytic pathways (secondary haemostasis) → haemorrhage in deep tissues.

Disorders of 1° haemostasis

- *Vascular purpura:* causes include infections, long-term steroid therapy, and vasculitis. In immunocompromised patients, HSV, VZV, and arboviruses (O'nyong-nyong, chikungunya) can cause fatal haemorrhage.
- *Defective platelet function:* can result from drugs (e.g. NSAIDS, aspirin) and complicate some of the haemorrhagic fevers (e.g. Lassa, dengue, Marburg, Ebola), alcoholism, hepatic cirrhosis, uraemia, paraproteinaemias, leukaemias, and myeloproliferative disorders.
- *Thrombocytopenia:* may result from defective production, ↑ destruction/consumption, and splenic pooling.

Onyalai: means 'blood blister' and is a disorder of unknown aetiology that occurs in central southern Africa. *Clinical features:* recurrent haemorrhagic bullae on mucous membranes and less frequently skin, epistaxis, and cerebral haemorrhage. Mortality is 3–10% due to haemorrhagic shock and cerebral haemorrhage. *Management* includes blood product support.

Management of bleeding due to thrombocytopenia/defective platelet function

- Treat underlying causes of thrombocytopenia.
- Desmopressin for uraemic platelet dysfunction.
- Anti-fibrinolytics (e.g. tranexamic acid) for mucosal bleeding.
- Immune thrombocytopenia can be treated with intravenous immunoglobulin (0.4 mg/kg over 5 days or 1 mg/kg over 2 days) or prednisolone (1 mg/kg od for at least 4 weeks).
- Platelet transfusions may be necessary for acute bleeding but the effect only lasts a few days and they may be ineffective if peripheral consumption is the cause of thrombocytopenia.

Disorders of 2° haemostasis

These can be congenital such as haemophilia A (factor VIII deficiency), haemophilia B (Christmas disease, factor IX deficiency), and von Willebrand's disease (deficiency or abnormality of von Willebrand factor) or acquired 2° to malabsorption (causing vitamin K deficiency), liver disease, disseminated intravascular haemolysis (DIC), and snake envenoming.

Causes of thrombocytopenia

| ↓ Production | Infections (e.g. typhoid, brucellosis, rubella, mumps, hepatitis C, HIV), megaloblastic anaemia, alcoholism, marrow infiltration or failure (e.g. leukaemia, aplastic anaemia, drugs/chemicals) |
| ↑ Peripheral consumption | Infections (e.g. malaria, trypanosomiasis, dengue and other arboviruses, EBV, CMV, Marburg virus), hypersplenism, pregnancy, chronic hepatic disease, DIC, microangiopathic haemolytic anaemia, ITP, onyalai, acute viral infection, AIDS, drugs (e.g. quinine, penicillin, valproate), lymphomas, CLL |

Congenital disorders

Clinical features

Haemophilia is sex-linked and boys may present with haemorrhage after circumcision or other surgical interventions. Other clinical features include spontaneous bleeding into joints and muscles (especially if factor level is <1%) which produces crippling arthropathy and deformity of the limbs. Cerebral haemorrhage and spontaneous intra-abdominal or upper respiratory tract bleeding may also occur. The presentation of von Willebrand's disease is usually with bleeding from mucous membranes (as occurs in disorders of primary haemostasis) because of the central role of von Willebrand factor in mediating activation and aggregation of platelets at the site of vascular damage.

Management

Requires referral to a specialist. NSAIDS and IM injections should be avoided. Spontaneous musculoskeletal bleeds can be managed with rest, ice, elevation, analgesia, and gentle physiotherapy once the acute symptoms have settled. Tranexamic acid 25 mg/kg PO tds can be helpful for mucosal bleeding. Vaccinate against hepatitis B, screen regularly for other TTIs if the patient is receiving plasma-based products.

Desmopressin (0.3–0.4 mg/kg/q12–24 h IV in 50 ml 0.9% saline over 20 mins) raises factor VIII and may be effective in patients with mild/moderate haemophilia A. Haemophilia B is best treated with virus-inactivated factor IX concentrate though cryosupernatant (or FFP can be used). Desmopressin is generally effective for von Willebrand's disease but cryoprecipitate (for factor VIII replacement) and platelet transfusions may be required in severe cases.

Acquired coagulation disorders

Vitamin K is a co-factor for coagulation factors II, VII, IX, and X and the anticoagulant proteins C and S. These factors are produced in hepatocytes and deficiency of vit K as well as hepatic dysfunction can lead to coagulopathy. Vit K deficiency results from small bowel fat malabsorption, biliary or pancreatic dysfunction, starvation, or prolonged antibiotic use.

Haemorrhagic disease of the newborn (HDN): Neonates are vitamin K-deficient because of poor placental transfer and ↓ hepatic synthesis. This can lead to bleeding (e.g. intracranial haemorrhage) in the 1st week of life in premature infants and infants of mothers on anti-TB therapy, anticonvulsants, or warfarin. Some advocate the use of vitamin K 10 mg/day PO from 38 weeks' gestation in patients on anticonvulsants. The treatment of HDN is with parenteral vitamin K and FFP if there are bleeding complications. Vitamin K levels are low in breast milk. Breastfed infants may present with HDN between 1–3 months of age which can be prevented with vitamin K 1 mg IM at birth.

Vitamin K antagonism: Warfarin is a competitive inhibitor of vitamin K. Overdose, sepsis, poor vitamin K intake/absorption, or simultaneous administration of potentiating drugs may cause bleeding. If the PT is >5x the normal range and the patient is bleeding, give vitamin K 10 mg IV and fresh frozen plasma (FFP; 15 mls/kg). Vitamin K permanently reverses warfarin anticoagulation, but takes >6 h to have an effect. It may take several weeks to re-anticoagulate, so if it is important to maintain some anticoagulation, smaller doses (e.g. 0.5–1 mg) may be given with FFP cover.

Bleeding in liver disease is due to a combination of ↓ clotting factor synthesis, thrombocytopenia, platelet dysfunction, vitamin K deficiency, DIC, and dysfibrinogenaemia and should be treated by parenteral vitamin K, FFP, and cryoprecipitate if fibrinogen is low.

Disseminated intravascular coagulation (DIC): Results from generalized activation of coagulation pathways in the vasculature and a cycle of consumption of coagulation factors and their inhibitors (see box). It may be asymptomatic or associated with bleeding, skin purpura, microangiopathic haemolytic anaemia, and arterial or venous thromboses. There is depletion of all coagulation factors leading to prolongation of APTT and PT, ↓ fibrinogen and platelets, and RBC fragmentation on the blood film. Management consists of treating the underlying condition, careful monitoring, and supportive care (e.g. blood products) as required. If there are predominantly thrombotic complications, consider cautious anticoagulation with IV heparin.

Laboratory issues

This section covers some principles and tests which are useful in evaluating haematological disease.

The role of primary level health centres in diagnosis and management of common conditions such as TB and malaria means they usually have a light microscope. This enables provision of several important investigations (e.g. WBC and platelet count, RBC morphology, differential WBC%). However, the microscopist should spend <4 h/day looking down the microscope if fatigue and poor quality reporting are to be avoided.

Reducing sources of error in laboratory tests

The following principles can reduce errors in several tests:
- Use accurate volumes.
- Check date, dilution, and storage of reagents.
- Keep instruments and cuvettes clean and grease/dust free.
- Keep colorimeters away from sunlight.
- Collect capillary or venous blood samples correctly and use appropriate amount of anticoagulant.
- Use correct centrifuge times and speeds.
- Filter stains/diluting mixtures; check for particles and use correctly buffered water.
- Run samples in duplicate.
- Use clean, dry slides.
- Fix slides with water-free methanol when completely dry.

To reduce specific sources of error, consult the laboratory's standard operating procedures for each test.

Some basic principles of laboratory management

1. Range of tests
It is generally better to provide a limited number of essential tests performed to high standards than to provide a wide range of poor-quality tests. Test selection should take into account sensitivity and specificity of tests, as well as positive and negative predictive values (influenced by the disease prevalence in the local population), reliability, availability of reagents and consumables, cost, safety, sustainability, and the skills of laboratory staff.

2. Management and operation of equipment
Involves regular maintenance and appropriate servicing contracts, availability of manuals, adequate space and light, minimization of dust and heat damage, and systems for reliable supplies of consumables and reagents. Laboratory staff using equipment should be appropriately trained and supervised and the tests they are asked to carry out should be appropriate for their skills and knowledge.

3. Ensure good quality results
Clinicians and laboratory staff need to have confidence in the accuracy and reliability of test results. Demonstrating the result of a particular test is correct is difficult in developing countries because laboratories lack access to reference samples.

Simple ways of promoting confidence in test results include:
- independent re-analysis of selected slides or samples within one laboratory.
- regular exchange of samples with neighbouring laboratories.
- including known samples within a batch of tests to demonstrate that the test is working (e.g. a blood sample known to contain HbS can be included in each batch of sickle-cell screening tests).

Other factors that are important in ensuring high-quality results are:
- appropriate collection and storage of specimens.
- use of standard operating procedures for each test.
- supervision and regular training of laboratory staff.
- maintenance of equipment and good-quality reagents.

4. Standard operating procedures (SOPs)

These are detailed descriptions of laboratory tests designed to prevent errors and ensure consistent results. They must be designed for the local situation, kept up-to-date, and adhered to by all staff. SOPs provide an excellent teaching resource. For each test, they should include:
- the principle of the test and valid reasons for requesting it.
- details of the specimen required and how it should be collected.
- the equipment and reagents needed, as well as information on how to maintain, procure, and store them.
- the method of the test.
- quality control measures and sources of error.
- safety considerations.
- the procedure to be followed in reporting the results (e.g. units to be used).

Endocrinology

Section editor   **Theresa Allain**

Diabetes mellitus

Diabetes mellitus (DM) is a syndrome caused by the lack, or diminished effectiveness, of endogenous insulin. DM is characterized by hyperglycaemia and deranged metabolism. Several forms of the disease exist and their prevalence throughout the world varies greatly.

Type I DM

An autoimmune disease, predominately of Caucasians, with highest prevalence in northern Europe. It is usually of juvenile onset and is the most common form of childhood DM; however, the increasing prevalence of type II diabetes in children and adolescents may reverse this order within a few decades. Type I DM may be associated with other autoimmune diseases in the patient or family. Environmental factors may be important, since a seasonal variation in onset has been noted and migrants tend to assume the risk of the country to which they have migrated. Patients always need insulin and are prone to ketoacidosis.

Type II DM

Accounts for more than 90% of global cases of DM. Its prevalence is increasing massively worldwide due to the changes in diet and lifestyle accompanying globalization and is directly associated with increases in obesity. The number of cases of DM is expected to double by 2025, this increase being most marked in developing countries. The worldwide diabetes epidemic is associated with an early age of onset of type II DM, some even presenting in childhood. 20% of type II diabetics eventually need insulin treatment.

Maturity onset diabetes of the young (MODY): presentation similar to type II DM.

Malnutrition-related DM (MRDM)

Accounts for 1% of diabetes presenting in a tropical setting. The WHO subdivides this disease into two classes:
• Protein-deficient pancreatic diabetes (PDPD).
• Fibrocalculous pancreatic diabetes (FCPD).
Both occur in young patients of low body weight. High doses of insulin are required, but ketoacidosis does not occur. Tropical calcific pancreatitis (see 🕮 p 244) may be a cause of FCPD. Another theory is that consumption of cyanide-containing foods (e.g. cassava/manioc/tapioca, ragi in India, and kaffir beers in Africa) on a background of protein-calorie malnutrition leads to build-up of toxic hydrocyanic acid, resulting in direct damage to the pancreas. Conversely, some believe that the malnutrition is a result and not a cause of the diabetes.

Other types of DM

• Gestational.
• Secondary — due to drugs (steroids, thiazide diuretics); pancreatic disease (chronic pancreatitis, TCP, post-surgery); endocrine disease (Cushing's, acromegaly, phaeochromocytoma, thyrotoxicosis).

Clinical presentation

- *Acute:* ketoacidosis, weight loss, polyuria, polydipsia. (Differential diagnosis of polyuria and polydipsia includes hypercalcaemia (📖 p 676) and diabetes insipidus (📖 p 522). Consider these causes if blood glucose normal.)
- *Subacute:* as acute but occurring over a longer time, plus lethargy, infection (pruritis vulvae, boils).
- *Chronic:* may present with complications: infection, cataract, microangiopathy (retinopathy, neuropathy, nephropathy) and macroangiopathy (MI, claudication), foot ulcers.

Diagnosis

- *Diagnosis of DM* requires demonstration of an abnormal blood glucose level on two separate occasions (if asymptomatic), or on one occasion if symptomatic.
- *An abnormal blood glucose level is defined as:*
  - either a fasting venous plasma glucose level ≥7.0 mmol/l *or*
  - a random plasma glucose level ≥11.1 mmol/l.
- Always check urine ketones on diagnosis.
- *The following features favour type I DM:* non-fasting ketonuria, short history, marked weight loss (from any weight), family history of type I DM, personal/family history of autoimmune disease. (Age and glucose level are not predictive.)
- *Diagnosis of PDPD* also requires the following: onset at <30 yrs of age, BMI <19, a history of childhood malnutrition, and the absence of keto-acidosis. Such patients will often require >60 units of insulin per day.
- *Diagnosis of FCPD* requires the following additional criteria: recurrent abdominal pain; and evidence of pancreatic calculi in the absence of alcoholism, gallstones, or hyperthyroidism.

Impaired fasting glucose

This is defined as a fasting plasma glucose 6.0–7.0 mmol/l and is associated with ↑ risk of ischaemic heart disease (IHD) and progression to diabetes. Management involves monitoring fasting glucose annually for progression to DM, and addressing other risk factors for IHD (e.g. weight loss, lipids, smoking, aspirin).

The oral glucose tolerance test (GTT)

This should only be used for epidemiological research and diagnosing gestational DM. The patient must be on a normal carbohydrate intake prior to the test. Fast the patient overnight, then take a plasma glucose (fasting sample).

Give 75 g oral glucose in 300 ml water (children 1.75 g/kg, max 75 g) and measure plasma glucose 2 h afterwards. DM is diagnosed if the fasting venous plasma glucose is ≥7.0 mmol/l and/or the 2 h sample is ≥11.1 mmol/l.

Screening for glycosuria is not a cost-effective way of diagnosis in the general population. However, this is an appropriate method of screening for gestational DM. If glycosuria is present, proceed to GTT.

Management of diabetes mellitus

Patient education and motivation are the key to success. Aim of treatment is to restore normoglyaemia and avoid complications. If home monitoring of control not feasible, aim for absence of symptoms of hyper- or hypo-glycaemia. Children are more likely to develop ketoacidosis. Glycaemic control important during pregnancy: hyperglycaemia in the 1st trimester carries a 3-fold ↑ risk of foetal abnormality/birth complications.

Education

Diet and adherence crucial. Teach monitoring of blood/urine glucose levels. If on insulin or sulfonylureas, advise patient to carry sweets at all times; alert patient/family/colleagues to signs of hypoglycaemia. Diet should avoid rapidly absorbed carbohydrate (e.g. sugar, sweets, fizzy drinks), but include regular meals of complex carbohydrate. Avoid long periods of physical activity without food. Explain importance of foot care. Where possible, arrange appointments with dietician and chiropodist. Stress need for regular follow-up.

Conservative management

Treatment should always include a healthy diet: low in fat, sugar, and salt; high in starchy carbohydrate and fibre; with moderate protein; eaten at regular times. Fruit and fruit juice contain a lot of natural sugar. In urban areas, processed foods may be favoured but should be avoided. Obese patients should lose weight. CVS risk factors should be minimized (i.e. smoking, hypertension, cholesterol, exercise).

Drug therapy

Treatment depends on the type of DM and drug availability. In uncompli-cated, newly diagnosed type II DM, try 3-month trial of diet and exercise. If glycaemic control not adequate by 3 months, start metformin if over-weight or a sulfonylurea if slim. Sulfonylureas stimulate insulin secretion and sensitivity and cause hypoglycaemia; tolbutamide (0.5–1.0 g bd) is short-acting and preferred. Gliclazide (40–160 mg od) and glibenclamide (2.5–15 mg od), longer-acting and cause hypoglycaemia in elderly. Metformin (500 mg–1 g 2–3 × daily with food) does not cause hypoglycaemia but may cause anorexia, diarrhoea, and lactic acidosis. It should not be used in patients with renal, heart, or liver failure. The above drugs may be combined. Thiazolidinediones (rosiglitazone and pioglitazone) reduce peripheral insulin resistance. Their maximum hypoglycaemic effect takes 2–3 months to take effect; should not be used as first line but can be used as an alternative to metformin or a sulphonylurea when 2 agents required.

Combining all 3 oral drug classes not recommended — patients still hyperglycaemic despite 2 oral agents require insulin. Insulin should always be used in a patient on maximal oral treatment who is losing weight. Oral drugs can be supplemented with daily injection of long-acting insulin; however, it may be simpler (and cheaper) to change completely to insulin. In obese patients who require insulin, metformin reduces weight gain.

Insulin

Soluble insulin (100 units/ml) is short-acting, peaking at 2–4 h and lasting up to 8 h. Medium-acting insulins are suspensions, peaking at 4–6 h and lasting up to 16 h. Long-acting insulins last up to 32 h. Human insulin analogues are available in soluble/short-acting, medium, and long-acting forms. They have faster onset, quicker offset, and associate with less hypoglycaemia than other insulins. Treatment regimes vary, and depend upon type of DM, availability of insulins, access to home monitoring, and lifestyle. Most require 20–60 units per day (pre-pubertal children 0.6–0.8 units/kg per day). Type I DM requires insulin action throughout 24 h of the day, whereas insulin-treated type II DM can often be controlled with a single injection of medium-acting insulin once/day. For type I DM there are 2 widely used regimes:

- **Two injections/day** Start with 0.5 units/kg/day, 2/3 given in morning and 1/3 in evening. Make 1/3 short-acting and 2/3 long-acting. The insulin injections should be given 20 mins before breakfast and evening meal. Avoiding hypoglycaemia relies on 3 regular meals a day and 2 snacks, one mid-morning and one before bed (Fig 12.1).
- **Basal bolus** Single injection of long-acting at bedtime (basal) and 3 injections of soluble during the day (bolus) before each meal. Test glucose before each meal and adjust the insulin dose 2 units at a time.

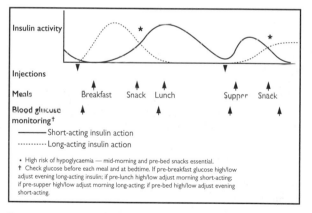

Fig. 12.1 Balancing insulin action and meals. How to monitor and adjust insulin doses with a typical twice-daily regime of short- and long-acting insulin suitable for a type I diabetic.

Diabetic treatment with intercurrent illness

Never stop insulin in type I diabetics even if they are unable to eat or drink. The stress of illness increases insulin requirements. However, oral intake is often reduced so it is important to monitor blood sugar levels, four times a day if possible. Drink plenty of water and, if unable to eat, replace meals with nutritious drinks e.g. soups or milky drinks. If calorie intake reduced, decrease long-acting insulin (e.g. by ~20%). Dose of short-acting insulin may need to be altered depending on blood glucose levels (e.g. if blood glucose 11–17 mmol/l, give 4 extra units; if 17–28, give 6 extra units; if >28, give 6 extra units and/or consider infusion).

IV insulin regimes

IV insulin may be required in certain circumstances e.g. DKA (see 🕮 p 508) or acutely unwell patients unable to take/absorb oral hypoglycaemics or whose blood glucose is too unstable to control with regular SC insulin. There is also evidence that careful control of blood glucose with IV insulin may improve the outcome of critical illness including acute coronary syndromes. IV insulin may be given either as a sliding scale or as a GKI (glucose-K⁺-insulin) infusion.

Insulin sliding scale infusion

- Make 50 units of soluble insulin up to 50 ml with normal saline (i.e. 1 unit/ml solution) and infuse at a rate according to the blood glucose as follows:*

Blood glucose (mmol/l)	Units/hour
≤5.0	1
5.1–12.0	3
12.1–20.0	4
>20.0	6

*This sliding scale regimen is only a guide — individual scales may vary between institutions, and may need to be adjusted for individual patients.

- Give IV fluids through separate vein/IV line: normal saline if blood glucose ≥11 mmol/l and 5% dextrose when blood glucose <11 mmol/l; give maintenance and replacement K⁺ according to blood K⁺ levels. In DKA, the initial K⁺ is often high but falls rapidly after insulin is started. If rapid access to K⁺ measurement is not available, give 20 mmol K⁺ per litre in the first 2 bags of fluid and then maintenance and replacement K⁺ according to blood levels.

GKI infusion

Add 15 units of soluble insulin to 500 ml 10% dextrose with 10 mmol K⁺. Infuse at 100 ml/h and check the blood glucose hourly. Make up new bottles with altered insulin units as shown below. Unless the blood glucose is quite stable, the GKI regime tends to be more wasteful as new bottles need to be made up frequently.

Blood glucose (mmol/l)	Insulin in bottle (units)
<5	6
5–15	15
>15	25

Diabetic follow-up

Diabetes is an increasing problem, even in tropical, rural areas. The complications of diabetes can be devastating but simple measures, such as good blood pressure control, are effective in reducing complications. Some complications, such as cataract, can be easily identified and addressed. It is therefore essential to establish locally accessible diabetic clinics in which patients can be regularly reviewed. Follow-up is necessary with all diabetic patients, in order to:

• Identify and resolve problems with treatment.
• Encourage adherence with treatment and maintain education.
• Monitor foot care.
• Prevent and monitor the development of long-term complications.

Frequent follow-up and tight control are essential during pregnancy.

Prevention of complications

Diabetics are at increased risk of microvascular and macrovascular complications, including stroke (relative risk, RR 2–3 × that of non-diabetics), MI (RR 2–5), blindness (RR 20), renal failure (RR 25), and limb amputation (RR 40).

• *Good glycaemic control*: use the following to assess glycaemic control:
  • Symptoms.
  • Home urine testing (aim for 0–0.25%).
  • Home glucose records (aim for 4.5–6.5 mmol/l).
  • History of hypoglycaemic attacks.
  • Glycosylated Hb (HbA$_1$c; indicates mean glucose level over the last 8 weeks — aim for <7%.
• *Control of hypertension* is more effective at preventing complications than good glycaemic control; target BP is 140/80 mmHg (125/75 mmHg if persistent proteinuria). ACE inhibitors are the drug of first choice but all antihypertensive drugs are probably effective.
• *IHD risk factor modification*: stop smoking, control of hyperlipidaemia, aspirin for those with hypertension or vascular disease.

Clinic checklist

Ideally every 6 months check:

1. Treatment and glucose control.
2. Blood pressure.
3. Injection sites.
4. Feet: pulses, numbness, sores, nail care.
5. Both eyes:
• Check acuity (with glasses if worn, otherwise use pin hole).
• If acuity ↓, check for cataracts; if no cataracts, maculopathy is likely (more common in type II DM).
• Check fundus for retinopathy — if cotton wool spots or new vessels are present, refer for laser treatment.
6. Urine dipstick for albumin — albuminuria or a rise in BP may indicate nephropathy. Exclude UTI; check serum creatinine. Albuminuria warrants aggressive treatment of BP.
7. If macrovascular disease or nephropathy is present, check lipids.

Diabetic ketoacidosis

Without insulin, glucose is unable to enter cells and the body is forced to make alternative substrates for metabolism, in the form of ketones produced in the liver. Lack of insulin eventually leads to hyperglycaemia and a build-up of acidic ketones. This may be precipitated by infection.

Clinical features: deterioration is often gradual over several days. There may be hyperventilation (with sweet, ketotic breath), vomiting, hyperglycaemia, and coma.

Investigations: FBC, U&Es, bicarbonate, blood gases, infection screen (urine and blood cultures, CXR). Test the urine for ketones. *Blood glucose may not be very high.* The seriousness of the condition is governed by pH, bicarbonate (HCO_3) levels, and the level of ketones.

Management

- Urgently correct dehydration (may be life-threatening) e.g. normal saline 1.5–2 litres/h for the first 2 h.
- Give soluble insulin 6 units/h IV until the blood glucose is <12 mmol/l. Then *either* switch to a GKI or sliding scale regimen (📖 p 504), *or* (if neither are available) halve the rate of infusion to 3 units/h IV.
- If facilities for IV infusion not available, give 20 units IM, then 6 units per hour until blood glucose <10 mmol/l, then 6 units IM every hour.
- Measure K^+ hourly. Initial K^+ often high but falls rapidly with insulin: if rapid K^+ measurement not available give 20 mmol K^+ per litre in the first 2 litres of fluid (unless oliguric, when K^+ may need to be withheld), and then maintenance and replacement K^+ according to blood levels.
- Monitor vital signs and blood glucose every hour.
- Prevent complications, including aspiration, DVT. Pass an NG tube to decompress stomach. Be alert to shock, cerebral oedema, and DIC.
- If immobility prolonged, give 5000 IU heparin SC bd.
- Giving bicarbonate is unnecessary — insulin and fluid will correct acidosis provided the underlying cause (e.g. infection) is treated. If there is gross acidosis without ketosis, consider aspirin overdose, or lactic acidosis in elderly diabetics.
- Identify and manage the precipitant e.g. poor compliance with treatment, intercurrent illness. Educate to help avoid recurrent DKA.

Hyperglycaemic hyperosmolar non-ketotic coma (HONK)

HONK generally affects older, type II diabetics. There is usually a more gradual history with intense dehydration and severe hyperglycaemia (>35 mmol/l). There is no acidosis or ketosis and the plasma osmolality may be >340 mmol/kg. (Plasma osmolality may be estimated by the formula: osm = $2[Na^+ + K^+] + [urea] + [glucose]$ mmol/l.)

Treat as for ketoacidosis, but correct the osmolality slowly (over 2–3 days) using half normal or normal saline to avoid cerebral oedema after large fluid shifts. DVT is more likely, so use heparin prophylaxis from the outset. Always consider and look for a precipitant e.g. infection, silent MI.

Hypoglycaemia

This is usually due to administration of excess insulin, sulfonylureas, or thiazolidinediones. It presents with altered (often aggressive) behaviour, sweating, tachycardia, and, rarely, fits and coma of rapid onset. If the patient is unable to take sugar orally, give IV e.g. 25–50 ml of 50% dextrose followed by a saline flush to avoid damaging the vein (may also use 10% or 20% glucose, but larger volumes may be required); improvement should be rapid. This should be followed quickly by feeding with complex carbohydrate. If IV access fails, try glucagon 0.5–1 mg IM (500 mcg for children <8 y old or <25 kg) to attempt to promote conversion of hepatic glycogen to glucose (repeated doses of glucagon become less effective as glycogen stores become depleted). If a long-acting insulin or oral agent has been taken, the patient will need monitoring and may require further IV dextrose for 48 h. In prolonged resistant hypoglycaemia, give dexamethasone 10 mg IV stat then 4 mg IM 6 h to combat cerebral oedema.

Diabetic nephropathy

Early disease is manifested by microalbuminuria; this may progress to frank proteinuria (detected by dipstix) and a gradual decline in renal function, leading over 10–15 yrs to end-stage renal failure. In type I DM, nephropathy develops ~7–10 yrs after onset; in type II it may be present at diagnosis. Retinopathy is usually present in both type I and II diabetics with nephropathy.

Management
- Good glycaemic control: careful monitoring is essential since requirements for insulin and oral hypoglycaemics tend to fall in CRF, due to reduced renal excretion and reduced insulin resistance. Avoid glibenclamide (risk of hypoglycaemia) and metformin (risk of lactic acidosis).
- Control blood pressure to prevent progression of renal damage. Target BP is 125/75. Patients are at high risk of hypertension since salt and fluid loads are less well handled. There may be a need for massive diuretic therapy, unless dialysis is possible.
- ACE inhibitors slow progression of nephropathy, even in normotensive diabetics with microalbuminuria.
- Control hyperlipidaemia.

Nephropathy in the diabetic patient is strongly correlated to the risk of coronary disease and cardiovascular death. Aggressive management of vascular risk factors is also required (smoking/BP/lipids/aspirin). Watch for the abrupt onset of pulmonary oedema or congestive heart failure, which may be the first signs of severe ischaemic heart disease.

Thyroid disease

The gland may become enlarged either diffusely (goitre) or in single or multiple nodules and, in each case, the patient may be euthyroid, hypothyroid, or hyperthyroid.

Hypothyroidism (myxoedema)

Clinical features: include weight gain, lethargy, constipation, dislike of cold, menorrhagia, infertility, dry skin, hoarse voice, depression, dementia, cerebellar ataxia, myopathy, angina, galactorrhea, and vitiligo. Examination may reveal coarse features, bradycardia, goitre, CCF, non-pitting oedema, ascites, pleural effusion, delayed reflexes, loss of the outer third of the eyebrows.

Diagnosis: ↑TSH, ↓T_4 (and T_3). FBC may show macrocytic anaemia (check B_{12}/folate) or iron deficiency (menorrhagia); ECG may show bradycardia and ischaemia; cholesterol and triglycerides may be ↑. Positive antithyroid antibodies suggest an autoimmune cause.

Management: T_4 50–150 mcg od, adjusted according to clinical state (aim to keep TSH <5 mU/l). In the elderly/those with ischaemic heart disease, begin with 25 mcg/day and monitor for angina or tachycardia (propranolol may be needed e.g. 10–40 mg 3–4 times daily). Usually required lifelong;
if De Quervains thyroiditis is suspected, withdraw thyroxine after 6 months and monitor. If area is iodine-deficient, use Schiller's iodine (1:30 diluted Lugol's iodine) 2 drops od for 6–12 months.

Myxoedema coma

Very rare, with 50% mortality. Often precipitated by infection, MI, CVA, or trauma. Look for hypothermia, hyporeflexia, bradycardia, paralytic ileus, and fits.

Investigations: T_3, T_4, TSH, FBC, U&E (may have hyponatraemia), glucose, cultures, and ABG (hypoxia and hypercapnia).

Management: give O_2 and treat any precipitating cause.
- If available, give 5–20 mcg T_3 by slow IV injection, repeated 6–12 h.
- Give hydrocortisone 100 mg q8 h IV (especially if pituitary hypothyroidism suspected).
- Pass NG tube and, unless there is paralytic ileus, administer T_4 300 mcg od.
- Rehydrate with normal saline, avoiding CCF. Hyponatraemia is usually due to water retention so fluid restriction may be necessary.
- Correct hypothermia and hypoglycaemia.
- Monitor for pancreatitis and arrhythmias.
- After 3 days, start thyroxine PO od at the usual dose.

Compensated/subclinical hypothyroidism

Raised TSH, normal T_3 and T_4, clinically euthyroid. Usually follows treatment for thyrotoxicosis or at an early stage of autoimmune hypothyroidism. Measure thyroid auto-antibodies. Treat with T_4 if antibody-positive, hypercholesterolaemia, or subfertility. Otherwise, monitor TFT 6 monthly.

Causes of goitre or thyroid nodules

- Physiological: endemic (iodine deficiency) or sporadic (pregnancy/puberty).
- Diffuse, autoimmune (Graves' or Hashimotos).
- Thyroiditis (Acute De Quervains).
- Goitrogens.
- Dyshormonogenesis.
- Nodular goitre (single or multi-nodular — euthyroid or thyrotoxic).
- Tumours (benign and malignant).

Causes of hypothyroidism

- *Autoimmune hypothyroidism:* usually occurs in women. If a goitre is present, diagnosis is Hashimoto's thyroiditis; if none, diagnosis is atrophic hypothyroidism. Associated with previous Graves' disease, IDDM, Addison's disease, pernicious anaemia; rarely with thyroid lymphoma.
- Post thyroidectomy or radioiodine treatment.
- *Drug-induced:* anti-thyroid drugs, amiodarone, lithium, iodine.
- *Post-viral thyroiditis (De Quervains):* often follows 6 weeks after a viral prodrome. Goitre is tender. Inflammatory markers are raised. Can be hypo-, hyper-, or euthyroid. Self-limiting illness; usually lasts 6 months but may require treatment in interim.
- *Iodine deficiency:* ([] p 658). Previously widespread (e.g. >50% of countries in Africa). May be endemic, especially in mountain areas, or sporadic (pregnancy/puberty). Iodination programmes have improved the situation but endemic goitre is still seen in many adults.
- *Dyshormonogenesis:* a number of defects, all autosomal recessive.

Abnormal TFTs in non-thyroidal illness

'Sick euthyroid syndrome'. Seen in severe illness, starvation, or fasting. TSH↓ or normal, T_3↓, T_4↓ or normal. Patient may be clinically hypothyroid. Does not require treatment; abnormalities correct when the underlying problem is treated. If abnormalities persist, consider hypopituitism.

Amiodarone-associated thyroid abnormalities

Abnormal TFTs are common on amiodarone as well as true thyroid dysfunction. The drug blocks conversion of T_4 to T_3, so may see raised T_4, normal/↓T_3, and normal/↑TSH. True thyroid dysfunction more likely if thyroid auto-antibody positive. Only treat if clinical hypo-/hyperthyroidism supported by TFTs.

Hyperthyroidism (thyrotoxicosis)

Occurs more commonly in women

Clinical features: weight loss, diarrhoea, oligomenorrhoea, tremor, emotional lability, heat intolerance, sweating, itch, fatigue, hair thinning, and eye protrusion. Examination may reveal tachycardia, AF, fine tremor, eye disease, goitre/nodule(s), thyroid bruit, myopathy.

Complications: include heart failure, AF, osteoporosis, gynaecomastia.

Diagnosis: suppressed TSH, $\uparrow T_3$ and/or T_4. Nuclear thyroid scanning is best way to differentiate toxic nodules and multinodular goitres from Graves' disease (diffuse increased uptake) and hyperthyroid thyroiditis (decreased uptake). Scan can be done while taking antithyroid drugs. USS, thyroid auto-antibodies, ECG, FBC, U&E also useful. Test the visual fields and acuity.

Management

1. Gain rapid symptom control with propranolol 40 mg qds.
2. Start carbimazole at 40 mg od for 4–6 weeks (may have to increase to 60 mg if not achieving control). Propylthiouracil is an alternative.
  - In Graves' disease, options are then to either reduce the dose according to TFTs and maintain on 5–10 mg od for 12–18 months before stopping, *or*
  - 'Block and replace' — leave on carbimazole 40–60 mg od and once TSH starts to rise add levothyroxine 50–150 mcg od for 18 months.
  - Block and replace is simpler as it does not require regular monitoring of TFTs and may be associated with lower relapse rates.
  - With both regimes ~50% will relapse, usually in the next 18 mths.
  - If carbimazole is used to treat toxic nodules/multinodular goitres, the lowest effective dose should be used and treatment is usually lifelong.
  - N.B. in the West 0.1% have agranulocytosis on carbimazole; therefore tell the patient to return if they have a severe sore throat after starting treatment; check the FBC.
3. Radioiodine is best treatment for toxic nodule or multinodular goitre. A single treatment should lead to cure with minimal risk of hypothyroidism. Radioiodine can be used for Graves' (usually reserved for relapsed cases) but occasionally inadequate treatment requires a repeat dose and post-treatment hypothyroidism is common.
4. Surgery is useful for large goitres but runs similar risks of over- and under-treatment as radioiodine in Graves' disease.
5. Patients should be made euthyroid with drugs before surgery or radioiodine to avoid thyroid storm.

In pregnancy, lowest dose of antithyroid drug should be used and the foetus should have US scan for goitre before delivery.

Subclinical hyperthyroidism

Suppressed TSH, normal T_3 and T_4. Found in multinodular goitre and after treatment for Grave's. Patients are usually clinically euthyroid. Not thought to require treatment but may be associated with increased cardiovascular morbidity and mortality.

Causes of hyperthyroidism

- *Toxic multi-nodular goitre:* common in areas of recently treated iodine deficiency.
- *Graves' disease:* genetic predisposition leads to antibodies to TSH receptors and a diffuse goitre. There may be ophthalmopathy, pre-tibial myxoedema (oedematous swellings on shins), anaemia, ↑ESR, ↑Ca^{2+}, and abnormal LFTs. It is associated with other autoimmune diseases in the individual or their family.
- *Toxic adenoma:* nodule producing T_3/T_4.
- *Thyroiditis:* post-partum or triggered by viral illness (mumps, coxsackie). The goitre may be painful. Self-limiting condition.
- *Others:* medication, follicular carcinoma of the thyroid, choriocarcinoma, struma ovarii (ovarian tumour secreting T_3 & T_4).

Thyroid eye disease

All patients who are thyrotoxic can have lid retraction and lid lag due to autonomic overactivity. Patients with autoimmune thyroid disease (hyper- and hypothyroidism) can develop autoimmune ophthalmopathy. This occurs in the presence of specific auto-antibodies causing retro-orbital inflammation and lymphocyte infiltration. It may precede thyrotoxicosis.

Clinical features: gritty sore eyes, blurred vision, double vision, eye pain, and/or protrusion. Ophthalmopathy is worse in smokers and in those in whom hypothyroidism occurs during the course of treatment. Examination may reveal lid retraction and lid lag, proptosis, conjunctival oedema, corneal ulceration, papilloedema, optic atrophy, impaired colour vision (earliest sign of optic nerve compression), ophthalmoplegia.

The main risks to sight are exposure keratitis and optic nerve compression; ask the patient to shut his/her eyes and check eye closure is complete. Where available, a CT scan or US may be used to demonstrate thickening of rectus muscles and optic nerve compression.

Management: stop smoking. Pay close attention to maintaining the euthyroid state. Protect the cornea: wear sunglasses at all times to keep out dust/wind, tape eyelids shut with micropore in bed, consider tarsorraphy. Try hypromellose eye drops for lubrication. Use an eye patch for diplopia. Steroids (80 mg od prednisolone) work but systemic side-effects of the doses required are unacceptable for long-term use. Orbital radiotherapy and surgical decompression are effective. These options should be reserved for situations where sight is threatened; seek expert advice.

Cushing's syndrome

Cushing's syndrome is due to chronic glucocorticoid excess. The most common cause is corticosteroid treatment. It is important to differentiate this cause from endogenous overproduction of cortisol. Cortisol is normally released after ACTH stimulus from the hypothalamo-pituitary axis and Cushing's syndrome is classified as either ACTH dependent (i.e. excess stimulus) or ACTH independent (i.e. ↑cortisol without ↑ACTH). Also consider alcoholic pseudo-Cushing's, depression, and ectopic ACTH from carcinoma.

Clinical features: moon face, obesity, impaired glucose tolerance, hypertension, hypogonadism, osteoporosis, purple striae, limb wasting and myopathy, hirsutism, thin skin, bruising, peripheral oedema, ↑infection, poor wound healing, hypokalaemia, psychological change (depression/mania/psychosis). Increased pigmentation if ACTH high.

Diagnosis: Investigation has two phases: (1) to establish the presence/absence of Cushings syndrome and (2) to establish the cause (pituitary/adrenal/ectopic). Do an overnight dexamethasone (DXM) suppression test (screening test); give DXM 1 mg PO at 11 p.m. Take blood for plasma cortisol at 9 a.m. (normal <170 nmol/l: higher in Cushing's syndrome; N.B. the OCP gives false high values). If this tests abnormal proceed to 2 or more of:

- 24-h urinary free cortisol (normal <700 nmol/24 h). Occasionally patients with Cushing's have normal values.
- 9 a.m. and midnight cortisols — loss of diurnal variation.
- 48 h (low-dose) DXM suppression test: give DXM 0.5 mg 6 h for 2 days then check 9 a.m. serum cortisol on the second day (should be <50 nmol/l). If not suppressed, a diagnosis of Cushing's can be made.

For differential diagnosis, consider pituitary/adrenal imaging (CT or MRI), CXR, high-dose dex. suppression test. As above but give 2 mg DXM 6 hrly for 48 h. Pituitary ACTH-driven Cushing's will show some suppression; adrenal or ectopic ACTH will not.

Expert help is required for investigation and management.

Management of Cushing's syndrome

ACTH-dependent

- Iatrogenic (ACTH or synacthen treatment) — treat by ↓ dose.
- Cushing's disease; ACTH-producing pituitary adenoma — treat with surgery, radiotherapy, or medically, with metyrapone. Check for deficiency of other pituitary hormones and replace if necessary. Consider bilateral adrenalectomy if pituitary surgery not possible but may develop Nelson's syndrome.
- Ectopic ACTH (or rarely, CRH) production from tumours, especially small-cell bronchial Ca — treat the cause. Also consider metyrapone/ketoconazole or adrenalectomy if prognosis warrants.

ACTH-independent

- Iatrogenic (prednisolone or dexamethasone treatment) — ↓ dose.
- Alcohol excess — reduce alcohol intake.
- Cortisol-producing tumours (adrenal adenoma or Ca) — remove tumour. Medical treatment as above.

Addison's disease

Adreno-cortical insufficiency, leading to ↓ gluco- and mineralocorticoids.

Clinical features: weakness, apathy, anorexia, weight loss, abdominal pain, oligomenorrhoea. There may be hyperpigmentation, vitiligo, hypotension, and sexual dysfunction. Dehydration in crises.

Investigations: synacthen tests. Check for hyperkalaemia, hyponatraemia (may be SIADH), uraemia, acidosis, hypercalcaemia, and eosinophilia. Get a CXR (looking for signs of TB) and AXR.

Causes: idiopathic (probably autoimmune, associated with other such diseases), adrenal TB, adrenal metastases, HIV, fungal infection, ketoconazole treatment.

Management: treat cause. Replace steroids with PO hydrocortisone, 20 mg in morning, 10 mg at night, and adjust the dose according to plasma cortisol (aim for 700–850 nmol/l) and clinical symptoms (↑ if postural hypotension, ↓ if patient becomes Cushingoid). Warn the patient about not stopping steroid treatment abruptly and, if possible, give syringes to give the hydrocortisone IM if vomiting prevents oral therapy. Explain that they need to take more hydrocortisone during intercurrent illnesses. There should be 6-mth follow-up.

Addisonian crisis

Hypotension and shock in a known Addisonian patient or someone on long-term steroids who has omitted their tablets. Often there is preceding infection, trauma, or surgery.

Management

- Take bloods for urgent ACTH and cortisol.
- Resuscitate with colloid then crystalloids.
- Give 100 mg hydrocortisone IV stat, then q6–8 h.
- Culture blood, urine, and sputum.
- Give a broad-spectrum antibiotic.
- Monitor for hypoglycaemia.
- If stable after 72 h, change to oral hydrocortisone 3 times daily e.g. 10 mg/5 mg/5 mg (note oral and IV hydrocortisone doses NOT equivalent).

Hyperaldosteronism

Excessive aldosterone production independent of the renin angiotensin system. Typically, there is hypertension, hypokalaemia, alkalosis, and mild hypernatraemia. May be present in 1–5% of patients with 'essential' hypertension. Suspect if K^+ low before treatment of BP or persistent hypokalaemia on thiazides. Check plasma K^+, aldosterone ($\uparrow$), and renin ($\downarrow$). Most cases are due to adrenocortical adenoma (Conn's syndrome); rarely, adrenal hyperplasia and CA. In 2° hyperaldosteronism (e.g. heart or liver failure, diuretic therapy), aldosterone and renin are both raised. Also consider elevated non-aldosterone mineralocorticoids in congenital adrenal hyperplasia — in which case both aldosterone and renin are low.

Management: can be medical with spironolactone 100–400 mg daily, glucocorticoids (e.g. dexamethasone 0.75 mg in morning, 0.25 mg at night), or surgical. Treat 2° disease by treating the cause. Give K^+ replacements.

Hypopituitarism

The pituitary produces ACTH, GH, FSH, LH, TSH, and prolactin. $\downarrow$ production of one or more of these is termed hypopituitarism and may be due to: infarction (Sheehan's syndrome post-partum haemorrhage or Russell's viper envenoming), cysts, granulomatous disease, abscesses, congenital defects, stroke, basal skull fracture, pituitary adenoma, hypophysectomy, and irradiation. There may be atrophy of the breasts, small testes, hair loss, thin skin, hypotension, visual field defects (bitemporal hemianopia, initially of upper quadrants). Investigate with lateral skull X-ray, assessment of visual fields, U&Es, FBC, TFT, testosterone/oestrogen, cortisol, CT head. Endocrine testing requires stimulation tests. A specialist centre is needed for treatment, which involves replacement of hydrocortisone, thyroxine, and oestrogen/testosterone.

Hyperprolactinaemia

Presents with amenorrhoea, infertility, galactorrhoea in women, and impotence in men. There may be visual field loss due to pressure effects. Causes may be physiological (pregnancy, stress), drugs (metaclopramide, haloperidol, methyldopa, oestrogens, TRH), or disease — pituitary disease (adenoma or stalk compression), CRF, hypothyroidism, sarcoid. Treat the underlying cause. If cause is pituitary adenoma, give bromocriptine (first line, often the only treatment required), surgery, and radiotherapy.

Acromegaly

Caused by ↑ secretion of GH from a pituitary tumour (in children, in whom epiphyseal plates have not yet fused, it results in gigantism). Adults have coarse features, prominent mandibles and hands and feet, large tongues, arthralgia, muscle weakness, and paraesthesiae (carpal tunnel syndrome). There is an increased risk of Ca colon, DM, HT, and cardiomyopathy. Diagnose by ↑ IGF1 levels or failure of GH to suppress during an oral glucose tolerance test. Treatment is usually a combined approach between medicine (bromocriptine or, preferably, somatostatin if available), surgery, and radiotherapy.

Diabetes insipidus (DI)

Results from a failure of antidiuretic hormone action either due to lack of production (cranial DI) or renal insensitivity (nephrogenic DI). There is reduced water resorption by the kidney, polyuria, and polydipsia.

- *Cranial causes:* head injury, metastases, sarcoid, meningitis, and surgery.
- *Nephrogenic causes:* ↓K$^+$, ↑Ca^{2+}, drugs (e.g. lithium), sickle-cell disease, renal failure, pyelonephritis, and hydronephrosis.

Diagnosis: by early morning urine osmolality (if >800 mosmol/l, DI is excluded), U&Es, water deprivation test.

Treatment: for cranial DI is DDAVP replacement. For nephrogenic DI, remove underlying cause. May take weeks to recover; thiazides and indometacin 100 mg/day may reduce urine output during this time.

Phaeochromocytoma

A tumour, usually in the adrenal medulla producing catecholamines. May be inherited as part of the multiple endocrine neoplasia syndrome (MENIIa) and associated with neurofibromatosis and medullary thyroid cancer. There is hypertension, cardiomyopathy, weight loss, hyperglycaemia, and crises of fear, palpitations, tremor, and nausea. Check 24 h urinary catecholamine excretion (raised in phaeochromocytoma); imaging (CT/MRI or meta-iodobenzylguanidine scan) may aid diagnosis, especially of extra-adrenal tumours. Cautiously reduce the BP with phenoxybenzamine 10 mg od (increased each day by 10 mg, up to 1–2 mg/kg in 2 divided doses). Once the pressor effects of excess catecholamines have been suppressed, beta blockade may be used to control tachycardia e.g. propranolol 20 mg tds. Add phentolamine 2–5 mg IV, repeated if necessary, during crises. Surgery provides the only cure.

Ophthalmology

Section editor   **David Yorston**

Sources:
J Sandford–Smith. *Eye diseases in hot climates.* Butterworth–Heinemann, Oxford 1990. E. Sutter. *Hanyane — A Village Struggles for Eye Health.* MacMillan, London 1989 International. Resource Centre. *Journal of Community Eye Health.* ICEH, 11 Bath St., London

Global blindness

The WHO estimates that 36 million people worldwide are blind (corrected visual acuity of less than 3/60 in the best eye). This figure is increasing every year because the world's population is both increasing and ageing. By far the majority live in the developing world. A further 124 million people have low vision (corrected acuity of less than 6/18 to 3/60).

Cataract is the most common cause of blindness worldwide, with an estimated 17 million blind people and over 100 million eyes justifying cataract surgery because of severe visual impairment. In 1999, an estimated 10 million cataract operations were performed worldwide. It is calculated that as many as 30 million cataract operations need to be performed annually if cataract blindness is to be controlled in the next 10 years.

With improvements in hygiene and primary health care, particularly in Asia, degenerative conditions, such as glaucoma, diabetic retinopathy, and age-related macular degeneration are the fastest growing causes of blindness. However, trachoma and vitamin A deficiency continue to be major problems in the most deprived communities.

Trachoma and onchocerciasis are blinding ocular infections responsible for approximately 5% of all blindness. Both occur in poor communities. Blindness can be prevented through relatively simple, low-cost interventions including the use of antimicrobials. Vitamin A deficiency is a major cause of blindness in children and again occurs in poor communities.

Visual loss due to refractive errors, particularly myopia, is an increasing problem especially in Asia. Refraction followed by the appropriate spectacle correction will restore sight, but for people living in isolated communities, the 'refractionist' and spectacles are often either unavailable or unaffordable.

These five diseases (cataract, trachoma, onchocerciasis, vitamin A deficiency, and refractive errors) are all avoidable (preventable or curable) and constitute at least 70% of all cases of blindness worldwide.

Presenting symptoms of eye disease

People attending with an eye complaint are usefully considered according to the main symptom:
- *Visual loss:* they cannot see in the distance with one or both eyes.
- *Red painful eye(s):* eye pain or discomfort, with or without a history of trauma.
- *Inability to read:* reduced near vision, despite good distance vision. This is due to presbyopia after 40 years of age.
- *Other symptoms:* e.g. watering eyes, flashing lights.

Visual loss

Examination
- Measure the visual acuity without and with a pinhole.
- Examine the cornea and pupil with a torchlight.
- After dilating the pupil, examine the optic disc and retina with an ophthalmoscope.

Refractive errors

There are five different types of refractive errors:
- *Myopia* — short-sightedness, causing poor distance vision but good near vision.
- *Hypermetropia* — long-sightedness, giving difficulty with near vision in young people. Uncommon in patients <40 yrs old.
- *Astigmatism* — due to a different refraction in two axes of the eye.
- *Aphakia* — severe hypermetropia due to removal of the lens.
- *Presbyopia* — poor accommodation leading to difficulty with reading and near vision after 40 years. It is treated with reading spectacles that usually have a strength of between +1.00 and +4.00 dioptres. In patients under 50 years, +1 to +2 is sufficient. Patients >70 will require +3 to +4.

Most people with poor distance vision due to refractive errors have myopia. Myopia can be diagnosed as follows:
- The distance vision improves with a pinhole.
- Near vision is good, despite poor distance vision.

Myopia can be corrected with minus lenses. In the absence of a trained refractionist, the following method will usually give an acceptable spectacle correction. If you have trial lenses available, test one eye at a time. Start with a −1 lens and gradually increase the stength by steps of −1, measuring the visual acuity with every lens. When increasing the power does not lead to any further improvement, choose the minimum power that will give the best visual acuity. Repeat the process for the other eye.

Aphakia is becoming less common as most cataract operations include insertion of an intraocular lens. It can be corrected with a +11.0 dioptre lens.

Testing visual acuity

All eye patients must have their vision measured. Any opacity of the lens or cornea, or damage to the central retina or optic nerve will reduce the visual acuity.

Only the distance acuity is measured; near vision will always be reduced in older patients who do not have reading glasses. Distance vision is measured at 6 metres. Each eye is tested individually, using the patient's own distance glasses, if they have any. The patient stands 6 metres from the chart and covers one eye. Literate patients read out the letters, starting at the top. Illiterate patients use an 'E' chart, indicating if it is pointing left or right, up or down.

Each line on the chart is labelled with a number. The top line is 60, the second is 36, etc. These numbers indicate the distance at which that line can be read by a normal eye. The 3rd line on the chart can normally be read at 24 metres, so if a patient can only read this line at 6 metres, the visual acuity is 6/24. The 6 identifies the distance at which the line was read and the 24 identifies the distance at which that line would be read by a normal eye. Normal vision is 6/6. In practice, most people can do most of their normal daily activities with a vision of 6/18.

If patients cannot see the top line at 6 metres, bring them closer. If they can read it at 3 metres, the acuity is 3/60. If they cannot see the top line, ask them to count your fingers, see your hand move, or see light. If they have no perception of light, it is probable that the eye is permanently blind and no treatment will restore vision.

Sometimes the visual acuity is reduced because the patient needs glasses. You can partially overcome a refractive error by using a pinhole. To make a pinhole, take some dark card (e.g. exposed X-ray film) and with a hot 21G needle, make a hole in the centre of the circle. The patient holds the film and looks through the hole in the middle. If the vision improves, the eye has a refractive error.

Cataract

Cataracts cause a gradual, progressive, and painless decrease in visual acuity. Because they progress very slowly, most patients who are blind from cataract never come to an eye clinic, since they accept their blindness as normal for their age. Elimination of cataract blindness requires community involvement to change attitudes and reduce barriers that block access to eye services.

Diagnosis: When complete, cataracts can be seen as a white opacity in the pupil, while younger cataracts give a grey-white appearance to the pupil. Examination of the fundus of the eye with an ophthalmoscope, after dilation of the pupil, shows an opacity in the red reflex with obscuration of fundus detail due to the lens opacity. The pupil reaction to light is normal in an uncomplicated cataract.

Management: There is currently no way to prevent cataracts forming. The only treatment is surgery to remove the lens and replace it with an artificial intraocular lens (IOL). Surgery is usually performed under local anaesthesia. Following surgery, 80–90% of eyes should be able to see 6/18 or better. The patient may then need corrective spectacles to obtain optimal vision.

Corneal opacity

Diagnosis: There is a white opacity on the cornea, which usually prevents a clear view of the pupil. This may follow a corneal ulcer, injury, or be due to trachoma, vitamin A deficiency, or leprosy. Most corneal scars are preventable by primary prevention (e.g. vitamin A deficiency) or by good management of the original condition (e.g. corneal ulcer).

Management: If both eyes have severe visual loss, then a corneal graft or optical iridectomy may be considered to try and improve the vision. Specialist care and very good follow-up are essential to obtain reasonable results.

Glaucoma

May be acute with a red painful eye, or chronic with gradual progressive loss of peripheral vision due to optic nerve damage. The patient is unaware of the loss of sight until visual acuity is impaired, which occurs only after most of the optic nerve has been destroyed.

Diagnosis: of chronic glaucoma is difficult. Detecting peripheral visual field loss requires expensive and complex equipment. Measuring IOP is simpler, but unreliable, as many patients with an elevated IOP do not have glaucoma, and some patients with glaucoma have a normal IOP. The most reliable method of diagnosis is observation of characteristic changes in the optic disc (increased size of the optic cup). However, this requires expertise.

Management: of glaucoma consists of lowering the IOP with filtration surgery or lifelong eye drops (e.g. timolol 0.25% bd). Treatment prevents progression and preserves the remaining vision, but does not improve vision, so patients who are already blind should not be treated.

Table 13.1 Common causes of poor distance vision

	Refractive error	Corneal opacity	Cataract	Diseases of optic nerve and retina
Causes	Myopia Astigmatism Aphakia (Hypermetropia)	Corneal ulcer Trachoma Vitamin A deficiency Leprosy	Usually age related. Also:- Eye injuries Diabetes Iritis	The glaucomas Optic atrophy Macula degeneration Diabetic retinopathy Hypertensive retinopathy Retinal detachment
Signs and symptoms	Vision improves with a pinhole.	White scarring of the cornea in a quiet white eye. Pupil difficult to see. Absent or poor red reflex.	White or grey pupil. Pupil reacts to light. Absent or poor red reflex.	Cornea and lens should be clear. Pupil may not react normally to light. Specific signs seen with an ophthalmoscope in the retina or optic nerve.
Management	Spectacles	Often no treatment. Surgery may be considered when both eyes are affected.	Cataract removal if the visual acuity is less than 5/60, or if the person's lifestyle is affected.	Management is directed at the cause.

Red eye

History and examination
- Ask about any known cause, particularly any injury.
- Measure the visual acuity.
- Carefully examine the eyelids, conjunctiva, cornea, pupil with a torch.

Injuries to the eye

First ask about any injury to or foreign body into the eye.

Corneal or conjunctival foreign bodies (FB)
The history is usually straightforward. The FB may be obvious or you may need to evert the upper eyelid to check the conjunctiva for objects scratching the cornea each time the patient blinks.
To remove the FB:
- Lie the patient flat.
- Apply local anaesthetic drops e.g. lidocaine 4% to the conjunctiva.
- Light the eye with a torch so that the FB is easily visible.
- Loupe magnification is useful.
- Lift off the FB with the corner of a thick piece of paper, or carefully with a needle.
- Give an antibiotic eye ointment or drops and eye pad for 1 day.

Corneal abrasion
This occurs when trauma removes some corneal epithelium. There is sudden severe pain and photophobia. To confirm the diagnosis, apply fluorescein which stains the cornea where there is no epithelium. Treat with an antibiotic eye ointment or drops until the pain has gone and the epithelium is completely healed.

Hyphaema
If there is a severe blunt injury (e.g. hit in eye by stone/fist), then bleeding may occur inside the eye. A blood level (hyphaema) may be visible between cornea and iris. This will usually resolve over a few days with rest. Avoid aspirin, as this may lead to further bleeding. If the eye is painful, give acetazolamide 250 mg qds for 3–7 days to lower the IOP and topical prednisolone 0.5–1.0% drops qds to reduce the inflammation. If the hyphaema has not resolved after 5 days, consult an eye specialist.

Penetrating eye injury
A penetrating injury (involving the full thickness of cornea or sclera) is very serious. Common causes include thorns, and splinters when chopping firewood. Be very careful examining the eye as pressure may aggravate the injury. Gently apply an antibiotic eye drop (not ointment), put an eye pad over the eye, and refer the patient to a specialist immediately. Systemic antibiotics (ciprofloxacin 750 mg BD) may reduce the ~30% risk of an intraocular infection. If immediate referral is not possible, then conservative treatment with antibiotics and an eye pad is probably better than a non-eye surgeon 'having a go'.

Table 13.2 Common causes of non-traumatic acute red eye

	Conjunctivitis	Corneal ulcer	Iritis	Acute glaucoma
Pain	Irritation	Moderate to severe	Moderate	Severe
Vision	Normal	Variable loss	Variable loss	Severe loss
Redness	Especially in the fornices	Around the cornea	Around the cornea	Around the corneal limbus
Cornea	Normal	Opacity on cornea	Keratic precipitates seen with magnification	Oedematous and hazy
Pupil	Normal	Normal	Constricted and irregular	Half dilated and fixed
Special features	Discharge, often bilateral	Stains with fluorescein	Irregular pupil may be more obvious as the pupil is dilated	Raised IOP
Treatment	Topical antibiotics	Topical antibiotics or antimicrobials	Dilate pupil and give topical steroids if certain of diagnosis	Acetazolamide 250 mg qds Drops to lower IOP Surgery is usually needed

Red eye with no injury

If there is no history of eye injury, then consider:
- Conjunctivitis.
- Corneal ulcer.
- Iritis.
- Acute glaucoma.

(See table on 📖 p 531).

Conjunctivitis

1. Infective conjunctivitis

Infection or inflammation of the conjunctiva is common in the tropics. Important causes and a way of differentiating them are given in Table 13.3.

Diagnosis: irritation of the eye with discomfort but normal vision. The eye is red with increased discharge. Severe disease may produce swelling of the eyelids (chemosis).

Management: give an antibiotic eye ointment or drops e.g. chloramphenicol 0.5–1%, initially q2 h, then qds for 5–7 days. Do not pad the eye.

2. Ophthalmia neonatorum

A specific conjunctivitis occurring in the first 4 weeks of life, usually due to *Neisseria gonorrhoeae* or *Chlamydia trachomatis* (see 📖 p 22). The lids are very swollen and covered with pus. Untreated, gonococcus infection causes a rapid progression with complete destruction of the cornea and permanent blindness.

Management: give appropriate systemic and topical antibiotics which will be effective against local strains of *Neisseria* (see 📖 p 609). Most cases of ophthalmia neonatorum may be prevented by irrigating the eyes of all newborn babies with 2.5–5% povidone-iodine solution immediately after delivery.

3. Chlamydial conjunctivitis (trachoma) — see below.

4. Epidemic haemorrhagic conjunctivitis

A highly contagious viral conjunctivitis usually due to enteroviruses. After a 1–2 day incubation period, multiple petechial haemorrhages occur. Most patients recover quickly.

Management: give an antimicrobial agent e.g. povidone-iodine 1.25% 1 eye drop qds, to help reduce transmission and reassure the patient.

5. Allergic conjunctivitis

Children and young adults may develop a chronic allergic conjunctivitis (vernal conjunctivitis). There is severe itching/irritation with a mucus discharge, sometimes with swelling and pigmentation around the cornea.

Management: treatment with topical steroids is effective but has serious side-effects. If possible, children with severe disease should be seen and treated by an eye specialist. In milder cases, parents should be reassured that the condition does not lead to loss of sight and is usually self-limiting — children 'grow out of it'. Symptoms may be reduced by bathing the eyes with cold clean water.

Table 13.3 Common causes of conjunctivitis

	Age and state of patient	Secretions	Special features	Treatment
Bacterial	Any	Purulent	Red and swollen Purulent discharge	Topical antibiotics for 5 days
Ophthalmia neonatorum	First 4 weeks of life	Purulent	Very red and swollen Purulent discharge	Systemic and topical antibiotics for 10 days
Viral	Any	Watery	May have corneal lesions	Symptomatic only
Chlamydial (trachoma)	Usually young children	Mucopurulent	Follicles and papillae on upper lid	Azithromycin tablets or tetracycline ointment for 6 weeks
Allergic (vernal)	Children	Stringy mucus	Very itchy, large papillae Infiltrate and pigmentation around cornea	Cromoglicate and possibly steroid eye drops for symptoms.

Corneal ulcers

A corneal ulcer may occur spontaneously or follow a corneal abrasion. There are many causes — the main ones are summarized in Table 13.4.

Diagnosis: there is usually severe pain, a watery discharge, and blurred vision. There is redness around the cornea, and the cornea is cloudy, often with a localized white or grey opacity, which stains with fluorescein. In severe cases, there may be a fluid level of pus inside the eye ('hypopyon'). If the ulcer is caused by infection, the organism may be identified by gram stain and culture of a scraping from the edge of the ulcer.

Management: depends on the cause, and is summarized in Table 13.4.

Snake venom ophthalmia

Spitting elapids have evolved modified fangs which enable the snake to eject a spray of intensely irritant venom into the eyes of an aggressor, causing intense pain, conjunctivitis, corneal erosions (and occassionally anterior uveitis). Secondary bacterial infection of corneal erosions may cause permanent scarring and blindness.

Management: Wash venom from affected eye or mucous membranes with copious amounts of water. Apply topical chloramphenicol or tetracycline ointment. 0.1% adrenaline eyedrops relieve the pain.

Uveitis

Inflammation of the uvea may involve both anterior uvea (iris and ciliary body) and posterior uvea (choroid). Causes include: infections (e.g. leprosy, onchocerciasis, toxoplasmosis, TB, syphilis) and systemic diseases (e.g. certain types of arthritis, sarcoidosis, Behcet's, inflammatory bowel disease). However, most cases, particularly of anterior uveitis, have no known cause, and multiple investigations are unnecessary.

Anterior uveitis (iritis, iridocyclitis)

Clinical features: the pain of iritis varies from mild to severe and is associated with photophobia and often some blurring of vision. Blood vessels around the margin of the cornea (the limbus) are dilated. The iris constricts and adheres to the front of the lens (posterior synechia), making the pupil irregular. These synechiae can lead to secondary glaucoma and cataract. When the pupil is dilated, adhesions may be seen before they break, leaving iris pigment on the front of the lens. Pus collecting in the anterior chamber can be seen with a slit lamp microscope.

Management: dilate the pupil to break any posterior synechiae (cyclopentolate 1% or atropine 1%); give anti-inflammatory agents (prednisolone 0.5–1.0% drops) to reduce the inflammation.

Posterior uveitis

Clinical features: presents with visual loss because of involvement of the overlying retina. Not usually painful but a severe attack may cause discomfort. A white inflammatory lesion may be seen in the retina. Once the inflammation has settled, characteristic scars occur with pigment atrophy and hypertrophy.

Management: requires treatment of cause.

Acute glaucoma

If the IOP increases suddenly over a few hours, the eye becomes red and very painful with severe loss of vision. Acute glaucoma is unusual in people <50 years. It may occur spontaneously or as a complication of a completely white cataract. The cornea appears hazy and the pupil is semi-dilated and does not react to light. The IOP is very high.

Management: give acetazolamide 500 mg stat and then 250 mg qds. Refer to an eye specialist since urgent surgery is usually required.

Table 13.4 Common causes of corneal ulceration

Cause	Predisposing factors	Clinical features	Treatment
Herpes simplex	Fever	Irregular branching ulcer	Aciclovir ointment
Bacteria	Trauma	Often severe pain and loss of vision; hypopyon may be present	Intensive topical or sub-conjunctival antibiotics
Fungus	Hot and humid areas, minor trauma	Often severe pain and loss of vision; hypopyon may be present	Antifungal agents
Vit A deficiency	Measles Malnutrition Malabsorption	Dry cornea. Central 'punched out' oval ulcer, often in a quiet eye	Vitamin A 200,000 iu stat immediately, then after 1 day, and 2 weeks
Exposure ulcer	Leprosy Facial burns	Eyelids do not close; lower third oval ulcer	Antibiotic ointment Tape eye closed Tarsorrhaphy

Trachoma

Trachoma is a chronic conjunctivitis caused by infection with *Chlamydia trachomatis*, serotypes A, B, and C. Inflammation from active infection leads to scarring of the upper conjunctiva and tarsal plate causing the eyelashes to turn in and scratch the cornea, producing ulceration, scarring, and blindness.

Transmission: the disease occurs particularly in poor dry areas of the world in which there is inadequate water supply and poor community sanitation. The classic trachoma environment can be described as:
- Dry: lack of water
- Dirty: lack of sanitation
- Discharge: lack of personal hygiene

Transmission of trachoma from child to child, and child to mother occurs through:
- Flies: flies go from individual to individual
- Fingers: direct contact with ocular discharge
- Family: within the family, child to child

Clinical features and diagnosis: see the 5-point WHO grading system opposite. TF and TI are found mainly in pre-school children; TS, TT, and CO occur more commonly in women than men, starting at around the age of 15 and gradually increasing in prevalence.

How to examine the eye for trachoma: use good light (sunlight or strong torch) and ×2–2.5 magnification. Examine each eye separately.
- Look for trichiasis (either inturned lashes or previously removed eyelashes). Push upper lid upwards slightly to expose lid margins.
- Check cornea for opacities.
- Check inside upper eyelid by everting it. Ask the patient to look down; gently take hold of eyelashes between thumb and first finger of left hand, and evert the upper eyelid using a glass rod or similar instrument in the right hand. Steady the everted lid with left thumb and examine the conjunctiva for follicles, intense inflammation, and scarring.

Management
- azithromycin 1 g PO as single dose (20 mg/kg if <45 kg) *or*
- for pregnant women, erythromycin 500 mg PO bd for 7 days *or*
- tetracycline 1% topical ointment both eyes bd for 6 weeks.

Studies are still evaluating the merits of treatment of whole communities vs. just affected individuals. Entropion and trichiasis will require surgery.

Prevention: of trachoma is considered under the acronym SAFE (see box opposite). Control requires first identifying a community with blinding disease. This can be done using the grading scheme and a survey of 1–10 year old children for TF and TI, and women over the age of 15 yrs for TT. A prevalence of TF in excess of 20%, or TT in excess of 1%, would identify a community with severe disease.

Trachoma grading (see colour plate 25)

Signs must be clearly seen in order to be considered present. Grading is important for community prevalence surveys to decide whether mass treatment is warranted.

- **Normal:** the normal conjunctiva is pink, smooth, thin, and transparent. Over the whole area of the tarsal conjunctiva, there are normally large deep-lying blood vessels that run vertically. The dotted line in colour plate 25(a) shows the area to be examined.
- **Trachomatous inflammation — follicular (TF):** the presence of five or more follicles in the upper tarsal conjunctiva. Follicles are round swellings that are paler than the surrounding conjunctiva, appearing white, grey, or yellow. Follicles must be at least 0.5 mm in diameter (see colour plate 25b).
- **Trachomatous inflammation — intense (TI):** pronounced inflammatory thickening of the tarsal conjunctiva that obscures more than half of the normal deep tarsal vessels. The conjunctiva appears red, rough, and thickened. There are numerous follicles, which may be partially or totally covered by the thickened conjunctiva (see colour plate 25c).
- **Trachomatous scarring (TS):** the presence of scarring in the tarsal conjunctiva. Scars are easily visible as white lines, bands, or sheets in the tarsal conjunctiva. They are glistening and fibrous in appearance. Scarring, especially diffuse fibrosis, may obscure the tarsal blood vessels (see colour plate 25d).
- **Trachomatous trichiasis (TT):** at least one eyelash rubs on the eyeball. Evidence of recent removal of inturned eyelashes should also be graded as trichiasis (see colour plate 25e).
- **Corneal opacity (CO):** easily visible corneal opacity over the pupil. The pupil margin is blurred viewed through the opacity. Such corneal opacities cause significant visual impairment (worse than 6/18 vision) and, therefore, visual acuity should be measured (see colour plate 25e).

WHO's 'SAFE' strategy for the global elimination of trachoma

- **S** Surgery for entropion and trichiasis
- **A** Antibiotics for infectious trachoma
- **F** Facial cleanliness to reduce transmission
- **E** Environmental improvements such as control of disease-spreading flies and access to clean water

Specific eye conditions

Vitamin A deficiency and xerophthalmia

Xerophthalmia is due to vitamin A deficiency, which may lead to corneal ulceration and blindness, particularly in association with measles infection. It is a medical emergency, as severe vitamin A deficiency has a high mortality — see 📖 p 648. Patients with acute corneal lesions should be referred, whenever this is possible, to a hospital for treatment of their general condition as well as their eye disease.

Ocular leprosy

Leprosy (📖 p 448) can affect the eyelids, cornea, or pupils by damaging the nerves to the eye or by causing iritis.

Eyelids: nerve damage may occur during a type 1 reaction and cause an inability to close the eye (lagophthalmos), with resulting corneal exposure, ulceration, scarring, and blindness. In the acute stages, systemic treatment of the leprosy reaction may restore nerve function.

Management: requires protection of the cornea when the patient is asleep by applying ointment and strapping the upper eyelid to the cheek. If severe and permanent, or if there is evidence of corneal ulceration, a tarsorrhaphy will be required to protect the cornea. This consists of sewing together the lateral third of the upper and lower eyelid margins.

Cornea: ophthalmic nerve damage results in corneal anaesthesia. The patient does not blink as much as usual and may be unaware of minor trauma to the cornea, causing ulceration, scarring, and blindness.

Management: prevent by early recognition of the problem and educating the patient to protect the cornea during the day by blinking and at night, with ointment and strapping of the eyelid to the cheek. If these measures fail, then a permanent lateral tarsorrhaphy is required.

Pupil: there may be acute anterior uveitis with a red painful eye, and small irregular pupil. This may occur as part of an erythema nodosum leprosum reaction. Leprosy also causes a chronic low-grade anterior uveitis in which the pupil is very small and irregular and will not dilate. The eye is usually white in chronic iritis.

Management: in acute anterior uveitis, the pupil should be dilated immediately and the patient kept on atropine and topical steroids. In chronic anterior uveitis, it is important to keep the pupil dilated and to maintain the patient on mydriatic eye drops for life.

HIV infection and the eye

The ocular manifestations of HIV infection include:
- Herpes zoster ophthalmicus.
- Squamous cell carcinoma of the conjunctiva.
- CMV retinopathy.

Herpes zoster

Presents initially with pain over one side of the head and face followed by a vesicular rash. The eyelids are always involved and there may be a keratitis and iritis, which can cause raised intraocular pressure. The disease is often blinding in HIV-positive patients with corneal involvement and severe intraocular inflammation. Treatment is with oral aciclovir 800 mg 5×/day. This is sometimes the first manifestation of HIV infection, and all patients should receive counselling and an HIV test.

Squamous cell carcinoma of the conjunctiva appears as a raised irregular white lesion, usually on the temporal conjunctiva, that grows to invade the fornices, lids, and cornea. Treatment is by wide surgical excision where possible.

Cytomegalovirus (CMV)

Infection of the retina is the most common opportunistic infection of the eye and a major cause of blindness in AIDS patients. It only occurs when the CD4 count is low (<100), so it occurs late in the disease. Where HAART is available, CMV retinitis has become rare. The appearance is one of red haemorrhages and pale necrotic tissue. It is bilateral in 50% of cases. It is slowly progressive and can destroy the whole retina. Treatment, if available, is with
- ganciclovir 5 mg/kg IV q12 h for 2–3 weeks, then 5 mg/kg/day, or
- foscarnet 60 mg/kg IV q8 h for 2–3 weeks, then 90–120 mg/kg/day.

However, both have severe side-effects and are expensive. Alternatively, ganciclovir can be given by weekly intravitreal injection. This requires much lower doses, with little risk of systemic toxicity, but does carry a risk of endophthalmitis and the inconvenience of weekly intraocular injections.

Onchocerciasis and the eye

Onchocerciasis is an infection of the skin and eye due to the filarial worm *Onchocerca volvulus* (see 📖 p 572). Inflammation can affect the:
- cornea, causing acute punctate keratitis which may lead to sclerosing keratitis and corneal scars.
- iris, causing anterior uveitis and posterior synechiae.
- choroid and retina, causing chorioretinitis, night blindness, and chorioretinal atrophy (most marked temporal to the macula).
- optic nerve, causing optic neuritis and secondary optic atrophy.

No treatment can restore vision that has been lost to onchocerciasis, but annual treatment with ivermectin prevents eye damage in endemic areas.

Dermatology

Section editor   **Terence Ryan**

Introduction

Skin function and failure

The skin is a large and visible organ at the interface of the body and the environment. When it fails, management is based on enhancing or supplementing its functions. These functions are:

1. Protection from the environment: effective barrier function relies on the skin's capacity to repair itself when damaged. Extensive skin damage e.g. burns or toxic epidermal necrolysis, may be fatal.
2. Perception: loss of protective sensation including pain may lead to injury or pressure ulcers. Disease itself may cause discomfort/pain.
3. Thermoregulation: control of cutaneous circulation and sweating prevents potentially fatal cooling and overheating.
4. Communication and display: healthy skin contributes a 'look good, feel good' factor; disease may cause stigma and worsen marriage prospects.

Common problems

Skin disease is among the top 3 reasons people seek health care. The most common problems are:

- Infestations and infections.
- Absent skin: burns and ulcers.
- Sexually transmitted infections affecting skin or mucosae.
- Dermatitis (eczema), psoriasis, and bullous disorders.

Management of skin disease with limited resources

Management of skin disease in low-resource settings is a world apart from the therapies available in private sector or developed world clinics. However, 'high tech' treatments are not essential to good skin care, which may be delivered using locally available resources at low cost.

Care of the skin demands attention to barrier function and, for this, most locally available emollients are usually satisfactory. It is essential to prevent further damage to diseased skin, both from infection (by keeping wounds clean and ensuring good hygiene) and from trauma. 'Off-loading' the skin is important in preventing pressure ulcers. Simple measures prevent further skin damage: well-fitting shoes help prevent foot trauma and hats provide protection from the sun; a blanket may provide warmth, shade, and cover from flies; and injury from fire may be reduced by education and safer cooking devices.

Consider the social aspects of skin disease which may significantly affect quality of life. Stigmatization may occur as a result of skin disfigurement, the unpleasant odour of chronic ulcers, albinism, leprosy, or the cutaneous manifestations of AIDS. The discomfort and disfigurement caused also fuel a market in ineffective remedies; this and overusage of cosmetics contribute to the cycle of poverty.

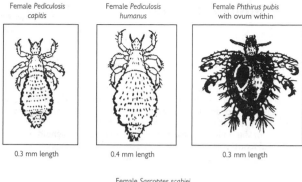

Female *Pediculosis capitis*

0.3 mm length

Female *Pediculosis humanus*

0.4 mm length

Female *Phthirus pubis* with ovum within

0.3 mm length

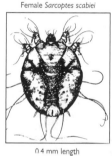

Female *Sarcoptes scabiei*

0.4 mm length

Fig. 14.1 Human head (*P. capitis*), body (*P. humanus*), and pubic (*P. pubis*) lice; and the mite causing scabies (*Sarcoptes scabei*).

Infections of the skin

📖 See Chapter 5.

Skin infestations

Arthropod contact or bites are the most common cause of itch. Papular urticaria and vasculitic lesions may result in sensitive individuals, and heavy infestations may occur in the immunocompromised. An itch–scratch cycle contributes to pyoderma, management of which must include treatment of the underlying infestation. Treatment of household contacts is also an essential part of effective management. Bites from gnats, blackfly, and midges are best prevented by thick clothing.

Lice

There are three species of medical importance: the head louse (*Pediculus capitis*), body louse (*P. humanus*), and pubic or crab louse (*Phthirus pubis*). The body louse is also important as the vector of epidemic typhus (*Rickettsia prowazeki*), relapsing fever (*Borrelia recurrentis*), and trench fever (*Bartonella quintana*).

Transmission is by close personal contact, increased by poverty, over-crowding, and poor hygiene. The lice pierce the skin to take a blood meal, injecting saliva and defecating at the same time. A rash occurs due to a hypersensitivity reaction to the saliva. Blue macules <1 cm in diameter occur during pubic louse infection possibly due to injection of an antico-agulant. Body lice live in the host's clothes, passing onto the skin only to take a blood meal. Head and pubic lice infest the skin directly. Eggs ('nits') are laid and firmly glued to hairs.

Management: For body lice the focus is on laundering. Lice are easily dislodged and readily lay eggs in bedding, towels, and clothing. Clean clothes in a very hot wash, then iron the seams; or dust clothes with 1% malathion powder. For head and pubic lice, apply 0.5% malathion liquid on the affected parts, allow to dry naturally, and remove by washing after 12 h. (Alternatives to malathion in case of resistance: carbaryl 0.5–1%; permethrin 5%; phenothrin 0.2–0.5%.) Detailed information on head lice detection and management is available at *www.health.wa.gov.au/headlice*.

Scabies

Sarcoptes scabiei is transmitted by close personal contact. The female burrows into the epidermis to lay eggs; burrows can be seen as 0.5–1.5 cm long irregular tracks. Sensitization to mite faeces and saliva occurs within a few weeks of 1° infestation. Re-infestation results in almost immediate irritation and, in some cases, a generalized urticaria.

Itchy papules and linear burrows occur in a symmetrical distribution, particularly in the finger webs and on the flexor surface of the wrists (frequent hand washers have fewer lesions on the hands). Other sites commonly include elbows, axillae, genitalia (particularly scrotum), peri-umbilicus, and breasts. Head infestation is common in infants, but unusual

in older age groups. Macules and pustules occur. Scratching results in 2°
bacterial infection. Severe, hyperkeratotic ('Norwegian') scabies is seen in
immunocompromised (e.g. HIV +ve) patients.

Management: Apply malathion 0.5%, permethrin 5% cream, or benzyl-
benzoate 25% to the body and leave on for 24 h before washing off.
Malathion and permethrin are applied twice, 1 week apart. Benzyl benzoate is applied on 3 consecutive days and may require repeated applica-
tions to penetrate the crusts. Sulphur 2–8% creams may be used to
soften the crusts (also safe in babies). Ivermectin 200 mcg/kg PO stat is
an alternative for scabies complicating other skin diseases, for Norwegian
scabies, or for communities such as prisons. All clothing worn the previous day, and the day of the treatment, and all bedding, must be washed.
Iron the laundry or dry for an hour in a hot dryer. Place any un-washable
items into a closed plastic bag for 2 weeks. The eggs will hatch in about
10 days, but scabies aren't able to live away from human skin for more
than 24 h, so the mites will die. Asymptomatic infection is common, so
treat the whole household. *Note:* itching may persist for some days but
does not usually indicate treatment failure.

Trombiculid mites (Chiggers)

Chiggers are the larvae of trombiculid mites, several species of which
may cause an itchy dermatitis. The tiny larvae assemble at the tips of
grass stems and other foliage and then attach to passing mammals and
birds including humans, feeding on the host tissues. Typically, an itchy
dermatitis occurs within a few hours of walking through long grass or
other vegetation. Application of repellents e.g. diethyltoluamide (DEET)
to skin and clothing will help prevent chigger attack.

Ulcers

Ulcers represent the absence of surface layers of skin. They invite infection and require a greatly enhanced blood supply for repair. Reasons for delay in healing may be local (in the wound), general ill health, and/or lack of access to care.

Neuropathic (pressure) ulcers are due to lack of awareness of prolonged compression of blood supply. They occur in the sick and elderly, and in patients with neurological deficits such as paraplegia, diabetic neuropathy, or leprosy. They are preventable with a little knowledge about who is at risk, frequent off-loading, and by encouraging movement. Skin care with washing and emollients and gentle movement is always beneficial since it restores barrier function, reduces entry points for bacteria and irritants, and switches off repair requirements. The skin that is in repair mode is hugely demanding on its blood supply.

Venous ulcers are a consequence of impaired venous emptying, often due to damage to venous valves by trauma or thrombosis. Risk factors include obesity, upright posture, advanced age, and immobility. They occur less commonly in those who frequently sit on the ground in a cross-legged posture or actively use their legs. Their prevalence is increasing.

Arterial ulcers occur due to peripheral vascular disease. Risk factors are those for atherosclerosis, including smoking, diabetes, and advanced age.

Tropical ulcer is a term given to ulcers of the lower leg which commonly occur in persons (especially young men) exposed to the humidity and mud of a prolonged rainy season. They are attributed to mixed aerobic and anaerobic bacterial infection of superficial wounds, usually following minor trauma. A small, round, painful ulcer forms which may then spread rapidly, even exposing the underlying muscles and tendons. The patient may be febrile. After a few weeks, the ulcer stops spreading as the inflammation reduces and the pain diminishes. Some ulcers heal spontaneously leaving a scar; others become chronic and may persist for years.

Sickle cell disease contributes to ulceration of the leg, especially of the ankle after mild trauma, often beginning in early adolescence.

Other causes of ulcers include Buruli ulcer, cutaneous diphtheria, cutaneous leishmaniasis, leprosy, tuberculosis, sexually transmitted infections, non-venereal treponematoses, actinomycosis, chronic osteomyelitis, dracunculiasis, trypanosomal chancre, and the eschars of rickettsiae and anthrax.

Management of ulcers

Management must address the specific causes of ulceration. In addition there are some general principles for management of all ulcers.

Ulcers need covering and should be kept moist. Remove any pus or slough and clean with 1–6% hydrogen peroxide or dilute sodium hypochlorite solution (≤0.5% available chlorine) at each dressing change. Apply clean dressing using short pieces of bandage or well-washed linen that do not completely encircle the leg. Wet dressings with saline or impregnate with honey or coconut oil, and cover to prevent evaporation;

this will soften crusts and encourage healing. Hydrocolloid dressings may be available in some settings. Avoid adherent dressings that remove with them any new epidermis growing in the ulcer base. Beware evaporation during dressing changes, which may cool the ulcer below the optimum temperature for cellular repair. Wash and apply emollient to surrounding skin.

Blood supply to the ulcer should be maintained and optimized by off-loading pressure and encouraging exercise. When the arterial system is healthy, veins must be emptied by elevation and compression. Treat any deep infection (surface contamination does not require antibiotics). Optimize other conditions contributing to poor healing (see box).

Most other causes of delayed healing despite adequate care are to be found in the ulcer. Foreign bodies, pus, necrotic tissue, and sequestra must be removed and oedema treated. Dead tissue can be excised without pain. Maggots, if present, are a cheap and effective way of debriding an ulcer. Green bottle (*Lucilla sericata*) maggots are commercially available in many places; packaged in tea bags their secretions are an effective debriding agent. Large or chronic ulcers may require excision and/or grafting. Local application of *Aloe barbadensis* (Aloe vera) promotes wound healing but, in general, herbal remedies should be avoided in the absence of evidence for their efficacy.

Tropical ulcer: in addition to above measures, give antibiotics to eradicate infection e.g. procaine benzylpenicillin 0.6–1.2 g IM daily for 3–7 days.

Conditions contributing to poor ulcer healing

- Malnutrition
- Vitamin or mineral deficiency.
- Anaemia.
- Systemic infection.
- Steroid therapy, cancer, chemotherapy.
- Diabetes mellitus.
- Heart, renal, or liver failure.
- Immune dysfunction.
- Immobility.
- Smoking.
- Depression, anxiety, and belief in sorcery.

Buruli ulcer

Buruli ulcers are a chronic necrotizing skin disease of tropical forest areas caused by infection with *Mycobacterium ulcerans*. Cases have been reported in east, central, and west Africa, Asia, central and south America, Papua New Guinea, and Australia. The mode of transmission is unknown but possibilities include inoculation by minor trauma, biting insect, or contaminated aerosols of water.

Lesions start as a painless nodule which may be itchy. Some resolve spontaneously, but many enlarge and break down to form a relatively painless ulcer with edges that may be undermined for 5–15 cm. Mycolactone, a bacterial exotoxin, contributes to necrosis and ulcers may spread rapidly to become very large and disfiguring. There are few systemic signs (although lymphadenopathy and lymphoedema may occur). Complications include 2° bacterial infection and tetanus. Without treatment, many lesions eventually slowly heal after a few years, often causing severe scarring, contractures, and deformities.

Diagnosis is based on a typical clinical picture and/or demonstration of acid fast bacilli in the ulcer's base.

Management relies on encouraging early presentation in endemic areas, surgical excision (where possible), and prevention/management of complications. Chemotherapy with anti-mycobacterial agents is generally ineffective. Completely excise nodule if recognized early. At the ulcer stage, treat any 2° infection, irrigate ulcer with saline, and, if resources allow, excise all diseased tissue and cover the wound by skin grafting. To prevent severe contractures every effort should be made to maintain a position of function by massaging with oils and keeping the legs extended for standing and the arms flexed for feeding.

Blistering disorders

Causes of blisters include burns, acute dermatitis from irritants or allergens, infections (e.g. impetigo, fungal infections of the foot), drugs, autoimmune diseases (pemphigus, pemphigoid, dermatitis herpetiformis), genetic disorders (e.g. epidermolysis bullosa), porphyria.

Pemphigus causes fragile, intra-epidermal blisters in adults, usually also affecting the mucosa of the mouth. An increased incidence of its most superficial form (foliaceious pemphigus) has been described in a community in Brazil, occurring as an autoimmune response to insects. Treatment is with high-dose steroids (prednisolone 60–100 mg daily), which may gradually be reduced as the blistering resolves.

Pemphigoid causes sub-epidermal blisters, frequently partially blood-filled. It is seen most commonly in the elderly. It responds well to systemic steroids; mild cases with only a few blisters may respond to topical steroid creams.

Dermatitis herpetiformis causes an itchy papules and vesicles over extensor surfaces and is associated with coeliac disease. Treatment is with dapsone.

Porphyria cutanea tarda is rare. It causes skin fragility (blisters from minor knocks) and blisters in light-exposed sites. Causes include liver disease (including chronic hepatitis C infection) and alcohol abuse.

Stevens–Johnson syndrome is a severe form of erythema multiforme complicated by severe blistering of skin and mucosae including the mouth, eyes, and genitalia, and accompanied systemic features such as fever. The target lesions of erythema multiforme may be evident, but in its most severe form, toxic epidermal necrolysis (TEN, associated with a positive Nikolsky sign) causes widespread blistering of the skin. Other complications include diarrhoea, anterior uveitis, pneumonia, renal failure, and polyarthritis. A wide variety of triggers may be responsible, including drugs (e.g. sulphonamides; thiacetazone in HIV +ve patients), streptococcal infections, viral infections (e.g. HSV Orf), malignancy, and some systemic diseases (e.g. SLE). *Management*: Stop any potential drug trigger. Nurse patients as for extensive burns, with careful attention to fluids, nutrition, and prevention of 2° bacterial infection. In the absence of good nursing care and attention to fluids, the mortality from fluid loss is high. The role of steroids is controversial: they reduce progression but also significantly increase the risk of infection. IV immunoglobulins are sometimes used but large controlled trials are required to confirm their benefit. TEN is associated with a high mortality.

Drug eruptions

Adverse reactions may follow both conventional drugs and alternative remedies. Drug rashes tend to be symmetrical and are commonly erythematous, urticarial, purpuric, or ischaemic. Exfoliation or vesiculation are rare. Drugs are an important cause of Stevens–Johnson syndrome. A fixed drug eruption occurs at the same (fixed) site following a particular drug (e.g. sulphonamides, tetracyclines). It may blister within a few hours of intake and it leaves an annular pigmented mark.

In general, most drugs take >5–10 days to initiate a reaction unless the drug has previously caused a reaction or an infection has 'primed' the body to a medicine (e.g. cough mixture or antibiotics). Drug eruptions occur more commonly in HIV/AIDS.

Management of drug eruptions
- Ask the patient about previous reactions to drugs.
- Stop all drugs likely to have caused the reaction.
- Give prednisolone 1 mg/kg if the reaction is acute and severe.
- In less severe cases, it is possible to restart the drugs one by one to identify the causative drug, but there is a high risk of morbidity and only essential drugs should be restarted. **Do not reintroduce drugs that have caused anaphylaxis, TEN, or severe exfoliative dermatitis**.

Rashes

Basis of rashes

- The skin varies in thickness and quantity of hair or sebaceous glands. Rashes affecting only one component of the skin will have a distribution which reflects this component (e.g. hair follicles in folliculitis or dermatomes in shingles).
- The lesions differ according to the depth of the inflammation. Near the surface it causes vesiculation and scaling, while deep dermal or subcutaneous inflammation results in nodule formation.
- The rate of development is determined by the type of inflammatory response. Erythema, wheals, and blisters are more acute; white cell infiltration, purpura, and pustules take longer; while ischaemic necrosis and exfoliation are more chronic responses.
- The distribution of the lesion may be typical — see Fig. 14.2.
- Endogenous rashes tend to be symmetrical; in contrast, a biting insect produces asymmetric lesions. Unlike the rashes of 2° syphilis, the site of the 1° chancre is not influenced by host symmetry. Fungus infections tend to be more obvious on one side of the body, whereas psoriasis is usually exactly symmetrical.

Pityriasis rosea

Pityriasis rosea is a viral infection of young adults. It begins with a single annular erythematous and scaling lesion on the trunk known as a herald patch; this is followed within a week by an erythematous and usually pruritic rash of the trunk with variable centrifugal spread. The rash resolves spontaneously within a few weeks and does not recur.

Lichen planus

The rash of lichen planus is composed of itchy, flat-topped, shiny, purplish papules which may have fine white 'Wickhams's striae' on the surface; lacy white lesions may also occur on the buccal mucosa. It usually resolves spontaneously over months; topical steroids may reduce irritation.

Common rashes

Maculopapular rashes

Extensive
- Scabies.
- Rubella.
- Measles.
- Body lice.
- 2° syphilis.

Sparse
- Typhoid rose spots.
- Flea bites.
- Gonococcal.
- Lichen planus.

Hypopigmentation
- Post-inflammation.
- Tinca versicolor.
- Vitiligo.
- Pityriasis alba.
- Pinta.
- Post-kala azar dermal leishmaniasis.
- Leprosy.
- Yaws.

Nodules
- Onchocerciasis.
- Fungal infections.
- Erythema nodosum.
- Leprosy.
- KS.
- Cutaneous leishmaniasis.
- Gouty tophi.

Plaques/crusts
- Fungal infections.
- KS.
- Cutaneous leishmaniasis.
- Psoriasis.
- Trypanosomal chancre.
- Impetigo.
- Pinta.
- Eschar (Rickettsia).

Urticaria
- Drugs.
- Gnathostomiasis.
- Strongyloidiasis.
- Schistosomiasis (Katayama fever).
- Loiasis.

Vesicles
- Chickenpox.
- Herpes zoster.
- Herpes simplex.
- Monkey pox.
- Papular urticaria.
- Orf.
- Vasculitis.

Pustules
- Bacterial infection.
- Gonococcaemia.
- Psoriasis.
- Irritant folliculitis.

Petechiae
- Meningococcaemia.
- Typhus.
- Viral haemorrhagic fevers.
- Causes of DIC.

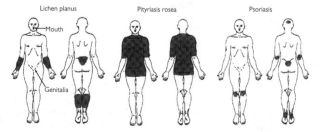

Fig. 14.2 Characteristic distributions of lichen planus, pityriasis rosea, and psoriasis.

Dermatitis (eczema)

An inflammatory reaction of the skin that may occur as a (usually asymmetrical) response to an external irritant or as a symmetrical endogenous response to a stimulus (atopic eczema).

Irritant dermatitis: The most common form of dermatitis, generally affecting the hands following contact with industrial irritants at work. It also affects the feet of barefoot agricultural workers. The skin is dry and unsupple with deep cracks which may become infected. Previously damaged skin is more susceptible to irritants.

Contact allergic dermatitis: Sensitization to an allergen, normally over months or years, results in the onset of dermatitis within hours of subsequent exposure to the allergen (e.g. cosmetics, nickel in zips, buttons, stainless steel watches, or jewellery, food, plants, medicines, metals). Irritant dermatitis is a risk factor for contact dermatitis. Patch testing identifies the specific allergen: suspected allergens are applied to normal skin, usually on the back, and examined at 48 h for redness, swelling, or vesiculation that identifies an allergen.

Atopic eczema: Atopy, which includes asthma and hayfever, is due to an IgE response to foods or environmental agents. Atopy affects up to 15% of children in developed settings, possibly due to altered immunity as a result of increased environmental hygiene and fewer helminths; or increased pollution; or changes in housing encouraging house dust mites. In atopic eczema, the skin is very itchy and dry and it becomes damaged by repeated scratching. 2° bacterial infection frequently occurs, associated with regional lymphadenopathy.

Psoriasis

The classic lesion of psoriasis is a sharply demarcated silvery plaque, often more active at the edge with a clear centre. Initially, or as plaques resolve, they may be atypical (e.g. scaleless, exudative, red). Plaques occur most commonly on knees, elbows, scalp; also navel, natal cleft, hairline. Lesions in flexures have decreased scale and are red, shiny, and liable to crack and macerate. Distinct forms occur:

- *Guttate psoriasis:* small, poorly defined lesions (often red with little silvery scale) that occur across the whole body; often in children after streptococcal sore throat or vaccination.
- *Palmar/plantar psoriasis:* lesions develop deep cracks and sterile pustules; nails often involved. Differentiate from fungal infection.
- *Generalized pustular psoriasis:* fever, arthropathy, bright red erythema followed by the development of multiple pustules. Can occur after stopping prolonged potent steroid therapy. Resolves spontaneously.

Psoriatic arthritis occurs in ~10% patients. 5 patterns are recognized: a small joint arthritis of hands and feet with distal interphalangeal joint involvement (most common); seronegative rheumatoid-like arthritis; large joint mono- or oligo-arthritis; spondylitis; and arthritis mutilans.

Management of dermatitis (eczema)

- Eliminate or avoid known irritants or allergens.
- Avoid soaps (these dry the skin); wash instead with emollients to keep the skin moist.
- Apply steroid creams to affected areas 1–2 times daily. Use the least potent steroid that works, for short periods of time only. Avoid strong steroids in children. A weak steroid (e.g. hydrocortisone 1%) can be used for short periods on the face or in flexures.
- Severe chronic allergy can be relieved by prednisolone and other steroid-sparing immunosuppressive drugs (e.g. azathioprine).
- Treat 2° bacterial infection vigorously.
- Breastfeeding may reduce the risk of atopic eczema. This is worth emphasizing for infants with a family history of eczema.

Management of psoriasis

This is a chronic condition, partly responsive to agents that depress cell turnover and partly responsive to immunosuppressive therapy. Treatment options are:

- Mild cases require reassurance alone.
- Emollients help to restore and maintain barrier function.
- Coal tar derivatives and dithranol ointments and creams are cheap but cosmetically unpleasant. Apply to lesions, starting at a low concentration and gradually increase the concentration.
- Systemic therapy may be required occasionally for generalized illness, particularly in the elderly. Options include methotrexate or ciclosporin. In general, systemic corticosteroids should be avoided.

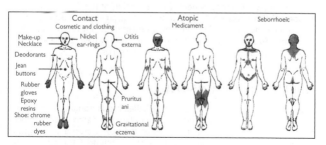

Fig. 14.3 Common patterns of dermatitis/eczema.

Vasculitis

Cutaneous vasculitis may occur in isolation, but often represents similar damage to blood vessels in other organs. Vessel wall damage presents as a range of morphologically distinct skin manifestations, including urticaria, palpable purpura, ulcers, necrosis, livedo reticularis. Superficial lesions may be vesicular/blistering; deep lesions may be nodular (e.g. erythema nodosum) and occasional suppurating. Urticaria occurs more commonly in infants, necrosis more commonly in adults. (*Note*: bruising and non-palpable purpura are more characteristic of platelet deficiency.)

Vascular damage may be mediated by several mechanisms. Commonly, immune complex deposition triggers complement activation and neutrophil infiltration and disintegration, causing a leucocytoclastic vasculitis. Lymphocytic vasculitis is also a common cause, and occurs due to cell-mediated immune responses to e.g. drugs and infections (viruses, bacteria, rickettsia). Antigen excess most commonly occurs in the context of overwhelming acute disease (e.g. streptococcal or meningococcal infection, autoimmune diseases such as SLE, malignancy) or drugs (including herbal remedies). Circulating noxious agents usually localize to the venular bed; arteriolar damage causes infarcts and embolic phenomena. Arthritis is a common, non-threatening association, classically described in Henoch-Schönlein purpura in children (see box).

Prognosis depends on vital organ involvement. Monitor regularly for haematuria as a sign of renal involvement.

Management

- Antibody 'excess' occurs as a physiological mechanism for removal of antigen, and vasculitis frequently resolves spontaneously, particularly in children.
- NSAIDs may help (caution in renal impairment).
- Treatment of infection or severe tissue breakdown eliminates triggers.
- Persistent leg vasculitis benefits from elevation of the limb.
- Consider corticosteroids if multi-organ involvement and fever (caution in severe infections). Mild renal involvement does not require specific therapy. Azathioprine or cyclosphosphamide may have a role in severe disease e.g. URT involvement with necrosis.

Erythema nodosum

This presents as symmetrical, tender, erythematous nodules on the shins or forearms, representing a nodular panniculitis associated with a lymphocytic vasculitis. Some causes are shown in the box opposite. Investigation is directed at underlying causes. It is usual to exclude TB, sarcoid, streptococcal sore throat, and inflammatory bowel disease, but most infections can be an infrequent cause. Treatment is symptomatic (analgesia). Most lesions resolve spontaneously over several days.

Henoch-Schönlein purpura

Henoch-Schönlein purpura is the name given to a syndrome of vasculitis (usually manifest as palpable purpura affecting the legs and buttocks), arthralgia, peri-articular oedema, abdominal pain, and glomerulonephritis, most commonly seen in children. It is an immune complex phenomenon, thought to be due to an environmental precipitant (e.g. streptococcal sore throat) in genetically susceptible individuals. Complications include GI bleeding (due to involvement of the GI mucosa), intussusception, nephritic syndrome; rarely, it may cause a protein-losing enteropathy, orchitis, or CNS involvement. The condition is usually self-limiting. Severe renal involvement may require immunosuppressive therapy.

Causes of erythema nodosum

Infections
- Streptococci
- Tuberculosis
- Chlamydia
- Yersinia
- Histoplasmosis
- Leprosy*

Drugs
- Sulphonamides
- Sulphonylureas
- Oral contraceptive
- Aspirin
- Phenytoin
- Dapsone

Sarcoidosis

Inflammatory bowel disease

Rarer causes include: Behçets disease, rheumatic fever, pregnancy

* See p 451 for erythema nodosum leprosum (ENL)

Causes of erythema multiforme

Infections
- Herpes simplex.
- Mycoplasma.
- Orf.
- Mumps.
- Streptococci.
- Viral hepatitis.

Drugs
- Sulphonamides.
- Sulphonylureas.
- Tetracyclines.
- Thiazides.
- Aspirin.
- Phenytoin.
- Carbamazepine.

Connective tissue diseases (e.g. SLE)

Malignancy

Radiotherapy

Urticaria

Urticaria is characterized by transient wheals (swelling and flushing of the skin) which are often itchy. Individual lesions last 30 minutes to 24 h, although new lesions may continue to develop. The reaction may be accompanied by joint pains, stomach aches, and fever. It occurs when allergens (e.g. food, drugs, helmiths) bind IgE to stimulate the release of inflammatory mediators, such as histamine in the skin, causing dermal oedema. Other triggers include immune complex disease and complement activation (e.g. due to antivenom, penicillins, infections), and the direct effect of some molecules to cause release of histamine in the skin (e.g. drugs such as morphine, shellfish). Urticaria may be a manifestation of vasculitis (e.g. in meningococcal septicaemia), when lesions may be delayed in onset, last many hours, and become purpuric.

- In angioedema, the oedema extends into the subcutaneous tissues. Larger, more solitary lesions lasting 4–48 h may occur, and there may dramatic swelling of the eyes, lips, and oropharynx.
- *Chronic urticaria:* recurrent urticaria over >3 months. Causes include helminth infection, food additives. Often no single aetiology identified.
- *Papular urticaria:* itchy and persistent papules following damage to epidermis, often by insect bite. Lesions intensely pruritic and often blister.
- Dermographism is a common exaggerated response in which a linear wheal surrounded by a flare occurs immediately following a scratch.

Urticaria may be life-threatening when:
- It is part of an anaphylactic reaction.
- Angioedema compromises the airway.
- It is part of a severe systemic disease (e.g. septicaemia, SLE).

Management

Identify and remove/treat the stimulus (check for intestinal helminths, trichinosis, onchocerciasis, dracunculosis, lymphatic filiariasis, strongyloidiasis). Give antihistamine (e.g. Chlorphenamine 4 mg PO 4 hrly; promethazine 10–20 mg tds or 25 mg bd is more sedative). Steroids may help reduce airway inflammation in angioedema. Treat anaphylaxis as on 📖 p 351.

Erythema multiforme

As the name suggests, lesions of erythema multiforme take a variety of forms, including characteristic 'target lesions' — round, erythematous areas with a pale or dusky and sometimes vesicular centre. The rash is symmetrical and typically involves extensor surfaces and the palms and soles. Recognized triggers are summarized in the box on 📖 p 555. It is usually self-limiting.

Disorders of pigmentation

Skin pigmentation is mainly due to melanin ± other endogenous pigments (e.g. bilirubin). Some common causes of hyper- and hypopigmentation are given in the boxes opposite.

Hypopigmentation

Melanin is produced by melanocytes and transferred to keratinocytes in melanosomes. Loss of keratinocytes (exfoliation) therefore causes hypopigmentation, so skin is often paler following inflammation. When due to a mildly dry skin, chapping, or eczema, it is termed **pityriasis** (meaning branny) **alba.** This typically occurs on the face and limbs in children.

Pityriasis versicolor is due to *Pityrosporum* yeasts, themselves slightly brownish, which cause slightly scaly patches of hypopigmentation, especially of the upper trunk. The effect is most marked following sun exposure. In light-skinned individuals, the patches may look hyperpigmented. *Treatment*: regular application of selenium sulphide shampoo for 2–3 weeks; or itraconazole 200 mg daily for a week.

Depigmentation due to tuberculoid leprosy is more chronic, and scale, if present, is more adherent and does not usually exfoliate easily. Hypopigmented patches due to leprosy will be anaesthetic to pinprick.

Vitiligo

Vitiligo is the most important cause of hypopigmentation. Melanocyte death causes patches of complete depigmentation, often in a symmetrical distribution, which may occasionally become generalized. It affects ~2% of the world's population, and can be very disfiguring in those with pigmented skin, triggering unjustified fears of contagion and genetic transmission. There is often a personal or family history of associated autoimmune disease (e.g. thyroid, pernicious anaemia, diabetes). There is some evidence that free radicals mediate melanocyte injury, and lesions may be triggered by minor injuries such as knocks and abrasions.

Treatment is so unsatisfactory that patients should be protected from spending all their income on a search for cures. Early lesions may respond to strong topical steroids but the risk of skin atrophy discourages long-term use. Sun exposure may help, although areas of vitiligo will not tan. PUVA (phototherapy in combination with topical or systemic psoralens that sensitize the skin to ultraviolet radiation) may be more effective. Camouflage with sweat- and seawater-proof creams is tedious to apply but safe and effective. It is a self-help remedy that assuages frequent anger that 'nothing can be done'. For small, disfiguring facial lesions, cosmetic surgical transplantation of epidermis carrying healthy melanocytes is recommended for patients able to afford it.

Albinism

Albinism is caused by genetic defects in the enzyme tyrosinase, which is required for melanin synthesis. Tyrosinase may be either defective (less severe clinical features) or completely absent. Lack of melanin leads to white skin and hair, with red eyes due to a lack of iris pigmentation. Those affected develop potentially fatal squamous cell skin cancers in early adult life. Absence of retinal pigment impairs vision and schooling. In some communities significant stigma is attached to the condition. In certain areas (e.g. Tanzania), special programmes exist to educate communities to manage those affected.

Causes of hyperpigmentation

- Post-inflammatory hyperpigmentation.
- Addison's disease.
- Liver disease.
- Haemochromatosis.
- Acanthosis nigricans.
- Chloasma (melasma).
- Renal failure.
- Drugs (e.g. amiodarone, clofazimine).
- Naevi.
- Melanoma.
- Congenital (e.g. neurofibromatosis, Peutz–Jeghers syndrome).

Causes of hypopigmentation

Congenital
- Albinism.
- Phenylketonuria.
- Tuberous sclerosis.

Acquired
- Post-inflammatory hypopigmentation (including onchocerciasis).
- Pityriasis alba.
- Pityriasis versicolor.
- Vitiligo.
- Tuberculoid leprosy.
- Lichen sclerosis et atrophicus.
- Drugs (e.g. skin-lightening creams).

Skin cancers

The most important risk factor for cutaneous malignancy is sun damage, either long-term exposure to strong sunlight (most skin cancers) or sun burn (melanoma). Melanin pigment protects against sun damage, so lack or loss of melanin in albinism, white-skinned individuals, or depigmenting conditions increases cancer risk. Pale-skinned people should be encouraged to seek shade, use sunscreens on sun-exposed parts of their body, and to wear a hat outdoors. Infants should be protected from sunburn.

Actinic (solar) keratoses

These are pre-malignant, hyperkeratotic, adherent scaly lesions on an erythematous base, which occur post middle age in pale-skinned persons with long-term exposure to the sun. May resolve spontaneously or develop into SCC or BCC. Treat before become malignant. Many respond to emollients. Persistent lesions should be destroyed by curettage, cryotherapy, or daily application of topical fluorouracil cream.

Squamous cell carcinoma (SCC)

SCCs occur in sun-exposed areas. They may develop from actinic keratoses or at the edges of chronic ulcers and areas of inflammation (marjolin's ulcer). Oral lesions occur in long-term smokers. Usually a fleshy dry nodule breaks down to form an ulcerating lesion with hard raised edges. They are locally very invasive. Systemic metastasis rarely occurs. *Management*: early, wide, local excision is essential; local infiltration is often more extensive than is apparent. Removal at visibly obvious margins is often associated with recurrence.

Basal cell carcinoma (BCC)

BCCs occur in sun-exposed areas on the face. A slow-growing papule usually breaks centrally to form an ulcer with a rolled 'pearl-coloured' edge. Local infiltration may gradually cause extensive tissue damage and disfigurement, but they do not metastasize. *Management*: curettage, cauterization, or cryotherapy. (*Note*: the tumour's tendency to spread intradermally beyond the margins visible at the surface.) Fluorouracil cream may be used after surgery. Radiotherapy is also effective.

Melanoma

Any pigmented lesion that is variably coloured, changes shape, thickness, or colour, starts to bleed, or ulcerates, should be considered a potential melanoma. Pigmented satellite lesions around a mole also suggest a melanoma. They frequently originate in moles and are more common in people with many moles, who should be encouraged to examine these regularly and report changes to a doctor. Prognosis depends on the depth and degree of invasion. Melanoma is extremely invasive and may only be recognized following metastasis to the CNS or other sites. The original lesion may be quite innocuous. Management: is immediate, wide local excision.

Common cutaneous viral infections

Herpes simplex

Herpes simplex viruses (HSV-1 and HSV-2) cause various clinical syndromes including mucocutaneous disease, keratitis, encephalitis, and aseptic meningitis. Transmission is by direct contact through mucosal surfaces (oral or genital) or skin abrasions. 1° mucocutaneous disease, incl. gingivostomatitis, pharyngitis, herpes labialis (cold sores), and genital herpes, may be due to either viral subtype, but *recurrent* oral and genital herpes are more commonly due to HSV-1 and HSV-2 respectively.

Typical lesions are initially red and itchy but begin to vesiculate within 24 h. Fever, malaise, and lymphadenopathy are particularly associated with primary infection. A severe form with widespread vesiculation particularly affecting the face (eczema herpeticum) may occur in patients with atopic eczema. HSV may also cause erythema multiforme.

Management: treat herpes labialis with topical aciclovir and more severe infections with oral (200–400 mg 5 times a day) or iv (5–10 mg/kg tds) aciclovir for 5–10 days. Frequent severe recurrences warrant aciclovir prophylaxis (400 mg bd PO for 6–12 months).

Verruca vulgaris (common warts)

Flat, filiform, or verrucous warts caused by human papilloma virus (HPV); often regress spontaneously. They may be troublesome in HIV/AIDS.

Treatment: wart paints (e.g. topical salicylic acid), curettage, cryotherapy.

Poxvirus infections

Molluscum contagiosum

Molluscum contagiosum, caused by a poxvirus, produces 0.2–0.4 cm smooth 'warts' with central umbilication. It is common in children, in whom spontaneous resolution is the rule. Widespread lesions may occur in HIV/AIDS.

Treatment: includes local application of e.g. phenol or trichloracetic acid spiked into the centre of the lesion; cryotherapy.

Smallpox

Smallpox was eradicated in 1976, but is a potential agent of bio-terrorism. Control relies on isolation of cases and vaccination of contacts; there is no effective treatment. It carries ~50% mortality.

Monkeypox and tanapox

These poxviruses, closely related to smallpox, still cause occasional infections. The rash (1 or 2 lesions in tanapox; many covering the whole body in monkeypox) is preceded by a 2–3 day prodromal period with fever and other systemic signs. Lymphadenopathy occurs in monkeypox, characteristically involving both femoral and inguinal nodes. Unlike chickenpox, the lesions are always at the same stage and the peripheries are involved early. Both infections tend to resolve without treatment. Human–human transmission has been reported within households with monkeypox.

Varicella zoster virus

This herpes virus causes chickenpox (varicella) following 1° infection, and shingles (herpes zoster) following reactivation of latent virus in sensory ganglia. Transmission is by respiratory droplet inhalation or contact with vesicular fluid.

Chickenpox is generally a mild infection of children; it may be severe in neonates, adults (especially in pregnancy), and the immunocompromised. There is prodrome of fever, headache, and malaise followed by an itchy erythematous eruption involving the scalp and face and moving distally to involve the trunk. Daily 'crops' of lesions progress from papules to vesicles, pustules, and scabs and all stages may be present at once (cf. poxviruses). *Complications:* 2° bacterial infection is common in children and may cause scarring; pneumonitis (mainly seen in adults, especially smokers); mild encephalitis (ataxia); thrombocytopenia.

Herpes zoster usually occurs only once, often in the elderly or immunosuppressed, affecting just one sensory ganglion and associated dermatome. Scanty distant vesicles may occur due to haematogenous spread, and rarely disseminated zoster may occur in the immunocompromised. Paraesthesia and shooting pains can occur in the affected dermatome for several days before the appearance of a vesicular, erythematous rash and mild fever. The vesicles scab after 3–7 days. Zoster (or zoster scars) in patients <40 years old or in >1 dermatome suggests impaired cell mediated immunity, most commonly due to HIV. *Complications* include:

- Postherpetic neuralgia: may be very painful and difficult to treat. Opiates and/or amitriptyline (10–25 mg nocte) may help.
- Herpes zoster ophthalmica (of the 1st division of the Vth cranial nerve) may be complicated by conjunctivitis, keratitis, and periorbital swelling.
- HIV-associated herpes zoster can be more severe and prolonged, and affect >1 dermatome. Chickenpox is not a feature of HIV.

Management

Antiviral therapy is indicated for herpes zoster and for chickenpox in adolescents, adults, the immunocompromised, and patients with complications; it may be considered for chickenpox in high-risk patients e.g. those with chronic cardiovascular, respiratory, or skin conditions. Treatment should be initiated early, within 72 h of onset of the rash and continued for 7–10 days. Give acyclovir 800 mg PO 5 times daily or 5 mg/kg IV tds in severe infections (10 mg/kg in the immunocompromised). Alternatives for herpes zoster are valaciclovir (1 g PO tds) or famciclovir (500 mg PO tds). Steroids may speed resolution of herpes zoster and reduce incidence of post herpetic neuralgia (controversial).

Chickenpox in children: treat symptoms (paracetamol, topical antipruritics). Cutting fingernails and attention to hygiene ↓ risk of 2° bacterial infection. *In neonates/high-risk groups:* acyclovir may ↓ duration and complications (Oral: 200 mg qds if age <2 y; 20 mg/kg (max 800 mg) qds if ≥2 y. IV: 10–20 mg/kg if age <3 m; 250 mg/m² if 3 m–12 y.)

Cutaneous leishmaniasis (CL)

A widespread disease, caused by different species of Leishmania parasites, that manifests in slightly different ways. *L. tropica* is anthroponotic; the *L. mexicana* and *L. braziliensis* species complexes (New World) and *L. major* (Old World) are zoonoses of rodents, dogs, or other mammals. Transmission occurs following the bite of *Phlebotomus* and *Lutzomyia* sandfly vectors, following which the parasite multiplies in skin macrophages, causing local tissue damage.

Clinical features

Weeks to months after a bite, a nodule develops at the bite site. This grows slowly (up to 5 cm), becomes ulcerated, and is covered by a crust which may drop off to expose a relatively painless ulcer — pain often indicates 2° bacterial infection. The ulcer may be dry or exudative, depending on the species. It heals over months or years, leaving a 'tissue paper' scar. Satellite lesions may occur. 2° infection is uncommon. *L. mexicana* classically causes lesions of the pinna ('chiclero ulcer') that take years to heal, often destroying the pinna.

Certain forms do not resolve spontaneously, but are uncommon compared to the vast numbers of classical CL:

• **Mucocutaneous leishmaniasis (MCL)** only occurs in New World CL. *L. braziliensis* is the most important cause (also occurs with *L. guyanensis*, *L. panamensis*). 2° mucocutaneous lesions develop months to years after 1° lesion has healed. Starting on the upper lip or nostril edge, MCL eventually destroys the mucosa and cartilage of the nasopharynx, larynx, or lips.

• **Disseminated cutaneous leishmaniasis (DCL)** is usually caused by *L. mexicana* or *L. aethiopica*: The 1° nodule spreads slowly without ulceration while 2° lesions appear symmetrically on limbs and face. In individuals unable to mount an appropriate immune response, infection continues to spread and responds only transiently to chemotherapy (anergic DCL).

• **Recidivans leishmaniasis** is usually caused by *L. tropica*, often on the cheek. The lesion heals in the centre but nodules with scanty parasites persist at the edges for years.

Diagnosis

Clinical, supported by identification of Giemsa-stained parasites in skin smears taken from the edge of active ulcers.

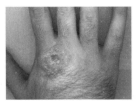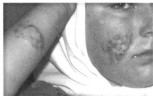

Fig. 14.4 Cutaneous leishmaniasis of the hand due to *L. tropica* (left) and Leishmania recidivans of the face and arm (right).

Local treatments for CL

Suitable for Old World CL (*L. tropica* and *L. major*) and *L. mexicana* as there is no risk of these causing later MCL.

- Intra-lesional infiltration of sodium stibogluconate or meglumine antimoniate is widely used: 1 ml of undiluted antimonial is injected into the base and edges of the lesion This is repeated 2–3 times weekly for 2–3 week. If the injections are very painful, lignocaine 2% can be mixed in the syringe.
- *Leishmania* are killed at 40–42°C, so heating the wound by radiofrequency or heat pads improves healing.
- Cryotherapy is successfully used in Old World CL, either alone or combined with intra-lesional antimonial.
- Topical treatment with paromomycin 15% ointment is effective in *L. major* and *L. mexicana*.

Systemic therapy for Old World CL

L. tropica and *L. major* cause Old World CL, do not cause MCL, and usually self-heal without problems. Only need systemic treatment if:

- Sores too large or badly sited for local therapy.
- Ulcerated or severely inflamed sores, or overlying a joint.
- Disease with lymphatic spread.
- Lesions with involvement of cartilage.

Treatments

- Oral fluconazole 200 mg od for 6 weeks Is effective in *L. major* CL.
- Miltefosine or injections of antimonials or amphotericin B — see below.

Systemic therapy for New World CL

CL from Central or South America could be caused by *L. braziliensis*. If in doubt, consider all New World CL to be *L. braziliensis*, because differentiation from *L. mexicana* is usually impossible geographically, clinically, or parasitologically unless PCR available. Systemic treatment of *L. braziliensis* CL should prevent subsequent MCL.

Treatments

- 10–20 mg/kg/day sodium stibogluconate by IM or slow IV route, or meglumine antimoniate by deep IM for a minimum of 4 weeks, or until lesion healed.
- Pentamidine isethionate 4 mg/kg once or twice weekly until lesion is no longer visible.
- Miltefosine 100 mg/day × 28 days has been successful in many cases.
- MCL responds better to amphotericin B: give initial 1 mg test dose, then 5–10 mg, increasing by 5–10 mg daily up to maximum of 0.5–1 mg/kg administered on alternating days (total cumulative dose of 1–3 g usually required).

Treatment of diffuse CL

- DCL is almost impossible to cure: give sodium stibogluconate or meglumine antimoniate 20 mg/kg IM od for several months after clinical improvement; relapse is common.

Lymphoedema (elephantiasis)

Lymphoedema is caused by obstruction to lymph flow causing regional accumulation of lymph in the soft tissues. There is increased susceptibility to soft tissue infection which causes further lymphatic damage and a vicious cycle of worsening lymphoedema. In some conditions (particularly lymphatic filariasis), chronic trophic skin changes including hyperkeratosis, nodular fibrosis, and excess adiposity may lead to the characteristic appearance of elephantiasis of the affected limb or body part. Causes of lymphoedema include:

- Lymphatic filariasis (see below).
- Malignancy (including lymphatic involvement, radiotherapy, surgery).
- Chronic oedema (e.g. congestive cardiac failure).
- Lymphatic blockage due to TB, leprosy, or KS.
- Podoconiosis.
- Congenital (Milroy's disease).

Management

Involves treating the underlying cause and general measures to promote lymph flow and prevent disease progression and complications (see box).

Lymphatic filariasis

Lymphatic filariasis is caused by 3 geographically distinct species of filarial worm, *Wuchereria bancrofti*, *Brugia malayi*, and *B. timori* (Fig.14.6, 🔲 p 571). Transmission occurs via the bite of mosquito vectors. Infective larvae enter the host during a blood meal and migrate to lymphatics, particularly around the groins and axillae, where they develop into adult worms which may survive >10 years. Females grow up to 10 cm in length (males ~4 cm) and produce microfilaria (~260 μm) which enter the blood stream. Onward transmission occurs when microfilaria are taken up by a mosquito during a blood meal. Host pathology is thought to be due to the immune response to adult worms and endosymbiotic *Wolbachia* (see box). Microfilariae are responsible for tropical pulmonary eosinophilia. In endemic areas, asymptomatic microfilaraemia is common, as are asymptomatic seropositive patients without microfilaraemia.

Acute lymphatic filariasis ('filarial fever') is usually recurrent, most commonly affects the limbs, spermatic cord/testes (funiculitis/epididymo-orchitis ± hydrocoele), and breasts, and encompasses 2 syndromes:
- **Acute filarial lymphangitis (AFL)** caused by death of adult worms leads to a local inflammatory nodule / lymphangitis which spreads *distally*, accompanied by systemic symptoms including fever, rigors, headache, myalgia, arthralgia ±delirium.
- **Acute dermatolymphangioadenitis (ADLA)** due to 2° bacterial infection causes ascending lymphangitis with associated soft tissue infection/inflammation (cellulitis) and systemic upset. Lymphatic damage from recurrent attacks probably causes chronic lymphatic filariasis.

General measures in the management of lymphoedema

The basis of management is the promotion of lymph flow by reducing the gravitational venous load on the impaired lymphatics and preventing the cycle of inflammation and further lymphatic damage. The following simple measures may profoundly improve the outcome of lymphoedema by slowing down or halting disease progression. They also benefit patients with established severe lymphoedema/elephantiasis, as collateral lymphatic channels re-establish lymph flow if kept free from 2° infection, and prevention/treatment of infection reduces social stigma associated with foul smelling, chronically infected tissues.

Minimize risk of further lymphatic damage due to inflammation:
- Wash the affected part twice daily with soap and water.
- Use emollients to promote skin barrier function.
- Wear shoes; keep nails clean.
- Treat minor wounds or abrasions with topical antiseptics.
- Ensure early antibiotic treatment of soft tissue infections.

Promote lymph flow in the affected limb:
- Exercise.
- Raise the affected limb at night.
- Diuretics to reduce the venous load.
- Deep expiratory breathing e.g. chanting (increases venous return).
- Massage of the affected limb.

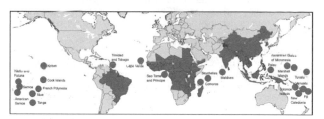

Fig.14.5 Global distribution of lymphatic filariasis which affects 120 million people in 83 countries. (Reproduced from the *Weekly Epidemiological Report*, No.22, 2006, with permission from the WHO.)

Chronic lymphatic filariasis: usually occurs as a result of lymphatic damage from recurrent acute attacks, which continue to complicate and exacerbate the chronic phase of the disease. Clinical features include:

- Hydrocoele, which may be massive and interfere with walking. Usually contains clear, straw-coloured liquid ± blood/lymph; may contain microfilariae. Repeated tapping of fluid causes fibrosis ± abscesses.
- Lymphoedema (elephantiasis) of the legs is common, usually asymmetrical, and starts distally.
- Chyluria and lymphuria are due to rupture into the renal pelvis or bladder of damaged lymphatics draining (i) intestines → fat in urine (chyluria) or (ii) other organs → lymph in urine. Associated haematuria may cause clot retention. Chronic chyluria may cause malabsorption.

Other complications: attributed to lymphatic filariasis, often in the absence of microfilaraemia, include arthritis (esp knee); endomyocardial fibrosis; skin rashes; thrombophlebitis; and nerve palsies.

Microfilarial periodicity: parasitaemia is periodic, peaking at the key biting time of the mosquito vector in a particular location. *W. bancrofti* and *B. malayi* usually exhibit nocturnal periodicity (peak parasitaemia around midnight); in the Pacific, *W. bancrofti* exhibits diurnal periodicity (peak about midday). Nocturnal and diurnal *subperiodic* forms also occur with less marked peaks of parasitaemia at night and day respectively.

Diagnosis: in endemic areas is largely clinical. Parasitological diagnosis relies on isolation of microfilaria from blood, so samples should be taken during peak parasitaemia. The poor sensitivity of stained blood films may be improved by membrane filtration techniques. Simple card tests to detect circulating filarial antigens (CFA) are available for *W. bancrofti* but not *Brugia* species. Serology has a role, particularly in travellers returning from endemic areas.

Management

- Albendazole 400 mg PO bd for 3 weeks kills adult worms but is more effective in combination with diethylcarbamazine (DEC) or Ivermectin.
- Albendazole 400 mg plus either Ivermectin 200 µg/kg or DEC 6 mg/kg, as a single oral dose repeated annually for 5 years, is now used for mass drug administration programmes.
- Avoid DEC in *O. volvulus* and Loa Loa endemic areas due to risk of Mazzotti reaction.
- Avoid DEC during acute attacks as macrofilaricidal activity ± release of *Wolbachia* endotoxins may exacerbate symptoms.
- Ivermectin monotherapy only kills microfilaria so needs to be repeated during the lifetime of the adult worms (may be up to >10 years).
- Doxycycline 100 mg PO bd for 6 weeks (against *Wolbachia*) has been shown to reduce filaraemia and improve lymphoedema.
- Surgical management is required for chronic severe hydrocele. The long-term benefit of surgery for elephantiasis is often limited.
- For general principles of lymphoedema management, see box, p 569.

Wolbachia endosymbionts in human filarial infections

Endosymbiotic *Wolbachia* bacteria (related to *Rickettsia*) live within filarial worms and are now recognized to be important in worm reproduction, development, and pathology. Release from adult worms of *Wolbachia* endotoxins is thought to play a major role in the inflammatory pathology of lymphatic filariasis and onchocerciasis. Early trials of anti-*Wolbachia* chemotherapy with doxycycline have shown significant benefits in both these diseases.

Prevention and public health strategies

- *Prevention*: education to reduce vector–human contact; personal protection from mosquito bites; vector control.
- *Mass drug administration*: is promoted by GAELF (Global Alliance to Eliminate Lymphatic Filariasis) for communities with >5% infection prevalence. The whole community is treated once yearly for 5 years with single-dose Albendazole 400 mg plus either DEC 6 mg/kg or Ivermectin 200μg/kg (avoid DEC in Loa loa or *O. volvulus* endemic areas). Addition of DEC to table salt has been used with success.

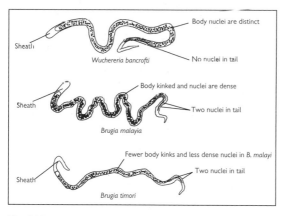

Fig. 14.6 Blood film appearances of the microfilariae lymphatic filariasis.

Onchocerciasis ('river blindness')

Onchocerca volvulus occurs in areas with fast-flowing rivers and biting *Similium* blackflies, the parasite's vector. In the west African savannah, it was a common cause of blindness until the Onchocerciasis Control Programme reduced its prevalence. It still causes blindness and skin manifestations in other areas. Clinical features include:

- Subcutaneous nodules containing adult worms, conspicuous over bony prominences (e.g. iliac crests, ribs, knees, trochanters).
- Cutaneous and eye manifestations due to host inflammatory reactions to dying microfilariae which migrate in the skin (see box) and eye. Ocular lesions include transient punctate keratitis and potentially blinding conditions e.g. sclerosing keratitis, iridocyclitis, and optic atrophy.

Forms of dermal onchocerciasis

- *Acute papular onchodermatitis:* small scattered itchy papules, ± vesicles and pustules, ± skin oedema, often on the trunk and upper limbs.
- *Chronic papular onchodermatitis:* larger itchy, hyperpigmented, often flat-topped papules ± areas of hyperpigmentation.
- *Lichenified onchodermatitis:* itchy, hyperpigmented papulo-nodules or plaques which become confluent. The itching is intense initially; the rash is asymmetrical, often affecting one or both legs.
- *Atrophy:* loss of elasticity with excessive wrinkles particularly on the buttocks; inelastic folds of inguinal skin form hanging groins, often filled with enlarged lymph nodes.
- *Depigmentation* (leopard skin): patches of decreased pigment or loss contrasted with normally pigmented skin around hair follicles.

Diagnosis: confirmed by finding microfliariae in skin snips or the eye. Ask the patient to put their head between their knees for >2 mins before examining the anterior chamber with a slit-lamp. If skin snip and eye examinations are both negative but onchocerciasis is still strongly suspected, perform the Mazzotti test: give DEC 50 mg PO; increased pruritis within 24–48 h indicates that the patient is infected.

Management

- Ivermectin 150 mcg/kg PO stat clears microfilariae from skin for ~6–9 months. Repeat the dose when patient is symptomatic (typically each 6–12 months) throughout the lifespan of the adult worms (15–20 yrs).
- Doxycycline 100 mg PO bd for 4–6 weeks (against *Wolbachia* endosymbionts) can reduce microfilariae in skin for 12–18 months.

Prevention: Ivermectin mass distribution programmes; vector control.

Mazzotti reaction: DEC may → severe adverse reactions in *O. voluvulus* infection due to an immune reaction to worm death. Local reactions include skin rashes, exacerbation of eye lesions; severe systemic reactions may occur with fever, myalgia, arthralgia, respiratory distress, and shock. Avoid DEC therapy in onchocerciasis endemic areas.

Loiasis (Loa loa)

Loa loa is transmitted in the central African rainforests by bites of *Chrysops* horse flies. As the injected filarial larvae mature, they migrate away from the site in the subcutaneous layers (producing itching, prickly sensations) or deeper fascial layers (pain, paraesthesia). Transient 'calabar swellings' of the limbs occur at intervals, lasting between a few hours and days, due to the host immune response to migrating adult worms; the overlying skin is slightly inflamed. Worms migrating beneath the conjunctiva may be clearly visible for minutes to hours, and produce acute eye irritation.

Diagnosis
Clinical or serological; microfilariae can also be found in filtered blood samples collected around mid-day.

Management
Oral DEC 1 mg/kg on day 1; 1 mg/kg bd on day 2; 2 mg/kg bd on day 3, and 2–3 mg/kg tds from day 4–21. Start persons with heavy microfilaraemia at a low dose and give steroid cover for first 2–3 days (risk of meningoencephalitis with dying microfiaria). Check for mixed infection with *O. volvulus* before using DEC — if present, use ivermectin as there is risk of Mazzotti reaction. Doxycycline 100 mg bd PO for 4–6 wks will produce a more gradual reduction of microfilaraemia by acting on endosymbiotic *Wolbachia* within the worms.

Prevention
Avoid vector contact; DEC 300 mg PO once weekly may provide effective prophylaxis; vector control.

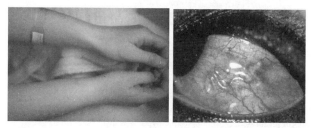

Fig.14.7 Loa loa: calabar swelling (left): this patient noted an uncomfortable swelling in his right forearm which moved up his arm over 3–4 days and then disappeared. A subconjunctival adult worm (right) of Loa loa is seen: this patient felt irritation in his eye and, when looking in the mirror, noted a moblie thread-like worm crossing the eye under his conjunctiva; it disappeared in about 1 hour.

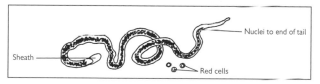

Fig. 14.8 Appearance of Loa loa microfilaria on a blood film.

Dracunculiasis (Guinea worm)

Dracunculus medinensis infection occurs following ingestion of unclean water containing its copepod crustacean vector. Released larvae migrate into body cavities where they mature and mate. Months later, adult females (50–100 cm long) migrate in the subcutaneous layers of the skin to the extremities where an ulcer forms and the tip of the worm protrudes. In contact with water, large numbers of larvae are released from a loop of the worm's uterus which prolapses to the skin surface.

Clinical features: include a systemic hypersensitivity reaction to infection. Protrusion of the gravid female causes a painful blister which may become 2° infected with bacteria. Some worms migrate to sites such as brain, joints, or eyes, resulting in cerebral/subdural abscesses, arthritis, or blindness. Diagnosis is clinical in endemic areas in sub-Saharan Africa.

Management: female worms can be removed before they form a blister by identifying them subcutaneously and making a small incision in the skin at their midpoint and pulling the worm out with careful traction and massage along its track. Metronidazole for 1 week reduces inflammation and eases the removal. After a blister has burst, analgesics will be needed before the worm can be pulled out. Keep the blister clean and covered.

Prevention: involves improving the water supply or filtering drinking water through cloth to remove the crustaceans. The Guinea worm eradication programme has reduced transmission to scattered foci within affected countries.

Other parasites that invade the skin

Cutaneous (furunculoid) myiasis

This is an infestation of the skin with fly larvae (maggots). *Dermatobia hominis* (the tropical botfly) is endemic in Central and South America. Female flies attach their eggs to mosquitoes and other blood-sucking arthropods, which deposit the eggs during a blood meal. Warmth from the host causes the eggs to hatch and larvae penetrate the host skin. In sub-Saharan Africa, female *Cordylobia anthropophaga* (tumbu) flies lay their eggs in shaded soil or clothing hung out to dry (particularly if contaminated by urine); larvae hatch in 2 days and penetrate the skin. In both cases, as each larva grows subcutaneously, a 'boil'-like lesion with a central punctum develops.

Management: removal of the larvae. Occluding punctum with Vaseline or fat may allow larva to be grasped as it emerges for O_2. Surgical removal is sometimes required. Treat any 2° bacterial infection.

Prevention: insect repellents, clothing and mosquito nets for *D. hominis*; ironing clothing (incl. underwear) destroys the eggs of *C. anthropophaga*.

Tungiasis (*Tunga penetrans*, the Jigger Flea)

The 1 mm female pig flea burrows into the skin, usually of the toe webspaces, and grows to about 1 cm in 2 weeks. The female discharges its eggs on the surface and its collapsed carcass is extruded.

Management: careful removal of the flea and its eggs. Avoid 2° bacterial infection.

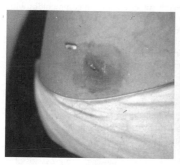
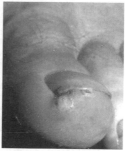

Fig. 14.9 (a) Furunculoid myiasis: this traveller developed a 'boil' on her buttock soon after return from Africa from which the larva of *Cordylobia anthropophaga* (the 'tumbu fly') was extracted. (b) Tunga penetrans (the 'jigger flea'): two lesions are seen at the edge of the toenail.

Cutaneous larva migrans

Infection with filariform larvae of canine hookworms (*Ancylostoma caninum* or *A. braziliense*) for whom humans are accidental hosts. Larvae migrate 1–2 cm per day in the skin, leaving an intensely itchy, red irregular track, before they eventually die.

Management: single-dose albendazole 400 mg by mouth. Thiabendazole cream or 10–15% suspension can also be applied topically. Untreated, the rash will eventually resolve spontaneously.

Larva currens

A cutaneous eruption resulting from autoinfection into the skin (often of the buttocks/perianal area) by *Strongyloides stercoralis*. The urticarial wheals are linear and move ~1–2 cm per hour; the abdomen and buttocks are most affected.

Podoconiosis

Podoconiosis is a cause of lymphoedema in certain highland areas of east and central Africa rich in volcanic soils. Microscopic mineral particles penetrate the dermis of the sole of the foot and cause chronic lymphatic damage, especially in young adults who habitually walk barefoot.

The non-venereal treponematoses

These disfiguring conditions primarily affect children in communities with poor hygiene. Like syphilis, they have three stages, with a long period of latency before the manifestation of 3° disease. Unlike syphilis, the 3° lesions are infective, which causes problems for their eradication since it is difficult to identify latent carriers. Transmission is by direct contact, probably through abrasions (spirochetes cannot penetrate intact skin).

Clinical features

- **Yaws:** the 1° lesion is a papule which develops into a round/oval 2–5 cm painless, itchy papilloma. It normally heals in 3–6 months. Weeks to years after this lesion resolves, multiple 2° lesions occur in crops on any part of the body and last up to 6 months. They are papules or papillomas of various shapes; they may ulcerate and form yellow-brown scabs. Other lesions include dermatitis or hyperkeratosis of palms and soles; local lymphadenopathy; dactylitis; long bone swelling; rarely, osteitis of nasal bones. After a latent period, the disease reappears with necrotic destruction of skin and bones (gummas). Other clinical features include hyperkeratosis; palatal destruction and 2° infection; sabre tibia; bursitis.
- **Endemic syphilis (bejel):** 1° lesion is rarely seen. The first lesions are usually painless ulcers of lips and oropharynx. There is osteoperiostitis of long bones, condylomata lata, angular stomatitis; rarely a 2° syphilis-like rash; and generalized lymphadenopathy. Late lesions include bone destruction (as in yaws), skin ulcers, and palmar and plantar keratosis.
- **Pinta** primarily affects the skin. Satellite lesions surround the 1° papule; there is regional painless lymphadenopathy. 2° stage plaques appear within a few months anywhere on the body. The 3° disease involves depigmentation and atrophy of the skin.

	Yaws	Bejel	Pinta
Organism	*T. pertenue*	*T. pallidum*	*T. carateum*
Age group	15–40	2–10	10–30
Occurrence	Africa	Africa	Latin America
	S. America	Middle East	
	Oceania	Asia	
Climate	Warm, humid	Dry, arid	Warm

Diagnosis

Motile spirochaetes can be seen on dark-field microscopy of lesion exudates. There are no serological or morphological features that differentiate syphilis-causing *T. pallidum* from the other treponemes. The precise diagnosis is clinical.

Management

A single dose of benzathine penicillin G 0.9 g IM (alternatives: erythromicin 250–500 mg PO qds or amoxicillin 500 mg tds for 15 days).

Prevention: identification of active cases, followed by treatment of all contacts. If >10% in a community are actively infected, all should receive penicillin.

Bone, joint, and soft tissue infections

Section editor   **Tony Berendt**

Infections of skin

Skin infections can be divided into:
- Pyodermas: pus is formed within the skin; a localized infection.
- Spreading infections: diffuse infection spreading along tissue planes.

Pyodermas

1. Impetigo
Superficial infection of the epidermis, often at sites of skin damage (e.g. cuts, eczema, chickenpox, scabies, insect bites). A golden-yellow vesicle quickly bursts to become an area of epidermal loss, which crusts over and enlarges. There may be a little pus under the edges of the lesion. Impetigo is highly contagious: 1° lesion → satellite lesions elsewhere on the skin (spread by patient's own fingers) → infection of contacts. *Staph aureus* and *Strep pyogenes* are most commonly found, often together.

Management
- Give systemic antibiotics (see Table 15.1).
- Apply topical antiseptics (e.g. Gentian violet or chlorhexidine).
- Soak off crusts in saline or weak antiseptic.

2. Furuncles (boils), carbuncles, and abscesses
Staph aureus causes abscesses in the dermis or subcutaneous fat. A furuncle (boil, pimple) is pus collecting in a hair follicle or a sebaceous/sweat gland in the skin. Carbuncles are furuncles that have spread deeper (often 2° to patient squeezing or sitting on the furuncle), so multiple points of pus occur. An abscess is a collection of pus at a deeper level — indicated by swelling, erythema, warmth, and fluctuance. Tenderness is common in all skin infections, but pressure on an abscess is very painful.

Management
- Drain pus and remove necrotic tissue and debris. The abscess cavity should be packed and left to heal by 2° intention — do not suture or allow the opening to close until the interior has healed.
- If the infection spreads in the surrounding soft tissues, give 1–2 wks of antibiotics (see Table 15.1). If antibiotics are unavailable or in short supply, drainage and good wound care alone may suffice.

Spreading infections
These are more commonly caused by beta-haemolytic *Streptococci* (BHS) (e.g. Group A BHS, also known as *Strep pyogenes*) than by *Staph aureus*, except when surrounding a staphylococcal abscess.

1. Erysipelas
Spreading infection in the epidermis, producing a large area of red, shiny, tender skin. The patient is unwell and febrile. The involved area is sharply demarcated from normal skin because the dermo-epidermal junction limits the spread of the inflammatory response in a lateral direction. Erysipelas is common on the face. Severe infection produces skin blistering; necrotic tissue encourages toxin production so the infection becomes worse if the infection is not treated.

Management: antibiotics (see Table 15.1).

Soft tissue infections

Insect bites, reduced access to antibiotics, poverty, and malnutrition contribute to a high incidence of soft tissue infections in the tropics. Some conditions, such as pyomyositis (infection of muscle), are particularly common in the tropics compared to temperate zones.

Table 15.1 Causative organisms and antibiotic choices

Condition	Microbiology	Treatment choices	Duration
Superficial infections			
Impetigo Furuncles Abscesses Carbuncles Erysipelas Cellulitis Bursitis	Group A beta- haemolytic streptococci *Staph aureus*	1st flucloxacillin *or* co-amoxiclav 2nd cephalosporin 3rd erythromycin or clindamycin 4th co trimoxazole If associated chronic ulcer, wound, water contact, or trauma, add ciprofloxacin + metronidazole	Until clinical resolution, usually 5–14 days
Deep Infections			
Acute septic arthritis Osteomyelitis Pyomyositis Necrotizing fasciitis	*Staph aureus* Group A beta- haemolytic streptococci; Mixed flora	1st cephalosporin + clindamycin 2nd co-amoxiclav If associated wound, diabetes, ulcer, or water contact, add ciprofloxacin + metronidazole	>6 weeks or until clinically cured for >1 week or until ESR normal for >1 week

Usual adult doses

Intravenous route:
Benzylpenicillin 1.2–2.4 g IV q6 h
Flucloxacillin 1–2 g IV q6 h
Cefuroxime 750 mg–1.5 g IV or IM q6 h to q8 h
Co-amoxiclav 1.2 g IV q8 h
Erythromycin 500 mg–1 g IV q6 h
Clindamycin, ciprofloxacin, erythromycin, and metronidazole are all very well absorbed PO and seldom require IV administration

Oral route:
Oral flucloxacillin and cefuroxamine have incomplete bioavailability; not advised for severe infection. Penicillin is incompletely absorbed, so choose amoxicillin 0.5–1 g PO tds or ampicillin 0.5–1 g PO qds
Flucloxacillin 500 mg–1 g PO qds
Cefuroxime 250 mg PO bd
Co-amoxiclav 625 mg PO tds
Erythromycin 500 mg PO q6 h
Clindamycin 300 mg PO q6 h
Ciprofloxacin 500 mg PO bd
Metronidazole 800 mg PO initially, then 400–500 mg PO tds; or Ig tds PR

2. Cellulitis

Infection involves the dermis and usually subcutaneous fat as well. There is obvious diffuse swelling and the erythematous area is not so clearly demarcated from uninvolved skin as it is in erysipelas. It commonly involves the lower leg, spreading from breaks in the skin: minor injuries, fungal infection (eg. athlete's foot), scabies, or insect bites which have been scratched. Always bear in mind an underlying abscess, which may form within cellulitis, especially in the hand. When cellulitis is near the knee or elbow but spares the extremity, consider an underlying prepatellar, pretibial, or olecranon bursitis.

Management: see box
Scaling and desquamation are normal after some days of infection; blisters may require aspiration but generally protect the lesion and should be left intact in most cases. Subcutaneous abscesses can develop despite antibiotics. Recurrence is relatively common: if multiple recurrences occur, prolonged courses of treatment, long-term prophylaxis, or standby antibiotics to take at the onset of symptoms can be helpful.

3. Bursitis

Bursitis most commonly involves the elbow or the knee, and presents as cellulitis over the joint, or as a red painful swelling. The pathogens are usually BHS or *Staph. aureus*. Although bursitis often restricts the movement of the joint, this is related to the mechanical effects of the swelling and the associated tenderness of the soft tissues, and careful examination can usually distinguish bursitis from the much more serious condition of septic arthritis.

Management: (see box)
In chronic bursitis, suspect TB, underlying osteomyelitis (erosion of bone detectable on X-ray), or chronic septic arthritis.

4. Necrotizing fasciitis

Necrotizing fasciitis is a medical and surgical emergency with high mortality. The most common cause is Group A BHS, but other organisms (e.g. *Vibrio vulnificus* acquired from contact with water, or mixed aerobe/anaerobe infections following abdominal or perineal wounds) can also cause necrotizing fasciitis.

Infection spreads very rapidly in the loose connective tissue adjacent to the fascial plane, leading to necrosis of subcutaneous tissues and thrombosis of blood vessels that supply the skin or muscle. The pace of spread and severity of the underlying process are greater than the time it takes devascularized skin to necrose. As a result, necrotizing fasciitis typically causes severe systemic upset (often with high fever and shock) and pain that seem disproportionate to the local physical signs.

Management: see box
Development of fixed tissue staining, echymoses, superficial blistering (early in disease, not late as in cellulitis, and on obviously unhealthy skin) makes the diagnosis probable.

MRSA

Methicillin resistance occurs in clones of *Staph aureus* that have a mutation in the penicillin binding protein on their surface. Methicillin resistance indicates resistance to all beta lactam antibiotics, including flucloxacillin and co-amoxiclav. Methicillin-resistant *Staph aureus* (MRSA) is becoming more common in developing countries and, in particular, in large centres. By 2006, >20% of *Staph aureus* isolates in large urban hospitals in South America, India, Sri Lanka, Kenya, South Africa, Nigeria, and Cameroon, and in many other countries were MRSA. In rural settings, the prevalence of MRSA is far lower — but increasing. Thus, whilst flucloxacillin, co-amoxiclav, and cephalosporins are still recommended as 1st line treatment for bone, joint, and soft tissue infections, it should always be borne in mind that poor clinical response may indicate MRSA. In centres in which MRSA is prevalent, empiric treatment for *Staph aureus* infections is with vancomycin or teicoplanin. In most areas, doxycycline has high activity against MRSA, and in many areas chloramphenicol and fucidic acid are effective. Rifampicin, although effective against most MRSA strains, is generally restricted for use in TB.

It is important to establish whether MRSA is prevalent in the locations you are working; whether specimens can be sent for culture and sensitivity; and what antibiotics remain effective against the local strain of MRSA.

Management of cellulitis
- Antibiotics for 1 week or longer.
- If cellulitis is 2° to a chronic ulcer, in a diabetic, or follows water contact, broaden the antibiotic cover to include Gram −ve rods and anaerobes.
- Consider wound debridement and cleaning.
- Drain underlying abscesses (esp. in the hand).
- Rest and elevate the limb.

Management of bursitis
- Antibiotics for 2–3 weeks.
- Needle aspiration to remove some pus without surgery — this is useful for diagnosis and symptom relief.
- Avoid incision and drainage where possible: the synovial fluid produced in the bursa produces high-volume wound drainage, can delay healing, and sometimes produces a synovial fistula.

Management of necrotizing fasciitis
- Early surgery is mandatory: explore the fascial plane and excise the affected area back to bleeding tissue.
- Broad-spectrum antibiotics: high-dose penicillin plus gentamicin plus metronidazole is a good 1st choice. Where available, add clindamycin (beneficial in animal models of necrotizing fasciitis). Adjust antibiotics when cultures are available from surgical samples.
- Intensive care support and reconstructive surgery — without these, prognosis is poor.

Infections of muscle

Pyomyositis

Also called 'tropical pyomyositis', it is a 1° bacterial infection of striated muscle that is common throughout the tropics and subtropics, particularly in young men.

Clinical features

There are three characteristic phases:

1. *Woody phase*: the affected muscle is painful, hard, and woody on palpation. The patient may have little systemic illness; this phase may last for days–months. The condition is difficult to diagnose, and can sometimes be mistaken for a tumour.
2. *The muscle liquefies* → intramuscular abscess, with a very tender swollen muscle. Ultrasound shows intramuscular collections; for psoas abscess, CT or MRI scanning may be necessary. (Note: psoas abscess is also a complication of lumbar spinal infections and does not always represent 'pure' pyomyositis.) Gram stain and culture of pus usually reveals *Staph. aureus* (rarely BHS).
3. A bacteraemic illness ± ?multiple abscesses in different muscles.

Management

- Antibiotics for >3 weeks.
- Drain abscesses surgically or percutaneously, depending on circumstances.

The overall prognosis is generally good.

Gas gangrene

A spreading and necrotizing infection within muscle, characterized by severe systemic illness, muscle pain, and crepitus due to gas formation. Gas gangrene is generally caused by *Clostridium perfringens*, which produces toxins that cause muscle necrosis. The infection is acquired through environmental (particularly soil) contamination of deep wounds involving muscle.

Management

- For established gas gangrene, extensive surgical removal of dead tissue is needed, often with excision of massive areas of muscle (for trunk wounds) and early amputation (for limb infection).
- The effect of the toxin on the whole body means that without successful treatment, the infection is fatal.
- High-dose penicillin is important, but unlikely to be effective without surgery.

Prevention

Through good wound care/wound debridement.

Septic tenosynovitis

Infections of the tendon sheath occur predominantly in the hand and the traumatized foot (including the chronically ulcerated).

Aetiology: as well as common bacteria, tenosynovitis in the non-traumatized hand can be caused by atypical mycobacteria such as *M. marinum*, *M. cheloniae*, and *M. kansasii*, and environmental fungi such as *Sporothrix schenkii*. If related to trauma or ulceration, a wide range of organisms may be involved. It can also occur 2° to disseminated gonococcal infection, sepsis with other bacteria, or *M. tuberculosis*.

Clinical features: swelling of one or more fingers, palm, or dorsum of the hand. Swelling in the foot can be minimal if fluid drains via an ulcer.

Diagnosis: can be clinical, confirmed by surgery, or made with ultrasound or MRI.

Management
- Generally requires drainage of the involved tendon sheath — to control the infection and to prevent adhesions and long-term stiffness.
- Tendons heal slowly if exposed — soft tissue or skin cover is important.
- See Table 15.1 for antibiotics: for pyogenic infections, treat for 2–4 weeks; for mycobacterial or fungal infections, use standard courses for the pathogen.

Septic arthritis

Bacteria infect the joint by blood spread or by direct inoculation (trauma, ulceration, or iatrogenic). Bacterial multiplication in the joint leads to acute inflammation — this causes destruction of articular cartilage and resorption of exposed bone, resulting in deformity, chronic osteomyelitis, and even joint fusion. Bacteraemia and septicaemia may occur. If pus tracks and discharges externally, a sinus is formed.

Clinical features

Although most cases of acute or chronic infection involve a single joint, multiple joint involvement occurs in 5–10% of cases.

- *Acute septic arthritis*: fever, pain, and loss of function. The joint is highly irritable; the patient resists both active and passive movement. Usually, the joint is obviously swollen, warm, and tender to touch, with little or no erythema unless accompanied by bursitis or cellulitis.
- *Chronic septic arthritis*: swollen and painful joint, but little systemic illness. There may be obvious deformity or crepitus from gross joint destruction.

Complications

Without timely and effective treatment, joint destruction ensues. There may be osteomyelitis, septicaemia, and — in the young child — growth plate disturbances leading to deformity or limb length discrepancy. Complications are much more likely if treatment is delayed.

Diagnosis

FBC, CRP, ESR, and biochemistry assess patient's general state but lack specificity. Plain X-rays determine extent of joint damage. MRI reveals the extent of bone and soft tissue infection, and aids surgical planning. Blood cultures are positive in <50%. Microscopy of aspirated synovial fluid shows neutrophils; bacteria may be seen on Gram stain; cultures often positive if antibiotics have not been previously given.

Management

- Systemic antibiotics penetrate inflamed joints well. For uncomplicated infections of normal joints, treat for 2 wks for streptococci and 3 wks for staphylococci and Gram −ve bacteria. Even shorter durations of therapy can be used for gonococcal arthritis. In joints with extensive pre-existing arthritis and exposed bone, or in compromised hosts (rheumatoid arthritis is a good example of both), treat for longer.
- Infections of the hip and shoulder joints require arthrotomy or arthroscopic washout.
- Infections in other joints can often be managed by a diagnostic tap before antibiotic therapy, followed by daily aspirates. Proceed to surgery if it fails to settle within 5 days. There is no place for continuous irrigation of the joint: this carries the risk of introducing antibiotic-resistant bacteria (e.g. *Pseudomonas*).
- Chronic septic arthritis generally requires surgery.

Causes of bone and joint infections

- Skin infections can seed via the bloodstream to give septic arthritis and acute osteomyelitis.
- If ineffectively treated, these acute conditions become chronic (e.g. when surgery is unavailable and prolonged courses of antibiotics are unaffordable).
- Major cause is injuries on roads and in factories, armed conflict, and landmine injuries.
- Some 1° infections of bone and joint are more common in the tropics: TB, brucellosis, melioidosis, histoplasmosis, and blastomycosis.

Organisms causing acute septic arthritis

- *Staph. aureus* — most common in all age groups and all countries.
- *Haemophilus influenzae* — in populations without access to HIB vaccine.
- Beta-haemolytic streptococci of all groups (including Group B in pregnancy, neonates, and diabetics).
- Enterobacteriaciae (e.g. *E. coli*) — in neonates and elderly.
- *N. gonorrhoeae* — in sexually active individuals.

Organisms causing chronic septic arthritis

- The same organisms as acute septic arthritis, plus:
- *M. tuberculosis*.
- *Brucella*.
- Occasionally, fungi (e.g. *Sporothrix schenkii*).

Osteomyelitis

Acute 1° haematogenous bone infection presents in a similar fashion to acute septic arthritis. Chronic osteomyelitis may follow septic arthritis, but is also seen in spinal infections (discitis and vertebral osteomyelitis), fracture-fixation infections, and the diabetic foot. Organisms causing acute osteomyelitis are largely the same as those causing acute septic arthritis.

Clinical features

- *Acute osteomyelitis*: fever, localized bone pain, and loss of limb function. Osteomyelitis can cause septic arthritis, especially in young children.
- *Chronic osteomyelitis*: chronic drainage from wound or sinus tract, pain, flares of intercurrent acute infection, impaired function, and/or chronic ill health. Visible or palpable bone in a wound makes osteomyelitis highly likely. An orthopaedic implant or an open fracture with a chronically draining wound is almost certainly infected.

Diagnosis: anaemia, ↑WBC, ↑CRP, ↑ESR indicate the ill health of acute or chronic infection.

- *X-rays*: become abnormal after 7–10 days, as involved bone is demineralized (lytic areas), attempts to heal (periosteal reaction), and in parts dies (sclerotic areas). Changes evolve over a few weeks; the process is aggressive. There may be evidence of loosening of metalware.
- *Other imaging:* US can show abscesses adjacent to bone and delineate sinus tracts. CT is useful for assessing bony union, bone destruction, and sequestrum formation and soft tissue collections. MRI detects marrow oedema, cortical breaches, sinus tracts, and soft tissue collections, but is less useful in patients with extensive metalware or recent surgery.

Treatment

- For acute osteomyelitis: give antibiotics (see Table 15.1) for >4 weeks. Use IV, then perhaps oral route. Evaluate need for surgery.
- For chronic osteomyelitis: evaluate surgery, patient's general fitness, and goals of treatment.

Control of intermittent flares — esp. if flares infrequent and respond to antibiotics. Monitor for progression of bone involvement.

Suppression with long-term antibiotics — if surgery impossible for technical reasons, unaffordable, or worse than disease. Long-term antibiotics can lead to drying of sinuses, improvements in general health, and reductions in pain.

Surgical exploration, debridement, and excision — with subsequent antibiotics. Aim to remove all dead bone, ensuring the skeleton is stable and soft tissue covers the bone at the end of surgery. Dead space inside debrided bone can be filled with muscle, cancellous bone graft (usually delayed until infection is arrested), or antibiotic-laden carriers. Antibiotics added to acrylic bone cement will generate very high local levels. With expert surgery, >90% of cases can be arrested. However, even without surgery or antibiotics, spontaneous long-term arrest can occur if sequestra discharge spontaneously. Many patients can live with their bone infection for long periods; in some situations, this may be the best that can be achieved.

Spinal infections

Common causes are *Staph. aureus*, *Brucella* spp, and TB. Initial blood-borne seeding to disc space is followed by involvement of adjacent vertebral bodies. Paraspinal muscles may also become involved, with collections (e.g. psoas abscesses). Retropulsion of disc and inflammatory tissue, or spinal epidural abscess, may compress the spinal cord, resulting in paralysis.

Clinical features: unusually severe backache, especially night pain; sudden paraparesis on a background of back pain and/or fever.

Diagnosis: plain X-rays may show irregularity and destruction of end-plates adjoining the infected disc space (which becomes reduced in height). MRI is best investigation. CXR or sputum examination may provide evidence of TB; the organism may be cultured from blood, aspirate of paraspinal or disc space abscesses, or guided biopsy of the disc.

Management
- Antibiotics (see Table 15.1). Treat pyogenic infections of the spine for 6–12 weeks.
- Surgery is reserved for cases with acute spinal epidural abscess, persistent pain, mechanical instability, recurrent infection with abscess formation, or cord compression.

Patients with spinal TB infection may recover neurologically on anti-TB medication, even if presenting with paralysis.

The diabetic foot

The dramatic worldwide increase in type II diabetes has brought an increase in patients with foot complications. These arise from diabetic peripheral neuropathy, with or without ischaemia, plus impaired systemic resistance to infection. A foot ulcer precedes most amputations in diabetics; most patients undergoing amputation for non-traumatic causes are diabetic. Good long-term glycaemic control is important.

- Motor neuropathy leads to increased curvature and height of the arch of the foot, resulting in hyperextension and subluxation at MP joints, and clawing at the IP joints. This produces pressure on metatarsal heads, heel and clawed toes, the tips of toes, and over the PIP joints.
- These deformities co-exist with a sensory neuropathy which means that the patient does not perceive pain until too late (or not at all).
- The patient may also sustain penetrating injuries or burns without knowing.
- The autonomic neuropathy results in dry, fissured skin which is more susceptible to injury and infection.
- There is also impaired white cell function.
- Peripheral vascular disease, if present, further impairs healing of ulcers.

Clinical features

Soft tissue infection and loss, draining sinuses with exposed bone, sometimes necrotizing fasciitis or septicaemia. Purulent drainage suggests infection, as does erythema, swelling, pain (which often occurs to some extent, despite neuropathy), and systemic symptoms.

Diagnosis: Blood tests may show ↑WBC, ↑CRP, ↑ESR, ↑glucose, and ↑creatinine. Plain foot X-rays may show gas in the soft tissues, bone destruction, and/or changes consistent with infection or diabetic osteopathy. Serial X-rays may show progressive changes over weeks. MRI is best imaging.

Management

- Assess fever, cardiovascular stability, hydration, and diabetic control.
- Examine sensation, peripheral perfusion (Buerger's test, palpation of pulses, and Doppler assessment including ankle-brachial pressure indices), and presence of cellulitis, necrosis, swelling, or crepitus.
- Debride the ulcer to determine its extent. If possible, probe with a sterile metal probe: palpable bone suggests underlying osteomyelitis.
- See Table 15.1 for antibiotics. Durations: (a) 72 h for amputation through healthy tissue; (b) 1–2 wks for amputation through infected soft tissue, without residual infected bone; (c) 4 wks for amputation or surgery through ischaemic or severely infected soft tissues, including deep tissue involvement (e.g. tendon sheaths); (d) 4–6 wks for osteomyelitis, fully resected, with restoration of soft tissue cover; (e) 6–12 wks for osteomyelitis with residual infected or dead bone.
- Surgery for significant soft tissue necrosis, abscess drainage, or bone death.
- Vascular surgical input if ischaemic; may be able to avoid amputation.

Prevention

Diabetic foot ulcers often recur without special attention to foot care and footwear. Appropriate long-term care, with offloading of pressure points, is also essential to obtain 1° healing of ulcers, even if not infected. Improve glycaemic control, stop smoking, and control blood pressure.

Fungal skin infections

Cutaneous infections

Dermatophytoses (tinea): common skin infections caused by fungi, particularly *Trichophyton* and *Microsporum* spp. They cause scaling or maceration between the toes (tinea pedis); itchy, scaly, red rash with definite edges in the groin area (tinea cruris); annular lesions with raised edges (often itchy) anywhere on the body (tinea corporis); scaling and itching of the scalp with loss of hair (tinea capitis). Treat with local application of Whitfield's ointment (benzoic acid compound) or clotrimazole for 2–4 weeks; for severe cases and nail involvement, use 4–6 weeks of griseofulvin 10 mg/kg PO (alternatives: terbinafine or itraconazole).

- *Pityriasis versicolor:* a superficial, hypopigmented, macular rash normally of the upper body. If extensive, can indicate a cause of chronic sweating (e.g. TB or AIDS). Treat with 2% selenium sulfide shampoo, Whitfield's ointment, or itraconazole 200 mg PO od for 5 days.
- *Superficial candidosis:* in addition to vaginal and oral infection, *C. albicans* can infect moist folds of skin (groin, under breasts, nappy area of baby) producing a very red rash and skin damage. Treat with topical nystatin or clotrimazole and keep dry.

Subcutaneous infections

1. *Mycetoma (Madura foot):* chronic infection of subcutaneous tissue, bone, and skin that is due to environmental organisms, either fungi (eumycetes, producing eumycetomas) or bacteria (actinomycetes or *Nocardia* spp. producing actinomycetomas), probably introduced into deep tissue by a thorn. The infecting organisms grow very slowly, typically forming 'grains' that are macroscopic colonies of fungi or bacteria. Mycetomas commonly occur on the foot or leg, but may occur anywhere. They start as an area of hard swelling; infection eventually spreads from subcutaneous tissues to invade and destroy bone. There is considerable swelling and usually multiple sinus tract formation, through which grains may discharge, but pain is rarely severe.

Diagnosis: On X-ray, underlying bone is expanded, eroded, and ultimately destroyed. There is some local lymphatic involvement. The cause needs to be determined by microscopy of the sinus discharge.

Management: fungal mycetomas rarely respond to systemic antifungals and frequently require amputation. Actinomycetomas may respond to streptomycin or rifampicin for 2–3 months plus cotrimoxazole for many months until there is clinical improvement.

2. *Sporotrichosis: Sporothrix schenckii* probably enters the subcutaneous tissue through an abrasion. It may present as a single ulcer or nodule. In the lymphangitic form, the fungus spreads down the lymphatics, forming nodules at intervals which may then ulcerate through to the skin. Chronic lesions may look like psoriasis or a granuloma.

Treatment: saturated aqueous solution of potassium iodide mixed with milk, 0.5–1 ml PO tds, increased in small increments to 3–6 ml tds, until 1 month after clinical resolution. (Alternative: itraconazole 100–200 mg od.)

Skin signs of systemic fungal infection

Systemic mycoses such as histoplasmosis, blastomycosis, coccidioido-mycosis, paracoccidioidomycosis, and other fungal infections in immuno-compromised individuals, often show skin signs. Such signs include purpura, ulcers, slow spreading verrucose plaques, nodules, papules, pustules, and abscesses

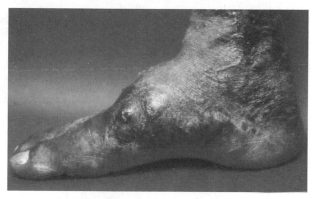

Fig. 15.1 Madura foot: fungal mycetoma caused by *Fusarium* species.

Sexually transmitted infections

Section editor   **Henrietta Williams**

Why are sexually transmitted infections important?

Sexually transmitted infections (STI) may cause both acute symptoms and long term consequences (including pelvic pain, infertility, tubal pregnancy, malignancy, pregnancy loss, neurological and cardiovascular disease, perinatal infections), that may have a significant impact on the health of both the individual and the population. The associated stigma may also affect psychological health and well-being. Prevalence is usually highest among the most vulnerable and marginalised groups in society, which, combined with the stigma, contributes to difficulties in accessing health care. Many STIs also increase the risk of HIV transmission.

Understanding the health consequences of STI for both the individual and society (including the association with HIV) is critical to the implementation of effective control policies. The recent increased understanding of the role of male circumcision in reducing the transmission of HIV and some STI is also likely to influence public health initiatives in the future.

Epidemiology and control of sexually transmitted infections

The May and Anderson equation encapsulates important factors in the epidemiology of STI. This states that:

$R_0 = BCD$, where:

R_0 is the reproductive rate and refers to the number of secondary cases resulting from an infected individual in a wholly susceptible community;

B is the probability of an infection being transmitted per sexual activity;

C is the rate of change of sexual partners;

D is the average duration of infectiousness.

Factors influencing these variables are listed in the table opposite. The success of public health interventions for control of STIs depends on reaching certain 'core groups' in the community in which a high STI prevalence is usually associated with frequent changes of partner and unsafe sexual practices. Such groups include commercial sex workers (CSW), men who have sex with men (MSM) and sexually active adolescents.

Variables influencing the reproductive rate (R_0) of an STI

Variable	Factors impacting these variables
Probability of an STI being transmitted (B)	• Condom usage. • Sexual practices e.g. 'dry sex'. • Treatment of other STI. • Circumcision. • Suppressive treatment e.g. HSV.
Rate of change of sexual partners (C)	• Safer sexual behaviour patterns. • Reduced partner change (especially concurrency of partners). • Delayed initiation of sexual intercourse.
Average duration of infectiousness (D)	• Education and awareness of STI. • Availability and access to diagnostic and treatment services. • Availability and access to syndromic treatment. • Screening of high risk individuals.

Challenges in controlling some sexually transmitted infections

Whilst the above model is effective for bacterial STI such as gonorrhoea, syphilis and chancroid, control of viral STI (e.g. HSV, HPV) is more challenging. A lack of curative treatment and poor accessibility to suppressive treatment results in symptomatic or asymptomatic viral shedding and ongoing transmission. This is highlighted by emerging evidence that HSV-2 is now a more common cause of genital ulceration than chancroid, even in those countries with high rates of ulcerative STI. The future development of vaccines is the only feasible option for effective control.

Other essential strategies for the control of STI include surveillance, legal policies and frameworks, available and accessible health services, anti-discrimination legislation and other measures to support those most vulnerable, research and evaluation, and targeted interventions.

Syndromic management of STI

Where resources allow, rapid, definitive diagnosis and treatment of STI, together with partner notification, are most effective in reducing further transmission and reinfection. Where this is not feasible, STI services focus on syndromic management, using treatment algorithms designed to cure the most common causes of defined clinical syndromes. Health care workers (HCWs) are trained to identify these syndromes by consistent groups of easily recognisable symptoms and signs.

Syndromic management is only aimed at symptomatic patients and treatment reflects local antibiotic resistance patterns. To maximise compliance, directly observed single dose treatment is used whenever possible. Syndromic management also includes partner notification and sexual health promotion.

Advantages of syndromic management
- prompt and rapid treatment at the point of presentation.
- does not need expensive or sophisticated laboratory resources.
- does not need highly trained laboratory staff.
- involves local trained health care workers.

This chapter outlines the management of the following STI syndromes based on WHO guidelines:
- urethral discharge.
- vaginal discharge.
- genital ulcer disease.
- inguinal buboes.
- scrotal swelling.
- lower abdominal pain in women.
- neonatal conjunctivitis.

http://www.who.int/reproductive-health/publications/rhr_01_10_mngt_stis/index.html

Urethral discharge in men

Urethritis is diagnosed if urethral discharge or an inflamed meatus is seen on examination, or dried discharge is seen on the penis. Most common presentation is urethral discharge and dysuria. In men with no definite signs of urethritis the urethra can be milked to detect the presence of a discharge. A gloved thumb is placed on the ventral surface of the base of the penis with the forefinger on the dorsum and gentle pressure is applied by moving the hand slowly towards the meatus.

Cause: The most common pathogens causing symptomatic urethritis in men are *Neisseria gonorrhoeae* and *Chlamydia trachomatis*. Less common are *Mycoplasma genitalium*, *Trichomonas*, HSV, *Adenovirus* and possibly *Ureaplasma urealyticum* (biovar 2). In 50% of cases, no causal pathogen can be identified. Recent evidence suggests sexual behaviour may predict aetiology, e.g. HSV and *Adenovirus* are commoner causes of urethritis in those practising insertive oral sex.

Diagnosis: If laboratory services are available, a sample of discharge can be air dried on a glass slide for microscopy and culture. Gram negative intra-cellular diplococci suggests *N. gonorrhoeae*. The presence of >5 PMNs in a Gram smear has traditionally been used to confirm the presence of urethritis but recent evidence suggests this may not be sufficiently sensitive and may therefore miss cases.

Management: includes treatment of the index case, partner notification, and treatment of contacts. If gonorrhoea cannot be reliably excluded by laboratory tests, treatment should be for both gonorrhoea and *Chlamydia* (📖 p 610), ideally with single dose treatment to aid compliance. The index patient should be asked to return if symptoms persist for >7 days. Persistence suggests failure of treatment or reinfection from an untreated partner. If reinfection likely, refer for laboratory investigations to identify less common causative pathogens; if no laboratory investigations are available treat for trichomoniasis.

Recommended treatment regimens
- Therapy for uncomplicated gonorrhoea (📖 p 609) plus therapy for uncomplicated *Chlamydia* (📖 p 611).

Alternative regimen if tetracyclines are contraindicated/not tolerated
- Therapy for uncomplicated gonorrhoea (📖 p 609) plus erythromycin 500 mg PO qds for 7 days.

Vaginal discharge

The usefulness of vaginal discharge as a symptom in the syndromic management of STI has recently been questioned. Personal and cultural factors may influence the subjective interpretation of vaginal discharge. particularly in Asia, so it is not always a reliable indicator of cervical infection. Vaginal speculum examination has therefore been added to the WHO algorithm to confirm the presence of discharge when feasible. Abnormal vaginal discharge is usually caused by vaginitis or vaginosis, although mucopurulent cervicitis (often caused by a sexually transmitted infection) is also a common cause and cannot be distinguished clinically. Cervical mucus or pus, the presence of cervical erosions, cervical friability and inter menstrual or post coital bleeding are more frequent in cervicitis, but do not reliably exclude vaginitis or vaginosis. Risk assessment has been shown to improve the specificity of the syndromic management of women with vaginal discharge by preventing over diagnosis of STI in low risk women. This assessment takes account of local STI prevalence as well as local sexual behaviour patterns.

Causes: Commonly bacterial vaginosis, candidiasis, trichomoniasis, and cervical infection caused by *Chlamydia* and gonorrhoea; these cervical infections are frequently asymptomatic. Non-infective causes of vaginal discharge usually present with a less acute history and include: malignancy, foreign body, atopic vulvovaginitis and cervical ectropion.

Diagnosis: History of the discharge and associated symptoms, as well as a risk assessment (see below). If microscopy is available, a Gram stain for *N. gonorrhoeae* from the cervix and a wet prep for *Trichomonas* from the vagina may be helpful.

Management: WHO guidelines suggest risk assessment in syndromic management of women with a vaginal discharge. If more than one of the following risk factors are present (and either partner is symptomatic) there is an increased risk of an STI:

- <21 years old.
- unmarried.
- >1 sexual partner in the last three months.
- new partner in the last three months.
- current partner with an STI.

All women are treated for endogenous vaginal infections and those at high risk of an STI are also treated for the common causes of cervicitis.

Recommended regimens

Cervicitis

- Therapy for uncomplicated gonorrhoea (📖 p 609) and *Chlamydia* (📖 p 611).

Vaginitis

- Therapy for bacterial vaginosis (📖 p 615) and *Trichomonas vaginalis* (📖 p 614), and, if indicated, for *Candida albicans* (📖 p 617).

Lower Abdominal Pain

Endometritis, salpingitis and pelvic inflammatory disease (PID) resulting from STI can present with lower abdominal pain (LAP) in sexually active women. PID may also occur in the absence of STI in sexually inactive women; in these cases the aetiology is often polymicrobial and may result from inadvertent introduction of flora from the lower genital tract during a gynaecological procedure.

Causes: of PID include *Chlamydia* and gonorrhoea and, less commonly, genital mycoplasmas (*Mycoplasma hominis* and *Ureaplasma urealyticum*). Non-sexually transmitted pathogens responsible for PID include *Actinomyces*, TB, anaerobes and *Mobiluncus*.

Diagnosis: In addition to LAP, PID commonly presents with fever, vaginal discharge, deep dyspareunia, menstrual disturbance, and less commonly nausea and vomiting. Signs include fever, lower abdominal tenderness, vaginal discharge, uterine tenderness, including pain with movement of the cervix (cervical excitation) and adnexal tenderness and/or adnexal masses. However clinical examination has low diagnostic sensitivity and specificity for PID and no reliable non-invasive investigations exist. A low threshold for treatment is advocated because delayed treatment increases the risk of long-term sequelae.

Management: Admit to hospital if severely unwell, for surgical emergencies (e.g. ectopic pregnancy, appendicitis), during pregnancy, if a pelvic abscess cannot be excluded, or if outpatient treatment has failed. Management should include treatment of all possible causes, and treatment of partners if a STI is likely or confirmed.

Recommended treatment regimens
Outpatient treatment
- Single dose therapy for gonorrhoea (📖 p 609) plus doxycycline 100 mg bd (or tetracycline 500 mg qds) plus metronidazole 400 mg bd for 14 days. Avoid alcohol with metronidazole and tetracyclines in pregnancy.

Inpatient treatment
- Ceftriaxone 250 mg IM od for 7 days, plus doxycycline 100 mg PO/IV bd (or tetracycline 500 mg PO qds) and metronidazole 400–500 mg bd PO/IV (or chloramphenicol 500 mg PO/IV qds) for 14 days; *or*
- Clindamycin 900 mg IV tds plus gentamicin 1.5 mg/kg IV tds; *or*
- Ciprofloxacin 500 mg PO bd (or spectinomycin 1 g IM qds) plus doxycycline 100 mg PO/IV bd (or tetracycline 500 mg PO qds) and metronidazole 400–500 mg PO/IV bd (or chloramphenicol 500 mg PO/IV qds).

For all of these regimens treatment should be continued until 2 days after symptoms have improved and then treatment should be continued for 14 more days with doxycycline 100 mg PO bd or tetracycline 500 mg PO qds
- If an IUD is present, remove once antibiotics started. Alternative contraception will be needed and should be discussed.

Scrotal swelling

Scrotal swelling is commonly due to epididymitis. In young, sexually active men this is usually due to a STI and often associated with testicular infection/inflammation (epididymo-orchitis).

Testicular torsion: should always be excluded in patients with a painful swollen scrotum. Acute torsion is usually accompanied by severe pain, which is worse when walking and is not relieved by supporting the testicle. Often there is associated nausea and vomiting. The testicle may be red and swollen. Urgent surgical exploration is needed as the testicle will not survive for more than 6 h with a compromised blood supply. Other causes of scrotal swelling include malignancy and trauma.

Causes: *Chlamydia* and gonorrhoea are the most common sexually transmitted causes of epididymo-orchitis. In men over 35 years of age non-sexually transmitted pathogens are more common, including *E. coli*, *Klebsiella* spp. or *Pseudomonas aeruginosa*. TB and *Brucella* infection may need to be considered. Associated urethral discharge strongly indicates a sexually transmitted pathogen.

Management

In addition to treatment for *Chlamydia* and gonorrhoea if suspected, management includes bed rest, support of the testicle and pain relief.

Recommended treatment regimens

Treatment of uncomplicated gonorrhoea (📖 p 609) plus treatment of *Chlamydia* (📖 p 611).

Genital ulcer

Causes: Genital ulcer disease often has multiple aetiologies. The commonest cause in a particular area is influenced by local prevalence of STIs and HIV. Ulceration caused by syphilis, lymphogranuloma venereum (LGV), granuloma inguinale, chancroid and *Herpes simplex* virus (HSV) cannot be accurately distinguished clinically. HSV-2 is commoner than previously realised, even in areas where other causes of genital ulceration are common. Unusual or atypical presentations are common in HIV infected patients and syndromic treatment therefore needs to cover HSV. Secondary bacterial infection of genital ulcers also frequently occurs.

Diagnosis: Patients should be offered serological testing for syphilis and HIV; laboratory diagnosis is otherwise not usually helpful.

Management: depends on local causes. Counselling includes advice on the window period for infectivity of HIV and syphilis, and the natural history of HSV and its transmission. Treatment should always cover syphilis, and treatment for HSV should be included where possible. Treatment for LGV, granuloma inguinale and chancroid depends on local prevalence rates. Advise patient to return for review if lesion not healed in 7 days. Individuals with HSV/HIV co-infection often have persistent multiple lesions and are at increased risk of transmitting HIV; conversely HIV negative patients with genital HSV are more susceptible to contracting HIV infection.

Recommended treatment regimens
- Therapy for syphilis (📖 p 606) *plus*
- Therapy for HSV if available (📖 p 616) *plus*
- Therapy for chancroid (📖 p 613) *or*
- Therapy for granuloma inguinale (📖 p 613) *or*
- Therapy for lymphogranuloma venereum (📖 p 611).

Inguinal buboes

Inguinal buboes are localised enlarged lymph nodes in the groin that are tender and sometimes fluctuant. LGV and chancroid are the most common causes. They are rarely the only signs of a STI and chancroid in particular is usually associated with a visible genital ulcer.

Recommended treatment regimens
- Ciprofloxacin 500 mg PO bd for 3 days plus *either* doxycycline 100 mg PO bd or erythromycin 500 mg PO qds for 14 days.

Treatment may need to be continued beyond 14 days. Fluctuant lymph nodes can be aspirated through clean skin but should not be incised or drained as this can delay healing. Biopsy is required for diagnosis if treatment fails.

Neonatal conjunctivitis

Causes: Neonatal conjunctivitis can be caused by gonorrhoea, *Chlamydia*, *Staphylococcus aureus*, *Streptococcus pneumoniae* and *Haemophilus* spp. *N. gonorrhoeae* is the most important cause as without appropriate treatment it can lead to blindness. It is the commonest cause of neonatal conjunctivitis in many developing countries.

Diagnosis: A red swollen sticky eye occurs 2–5 days after delivery in gonococcal conjunctivitis and at 5–12 days in chlamydial conjunctivitis. In practice treatment should cover both gonorrhoea and chlamydia.

Management
Treatment of gonococcal neonatal conjunctivitis
- Ceftriaxone 50 mg/kg (max 125 mg) IM stat.
Alternatively, if ceftriaxone not available:
- Kanamycin 25 mg/kg (max 75 mg) IM stat *or*
- Spectinomycin 25 mg/kg (max 75 mg) IM stat.

Treatment of chlamydial neonatal conjunctivitis
Erythromycin syrup 50 mg/kg PO daily in 4 divided doses for 14 days *or* Trimethoprin 40 mg with sulphamethoxazole 200 mg PO bd for 14 days.

Prevention: Neonatal infection with gonococcus can be prevented by washing carefully at the time of birth and applying 1% silver nitrate solution or 1% tetracycline ointment to the eyes. This is recommended for all babies born to mothers who are at high risk of gonorrhoea. This regimen however provides little protection from *Chlamydia*, which may also be present.

Syphilis

A worldwide disease caused by the spirochaete *Treponema pallidum*. The disease can be divided into four stages:

- Local primary infection.
- Dissemination, associated with 2° syphilis.
- A latent period during which infectivity is low (relapses into 2° syphilis may occur during the 1st 4 years after contact — the early latent period).
- Late syphilis, which occurs after many years with widespread gumma formation (granulomatous lesions with a necrotic centre and surrounding obliterative endarteritis) and long-term damage to the cardiovascular and central nervous systems.

Transmission: is almost exclusively through abraded skin at sites of sexual contact with infected persons. Other modes include congenital transmission (which produces severe disease in the infant) and infection by blood transfusion.

Clinical features

1° syphilis: 9–90 days after infection a primary genital ulcer or chancre forms. This is typically solitary, 'punched out', indurated, and painless, with a clear exudate. Atypical lesions occur and there may be multiple ulcers in HIV co-infected patients. Lesions, which are highly infectious, an resolve over a few weeks There is painless regional lymphadenopathy.

2° syphilis: coincides with the greatest number of treponemes in the body and blood, 1–6 months after contact. Specific features include:

- A transient, variable (but not vesicular) rash, particularly on the trunk, soles, and palms.
- In warm, moist areas where two skin surfaces are in contact (e.g. perineum), the papules enlarge and coalesce to form highly infectious plaques called condylamata lata.
- Silver-grey lesions with red periphery on mucosal surfaces called mucous patches (e.g. snail track ulcers in the mouth).

There is also:

- Low-grade fever.
- Malaise.
- Generalized lymphadenopathy.
- Arthralgia.
- Occasionally, focal involvement of eyes, meninges, parotid glands, or viscera (kidney, liver, GI tract).
- Symptoms of secondary syphilis generally resolve spontaneously within 12 months.

Late syphilis: Areas of local gummatous tissue destruction in skin, bones, liver, and spleen are most common. Other cardiovascular and CNS manifestations include:

- Ascending aortic aneurysm ± aortic regurgitation.
- Coronary artery stenosis.
- Chronic meningitis — cranial nerve defects, hemiparesis, seizures.

- CNS parenchymal disease (general paralysis of the insane, GPI) — psychoses, dementia, hyperactive reflexes, tremor, speech, and pupillary disturbances (Argyll–Robertson pupils).
- Tabes dorsalis — shooting pains in limbs, peripheral neuropathy, ataxia, Charcot's joints, positive Romberg's sign.

Congenital Syphilis

Transplacental infection may occur during any stage of syphilis, but is most likely during the early stages. Foetal infection may lead to late abortion or still birth (<10%). Neonatal features of congenital infection include rhinitis, a diffuse maculopapular, desquamative rash involving palms and soles (may be vesicular/bullous), hepatosplenomegally, lymphadenopathy, generalized osteochondritis/periostitis, CNS involvement, anaemia, jaundice, and thrombocytopaenia, although any organ may be affected and some newborns are asymptomatic. Death may occur e.g. due to pneumonia, liver failure, pulmonary haemorrhage or hypopituitarism.

In those children who survive the neonatal period, infection normally becomes latent, but there may be characteristic chronic signs and sequelae involving the bones (frontal bossing, saddle nose, protruding mandible, short maxilla, saber tibia), joints (recurrent arthropathy and effusions), teeth (peg shaped upper incisor's — 'Hutchinson's teeth'), eyes (interstitial keratitis), and neurological system (neurosyphilis, deafness).

Diagnosis
Diagnosis is often clinical, supported by routine bloods, Xrays (look for raised periosteum on plain X-rays of the long bones), VDRL/RPR on blood and CSF, ± specific serology and/or PCR if available. Test the mother. Treatment is cheap and safe, so all children born to infected mothers should be treated empirically, even if mother received treatment during pregnancy.

Treatment
Early congenital syphilis (≤2 years of age) and infants with abnormal CSF:
- *either* aqueous benzyl penicillin 100,000–150,000IU/kg/day administered as 50,000IU/kg IV bd for the first 7 days of life and then tds for a total of 10 days.
- *or* procaine benzylpenicillin, 50,000IU/kg IM od for 10 days.

Congenital syphilis of ≥2 years:
- aqueous benzylpenicillin, 200,000–300,000IU/kg/day, administered as 50,000IU/kg IV/IM every 4–6 h for 10–14 days.

Penicillin allergic patients: Penicillin is the treatment of choice in infants with congenital syphilis and alternatives should only be considered if there is a significant allergy to this antibiotic. An alternative (after the first month of life) is:
- Erythromycin 7.5–12.5 mg/kg PO qds for 30 days.

Diagnosis
- *Dark field microscopy* of lesion exudates for motile spirochaetes.
- *PCR* and *fluorescence staining* of exudates increasingly available —
  may be more appropriate for oral/GI specimens because of potential
  confusion with commensal spirochaetes on dark field microscopy.
- *Serology*: either treponeme-specific (FTA, TPHA) for exposure, or
  non-specific (VDRL, RPR) for active disease and screening. An enzyme
  immunoassay (EIA) to detect anti-treponemal IgG and IgM is also
  available: IgM usually detectable towards the end of 2nd week, and
  IgG in 4th or 5th week, of primary infection.
- *CSF examination* should be performed in any patient with neurological
  symptoms or signs. and in asymptomatic patients with syphilis for
  >2 years. The CNS can be involved in any stage of syphilis.
- *HIV testing* should be offererd to all patients with syphilis since
  dual infection is common and has implications for assessment and
  management.

Management
Early syphilis (stages 1 and 2 or latent syphilis of <2 years' duration):
- *either* benzathine benzylpenicillin 2.4 million IU IM stat (usually given as
  two injections into separate sites because of the large volume).
- *or* procaine benzylpenicillin 1.2 million IU, IM od for 10 days.
For penicillin-allergic patients alternatives include:
- *either* tetracycline 500 mg PO qds for 14 days.
- *or* doxycycline 100 mg PO bd for 14 days.
- *or* erythromycin 500 mg PO qds for 14 days for penicillin allergic
  pregnant patients.
Follow-up at 3, 6, and 12 months to assess treatment and possible
reinfection.

*Late syphilis (not neurosyphilis; includes latent syphilis of >2 years' or
indeterminate duration):*
- *either* benzathine benzylpenicillin 2.4 million IU IM (given as two
  injections into separate sites) once weekly for 3 weeks.
- *or* procaine benzylpenicillin 1.2 million IU IM od for 20 days.
For penicillin-allergic patients, alternatives include the following (however
penicillin is preferred therapy and should be given whenever possible):
- *either* tetracycline 500 mg PO qds (probably better).
- *or* doxycycline 100 mg PO bd, both for 30 days.
- *or* erythromycin 500 mg PO qds for 30 days.

Neurosyphilis
- *either* aqueous benzylpenicillin 2–4 million IU IV q4 h for 14 days.
- *or* procaine benzylpenicillin 1.2 million IU IM od plus probenecid
  500 mg PO qds for 10–14 days: ensure patient compliance with this
  outpatient regimen.
For penicillin-allergic patients, alternatives include:
- *either* tetracycline 500 mg PO qds for 30 days.
- *or* doxycycline 200 mg PO bd for 30 days.
Consult a neurologist if possible and follow up carefully.

Management of syphilis in pregnancy

Pregnant women should be treated with penicillin whenever possible. Pregnant women who are allergic to penicillin, but whose allergy is not manifested by anaphylaxis, may be given an extended course of a 3rd generation cephalosporin. Alternatives include erythromycin 500 mg PO qds for 14 days (early syphilis) or 30 days (other forms of syphilis). Note that the effectiveness of erythromycin is highly questionable, particularly for neurosyphilis, and many failures have been reported. Tetracyclines are contraindicated in pregnancy. The baby should be evaluated and treated soon after birth.

Gonorrhoea

Gonorrhoea results from infection with the Gram-negative coccus *Neisseria gonorrhoeae*. 1° infection through sexual contact usually involves the mucosal surfaces of the urethra, cervix, rectum, and oropharynx.

Without early effective treatment, both local and disseminated complications occur. Recent decades have seen the rise in strains resistant to penicillin, tetracycline, doxycycline, and other antibiotics. Conjunctival infection of neonates during vaginal delivery is a serious condition that may cause blindness if not treated early.

Clinical features: in **men**, urethral discharge and dysuria occur 2–5 days after infection. The discharge is initially mucoid, but becomes profuse and purulent (in contrast to non-gonococcal urethritis). Local complications include acute epididymitis, prostatitis, periurethral abscess, and urethral stricture. In **women**, infection produces signs of cervicitis (± urethritis) after ~10 days incubation period — vaginal discharge, dysuria, and intermenstrual bleeding. However, unlike men, many women are asymptomatic. Local complications include PID and peri-hepatitis. Frequency and urgency are uncommon symptoms in both men and women.

Haematogenous dissemination is a rare complication in untreated patients, which may → meningitis, endocarditis, osteomyelitis, sepsis, or acute destructive monoarthritis. Reactive polyarthropathy and papular/pustular dermatitis are recognized complications.

Diagnosis: Gram-negative intracellular diplococci in smears from the urethra in men (>90%) and endocervix in women (less reliable); culture.

Management: Resistance to pencillin, tetracyclines and the fluoroquinolones is increasing worldwide. As yet there appears to be no significant resistance identified to 3rd generation cephalosporins or spectinomycin. Local patterns of resistance must be considered when treating gonococcus. See box opposite for recommended regimens. Unless facilities available to exclude chlamydial infection, all patients should also be treated for *Chlamydia* since they often coexist. Treat sexual partners at the same time.

Locally recommended regimens:

1. Uncomplicated infection:
2. Pharyngeal infection:
3. Disseminated infection:
4. Gonococcal conjunctivitis:
5. Pregnant patients:

Recommended regimes

In uncomplicated genital and anal infection
- Cefixime 400 mg PO stat *or*
- Ciprofloxacin 500 mg PO stat (not during pregnancy) *or*
- Azithromycin 2 g PO stat *or*
- Ceftriaxone 125 mg IM stat *or*
- Spectinomycin 2 g, IM stat *or*
- Kanamycin 2 g IM stat *or*
- Co-trimoxazole 480 mg 10 tablets od for 3 days.

Always use the locally recommended regimen.

In disseminated infection
- Ceftriaxone 1 g IV/IM od for 7 days *or*
- Spectinomycin 2 g IM bd for 7 days.

Extend treatment to 14 days in meningitis, and 28 days in endocarditis.

Gonococcal conjunctivitis in adults is highly contagious. Manage with barrier nursing, frequent saline irrigation and antibiotics:
- Ceftriaxone 125 mg IM stat *or*
- Spectinomycin 2 g IM stat *or*
- Ciprofloxacin 500 mg PO stat
- (If above not available, alternative is kanamycin 2 g IM stat).

Neonatal gonococcal conjunctivitis (📖 p 22, 📖 p 603)
- Ceftriaxone 50 mg/kg (max 125 mg) IM stat
- [Alternative: Kanamycin 25 mg/kg (max 75 mg) IM stat]
- [Alternative: Spectinomycin 25 mg/kg (max 75 mg) IM stat]

Neonatal patients should be reviewed at 48 h.

Chlamydial infections

Chlamydia trachomatis is an obligate intracellular bacterium. Serovars D-K cause infection of the urethra, endocervix, or rectum and may → upper genital tract infection in women and epididymo-orchitis in men; less commonly these serovars can also cause conjunctivitis, arthritis and perihepatitis. Serovars L1-L3 cause Lymphogranuloma venereum. Serovars A-E are not sexually transmitted, but are an important cause of blindness worldwide due to trachoma (see chapter 13).

1. Uncomplicated urethritis/endocervicitis/proctitis

The D-K serotypes of chlamydiae have become the most common STI in the developed world. They are prevalent throughout the world, frequently coexisting with gonococcal infections, and are the most common cause of non-gonococcal urethritis (NGU) in men. Complications in men include epididymitis and (in homosexually active men) chronic proctitis. Infection in women is often subclinical or non-specific but may be associated with cervicitis, salpingitis, and endometritis, and is a major cause of female subfertility worldwide.

Screening asymptomatic women at risk of infection should reduce complications. Nucleic acid amplification tests that do not require cervical or urethral swabs are now widely available and a reliable way of case detection in asymptomatic infected individuals. These tests have now replaced culture and other testing techniques in many parts of the world, especially for screening purposes. Single dose treatment (directly observed where possible) for uncomplicated genito-urinary infection (azithromycin 1 g) is the preferred option in most situations. This eliminates the need for a test of cure as compliance is not an issue; effectiveness is excellent with cure rates as high as 90%, and resistance has not been documented.

2. Complicated Chlamydial Infections

Salpingitis, endometritis and other upper genital tract infection in women or epidiymo-orchitis in men resulting from *Chlamydia trachomatis* infection requires longer courses of treatment. Standard treatment is doxycycline 100 mg PO bd for 2 weeks ± azithromycin 1 g PO stat (see under syndromic management).

3. Lymphogranuloma venereum (LGV)

LGV is a chronic STI caused by the L1, 2, and 3 strains. The 1° lesion is a painless genital ulcer (rarely visible in women) that heals in a few days. After a latent period of days to months, acute, fluctuant inguinal lymphadenopathy (buboes) develops. With time, the buboes may spread locally and ulcerate → sinuses/fistulae. Subsequent chronic blockage of lymphatic drainage results in genital lymphoedema which is often quite severe in women. Although LGV has long been endemic in many parts of the world a recent epidemic has been seen amongst MSM in Europe and other developed countries. Most of these men have also been infected with HIV.

Diagnosis is by EIA, immunofluorescence (IF), DNA probe, PCR, or culture of bubo aspirate to demonstrate the organism, or by specific IF serological testing. Complement Fixation (CF) serological testing is helpful if there is a ≥4 fold rise in titre or a single titre of >1:64; a negative CF test rules out the diagnosis. Specific serovars responsible for LGV can be identified in some laboratories which may help with diagnosis.

Treatment doxycycline or tetracycline for 2 weeks (see box below). In LGV fluctuant lymph nodes should be aspirated through healthy skin. Incision and drainage or excision of nodes will delay healing and is contraindicated (late sequelae such as stricture/fistula, however, may require surgical intervention). Partner notification and treatment for all sexually transmitted infections is important.

Antibiotics regimens for chlamydial infection

Uncomplicated anogenital infection:
- Doxycycline 100 mg PO bd for 7 days **or**
- Azithromycin 1 g PO stat
- (Alternatives: amoxicillin 500 mg PO tds for 7 days **or** erythromycin 500 mg PO qds for 7 days **or** ofloxacin 300 mg PO bd for 7 days **or** tetracycline 500 mg PO qds for 7 days).

Uncomplicated anogenital infection during pregnancy:
- Erythromycin (base/ethylsuccinate) 500 mg PO qds for 7 days **or** amoxicillin 500 mg PO tds for 7 days.

LGV:
- Doxycycline 100 mg PO bd for 14 days **or**
- Erythromycin 500 mg PO qds for 14 days
- (Alternative: tetracycline 500 mg PO qds for 14 days).

Neonatal chlamydial conjunctivitis
- Erythromycin syrup 50 mg/kg per day in 4 divided doses for 14 days.
- (Alternative: co-trimoxazole 240 mg PO bd for 14 days).
Recommended regimens are those NOT in brackets.

Chancroid

An acute STI caused by *Haemophilus ducreyi* characterized by painful necrotizing ulceration and painful bubo formation; highly infectious and a common cause of genital ulcers in Africa and S.E. Asia. Chancroid is much more common in males, suggesting a female carrier state.

Clinical features: 3–7 days post-infection, painful papules form which rapidly develop into soft ulcers with undermined, ragged edges. Ulcers are haemorrhagic and sticky (often secondarily infected); if multiple they may become confluent; they occur at sites of trauma during intercourse (extra-genital ulcers are rare). 7–14 days later inguinal nodes may become involved: painful, matted, and tethered to erythematous skin = bubo. A discharging sinus may develop, in time becoming a spreading ulcer. Lesions heal slowly and commonly relapse.

Diagnosis: clean the ulcer with saline, then remove material from the undermined edge; or aspirate pus from bubo. Gram stain the smear. *H. ducreyi* are Gram −ve rods (fine, short, round-ended) sometimes seen in 'shoal-of-fish' or 'railroad track' formation. Beware contaminating organisms. Culture is difficult. PCR, immunofluorescence and serology may be available for diagnosis in some laboratories. Without treatment infectivity may continue for several months, but with appropriate antibiotic therapy (see box) lesions often heal in 1–2 weeks. Intercourse should be avoided until lesions have completely healed.

Granuloma inguinale (donovanosis)

Calymmatobacterium granulomatis causes chronic, destructive ulceration of genitals and surrounding tissues. Males are more frequently infected than females. It is not easily transmitted; patients' sexual partners are often uninfected.

Clinical features: 1–6 weeks following infection a painless indurated papule forms which slowly develops into a 'beefy' granulomatous ulcer with characteristic rolled edges. The lesion is elevated, well defined, and bleeds easily with trauma. Usual sites are in the anogenital region, thighs, and perineum; rarely vaginal (or rectal) lesions may present with PV (or PR) bleeding. Healing is uncommon without treatment; 2° infection can follow → painful, destructive lesions, as can squamous cell carcinoma. Inguinal nodes are not involved unless there is 2° infection. Subcutaneous granulomas form which may be mistaken for enlarged lymph nodes (hence the name 'pseudobubo') — they may also become an abscess, discharging via a sinus, or an infected ulcer. Elephantoid enlargement of genitalia may occur during healing.

Diagnosis: crush a piece of granulation tissue from the active edge of the lesion between 2 slides, air dry, and stain with Giemsa or Gram stains. Look for large mononuclear cells filled with Donovan bodies (intra-cytoplasmic Gram −ve rods that look like closed safety pins due to bipolar staining). Culture is difficult; PCR and serology are available in some research facilities. Treatment should be for at least 3 weeks or until all the lesions have epithelialized.

Management of chancroid

- Ciprofloxacin 500 mg PO bd for 3 days *or*
- Erythromycin 500 mg PO qds for 7 days *or*
- Azithromycin 1 g PO stat *or*
- Ceftriaxone 250 mg IM stat.

Single dose treatments may have higher failure rates than longer courses of antibiotics, so erythromycin is the treatment of choice. With HIV co-infection treatment is less effective. Co-infection syphilis and HSV may occur.

Management of granuloma inguinale (donovanosis)

- Azithromycin 1 g PO stat then 500 mg od.
- Doxycycline 100 mg PO bd.
- (Alternatives: erythromycin 500 mg PO qds *or* tetracycline 500 mg PO qds *or* co-trimoxazole 960 mg PO bd).

Duration of treatment: should be for atleast 3 weeks, continuing until all lesions have completely epithelialized.

Trichomoniasis

Vaginitis due to *Trichomonas vaginalis* produces an irritating, pruritic (rarely foul smelling) discharge 5–28 days post-infection, ± dyspareunia. Urethral infection with dysuria. The vaginal discharge is often copious, sometimes yellow or green, and pools in the posterior fornix. The vagina and ectocervix become inflamed; colposcopy reveals cervical haemorrhages in ~50% of symptomatic cases — 'strawberry cervix' (can be seen on speculum examination in >5% of women with trichomoniasis). Up to 50% of women with *Trichomonas* infection may be asymptomatic. Infection in men is usually asymptomatic but may cause urethritis.

Diagnosis in women is by wet prep microscopy of vaginal discharge for motile *Trichomonas vaginalis* (sensitivity 40–80%). Culture of vaginal discharge for has a sensitivity of ~80–90%. Pap smears often identify *Trichomonas*, but this is not a reliable method of diagnosis as there is a significant risk of both false negatives and false positives.

Diagnosis in men is not as easy. *Trichomonas* commonly results in urethritis in men but urethral swabs, urethral smears and first catch urine specimen are not sensitive in making a diagnosis. Often *Trichomonas* infection in men is only suspected and treated once other causes of urethritis have been excluded.

Management
- Metronidazole 2 g PO stat or 400–500 mg PO bd for 7 days works well (efficacy of a single dose is less clear).
- Tinidazole 2 g PO stat is an alternative.
- All sexual partners should be notified and treated.
- Patients should return after 7 days if symptoms persist. Failure can be due to resistance or reinfection. Patients often respond well to retreatment with the 7-day regimen.
- Refractory infections should be treated with metronidazole 2 g PO od plus 500 mg applied intravaginally each night for 3–7 days.
- During pregnancy, metronidazole may only be used at the minimum effective dose during the 2nd and 3rd trimesters (2 g PO stat).

Bacterial vaginosis

Bacterial vaginosis (BV) is a common cause of vaginal discharge. It is characterized by a reduction in hydrogen peroxide producing lactobacilli and an increase in other bacteria in greater amounts than are normally present in the vagina. These bacteria include *Gardnerella vaginalis*, *Mycoplasma hominis*, *Bacteroides*, *Mobiluncus*, peptostreptococci and a newly identified bacterium *Atopobium vaginae*. Clinically, most women complain of an offensive whitish discharge that tends to recur and may often seem worse after intercourse. There are usually no associated symptoms of vaginitis (itch or irritation). BV in non-pregnant women is associated with postpartum endometritis and surgical procedures e.g. hysterectomy, termination of pregnancy. In pregnancy, it can be associated with chorio-amnionitis and amniotic fluid infection, increased rates of foetal loss (all stages of pregnancy), premature rupture of membranes, low birth weight and preterm birth. BV increases susceptibility to and transmissibility of HIV.

Diagnosis is by microscopy and culture plays no part. Amsells criteria for diagnosis suggest 3 of 4 of the following need to be present for diagnosis: white homogenous vaginal discharge; vaginal pH >4.5; presence of clue cells (vaginal epithelial cells stippled with bacteria, >20%); and a fishy smell on addition of KOH to a sample of the vaginal discharge.

Management

- Metronidazole 400 mg PO bd for 7 days. A single dose of metronidazole 2 g is an alternative if adherence is likely to be poor.
- Clindamycin cream 2% intravaginally bd for 7 days can be used as an alternative.
- Partners are not routinely treated as it is a polymicrobial condition and not technically a STI.

Women often suffer from recurrence — up to 30% at 3 months and 90% at 9 months. The trigger for the reduction in hydrogen peroxide producing lactobacilli in the vagina of some women is not understood. There is no evidence on the optimal management of recurrent BV. For problematic, recurrent BV, expert opinion suggests 14 days of metronidazole and intravaginal clindamycin 2% followed by monthly 2 g doses of metronidazole and intravaginal acigel may be of benefit. Pregnant women who are symptomatic should be treated. It is unclear whether treating asymptomatic pregnant women improves pregnancy outcomes.

Genital herpes

Most genital herpes worldwide is caused by HSV-2, although primary genital herpes infections as a result of HSV-1 are increasing. Recurrent genital ulcers are due to reactivation of the latent virus from the dorsal root ganglia, and occur more frequently with HSV-2 than HSV-1 infection. Asymptomatic shedding is common and is an important cause of transmission: most infections are transmitted by people unaware they are infected. HSV seropositivity increases both the likelihood of transmitting HIV and susceptibility to HIV. Persistence of HSV ulceration and frequent recurrences are common in those who are immunocompromised, and acute episodes are more often prolonged, clinically atypical and severe.

Transmission occurs by direct contact with infected genital secretions. After an incubation period of 2–7 days, local infection and inflammation result in multiple vesicular lesions that rapidly ulcerate. The ulcers are greyish and extremely painful; they occur on the penis in men and the vagina, cervix, vulva, and perineum in women, often accompanied by a vaginal discharge. The ulcers may be present in the anus (usually in homosexually active men). 1° infection is accompanied by fever, malaise, and inguinal lymphadenopathy; extragenital involvement occurs in up to 20% of cases. Encephalitis is a recognized complication of genital herpes. Non-primary initial infection (e.g. HSV-2 infection with pre-existing antibodies to HSV-1) is often less severe clinically.

Diagnosis PCR, culture, direct immunofluorescence and serology are used. In many parts of the world where laboratory resources are accessible PCR has replaced culture and immunofluorescence as the primary method for diagnosis. Recent reliable Western blot type-specific serological tests are now available and may play a part in the diagnosis of genital ulcers. These tests may also be useful for discordant couples, as part of preconception counselling.

Management

- Analgesia and salt baths may help relieve discomfort and pain associated with primary infections.
- *In those with a first clinical episode* (take a careful history), aciclovir 200 mg PO 5 × daily for 5 days or valaciclovir 500 mg bd for 5 days reduces formation of new lesions, duration of pain, time required for healing, and viral shedding—but probably not the rate of future recurrence. Treatment should be started as soon as possible.
- *Recurrences* can be managed with either episodic treatment or suppressive treatment. Aciclovir 200 mg PO 5 × daily or valaciclovir 500 mg bd or famciclovir 125 mg bd, all for 5 days, can be used episodically. If >6 episodes per year give continuous oral suppressive treatment with aciclovir 400 mg bd, famciclovir 250 mg bd or valaciclovir 500 mg od; if >10 episodes per year use valaciclovir 1 g od. Recurrences become less common with increasing duration, so some experts recommend stopping antivirals after 1 year so that recurrence rates can be reassessed. The minimum continuous dose that will suppress recurrence should be determined empirically.
- Condoms can reduce transmission; long-term suppressive treatment with valaciclovir also appears to reduce transmission.

Candida vaginitis

Candida vaginitis is not an STI. It occurs due to overgrowth of the commensal vaginal yeast, *Candida albicans* (and less commonly other candida species). Antibiotic therapy, pregnancy, and immunosuppression all predispose to symptomatic candidiasis. Commonly there is vulvitis as well as vaginitis and intense vulval pruritus and erythema are characteristic. Discharge is thick, curd-like, and white (rarely it may only be scanty), and microscopy shows Gram +ve budding yeasts ± hyphae; visualization of the yeasts is made easier by the addition of 10% KOH to clear the epithelial cells.

Recurrent vulvo-vaginal candidiasis (RVVC) is defined as more than 4 episodes of microbiologically proven candida infection in a 12 month period. 5–8% of women in their reproductive life have RVVC. The majority of women have no demonstrable risk factors and it may be due to a cell mediated immunodeficiency at the vaginal mucosal level.

Men can suffer from candida balano-prostitis, but this is not as a result of transmission between partners, and treatment of partners is not generally helpful unless the male partner is symptomatic.

Management

- Miconazole or clotrimazole 200 mg intravaginally od for 3 days *or*
- Clotrimazole 500 mg intravaginally stat *or*
- Fluconazole 150 mg PO stat.
- (Alternative: nystatin 100,000IU intravaginally od for 14 days).
- Women with RVVC can be treated with a 2 week induction course of clotrimazole followed by weekly maintenance treatment with clotrimazole 500 mg as a pessary for 3–6 months.

Occasionally candida vaginitis may be caused by a strain of *Candida albicans* resistant to routine treatment, or to less common *Candida* species such as *C. glabrata* or *C. kruseii*.

Genital Warts

Genital warts are caused by infection with human papilloma virus (HPV) transmitted by skin to skin contact. There are more than 100 serotypes of HPV based on genomic DNA sequences and 35 serotypes preferentially infect the anogenital area. Serotypes 6 and 11 are typically responsible for warts and rarely insert themselves into the host genome. Infection with these types has no malignant potential. By contrast the oncogenic types (16, 18, 31, 33, 35 and 45) may integrate with the host genome and can eventually result in cervical squamous cell carcinoma if infection is persistent and other cofactors are also present. These oncogenic types do not cause genital warts.

Genital wart virus infection (GWVI) is common and prevalence rates amongst sexually active populations may be as high as 50%. However not all GWVI (even with low risk types) results in warts as many of those infected will have subclinical infection. There may be evidence of infection histologically or on colposcopy, however. HPV typing on clinical specimens is available in some countries.

Management

Genital warts are a cosmetic problem and, although the natural history is for them to resolve spontaneously, treatment is often requested. Treatment options include the following (application of topical treatments can often be done by the patient themselves):

- Cryotherapy ablation with liquid nitrogen.
- Surgical excision.
- Laser treatment.
- Podophyllotoxin cream or liquid (an antimitotic) can be applied to accessible warts twice daily in cycles of three days a week for a maximum of 4 weeks. Local irritation is a common side effect.
- Imiquimod is a new topical treatment that induces the production of local cytokines and is associated with a lower recurrence rate than other treatments. It should be applied once daily three times a week for up to 16 weeks.
- Cervical warts are best treated by cryotherapy after colposcopic examination. Warts can be resistant to treatment and cause problematic recurrences in pregnancy and in patients who are immunocompromised.
- Infection with oncogenic type HPV resulting in squamous intraepithelial lesions is best identified treated and followed up by colposcopy and regular Pap smears.

Prevention

Vaccines against HPV serotypes 16 and 18 (two of the commonest causes of cervical squamous cell carcinoma) are now available, and have shown excellent efficacy in preventing the 'precancerous' stage cervical intraepithelial neoplasia (CIN). One of the vaccines also targets serotypes 6 and 11 (together responsible for most genital warts).

Molluscum Contagiosum

Molluscum contagiosum virus infection produces raised umbilicated lesions or nodules with pearly caseous plugs. They are transmitted through skin contact and are common in immunocompetent children and adults but may be particularly severe in the immunocompromised. In children, lesions are usually non-genital and are transmitted through fomites or direct skin-to-skin contact. In adults, lesions can be in the genital region and more widespread. Treatment is usually for cosmetic reasons and can be difficult in those who are immunocompromised. Cryotherapy or immune modulators such as imiquimod or podophylotoxin can be used, or the lesion can be pricked with a sterile point and the contents expressed. Antiretroviral therapy usually leads to a marked improvement in HIV.

Scabies

Scabies is caused by infestation with the mite *Sarcoptes scabei*. Infection is from skin-to-skin contact and can affect any part of the body. In the genital region it is often papular and nodular, with crusting and excoriation. Intense itching at night is common. Scrapings from a nodule or burrow may produce mites that can be identified under the microscope. See 📖 p 545 for treatment. Repeat treatments may be required; bedding must be washed.

Pubic Lice

In *Phthirus pubis* infestation (see also 📖 p 544) eggs are attached firmly to pubic hair and the louse itself may be found on the abdomen, thighs, genital area or eyelashes. The louse is often difficult to see by the naked eye but can be placed under the microscope for confirmation of the diagnosis. Permethrin 1% applied to all affected areas is the treatment of choice. Lice in the eyelashes can be treated by application of petroleum jelly twice a day for 10 days. Bedding must be washed and contacts treated.

Chapter 17

Nutrition

Section editor   **Andrew Tomkins**

Malnutrition, health, and survival

Why does malnutrition occur?

Food insecurity, infections, and lack of care all contribute to malnutrition. Underlying exacerbating causes include trade tariffs, lack of political commitment, and political instability. Food insecurity may be acute, chronic, or seasonal. Socio-economics (poverty, cultural, civil unrest, disasters, social exclusion), climate, geography, agricultural factors (e.g. soil characteristics), and factors affecting animal husbandry and health all contribute. Seasonal availability of cereals, fruit, or vegetables affect dietary intake. Cultural preference, including gender inequality, determines who gets the best portions of food. Commercial marketing often affects food choice by children and adults. Certain cereals have characteristic limited bioavailability of micronutrients. Infection is frequently implicated. Pain, fever, sore mouth, breathlessness, and diarrhoea all ↓ appetite. Malnutrition develops due to a combination of anorexia, poor intake, malabsorption, ↑ nutrient requirements, and urinary and intestinal losses. Particularly important infections causing malnutrition are persistent diarrhoea, measles, pertussis, intestinal parasites, pneumonia, TB, and HIV/AIDS. Inadequate care often contributes and is exacerbated by short birth intervals, large family size, sick parents, and orphanhood.

Effects of malnutrition on health and survival

- *Immunity:* Malnutrition contributes to >50% deaths among children <5 years globally by suppressing host immunity (particularly cellular immunity), reducing antioxidant capacity, and slowing tissue repair after infection. Vit A and Zn deficiency are particularly important contributors to severe illness and mortality in childhood infection.
- *Growth and development:* Dietary as well as genetic factors affect growth. Better childhood diet → improved growth and development.
- *Organ function:* Individual nutritional deficiencies affect the eye (vit A), thyroid gland (iodine), brain (iron), respiratory and intestinal epithelia (vit A and Zn), and ovaries (anorexia).
- *Pregnancy outcome:* Maternal malnutrition affects maternal health, intrauterine development, birth weight, lactation, and infant/child health.
- *Foetal programming:* Intrauterine malnutrition causes ↑ risk of cardio-vascular diseases, hypertension, diabetes, and stroke during adulthood.

Whose responsibility is nutritional treatment?

Doctors often assume malnutrition is caused by parental ignorance or cultural preferences and that dietary advice is all that is necessary. Hospital administrators assume parents can bring the necessary nutritional diet to the ward. Nurses often focus on the medical aspects of treating the sick child. Economists assume that if incomes could be raised and food production could be increased, then malnutrition and disease would go away. In practice, there are many interventions needed if malnutrition is to be prevented and treated properly. The role of health professionals in advocacy for prevention of malnutrition is vital, but this section deals with the medical response only, requiring the same rigour of management as a microbial or metabolic illness. Nutritional treatment plans need careful prescription of specified amounts of food, medicines, and nutritional supplements with precise instructions on frequency of dosing.

Nutritional treatment strategies

Interventions include provision of nutritious, palatable foods, micronutrient supplements, demonstration of preparation of complementary foods in the home, improving household food security, and promotion of fortified foods. Ideally, involve a trained nutritionist; nutritional guidelines are also available from international agencies and NGOs (📖 p 663).

Nutrition & millennium development goals (MDGs)

The MDGs agreed by the UN are supposed to be achieved by 2015. Achieving adequate nutrition plays a key role in the majority of MDGs:

- *Goal 1: Eradicate extreme poverty and hunger:* Malnutrition erodes human capital, ↓ resilience to disease (esp infection), ↓ productivity, and prevents poverty reduction. Early child malnutrition has consequences for adult health, including an increased risk of chronic disease. Biological and social vulnerability overlap and compound each other.
- *Goal 2: Achieve universal primary education:* Malnourished children are more likely to perform poorly in school or not to enrol in school at all. Nutrition is critical for cognitive development so malnutrition reduces mental capacity. Malnutrition may also disable (blindness in vit A deficiency; impaired mental development in iodine deficiency).
- *Goal 3: Promote gender equality and empower women:* Gender inequality ↑ risk of female malnutrition. Dealing with malnutrition improves equality, and better-nourished girls are more likely to stay in school.
- *Goal 4: Reduce child mortality:* Malnutrition contributes to >50% child mortality, esp from infection. Breastfeeding, appropriate complementary feeding, and micronutrients (esp. vit A and Zn) are keys to child survival.
- *Goal 5: Improve maternal health:* Malnutrition contributes to maternal mortality. Deficiencies of several micronutrients (iron, vit A, folate, iodine, calcium, and Zn) are associated with pregnancy complications. Maternal stunting increases risk of cephalopelvic disproportion and obstructed labour.
- *Goal 6: Combat HIV/AIDS, malaria, and other diseases:* Among HIV +ve individuals, malnutrition ↑ disease progression, imortality, and ↓ resistance to opportunistic infections; it may ↓ the efficacy and safety of ART treatment. Malnutrition ↓ survival in malaria and TB.

Clinical assessment of malnutrition

Nutritional status is assessed by a combination of clinical features and anthropometric measurements, (📖 p 628).

Clinical syndromes

Most cases of severe malnutrition occur in children <5 y old; in older children or adults, suspect malnutrition 2° to underlying infection (e.g. HIV, TB) or malignancy. Classically, two syndromes of severe malnutrition are recognized in children: **marasmus** and **kwashiorkor** (see box, Fig.17.1 and Plate 21). These may be mixed: marasmic–kwashiorkor. It is unclear why some children develop oedema and others do not. Dietary deficiencies of energy, protein, and micronutrients are common to both syndromes. Zinc and selenium deficiency contribute to impaired anti-oxidant capacity.

Points in the history and physical examination

History

- Usual diet before current illness, complaints about lack of food or the quality of food, recent change in diet.
- Breastfeeding history: how long for? Mixed or exclusive BF? Is the child breastfeeding now?
- Is the mother ill or malnourished? Any evidence of TB or HIV/AIDS?
- Food and fluids taken in past few days; thirst?
- Recent illness (measles, diarrhoea, malaria, cough, etc).
- Behaviour and activity changes (crying, irritable, apathy, anorexia).
- Duration, frequency, and nature of any vomiting or diarrhoea.
- Recent sinking of eyes.
- Time when urine was last passed.
- Deaths of siblings or parent (esp from HIV/AIDS).
- Birth weight; whether a twin.
- Milestones reached (e.g. sitting, standing).
- Immunization and vit A doses up to date?

Physical examination

- General appearance, behaviour, mood (apathy, irritability), level of consciousness, facial appearance, signs of kwashiorkor/marasmus.
- Signs of shock: cold hands or feet, weak pulse, ↓capillary refill time, ↓ consciousness.
- Appetite for an offered portion of therapeutic food?
- Temperature — hypothermia/fever?
- Pulse and respiratory rate.
- Pallor, jaundice.
- Skin rash (e.g. post measles) or excoriation, cancrum oris.
- Oedema.
- Enlarged or tender liver, jaundice.
- Abdominal distension, tenderness.
- Signs of congenital syndrome (e.g. Down's syndrome).
- Anthropometric measurements (see 📖 p 628).

Clinical features of marasmus

- *Emaciated:* thin, flaccid skin ('little old man' appearance), fat and muscle tissue grossly reduced, prominent spine, ribs, pelvis.
- *Behaviour:* alert and irritable.

Clinical features of kwashiorkor

- *Oedema:* bilateral pitting limb oedema; periorbital oedema. Oedema may mislead observer into thinking child is plump and well, and makes assessment of dehydration much more difficult.
- *Skin changes:* desquamation, often in the flexures and perineum.
- *Hair changes:* dry, thin hair which may become depigmented appearing brown, yellowy-red, or white.
- *Hepatomegaly* is common.
- *Behaviour:* miserable, lethargic, and apathetic with sad facial expression.

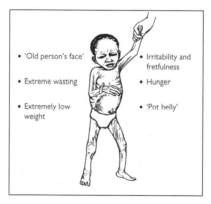

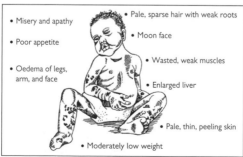

Fig. 17.1 Signs of marasmus (above) and kwashiorkor (below).

Pathophysiological consequences of severe malnutrition

Severe malnutrition is associated with impaired function of:
- kidneys (unable to excrete Na^+ load).
- intestine (villous atrophy; gut damage → bacterial translocation; gut enzyme deficiencies → malabsorption).
- circulation (easily develops fluid overload/CCF).
- thymus (atrophy → impaired immunity).
- brain (impaired intellectual impairment).
- liver (hypoglycaemia, abnormal drug metabolism).
- electrolyte homeostasis (K^+, Zn, and Mg deficiency).
- skin excoriation — source of local sepsis and septicaemia.
- body temperature control (hypothermia = sign of bad prognosis).

Specific nutrient deficiencies

Classical signs of specific nutrient deficiency occur in severe cases only. These include nutritional oedema (kwashiorkor), xerophthalmia (vit A deficiency), goitre (iodine), pellagra (niacin), scurvy (vit C), and rickets (vit D) — the clinical features and management of these conditions are described later in this chapter.

Laboratory measures

Where available, the following can be used in the assessment of nutritional status:
- Serum proteins (e.g. albumin, pre-albumin, transferrin).
- Micronutrients (e.g. serum retinol, plasma Zn, vit B12, folate, ferritin).
- Erythrocyte enzymes (e.g. erythrocyte glutathione reductase) indicating functional micronutrient deficiency.
- Urinary micronutrients (e.g. iodine).

However, plasma levels of several biomarkers change during inflammation (plasma Zn and vit A ↓; plasma ferritin ↑) making them difficult to interpret. Others are more stable e.g. transferrin receptor and Vitamin D. Plasma Na^+ levels are typically low (indicating dysfunctional Na^+ pumps rather than Na^+ deficiency). Plasma K^+ levels are typically low (indicating loss of muscle mass and intestinal losses of K^+ in diarrhoea).

Measuring malnutrition

Anthropometric indices

Anthropometry (body measurements) is used to quantify malnutrition by reference to international standards (see box). The following are commonly used:

- Weight for age (W/A): weight relative to the standard weight for a child of the same age.
- Height for age (H/A): height relative to the standard height for a child of the same age.
- Weight for height (W/H): weight relative to expected weight for a child of the same height.
- Mid upper arm circumference (MUAC).
- Body mass index (BMI): weight/(height)^2.

W/A, H/A, and W/H are expressed as % of the reference standard, or as multiples of the standard deviation (SD) from the mean of a reference population (see box) = 'Z score' (e.g. if weight is 2 SD below the mean weight of normal children of the same age, the Z score is −2).

Weight for age, height for age, and weight for height

Malnutrition may be classified using anthropometric measures as follows:

- Underweight:↓ W/A (Z score ≤1 mild; ≤2 mod; ≤3 severe).
- Stunting: ↓ H/A (Z score ≤1 mild; ≤2 mod; ≤3 severe).
- Acute malnutrition: ↓ W/H (wasting).
  - *Moderate* — ('*global acute malnutrition*' *or GAM*): W/H Z score ≤2 or W/H < 80%.
  - *Severe* — ('*severe acute malnutrition*' *or SAM*): W/H Z score ≤3 or W/H < 50% W/H or the presence of bilateral oedema.

If age is uncertain, height (65–110 cm) may be used as a proxy for age to identify children aged 6 months–6 yrs.

Mid upper arm circumference (MUAC)

MUAC is measured simply using a tape or marked plastic strip placed around the dominant upper arm. Between ages 1–5 years MUAC increases slowly, so simple cut-off values may be used for nutritional assessment (see box). A MUAC of <110 mm is equivalent to a W/H Z score of −3 (i.e. SAM requiring urgent nutritional rehabilitation) A MUAC of <125 mm is equivalent to a W/H Z score of −2 (i.e. GAM)

Body mass index (BMI)

BMI, defined as weight/(height)^2 (in kg/m^2) is only used for adults (not pregnant women, in whom MUAC is used). A BMI <18.5 is 'mild', 16–17 is 'moderate', and <16 is 'severe malnutrition'. A BMI >25 is 'overweight'; >30 is 'obese'.

Reference growth standards and growth charts

Traditionally, National Centre for Health Statistics (NCHS) growth standards were used for children aged 0–18 years.

In 2006, the WHO introduced new international growth standards for children aged 0–5 years, which are expected to be widely adopted in the near future.

For children aged 5–18 years, the WHO still recommends the use of NCHS standards. Both the NCHS and new WHO growth standards may be found at *www.who.int/nutrition*.

Example growth charts and a simplified WHO reference chart are shown on the following pages 630–1.

MUAC cut-off points for malnutrition in children, adults, pregnant women, and the elderly

Age group	Severe	Moderate	At risk
Children 1–5 yrs	<110 mm	110–125 mm	125–135 mm
Adults	<160 mm	160–185 mm	
Pregnant/lactating women	<170 mm	170–185 mm	185–210 mm
Elderly*	<160 mm	160–175 mm	

* MUAC is generally low among the elderly due to loss of muscle

Common mistakes with growth charts

- Writing January in the first box instead of the child's birth month.
- Writing the month in which the child was first weighed instead of his/her birth month in the first box.
- Missing out months.
- Writing the months as numbers and confusing them with ages.
- Forgetting to miss out blank boxes if the child has not been weighed for several months.
- Not using the calendar and estimating the child's age each time.
- Recording a child's weight in the wrong year.
- Putting the weight dot the wrong side of the kilogram line.

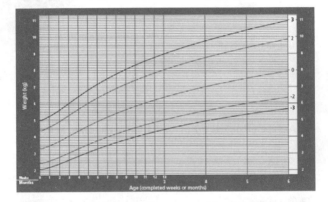

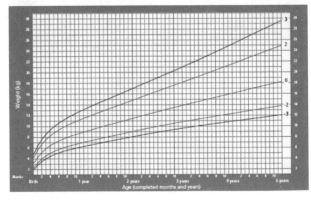

Fig. 17.2 Example growth curves for boys 0–6 mths (top) and girls 0–5 yrs (bottom). Each growth curve represents a Z score (see text) from –3 to +3. (Reproduced with permission of the WHO.)

Table 17.1 Chart for assessing degree of malnutrition (low weight for height) among children age 6–59 months using WHO/NCHS reference data[†]

Boys' weight (kg)					Length or height (cm)*	Girls' weight (kg)				
-4SD	-3SD	-2SD	-1SD	Median		Median	-1SD	-2SD	-3SD	-4SD
60%	70%	80%	90%	Median		Median	90%	80%	70%	60%
1.8	2.2	2.5	2.9	3.3	50	3.4	3	2.6	2.3	1.9
1.9	2.3	2.8	3.2	3.7	52	3.7	3.3	2.8	2.4	2
2	2.6	3.1	3.6	4.1	54	4.1	3.6	3.1	2.7	2.2
2.3	2.9	3.5	4 s	4.6	56	4.5	4	3.5	3	2.4
2.7	3.3	3.9	4.5	5.1	58	5	4.4	3.9	3.3	2.7
3.1	3.7	4.4	5	5.7	60	5.5	4.9	4.3	3.7	3.1
3.5	4.2	4.9	5.6	6.2	62	6.1	5.4	4.8	4.1	3.5
4	4.7	5.4	6.1	6.8	64	6.7	6	5.3	4.6	3.9
4.5	5.3	6	6.7	7.4	66	7.3	6.5	5.8	5.1	4.3
5.1	5.8	6.5	7.3	8	68	7.8	7.1	6.3	5.5	4.8
5.5	6.3	7	7.8	8.5	70	8.4	7.6	6.8	6	5.2
6	6.8	7.5	8.3	9.1	72	8.9	8.1	7.2	6.4	5.6
6.4	7.2	8	8.8	9.6	74	9.4	8.5	7.7	6.8	6
6.8	7.6	8.4	9.2	10	76	9.8	8.9	8.1	7.2	6.4
7.1	8	8.8	9.7	10.5	78	10.2	9.3	8.5	7.6	6.7
7.5	8.3	9.2	10.1	10.9	80	10.6	9.7	8.8	8	7.1
7.8	8.7	9.6	10.4	11.3	82	11	10.1	9.2	8.3	7.4
8.1	9	9.9	10.8	11.7	84	11.4	10.5	9.6	8.7	7.7
7.9	9	10.1	11.2	12.3	86	12	11	9.9	8.8	7.7
8.3	9.4	10.5	11.7	12.8	88	12.5	11.4	10.3	9.2	8.1
8.6	9.8	10.9	12.1	13.3	90	12.9	11.8	10.7	9.5	8.4
8.9	10.1	11.3	12.5	13.7	92	13.4	12.2	11	9.9	8.7
9.2	10.5	11.7	13	14.2	94	13.9	12.6	11.4	10.2	9
9.6	10.9	12.1	13.4	14.7	96	14.3	13.1	11.8	10.6	9.3
9.9	11.2	12.6	13.9	15.2	98	14.9	13.5	12.2	10.9	9.6
10.3	11.6	13	14.4	15.7	100	15.4	14	12.7	11.3	9.9
10.6	12	13.4	14.9	16.3	102	15.9	14.5	13.1	11.7	10.3
11	12.4	13.9	15.4	16.9	104	16.5	15	13.5	12.1	10.6
11.4	12.9	14.4	15.9	17.4	106	17	15.5	14	12.5	11
11.8	13.4	14.9	16.5	18	108	17.6	16.1	14.5	13	11.4
12.2	13.8	15.4	17.1	18.7	110	18.2	16.6	15	13.4	11.9

[†] Note these charts are being replaced by new WHO 2006 data which will be available on the WHO website http://www.who.int/nutrition/en/

* Up to 24 months, measure length of child lying down; 24–59 months, measure height of child standing

SD = standard deviation or Z-score; length is measured <85 cm

Managing malnutrition

Initial assessment should include a history, anthropometric measurements especially MUAC (📖 p 628), and examination for specific clinical signs of malnutrition (📖 p 624). Assess whether the child appears clinically well, or lethargic and unwell; if well, does he/she eat well when offered food? Use the algorithm below to classify the type of malnutrition and decide on type of treatment.

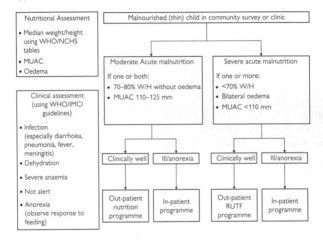

Fig. 17.3 Algorithm for categorization and management of children with malnutrition.

Outpatient therapeutic nutrition programme

The aim of an outpatient nutrition programme (see algorithm p. 632) is to identify the severity of malnutrition; plan a treatment regimen for those with GAM or SAM; decide where that regimen should be given (in paediatric ward, at home, or feeding centre); and give advice and treatment to carers of children with GAM and SAM.

1. Give nutritional guidance to improve dietary intake
- Give advice on specific feeding practices, including need to give extra food in convalescent phase of an illness and to improve the protein and micronutrient content of the traditional diet wherever possible.
- Advise on access to local programmes which increase food security (using local community development programme and/or a local programme of food supplements).
- Provide a 'take home' ration of food to provide protein, energy and micronutrients in a form which is palatable and can be stored safely without refrigeration (e.g. nutritional pastes).

2. Treat infection (many infections are subclinical in malnutrition)
- Treat all children with SAM for infection whether they have clinical signs or not (give antibiotics e.g. amoxicillin for 5 days).
- Give a single dose of albendazole 400 mg PO to all children >24 months to treat possible helminth infection.
- Give all children vit A (50,000, 100,000, and 200,000 iu for those <6 months, 7–12 months, and >12 months respectively, on days 1, 2, and 14 of the nutrition programme).
- Assess HIV status and treat.
- Diagnose and treat malaria.
- Consider TB as cause for poor nutritional response.
- Ensure the child is up to date with immunizations.
- Follow up the child every 2 weeks until weight gain is achieved.

Outpatient ready-to-use therapeutic food programme

The aim of this programme is to manage children with SAM at home provided they can eat adequate amounts of ready–to-use therapeutic food (RUTF, see box). This enables recovery of metabolic problems and promotes recovery of body mass and function.

1. Observe that the child eats offered portions of RUTF
2. Give sufficient RUTF till the next visit
- Follow up every 2 weeks until weight gain satisfactory (e.g. >5 g/kg/day).
- RUTF contains ~5.5 kcal/g; 200 kcals/kg body weight/day can → a daily weight gain of up to 20 g/kg body weight.
- Advise carer to give up to 100 kcal/kg body weight/day (using teaspoon equivalents of RUTF) until any oedema has resolved.
- If no oedema or once oedema resolved, give 150–220 kcal/kg body weight/day.

- Advise carer of need to feed frequently, to keep child warm (especially at night), and to come back to the clinic if the child develops an infection or consistently refuses RUTF.

3. Ensure the carer knows the ration is for the index child only

- RUTF is sometimes shared with other children, reducing the amount the index child receives. If the intake of RUTF falls to 100–150 kcals/kg body weight, daily weight gain to falls to ~5–10 g/kg body weight/day.
- Best to give cereal/legume supplement to carer of malnourished child to ensure other children in the family do not eat RUTF intended for the index child.

Ready-to-use therapeutic food (RUTF)

RUTF is a protein, energy, and micronutrient-rich food for severely malnourished children. Typically, RUTFs are very palatable, lipid-rich pastes, with a nutritional composition similar to F-100. RUTF does not require cooking, and the low water content makes it resistant to microbial contamination, so it can be stored safely at ambient tropical conditions for many months. Most severely malnourished children can take several teaspoonfuls of RUTF 5–7 times a day, achieving sufficient nutrient intake to achieve complete nutritional recovery. RUTF needs to be taken with water. Encourage breastfeeding. Other foods should not be encouraged until weight has been restored.

Production: RUTF can be produced locally. A typical recipe includes (by weight or volume): full-fat milk powder (30%), sugar (28%), vegetable oil (15%), peanut butter (25%), and mineral/vit mix (1.6%). Liquid milk is not suitable as it promotes microbial growth. Suitable oils include soya, cotton seed, rape seed, and corn oil. Sugar should be ground to 'icing sugar' quality to make the paste less 'gritty'. Peanut butter is made by roasting and grinding peanuts. The vit/mineral mix requires careful formulation; it cannot be provided from local markets and is best obtained as commercially prepared mixes (e.g. DSM, S Africa) Mechanical mixers should be used as hand mixing of ingredients is unlikely to disperse the micronutrients adequately. Two full-time workers can produce several hundred kgs of RUTF/week. Mixing/ingredient instructions are available on the WHO website (*www.who.int/nutrition/RUTF*).

Quality control: Avoid aflatoxin contamination by selecting out mouldy peanuts. Do not add water. Store in airtight containers to ↓ fatty acid oxidation. Locally produced RUTF has a shelf life of 3–4 months. If packaged in airtight, foil envelopes, in a nitrogen atmosphere, the shelf life is 24 months. Micronutrient levels in the feed can be measured by markers of individual components such as iron.

Cost and sustainability: Locally produced RUTF costs ~US$3.0 per kg (~$2.5 for raw materials + ~$0.50 for packaging, salaries, and storage.) Commercially produced RUTF costs more but lasts longer.

Inpatient therapeutic nutrition programme

Severely malnourished children who are clinically ill or anorexic should be admitted to hospital. Inpatient management aims to treat serious, life-threatening metabolic and infective complications of severe malnutrition and to establish the child on an adequate intake for nutritional recovery.

Nutritional rehabilitation

While this section concentrates on the management of severe malnutrition in young children, the principles of treatment are similar for all age groups, and combine therapeutic nutritional treatment with intensive medical care (📖 p 640). Management of infants is covered on 📖 p 644. Nutritional treatment may be divided into initiation, transition, and rehabilitation phases.

1) Initiation phase: Establish maintenance dietary intake using special feeds to enable metabolic disturbances to recover, and then ↑ to higher nutrient doses. Severely malnourished children cannot handle large quantities of dietary protein, fat, or Na^+. Start with a low-energy, low-protein intake to stabilize physiological and metabolic processes; this allows oedema to clear. Aim to provide 75 kcals/kg body weight and 1.0–1.5 g/kg protein per day using frequent small feeds of low osmolality.

- Prevent and treat complications of severe malnutrition (see 📖 p 640).
- Use a 'starter' feeding regimen containing of F-75 formula (see 📖 p 637).
- Give small amounts frequently — ideally 2 hourly, *at least* 4 hourly (see Table 17.2). Night feeding is required to prevent hypoglycaemia.
- If unable to take sufficient feed orally (<80 kcal/kg body weight/day), give via NG tube. Offer each feed by mouth and give remainder via NG. NG may be removed when child takes most of daily diet orally.
- Weigh child each morning before a feed; assess oedema daily.

2) Transition phase: Once appetite returns, oedema starts to clear and medical complications are treated (usually after ~3–7 days), child may enter transition phase in which dietary intake ↑ under close monitoring. Problems can occur with higher dietary Na^+ and osmolality. Need to intervene quickly if heart failure develops 2° to fluid overload: monitor vital signs. Key components of this phase:

- Switch to F-100 therapeutic milk (see 📖 p 646).
- Continue to feed regularly (e.g. 8 feeds in 24 h).
- Provided appetite remains good, increase successive feeds by 10 ml until refusal (likely to occur at ≥200 ml/day).
- Weigh daily but assess mean weight gain over 3 days.
  - If <5 g/kg body weight/day: ensure feeds being given properly; check.
  - for infection.
  - If 5–10 g/kg body weight/day: check if greater intake can be achieved.
  - If >10 g/kg body weight /day: anticipate early referral to rehabilitation phase.
  - Always monitor for heart failure (fast pulse/respiratory rate): ↓ feed if present.

Table 17.2 Volumes of F-75 per feed (ml) according to feed frequency

Child's weight (kg)	2-hrly feed	3-hrly feed	4-hrly feed	Child's weight (kg)	2-hrly feed	3-hrly feed	4-hrly feed
2.0	10	30	45	6.2	70	100	135
2.2	25	35	50	6.4	70	105	140
2.4	25	40	55	6.6	75	110	145
2.6	30	45	55	6.8	75	110	150
2.8	30	45	60	7.0	75	115	155
3.0	35	50	65	7.2	80	120	160
3.2	35	55	70	7.4	80	120	160
3.4	35	55	75	7.6	85	125	165
3.6	40	60	80	7.8	85	130	170
3.8	40	60	85	8.0	90	130	175
4.0	45	65	90	8.2	90	135	180
4.2	45	70	90	8.4	90	140	185
4.4	50	70	95	8.6	95	140	190
4.6	50	75	100	8.8	95	145	195
4.8	55	80	105	9.0	100	145	200
5.0	55	80	110	9.2	100	150	200
5.2	55	85	115	9.4	105	155	205
5.4	60	90	120	9.6	105	155	210
5.6	60	90	125	9.8	110	160	215
5.8	65	95	130	10.0	110	160	220
6.0	65	100	130				

3) Rehabilitation phase: Once able to tolerate larger quantities of food without complications, child enters rehabilitation phase, which aims to promote rapid growth. Preparations for discharge should include careful assessment of the physical, social, and economic environment of the child and family. The child should then be referred to an outpatient nutrition rehabilitation programme, such as the RUTF programme described above. Key issues during this phase include:

• Work towards increasing household food security.
• Provide support for families with serious social problems.
• Encourage regular visits to under-5 clinics, immunization, and regular vit A prophylaxis (200,000 m iu 3 times/year).
• Encourage sensory stimulation, using structured play therapy and physical activity to promote speech and motor development.
• Promote breastfeeding (see box).
• See child regularly (preferably every 2 weeks) until nutritional recovery is achieved (at least 85% weight/height is regarded as 'cure').

4) Follow-up after nutritional recovery
- See child every 2 weeks to check weight gain (after nutritional recovery child should grow at expected 1–2 g/kg body weight/day).
- Check for dietary/medical reasons for poor weight gain.
- Ensure child is integrated into clinic or community-based programme for monitoring progress of 'at risk' children.

Breastfeeding: key issues promoted by WHO/UNICEF

- Have a written breastfeeding policy that is understood by and routinely communicated to all health care staff.
- Train all health care staff in skills necessary.
- Inform all pregnant women about the benefits and management of breastfeeding.
- Help mothers initiate breastfeeding within a half-hour of birth.
- Show mothers how to breastfeed and how to maintain lactation even if they should be separated from their infants.
- Give infants no food and drink other than breast milk, unless medically indicated — exclusive breastfeeding up to 6 months if possible.
- Promote 'rooming in': mothers and infants should remain together 24 h a day wherever possible.
- Encourage breastfeeding on demand.
- Give no artificial teats or pacifiers (also called dummies or soothers) to breastfeeding infants.
- Foster the establishment of breastfeeding support groups.

Medical management within inpatient therapeutic nutrition programmes

Medical management aims to treat infections and metabolic problems that are especially common in severely malnourished children.

1) Hypoglycaemia: (blood glucose <3 mmol/l or <54 mg/dl) is often a result of infection and/or depletion of liver glycogen stores. If untreated, it can → lethargy, confusion, convulsions, coma, and death. Treat with 2–5 ml/kg 10% glucose IV upon admission, followed by 50 ml 10% glucose/sucrose PO/NG to prevent recurrence (1 rounded teaspoonful of sugar in 3.5 tablespoonfuls of water). Further glucose may be required; close monitoring is required. As consciousness recovers, begin feeding or give 60 g/l glucose/sucrose in water. Prevent hypoglycaemia by immediate and frequent feeding on admission and early treatment of infections.

2) Hypothermia: (rectal temp <35.5°C) usually occurs if ambient temperature drops (esp. during the night) and is often associated with infection and/or hypoglycaemia. It is a dangerous prognostic sign. Change wet nappies and bedding quickly and ensure child does not get cold during washing. Provide blankets/lamps/heaters to ensure child is nursed in warm environment, esp. at night. Encourage 'kangaroo' technique: mother lies supine with child on her chest, covered by her clothes and blankets. Cover child's head with a cap to ↓ heat loss.

3) Diarrhoea: is common on admission and during treatment; may be due to infection, excess osmolarity of the food, or premature transfer to the next feeding phase. If severe diarrhoea, go back to F-75. Milk intolerance is uncommon but may require non-milk-based feeds. Check that correct volumes of feeds are being given rather than large boluses which may cause diarrhoea. Severely malnourished children with HIV may have severe diarrhoea from *Cryptosporidium* or other intestinal parasites. Oral (and sometimes IV) rehydration is necessary for such children. Diarrhoea ± fever can be due to systemic infection (e.g. pneumonia, malaria, otitis media) Current WHO diarrhoea treatment regimes include the use of Zn preparations (10 mg daily); dysentery should be treated with antibiotics according to local policies in the light of microbial resistance — see 🕮 p 221.

4) Dehydration: is difficult to assess. It is easy and dangerous to overhydrate severely malnourished children — they cannot excrete Na^+ load and have impaired cardiac function. Assessment and management are described on 🕮 p 6 and 248–251. Children should be monitored carefully during rehydration. Monitor pulse/respiratory rate and urinary frequency. Useful signs of rehydration include return of tears, moist mouth, less sunken eyes and fontanelle, and improved skin turgor. Continue breastfeeding wherever possible.

5) Electrolyte abnormalities: Hyponatraemia is usually present but does not reflect a deficiency in total body Na^+; avoid giving too much Na^+ in oral or IV fluids. Hypokalaemia is common, especially in children with diarrhoea, and contributes to cardiac arrhythmias. Hypomagnesaemia may contribute to cardiac arrhythmias and muscle twitching. Phosphate levels are often low. K^+ and $Mg++$ should be added to feeds (📖 p 647). Children with severe malnutrition and diarrhoea need less sodium and more potassium than well nourished children. Use ReSoMal rather than standard oral rehydration solution (📖 p 248–251): give 5 mls/kg PO/NG every 30 mins for the first 2 h; aim to give 70–100 ml/kg over 12 h. Watch carefully for signs of fluid overload. Once rehydrated, replace volumes lost in stool. Reserve IV fluids for children in shock (📖 p 256).

6) Bacterial sepsis: is a common cause of death in severely malnourished children, particularly in the early stages of inpatient treatment. Poly-microbial infections are common and signs of infection such as fever and inflammation may be absent. All children with SAM should receive broad-spectrum antibiotics, even if there are no clinical signs of infection.

- Give amoxicillin 500 mg PO tds for 5 days (250 mg tds for children <10 yrs; 20–40 mg/kg daily in divided doses for children <40 kg; up to 15 mg/kg bd for infants <3 months) or chloramphenicol 25 mg/kg IM/IV tds for 5 days.
- If clinical signs of infection and child does not respond to above antibiotic regimen within 48 h, either add gentamicin 7.5 mg/kg IM/IV daily, or change to ceftriaxone (20–50 mg/kg daily by deep IM injection or by IV injection over 2–4 minutes).

Measles: Vaccinate all children aged 9 m–15 y against measles, unless proof of previous vaccination. Children immunized <9 m of age should be re-vaccinated as their previous immune response may be inadequate.

Malaria: Do blood film or rapid diagnostic test for malaria on admission and treat as necessary.

Intestinal helminths: Treat all patients with albendazole (400 mg once for children less than 2 years).

TB: Severely malnourished children are at ↑ risk of TB, but diagnosis is difficult as clinical features are non-specific and a definitive microbiological diagnosis is only possible in a minority of cases. Search for TB e.g. by aspiration of cervical glands or gastric washings. Consider the TB in children who do not respond quickly to standard nutritional and medical treatment, and in those with a history of household TB contact (see 📖 p 158).

Micronutrient deficiencies: are common, although classical clinical signs are often absent. Treat empirically: give oral vit A on admission (children <6 m 50,000 iu; 6–12 m 100,000 iu; >1 y 200,000 iu), and give the following daily for at least 2 weeks:

- a multivitamin supplement.
- zinc (2 mg/kg/day)*.
- folic acid (5 mg day 1, then 1 mg/day).
- copper (0.3 mg/kg/day)*.
- only once gaining weight, give ferrous sulphate 3 mg/kg/day.

(*Zinc and copper may be given as concentrated electrolyte/mineral solution (see below) added to feed.)

HIV/AIDS and malnutrition

Among severely malnourished children in sub-Saharan Africa, the prevalence of HIV is up to 15% in community treatment programmes, and up to 60% among those in paediatric wards where many are seriously ill with medical complications. Most severely malnourished HIV +ve children have low CD4 counts and need anti-retroviral treatment (ART). CD4 counts are not low in severely malnourished children without HIV.

Consider testing for HIV in any severely malnourished child. Testing might arouse fear and stigma because a positive test in the child reveals the mother is also HIV +ve (often previously unknown). The benefits of making the diagnosis include appropriate treatment of OIs, co-trimoxazole prophylaxis, and ART.

Specific issues in HIV +ve children include:
- Poor dietary intake due to weakness, painful oral lesions (e.g candida), anorexia due to fever/infections, and sickness of a parent or guardian (often also HIV+) → limited care and food provision.
- Malabsorption and chronic diarrhoea due to intestinal parasites (e.g. *Cryptosporidium*) cause nutrient losses from the intestine.
- Increased energy expenditure due to intercurrent infections.
- Severe weight loss and growth faltering, esp. stunting, are common.
- Micronutrient deficiencies (incl. vit A, Zn) are common.
- Anaemia is common in HIV +ve children, usually the result of chronic inflammation rather than micronutrient deficiency. Iron supplements may be harmful in HIV due to the increase in oxidative stress and HIV viral load.

Management
- Give the same nutritional therapy to HIV +ve as to HIV -ve children, but anticipate more dietary refusal due to infection. Ensure nutrition during OIs.
- Ensure best possible food and drinking water hygiene.
- Manage diarrhoea energetically. Give Zn supplements — see 📖 p 640 and 646.
- Treat infections and OIs vigorously (📖 p 83–103).
- Give co-trimoxazole prophylaxis.
- Refer to an ART clinic; measure CD4 count if resources allow.
- Prevent mother-to-child transmission — see 📖 p 132.
- Provide health care for the mother and/or carer, including HIV testing ± CD4 count to assess need for ART. A healthy mother/carer is crucial to the child's recovery.

Outcome: HIV greatly affects mortality in severe malnutrition. With adequate nutritional rehabilitation, the mortality among HIV –ve children should be <10%, but unless treated with ART, the mortality among HIV +ve children may be >30% despite all the above interventions.

Nutrition in people with HIV/AIDS

Good nutrition is essential for successful HIV/AIDS management, in order to maintain immune competence and strength and minimize the nutritional impact of infections. HIV/AIDS patients (even when asymptomatic) need an increased food intake:

- At least the recommended daily allowance (RDA) of vits A, B, C, E, and minerals (e.g. selenium, folic acid, Zn).
- More during recovery from an infection.

Nutritional education should start once a person is identified as HIV +ve. Focus on how to meet increased dietary needs and prevent OIs and improve hygiene. Support the entire family, including food security, hygiene, and psycho-social care of the HIV +ve patient.

To optimize intake: eat small, frequent meals; make food softer. Include body-building food (legumes, cereal, animal products), protective foods (fruits and vegetables, fortified food), and energy foods (sugar, starch and fat, staple foods).

Problems

- Nausea and vomiting: eat frequent small meals and avoid fatty food.
- Mouth sores: avoid hot and spicy foods; eat soft; mashed, liquid food.
- Anorexia: eat frequent small meals. Time ART to minimize impact of GI side-effects (e.g. nausea) on meals.

Severe malnutrition in infants

Feeding problems, including sickness or absence of the mother, insufficient breast milk (stress, war, drought), and inappropriate alternative infant feeding (unsafe bottle feeding), may cause malnutrition and illness in young infants. Diagnosis of severe malnutrition in young infants (who are <6 months old or <65 cm in length) is based on:

- W/H <70% (or −3 z scores)
  and *either*
- Weight loss or growth stagnation (for 1–2 weeks)
  or
- Poor clinical status (illness, apathy, etc.)

Breast feeding

Breastfeeding increases immunity, is hygienic, clean, and cheap, and there is usually a good supply, though mothers need support. Artificial feeding in circumstance of poverty carries risks of contamination (teats, bottles, milk left standing too long, unclean water) and dilution (no money to buy more milk, sharing with siblings). This can result in malnutrition through inadequate intake of artificial milk and repeated episodes of diarrhoea.

In times of insecurity, anxiety, and migration, breast milk might be reduced. Mothers often think they produce less breast milk because they are themselves malnourished. In practice, milk quantity is usually only reduced once maternal energy intake is <1600 kCal/day. Breast milk quality (especially of micronutrients) is quickly affected by the mother's diet. A mother's complaint that she does not have enough milk should be properly investigated. When the milk production is reported to be reduced or stopped, breastfeeding should be encouraged and the mother supported with nutritious food. Only if there is no other option should artificial feeding be used and then the mother (or caretaker) must be trained in using the milk safely.

Three-phase nutritional treatment

- *Initial phase* (1–15 days): supplement breast milk with specially diluted therapeutic milk (SDTM); total caloric intake (breast milk plus SDTM) should be 105 kCal/kg/day (140 ml/kg/day SDTM).
- *Transition phase* (2 days): when breast milk output increases after 10 to 15 days, SDTM can gradually be reduced to half the amount for 2 days (52 kCal/kg/day = 70 ml/kg/day SDTM), and then stopped completely.
- *Rehabilitation phase* (≥4 days): exclusive breastfeeding under close supervision.

Treatment for non-breastfed infants

Increase SDTM from 105 to 120 kCal/kg/day. Once infant has gained weight for 3 consecutive days in the initial phase, gradually replace SDTM with 'normal' breast milk substitutes. Ensure calorie intake gradually increases from 120 kCal/kg/day (normal intake) to 150 kCal/kg/day for extra growth.

Monitoring

Monitor weight gain on a daily basis. A special scale (10 g precision) is necessary. If an infant loses weight for 3 consecutive days, either the amount of food offered is not enough (breast milk plus therapeutic milk) or underlying medical or social problems must be addressed. Be alert for infections, including neonatal tetanus, which may cause poor suckling.

Medical treatment

Severely malnourished young infants require similar medical treatment regimes to older infants and children with severe malnutrition:

- Antibiotics — amoxicillin for at least 5 days (250 mg tds for children under 10 yrs; 20–40 mg/kg daily in divided doses for children <40 kg; up to 15 mg/kg bd for infants <3 months).
- Vit A (children <6 m 50,000 iu; 6–12 m 100,000 iu; >1 y 200,000 iu); mothers should receive 200,000 iu at or within 6 weeks of delivery.
- Folic acid 5 mg on admission followed by 1 mg daily.
- Ensure that the mother has her illnesses diagnosed and treated. Maternal depression affects infant feeding and growth.

Discharge

The following conditions should be met before discharge:

- Clinically well; no infections.
- Weight gain of ≥ 100–125 g/week without therapeutic milk supplementation for 7 days (min 5 g/kg/day, target 10 g/kg/day).
- Breastfed infants: active suckling; established breast milk production.
- Non-breastfed infants: supply of breast milk substitutes must be ensured and the caretaker should understand hygienic preparation and the dangers of artificial feeding.

Complications of severe malnutrition in infants

- *Hypothermia:* is a major cause of mortality in malnourished infants. Keep infants warm: skin-to-skin contact (kangaroo position); provide blankets and caps.
- *Dehydration:* use Re-So-Mal.
- *Malaria:* test on admission and as clinically indicated. Sulfadoxine-pyrimethamine (Fansidar®) should not be given to children <2 m old.
- *Anaemia:* iron is given as treatment for anaemia not as routine therapy. Give 2 mg/kg tds (preferably as a syrup e.g. Galfer or Fersamal) for >3 months, but only start after 14 days of nutritional treatment. When Hb is <5 g/dl, consider blood transfusion after careful evaluation.
- *Candidiasis:* is frequent in newborns — treat with nystatin.

Recipes and formulas for management of ill and severely malnourished children

Concentrated electrolyte/mineral solution (EMS)

This is used in the preparation of starter (F-75) and catch up (F-100) feeding formula and ReSoMal (low Na$^+$ oral rehydration solution [ORS], see 📖 p 250). Sachets containing these formulae are manufactured but if not available, prepare by disolving the following ingredients in cool, boiled water made up to 2500 ml solution. Store in sterilized bottles in the fridge to retard deterioration. Discard if turns cloudy and make fresh each month.

If possible, add selenium (28 mg of sodium selenate, $NaSeO_4.10H_2O$) and iodine (0.012 g of potassium iodide, KI) per 2500 ml.

Nutritional rehabilitation formulas F-75 and F-100

F-75 formula should be used for initial refeeding. Its low osmolality and low Na$^+$, energy, and protein load minimize the risk of severe metabolic disturbance during refeeding. Once appetite returns, oedema clears and medical complications are treated, F-75 is replaced by F-100 formula, which is higher in energy and protein to facilitate catch up growth. Ready made sachets of F-75 and F-100 are increasingly available but where these are not, they can be prepared using the following ingredients by mixing the milk, sugar, oil, and electrolyte mineral solution (EMS, see above) into a paste, and then slowly adding warm, boiled water to make up to 1000 ml. If available, use an electric blender or hand whisk.

Commercial packets of F-75 starter formula have an even lower osmolality because maltodextrins replace sugar.

Alternative milk ingredients

- If only whole dried milk (WDM) available, an alternative to F-75 may be prepared using 35 g WDM, 100 g sugar, 20 g oil, 20 ml EMS, and water up to 1000 ml. Similarly, to prepare an alternative to F-100, use 110 g WDM, 50 g sugar, 30 g oil, 20 ml EMS, and water up to 1000 ml.
- If only fresh cow's milk available, another alternative to F-75 may be prepared using 300 ml milk, 100 g sugar, 20 g oil, 20 ml EMS, and water up to 1000 ml. Similarly, to prepare an alternative to F-100, use 880 ml milk, 75 g sugar, 20 mg oil, 20 ml EMS, and water up to 1000 ml.

Specially diluted therapeutic milk (SDTM)

This is a 75% dilution of F-100 used for severely malnourished infants (see 📖 p 644). It is made by adding 350 ml water to 1 litre F-100 (Alternatively, mix 50 g dried skimmed milk, 75 g sugar, 25 g oil, and 850 ml of clean water.) It supplies 75 kCal/100 ml, 10 kCal % protein, 50 kCal % fat, and is isotonic with a medium Na$^+$ concentration.

EMS ingredients	Amt (g)	mol/20 ml
Potassium chloride: KCl	224	24 mmol
Tripotassium citrate	81	2 mmol
Magnesium chloride: $MgCl_2$, $6H_2O$	76	3 mmol
Zinc acetate: Zn acetate, $2H_2O$	8.2	300 μmol
Copper sulphate: $CuSO_4$, $5H_2O$	1.4	45 μmol
Water: make up to	2500 ml	

Nutritional rehabilitation formulas

Ingredients	F-75	F-100
Dried skimmed milk (g)	25	80
Sugar (g)	100	50
Vegetable oil (g)	27	60
Electrolyte/mineral soln (EMS, ml)	20	20
Water: make up to (ml)	1000	1000

Nutritional contents of F-75 and F-100

Contents per 100 ml	F-75	F-100
Energy (kcal)	75	100
Protein (g)	0.9	2.9
Lactose (g)	1.3	4.2
K^+ (mmol)	4.0	6.3
Na^+ (mmol)	0.6	1.9
Mg (mmol)	0.43	0.73
Zinc (mg)	2.0	2.3
Copper (mg)	0.25	0.25
% energy from protein	5	12
% energy from fat	32	53
Osmolality (mOsm/1)	413	419

Vit A deficiency

In developing countries, >80% vit A is derived from dietary carotenoids found in breast milk, dark green vegetables, and yellow and orange fruits. Margarine and meat (especially liver) are also sources. Vit A deficiency → ↑ morbidity and mortality among children and is a preventable cause of blindness from xerophthalmia.

Xerophthalmia is classified as follows:
- *Night blindness* (XN): individual bumps into objects in poor lighting.
- *Conjunctival xerosis* (X1a): dry conjunctiva has glazed appearance.
- *Bitot's spots* (X1b): white foamy spots on conjunctival surface, commonly at the corneoscleral junction on the temporal side.
- *Corneal xerosis* (X2): dry cornea, associated with the onset of visual impairment. Most common in children aged 2–4 yrs.
- *Corneal ulceration* (X3a): often worse in measles; central corneal ulceration may profoundly affect vision.
- *Keratomalacia* (X3b): severe destruction of the eye with blindness; occurs especially in severe malnutrition precipitated by measles.
- *Corneal scarring* (XS): follows healing after vit A replacement, often with permanent visual impairment.

Treatment:

For xerophthalmia, severe malnutrition, measles, and pneumonia/ diarrhoea in HIV-infected children:
- Give 3 doses of oral vit A at day 1, day 2, and in week 3.
- For xerophthalmia, also give topical antibiotic eye ointment (e.g. tetracycline 1% or chloramphenicol 1%) for 10 days.
- If cornea is involved, close the eye and gently cover with an eye pad.

Pregnancy: Vit A is teratogenic; high doses are contraindicated. A pregnant woman with xerophthalmia should receive vit A 5,000–10,000 IU PO od for ≥4 weeks. Vit A supplements should not be given to HIV +ve pregnant women as they increase perinatal HIV transmission.

Preventive and curative doses of vit A

0–6 months	50,000 IU
6–12 months	100,000 IU
>1 yr (including adults)	200,000 IU
Vit A-deficient pregnant women	10,000 IU

Prevention of Vit A deficiency   PUBLIC HEALTH NOTE

- Increase dietary vit A: carotenoids found in breast milk, spinach, carrots, sweet potatoes, mangos, papaya, milk, eggs, red palm oil, liver, fish liver oils.
- Prophylactic supplementation (200,000 iu) given 2–3 times a year to children aged 6 months–5 years in endemic deficiency areas.

Vit B₁ (thiamine) deficiency: beriberi

Thiamine is widely available but deficiency may occur when cereals such as rice are highly milled. Deficiency may also complicate alcoholism and nitrofurazone therapy for trypanosomiasis.

Clinical syndromes

- **Dry beriberi:** peripheral sensory and motor neuropathy: gradual onset of distal limb weakness and wasting with 'glove and stocking' sensory loss; foot drop and calf wasting common. Affected muscles may show oedema and painful contraction when hit. Reflexes and joint position sense are ↓ or lost; ataxia ± incontinence may develop in the later stages. Death occurs due to generalized and diaphragmatic paralysis.

- **Wet beriberi:** high-output cardiac failure. In typical wet beriberi, peripheries are warm with a bounding pulse, due to peripheral vasodilation In acute, fulminant beriberi, peripheries are cold due to poor cardiac output, but death occurs due to CCF.

- **Infantile beriberi:** occurs in infants breastfed from a vit B₁-deficient mother and is an important cause of infant mortality in parts of Asia. Irritability and oedema typically occur aged 2–3 months and may be confused with kwashiorkor; progressive heart failure occurs (± convulsions due to CNS involvement) and death is due to cardiorespiratory collapse.

- **Wernicke's encephalopathy** classically complicates thiamine deficiency in chronic alcohol abuse, but may also be precipitated by infections or by administration of carbohydrate (including IV dextrose) before thiamine replacement. Clinical features are confusion, ataxia, nystagmus, and ophthalmoplegia due to haemorrhagic degeneration in the midbrain and mamillary bodies. Korsakoff's psychosis may also occur in which there is profound loss of short term memory — this is reversible with thiamine replacement, unlike the other clinical features.

Diagnosis is usually clinical. CXR shows cardiolmegaly and pulmonary oedema in cardiac beriberi. Plasma pyruvate and lactate are ↑, red cell transketolase levels are low. Thiamine deficiency may be confirmed *in vitro* by ↑ activation of red cell transketolase after addition of thiamine.

Management:

- *Acute fulminant beriberi:* Thiamine 50–100 mg IV tds, followed by 10–25 mg/day PO.
- *Chronic beriberi:* Thiamine 10–25 mg/day PO for ≥6 weeks. Pain in limbs is relieved rapidly; peripheral neuropathy may take months to years to resolve.
- *Infantile beriberi:* Thiamine 25–50 mg given IV slowly followed by 10 mg IM daily for 1 week; then 3–5 mg/day orally for 6 weeks. Treat mother with thiamine 10 mg/day PO for 7 days, then 3–5 mg/day for 6 weeks.

Vit B₂ (riboflavin) deficiency

Riboflavin is found in meat, vegetables, milk, and wholemeal flour. Overt deficiency is uncommon. Some drugs e.g. phenothiazines and tricyclic antidepressants interact with riboflavin.

Clinical features: Angular cheilosis/stomatitis, sore red lips, atrophic glossitis. There may be plugging of sebaceous glands, giving a roughened appearance to the skin, and scrotal dermatitis. Anaemia occurs because riboflavin deficiency → poor iron absorption.

Management: Riboflavin up to 30 mg PO od. Usually rapidly cured.

Vit B₆ (pyridoxine) deficiency

Clinical signs of deficiency are rare, except as peripheral neuropathy during isoniazid therapy, and pyridoxine antagonists e.g. pyrazinamide and cycloserine may precipitate sideroblastic anaemia. Dietary sources include meat and plant foods.

Management: Pyridoxine 50–200 mg/day PO are widely used, but little evidence for efficacy. Doses up to 400 mg/day may be partially effective in idiopathic and hereditary sideroblastic anaemia. Give pyridoxine 10 mg/day during isoniazid therapy and to malnourished alcoholics.

Toxicity: Peripheral neuropathy is reported following prolonged high-dose pyridoxine. Improvement is limited even after stopping treatment.

Niacin deficiency: pellagra

Niacin and its precursor tryptophan are found in meat, fish, nuts, fruits, and vegetables are good sources of preformed niacin. Deficiency causes pellagra, and is common in communities where maize or sorghum are the staple, as bioavailability of niacin in maize is low, and high leucine levels in sorghum impair nicotinic acid and tryptophan metabolism; deficiency may be mitigated by sufficient dietary tryptophan e.g. in beans. Pellagra also occurs in malabsorption, isoniazid therapy alcoholism, and may contribute to diarrhoea, depression and skin disorders in HIV/AIDS.

Clinical features:
The classical triad is of dermatitis, diarrhoea, and dementia.

- *Skin:* a photosensitive, sunburn-like rash at sun-exposed sites; there may be a collar-like ring around the neck (Casal's necklace). Lesions are sensitive/inflamed, later becoming scaly and desquamates. Atrophic patches of skin remain between the fingers; the nails become brittle and atrophic.
- *Gastrointestinal:* gingival swelling ± bleeding; raw, fissured tongue; dysphagia; villous atrophy and malabsorption; diarrhoea and nausea.

- *Neurological:* insomnia, anxiety, depression, memory loss, photophobia; mania or psychosis (which may be permanent); pyramidal and extra-pyramidal signs; frontal reflexes. Confusion can precede death. Peripheral and cranial neuropathies also occur.
- *Eyes:* conjunctival oedema, corneal dystrophy, and lens opacities extending from the periphery to the centre.

Management: Nicotinamide 500 mg daily until complete recovery (at least 3–4 weeks).

Prevention: In confirmed outbreaks, consider vit B complex supplements for the entire population as a short-term measure: give nicotinamide 15 mg/person/day.

Vit B₁₂ deficiency

Vit B₁₂ is available in animal products including liver, fish, meat, eggs, and dairy products, but not in vegetables. Absorption depends on intrinsic factor from the stomach binding vit B₁₂ to facilitate uptake in the terminal ileum. Deficiency may be due to poor dietary intake (e.g. vegans), atrophic gastritis (pernicious anaemia), previous gastrectomy, and terminal ileal disease. Infection with *Diphyllobothrium latum* (fish tapeworm) has been implicated in Russia.

Clinical features
- *General:* Angular cheilosis, glossitis; hyperpigmentation of the hands and feet is noted in some populations.
- *Macrocytic anaemia:* see 📖 p 464.
- *Subacute combined degeration of the cord:* Dorsal column and cortico-spinal tract degeneration → sensory and both upper and lower motor neuron signs, classically with extensor plantars but absent knee and ankle reflexes, ± ataxia due to ↓ proprioception; pain and temperature sensation are preserved as spinothalamic tracts are not involved. May be precipitated by administration of high doses of folate to patients with combined B₁₂ and folate deficiency.
- *Other neurological sequelae:* peripheral neuropathy, optic atrophy, dementia, neuropsychiatric symptoms, neurodevelopmental delay.

Diagnosis: Low serum B12; macrocytosis; anaemia; low WBC and platelets (📖 p 464). Tests for pernicious anaemia: parietal cell/intrinsic factor Anti-bodies, Schilling test.

Management: Hydroxycobalamin 1 mg IM 3x/week for 2 weeks to replenish body stores, then 1 mg IM every 3 months (often needed for life); if neurological involvement, give 1 mg on alternate days until no further improvement, then 1 mg every 2 months.

Folate deficiency

Folate is heat labile and water soluble so is lost in prolonged cooking or boiling. Deficiency occurs in malabsorption, in pregnancy or haemolysis, and in patients on anti-folate drugs e.g. methotrexate or trimethoprim.

Clinical features: Blood changes are similar to vit B$_{12}$ deficiency (📖 p 464) but without the neurological sequelae. Deficiency in pregnancy ↑ risk of neural tube defects; intrauterine growth retardation, premature delivery, low birth weight.

Diagnosis: ↓ RBC folate; macrocytic anaemia (📖 p 464).

Management: Folic acid 5 mg PO od. Folic Acid is increasingly being added to flour as part of national government policies.

Vit C deficiency: scurvy

Vit C (ascorbic acid) is essential to collagen formation, promotes iron absorption, maintains healthy epithelial tissues, particularly of the mouth and skin, and promotes wound healing. It is found in fresh citrus fruit and potatoes but is easily destroyed by overcooking. Deficiency occurs in areas where fruit and vegetables are scarce, in the elderly, and in young children (who have ↑ requirements).

Clinical features:
- *General:* weight loss, stiffness, weakness, swollen painful large joints.
- *Skin:* dry skin, hyperkeratosis of hair follicles, 'corkscrew hairs', bruising, perifolicular petechial haemorrhages, poor wound healing.
- *Mouth:* gingivitis, bleeding gums, dental caries, loss of teeth.
- *Anaemia:* microcytic anaemia due to iron deficiency, and/or mega-loblastic anaemia as vit C is required for folate metabolism.

Treatment: Oral ascorbic acid, in divided doses per day for 2 weeks (Infants <1 m 50 mg/day; 1 m–4 y 125–250 mg/day, 4–12 y 250–500 mg/day, adults 500 mg/day).

Prevention: Avoid overcooking vegetables; eat citrus fruit, guavas. If necessary, supplement with tablets (children and adults 25–75 mg/day). Avoid artificial feeds without fortified vit C.

Scurvy in infants　　　　　　　　　**PAEDIATRIC NOTE**

Infantile scurvy typically presents at 6–12 months in premature or artificially fed infants. Erupting teeth cause bleeding of the gums. Subperiosteal haemorrhages cause limb pain and swelling, particularly in the long bones — most often palpable at the distal femur and proximal tibia; costochondral beading may also be palpable (scorbutic rosary). Occa-sionally, there is bloody diarrhoea. There may be a microcytic and/or megaloblastic anaemia. Plain X-rays of the long bones show epiphyseal changes and ground glass appearance of the shafts.

Vit D deficiency: rickets and osteomalacia

Vit D regulates calcium homeostasis by controlling intestinal absorption and renal excretion of Ca^{++}, and mobilizing Ca^{++} from bone. Vit D, also important in cell signalling, gene expression, platelet aggregation, and host immunity (esp. to TB). The best source of vit D is oily fish. Vit D_3 is rapidly formed in the skin by the action of UV light. Deficiency may occur due to dietary insufficiency, malabsorption, lack of UV exposure, liver disease, renal failure, or anticonvulsant therapy ($\uparrow$ Vit D metabolism 2° to enzyme induction). It causes rickets in children and osteomalacia in adults.

Clinical features
- Rickets is due to disordered bone mineralization at the growth plates of growing children, usually <2 years old. *Features*: irritability, hypotonia, painful wrists, and tender legs (which may be bowed once the child starts standing); swollen costo-chondral junctions ('rachitic rosary'), pigeon chest, indrawing of the lower ribs (Harrison sulcus), spinal deformities, bossing of the skull and craniotabes. Hypocalcaemia may → tetany and laryngeal spasm. Neurodevelopmental delay also occurs. Overt signs unusual in severe malnutrition, probably due to ↓ growth.
- Osteomalacia occurs in adults, often in women or in the elderly. It presents with acheing muscles and bones (pelvis, ribs, femora), pathological fractures, proximal myopathy (waddling gait).
- Vit D deficiency is also associated with susceptibility to infection including TB.

Diagnosis
Is clinical, aided by the following investigations:
- *X-rays:* Cupping and fraying of the metaphyses with widening of the epiphyses in rickets; osteopenia, Looser's zones (partial fractures without bony displacement e.g. of lateral scapular border, femur, or pelvis), biconcave deformity of the vertebrae.
- *Bloods:* low plasma 25-hydroxy vit D. Only in severe deficiency is there ↓ serum Ca^{++}, ↓PO_4^-, ↑ ALP.
- *Bone scanning* shows characteristic changes.

Management: Oral ergocalciferol (vit D_2): the daily intake for adults is 400–800 units, but deficiency should be corrected with a few days of high dose replacement: adults 40,000 units (1 mg), children <6 m 3,000 units; 6 m–12 y 6,000 units; 12–18 y 10,000 units daily. A single IM dose of 150,000 iu of vit D_2 in oil will protect for at least 6 months. Unless there is plenty of calcium in the diet or water, give calcium 500 mg PO od for the first 15 days of treatment. Specialist regimens are required if vit D deficiency due to renal disease or malabsorption.

Calcium deficiency and rickets   PAEDIATRIC NOTE

Rickets may also occur as a result of calcium deficiency in the absence of vit D deficiency, e.g. in African children fed a maize diet low in calcium. Clinical presentation is similar, but onset is usually later and hypo-tonia and bone pain tend not to be features.

Vit E deficiency

Vit E deficiency develops in patients with fat malabsorption (e.g. cholestatic liver disease) and in patients with congenital abetalipoproteinaemia who are unable to synthesis VLDL. Premature infants often have inadequate vit E stores → haemolytic anaemia.

Clinical features: Haemolytic anaemia, ataxia, and peripheral neuropathy.

Diagnosis: Plasma vit E (alpha-tocopherol) level.

Treatment: Few patients need treatment. Treat deficiency with Vit E in premature neonates (10 mg/kg PO od, or 20 mg/kg IM stat for neonates <1.5 kg), and children with severe fat malabsorption or abetalipoproteinaemia (100 mg/kg PO od).

Vit K deficiency

Vit K is essential for production of clotting factors II, VII, IX, and X, proteins C and S, and for bone growth. It is found in leafy green vegetables and is produced by intestinal bacteria. Deficiency occurs in poorly fed neonates and adults with malabsorption, and results in a bleeding tendency with ↑ prothrombin time. Neonates have low body stores, particularly those born prematurely, and deficiency causes 'haemorrhagic disease of the newborn'.

Treatment: Vit K (up to 10 mg PO/IV stat) in cases of haemorrhage. Dietary advice suffices in most non-bleeding cases. Haemorrhagic disease of the newborn is prevented by giving Vit K 1 mg IM stat to all newborns.

Iodine deficiency

Iodine is essential for thyroid hormone synthesis and brain development and function. Deficiency is usually due to low levels in soil and water, and most commonly occurs in mountainous areas (e.g. Nepal and Bolivia) and low-lying areas where flooding has washed iodine out of the soil (e.g. Bangladesh). Limited iodine availability can be worsened by eating brassicas, cassava, or soya beans. Deficiency causes goitre ± hypothyroidism; it is also the most common cause of preventable mental retardation ('cretinism') worldwide.

Clinical features
- *Goitre:* ↑ thyroid-stimulating hormone (TSH) from the pituitary → thyroid enlargement. Large goitres may cause dysphagia and hoarseness (recurrent laryngeal nerve compression). Patients may be euthyroid (most commonly) or hypothyroid. Not associated with ↑ risk of malignancy.
- *Endemic (neurologic) cretinism:* mental retardation, speech and hearing deficits, strabismus, spastic diplegia, and a characteristic apathetic facies with thickened features, May occur as a result of maternal hypothyroidism in any population, even in the absence of iodine deficiency.
- *Hypothyroidism:* clinical features are described on 📖 p 514. Severe hypothyroidism may → 'myxoedematous cretinism', characterized by short stature, ataxia, and mental retardation without hearing deficit.

Diagnosis

Is clinical, supported by ↑ TSH ± ↓T_4; urinary iodine measures of dietary iodine intake.

Treatment
- Iodized oil as a single dose repeated after 1–2 years (see box opposite).
- Lugol's iodine (often kept for sterilization) may also be given as 1 drop every 30 days, or 1 daily teaspoon of a solution containing 1 drop of Lugol's iodine in 30 ml of water.
- Surgery may be required for massive goitre.

Prevention of iodine deficiency   PUBLIC HEALTH NOTE

Visible goitre in >10% of the population indicates severe iodine deficiency and mass prevention should be undertaken with IM injections of iodized oil or oral iodine. Iodine should also be given to pregnant women in endemic areas to prevent cretinism due to congenital hypothyroidism.

- Iodized salt: Satisfactory iodization of salt can be tested using simple colour change kits based on starch/iodine interaction colours.
- Iodized poppy seed oil (IPSO) can be used in endemic areas where salt is not iodized: women should take IPSO 400 mg as a single dose, preferably before conception; children should receive 100 mg if <12 months, 200 mg between 1–5 years, and 400 mg between 5–18 years. In areas where intestinal parasites are endemic, give albendazole to ensure absorption. The dose lasts for up to two years.
- Over-replacement in endemic areas may → thyrotoxicosis.

Other micronutrients

Zinc

Zinc has antioxidant properties and is essential to several proteins and enzymes, including those regulating gene expression. Body stores are minimal so deficiency occurs quickly, especially in catabolic states or if intestinal losses are high. Zn is found in meat and fish; bioavailability from cereals is often poor because phytate binds Zn. Deficiency occurs in severe malnutrition (especially oedematous malnutrition) and low birth weight infants.

Clinical features: Failure to thrive, recurrent infections, persistent diarrhoea, scaly leasions (probably due to local candida) on the feet and buttocks, stunting, developmental delay. The classical rash of acrodermatitis enteropathica occurs rarely, usually due to a congenital disorder of Zn malabsorption. Plasma Zn is often ↓in individuals but single measurements are unreliable as they ↓ in acute infection.

Treatment: Zinc 10 mg/day reduces the frequency/severity of respiratory infections and diarrhoeal disease, including in HIV +ves, and improves wound healing. A 2-week course of zinc given for diarrhoea reduces mortality in the following 6 months.

Selenium

Several enzymatic processes require selenium. Dietary sources include cereals, meat, and nuts. Deficiency occurs where cereals are grown in low selenium soils → impaired antioxidant activity. This may contribute to coronary artery disease in some countries (e.g. Finland). Selenium stimulates immunity and has been advised in nutritional support for HIV.

Clinical features: selenium deficiency → cardiomyopathy in China where soils are deficient in selenium.

Treatment & prevention: selenium should be included in the electrolyte/mineral mix for treatment of severe malnutrition. Fertilizers help mitigate the effect of low selenium levels in the soil.

Copper

Copper is important for several enzymes with antioxidant properties and for development of collagen. It is widely available in shellfish, liver, kidney, nuts, and wholegrain cereals. Deficiency is uncommon and causes osteoporosis and leukopenia with ↑ risk of infection. Copper deficiency may be precipitated by high Zn doses → impaired copper absorption; Menke's disease is a rare cause due to defective copper metabolism. Dietary excess (± genetic predisposition) is implicated in Indian childhood cirrhosis (📖 p 303).

Treatment: Copper should be included in the electrolyte/mineral mix for treatment of severe malnutrition.

Fluoride

Fluoride is essential for mineralization of bones and teeth, and is present in the majority of foods and drinking water. Deficiency contributes to dental caries. Excess dietary fluoride may occur where the drinking water is very high in fluoride (e.g. Rift Valley in E Africa, the Punjab) causing clinical fluorosis.

Clinical features of deficiency include dental caries and softening of long bones with deformity. Conversely, fluorosis is characterized by excess fluoride deposition in teeth and bones, with chalky discolouration of teeth enamel, spinal rigidity, restricted joint movement, ectopic mineralization of tendons, ligaments, and occasionally muscles, ↑ bone density.

Prevention: Add fluoride to drinking water at source where fluoride levels low. Where fluorosis is endemic and fluoride levels in water are high, advise on alternative drinking water sources.

Iron

Iron deficiency is a common cause of anaemia (see 📖 p 460).

Multiple micronutrient supplements

While individual micronutrients have considerable impact on cellular immunity, antioxidant capacity and individual organ function, when several micronutrients are given together they may impair the absorption and metabolism of others. This is less likely if micronutrients are given together at one or two RDA doses.

At present, there is insufficient evidence that micronutrient preparations improve the health of individuals in a community regardless of their dietary intake, nutritional and disease status. However, there is evidence supporting multiple micronutrient combinations in HIV/AIDS and TB. There are insufficient data to recommend particular multiple micronutrient doses.

Multiple micronutrient preparations (up to 15 micronutrients in doses recommended by WHO/UNICEF) have been shown to improve outcome in pregnancy and ↑ birthweight. Benefits have also been shown in postnatal child growth, morbidity, and survival among children of HIV-infected mothers who receive supplementation with thiamine, riboflavin, niacin, folic acid, and vits B_6, B_{12}, C and E during pregnancy.

Obesity

The terms overweight and obese are interchangeable: a person is too heavy for their height compared with standard references. People become obese because they take in more calories in food and drink than they consume in metabolism and work. There is increasing evidence for diffrences between individuals in appetite, fat metabolism, and metabolic responses to a meal. There is a global epidemic of obesity among children in particular. Changes in patterns of dietary intake in recent years have been associated with reduction in physical activity.

Obesity tended in the past to be a disease of the prosperous and urbanization, but present epidemics of obesity affect the poor who buy cheaper, high-energy foods. Obesity ↑ risk of coronary heart disease, stroke, hypertension, type II diabetes, gallstones and other digestive disorders, back problems, arthritis of the knees and hips, accidents, fractures, and fatigue.

Diagnosis: A BMI >25 indicates probable obesity; >30 definite obesity. Children are obese if they weigh >97th centile on either the W/H or W/A curve (growth chart 📖 p 630).

Management: weight loss is difficult:
• Eat foods containing more fibre and less fat or sugar. Instead of high-energy snacks, eat fruit or maize cobs. Avoid sweets, chips, crisps, and cakes; ↓ alcohol.
• Exercise for >20 mins per day at a level sufficient to raise the pulse and respiratory rates.
• Be realistic and offer encouragement, not scorn.
• Advise stopping smoking to reduce cardiovascular risk.
• Avoid drugs which suppress appetite and metabolism — the evidence for these is lacking.

References/further information

Guidelines

- *MSF Nutrition Guidelines* (2004).
- *Valid International, Community Based Therapeutic Care* (2006).
- Waterlow, Ashworth, Tomkins, and McGregor, *Protein Energy Malnutrition* (2007).
- Rajabiun S et al. *HIV/AIDS: a guide for nutrition, care and support.* (FANTA project. Academy for Educational Development, Washington 2000).
- UNHCR/WFP, *Guidelines for selective feeding programmes in emergency situations* (1999).
- WHO (1999) *Management of severe malnutrition: a manual for physicians and other senior health workers.* WHO, Geneva.
- WHO, WFP, UNHCR, IFRC *The management of nutrition in major emergencies* (2000).
- Young H and Jaspars J (1995) *Nutrition matters. Part I.* Intermediate Technology Publication, London, pp. 3–24.
- Collins et al, Management of Severe Malnutrition in Children. *Lancet* 2006;368:1992–2000.
- Manary et al, Home Based Therapy for Severe Malnutrition with RUTF. *Arch Dis Child* 2004;89:557–561.

Multi-system diseases and infections

Section editors

Tania Araujo–Jorge (Chagas' disease)
Margaret Callan
(infectious mononucleosis)
François Chappuis
(African trypanosomiasis)
Cecilia P. Chung and Charles M Stein
(rheumatoid arthritis, osteoarthritis,
and SLE)
David Dance (plague, melioidosis)
Jeremy Farrar (influenza)
Stan Houston (prevention of infection
in the health care setting)
Michael G Jacobs
(sepsis, arboviruses, VHF)
Marc Nicol
(rickettsial infections, brucellosis)
Chris Parry (typhoid)
Yupin Suputtamongkol (leptospirosis)
David Warrell (relapsing fevers)
Syed Mohd Akramuz Zaman
(measles)

Differential diagnosis of fevers

Fever is a common presentation of infections (and, less commonly, inflammatory conditions or malignancy). The fever pattern does not reliably distinguish bacterial, viral, parasitic, fungal, or non-infectious causes of fever. Distinctive patterns of fever and pulse rate which were emphasized in the past (e.g. a step-wise increase in fever and relative bradycardia which were previously thought to be typical of typhoid) are now seldom emphasized. In fever from whatever cause, body temperature tends to rise in the late afternoon/evening and falls during the night. This gives rise to a sensation of being cold in the afternoon/evening and night sweats. Fever is often intermittent; it may be absent in the morning and absent if paracetamol, aspirin, or NSAIDs have been taken. Patients on steroids may have little or no fever.

A history of drenching sweats or rigors (chills or shivering, often uncontrollable and lasting for minutes) is always significant. Rigors are generally indicative of malaria or bacterial sepsis, and occasionally of severe viral infection (e.g. Dengue, Lassa fever). TB, kala-azar, and other chronic infections do not generally cause rigors, and nor do mild viral infections (e.g EBV or respiratory viruses), malignancy, or connective tissue diseases.

In view of the wide range of possible diagnoses, a detailed history and complete physical examination are essential. During the assessment, consider:

- Where is the site of infection?
- Which are the likely infecting organisms?
- Is this presentation unusual? Has it become more common recently? Might an epidemic be occurring?
- Is the patient immunocompromised (or might they be)? If so, consider the differential diagnoses for both immunocompetent and immunocompromised individuals.
- Serious infections such as meningococcal sepsis and malaria may have 'false localizing' symptoms and signs such as headache, breathlessness, vomiting, or diarrhoea.
- In the presence of localizing features, investigations are targeted towards the presumed cause. Specimens (blood, urine, CSF, etc.) for microscopy and culture, if available, are most useful.
- Treatment with antibiotics can be started based on a clinical diagnosis and the likely infecting organisms. Consult local guidelines for choosing antibiotics — if available.

Common infections with localizing features

• Pneumonia	Breathlessness, cough, sputum, pleurisy
• Pulmonary TB	Prolonged cough, haemoptysis
• Urinary tract infection	Urinary frequency, dysuria, haematuria, loin pain
• Infective enterocolitis	Vomiting, diarrhoea, abdominal pain
• Cellulitis	Red, hot skin
• Septic arthritis	Painful, swollen joint
• Osteomyelitis	Bone pain
• Meningitis	Headache, confusion, neck stiffness
• Streptococcal, EBV, or diphtheria infection	Sore throat, exudate over tonsils/pharynx
• TB lymphadenitis	Prominent cervical lymphadenopathy

Fever without localizing features

This is a challenging clinical problem. The following are helpful in determining the likely cause:
- Blood smears for microscopy for malaria.
- Total and differential white cell counts.
- Platelet count.
- Blood culture (where available).

The importance of malaria

In many tropical areas, malaria is the most common and important cause of fever and should be the first diagnosis considered. Patients generally have evening fevers, so may be afebrile in a morning clinic. In endemic areas, low-grade parasitaemia without symptoms is common in adults and older children (due the development of partial immunity to malaria). Thus, the finding of low-grade parasitaemia (or a positive rapid diagnostic test [RDT]) in an individual with fever does not prove that the fever is caused by malaria — always consider additional diagnoses. Febrile patients with no visible malaria parasites (or a negative RDT) should not be treated for malaria. It is false to assume that a patient can be ill, even severely ill, with malaria and have no malaria parasites detectable. However, blood films and RDTs may need to be repeated daily to be sure they are negative.

Blood counts in a patient with fever (see box opposite)

White cell counts and platelet count may give some useful clues to the cause of fever, although this must be considered in the context of careful clinical assessment of the patient.

Treatment of fever of unknown cause

Quite commonly, a positive diagnosis cannot be made after the initial clinical assessment and tests. The management then depends on:
- Your judgement of the most likely diagnoses.
- How severely ill the patient is.
- Available resources.

Patients who you judge to be (or at risk of becoming) seriously unwell should be given 'best guess' empirical antimicrobial therapy, using local guidelines if these exist.

Admission to hospital, if possible, is the best course if you are worried about the patient's condition. In time, the diagnosis is likely to become apparent, particularly if the patient is regularly reassessed.

Persistent fever despite antimicrobial therapy

- Antimicrobials chosen do not treat the infecting organism.
- Infecting organism is resistant to chosen antimicrobials.
- Inadequate drug concentration at site of infection — think about compliance, dose, absorption, drug penetration into special sites (e.g. CSF, collections/abscesses).
- Non-infectious cause of fever.
- Antibiotic-induced (drug) fever.

If total white cell count ↑, look at the differential WBC count

Differential white cell count	Common or important causes
• Neutrophilia	Bacterial infections (sepsis, focal infection, deep-seated abscess, leptospirosis, Borrelia infections), Amoebic liver abscess
• Lymphocytosis	Infectious mononucleosis (EBV), Whooping cough
• Eosinophilia	Invasive worm infections (e.g. acute schistosomiasis)

If total white cell count normal or low, look at the platelet count

Platelet count	Common or important causes
• Normal	Viral infections (including the prodrome of acute viral hepatitis), typhoid, rickettsial infection
• Low	Malaria, Dengue and other viral infections, HIV

Sepsis

The features of sepsis result from the interaction between the pathogen and host defences. Bacterial infections are the most common cause, but other serious infections (e.g. falciparum malaria, Lassa fever) can cause an identical clinical syndrome. Some non-infectious insults can produce an identical clinical syndrome (e.g. pancreatitis, chemical toxins, burns).

Definitions of sepsis and related disorders

Sepsis: Clinical evidence of infection, plus evidence of a systemic response manifested by 2 or more of:
- Temperature >38°C or <36°C.
- Heart rate >90 beats/min.
- Respiratory rate >20 breaths/min.
- WBC >12 or <4, or >10% immature forms.

Severe sepsis: Sepsis associated with organ dysfunction:
- Hypotension.
- Lactic acidosis.
- Oliguria.
- Confusion.
- Hepatic dysfunction.

Septic shock: Severe sepsis with hypotension despite adequate fluid resuscitation.

Management

The cornerstones of treatment are:
- IV fluid resuscitation.
- Antimicrobial therapy — 'best guess' empirical treatment should be started immediately (after blood cultures, if available).

In severely ill patients, a wide range of supportive measures (e.g. vasopressor therapy, IV hydrocortisone, mechanical ventilation, haemofiltration) might be indicated if available.

However, despite intensive treatment, mortality from sepsis remains high — overall, about 20–30% in sepsis, rising to 50% in patients with severe sepsis or shock, and over 80% in patients with multi-organ failure.

Pregnancy-related infections

The risk of maternal death varies from 7/100,000 in Scandinavia to 1000/100,000 in some parts of Africa and Middle East. The major causes of maternal death are:
- Sepsis.
- Hypertensive disorders of pregnancy.
- Haemorrhage.
- Complications of obstructed labour.

General principles of management
- Emptying the uterus is essential for a cure — deliver the baby or evacuate any retained products.
- Antibiotics should be started as soon as the diagnosis is made.
- A wide range of bacteria may cause these infections and there is often more than one organism — broad-spectrum antibiotic therapy should be used that includes cover for *Streptococci*, Gram −ves, and anaerobes.

Prevention
Are there any simple measures that could be introduced to prevent some pregnancy-related infections? Consider the major risk factors listed in the box. The most effective ways to reduce post-abortion infections are to make available:
- Contraceptives to prevent unwanted pregnancies.
- Medical abortions.

	Major factors increasing risk	Clinical features
Intrapartum chorioamnionitis	Pre-term labour Prolonged rupture of membranes Multiple vaginal examinations	Fever Maternal tachycardia Uterine tenderness Foetal tachycardia
Postpartum endometritis	Caesarean section (particularly after onset of labour or rupture of membranes) Use of unwashed hands or unsterilized instruments during delivery	Fever (usually 1–2 days postpartum) Tachycardia Lower abdominal pain Uterine tenderness
Post-abortion	Non-medical abortions Retained products of conception Operative trauma	Fever (usually within 4 days of procedure) Abdominal pain and tenderness Vaginal bleeding High risk of severe sepsis

Cancer

Cancer will become an increasingly important cause of premature mortality in the developing countries as populations expand and age, and as tobacco consumption increases and diets are westernized. Approximately 60% of global cancer occurs in developing countries: ~10 million new cases per year. This is likely to double by 2020; most of the increase occurring in developing countries. There is wide geographical variation in the prevalence of some cancers. Lung cancer is the most common cancer worldwide, followed by stomach, liver, colon and rectum, oesophagus, and breast. Breast cancer is the most common fatal cancer in women.

Cancer requires early intervention for therapy to be effective. Bearing this in mind, basic rules include:
- Cancer should be suspected in any unexplained illness, particularly in the elderly.
- An attempt should be made to get a histological or cytological diagnosis as soon as feasible.
- Once diagnosed, patients should start a planned regimen of treatment within days, not weeks. Tumours grow exponentially and there is no room for delay.

Signs and symptoms common to many forms of cancer
- *Pain*: due to direct effect of tumour (e.g. infiltration of nerves or compression), its treatment, or metastatic spread to the bones. Any patient with unexplained persistent pain should be suspected of having malignant disease.
- *Weight loss*: due to involvement of GI tract (obstruction, metastatic liver involvement), anorexia, or general cachexia due to a catabolic state. May be exacerbated by treatment.
- *Tumour mass*: often ignored by doctors but requiring early diagnosis by biopsy, preferably by fine needle aspiration.
- *Fever*: while normally caused by superimposed infection, fever may itself be a feature of cancers such as lymphomas, renal CA, and tumours metastasizing to the liver. Frequently occurs as drenching night sweats without rigors.
- *Anaemia*: normocytic normochromic (sometimes hypochromic) due to bleeding, malabsorption, or anaemia of chronic disease.
- *Hypercalcaemia*: due to widespread metastases to the skeleton or, more commonly, to paraneoplastic syndromes.

Paraneoplastic syndromes
These occur relatively commonly and are due to tumour-derived cytokines or hormones or to a tumour-induced immune response cross-reacting with normal tissue. The range includes endocrine, neurological, dermatological, musculoskeletal, and haematological syndromes. Paraneoplastic symptoms often improve on therapy. Most neurological problems are due to metastases, and most endocrine problems due to endocrine tumours themselves, not paraneoplastic syndromes.

WHO performance status

This is useful for grading the status of cancer patients and determining prognosis.

0 Able to carry out normal activity without restriction
1 Restricted in physically strenuous activity but walking about and able to carry out light work
2 Walking about and capable of self-care but unable to carry out any work; up and about >50% of waking hours
3 Capable of self-care; confined to bed or chair >50% of waking hours
4 Completely disabled; cannot carry out self-care; totally confined to bed or chair

Important complications of some tumours

- Spinal cord/cauda equina compression[†].
- Cerebral metastases and raised intracranial pressure[†].
- Carcinomatous meningitis — leads to headache and increased ICP
- Pleural and pericardial effusions.

[†] *Management* requires immediate administration of dexamethasone 8 mg bd IV. Neurological symptoms should settle quickly. Delay in the treatment of spinal cord compression will result in paraplegia.

Website: *http://www.inctr.org/about/develop.shtml*

General rules of cancer management

Whenever you see a patient known to have cancer, think of the following points:

1. **Could the patient have neutropenia?** Infection in a neutropenic patient often presents suddenly with sepsis, but without localizing features, and cultures are usually negative. Neutropenia commonly occurs if the patient has had chemotherapy, Normal bacterial flora from the mouth, digestive tract, respiratory tract, or skin are usually responsible, and indwelling lines and catheters may be the source. Any cancer patient who is feeling 'run down' must have their WCC checked immediately and not be sent home. Such patients can deteriorate quickly and be dead within hours.

2. **Could the patient have hypercalcaemia?** Unlike 1° parathyroid disease, the onset is rapid and there are none of the classical 'stones, bones, or groans'. Instead clinical features include: polyuria, thirst, confusion, fatigue, coma. Treatment of hypercalcaemia will produce a marked improvement in the patient's condition.

3. **Is the patient's pain controlled?** Use morphine — it is a very effective drug. The following regimen is useful:
   - Give morphine 10 mg q4 h at 07.00, 11.00, etc., until 23.00, at which point give a double dose so that the 03.00 dose can be missed out, offering the chance of a good night's sleep.
   - If pain breaks through, give an extra dose of morphine 10 mg (even if the next q4 h dose is only 10 mins away), continuing the q4 h dose as normal.
   - As more breakthrough doses are required, increase the regular q4 h dose (e.g. to 20 mg).
   - (If using long-acting morphine (e.g. MST 80 mg bd), take total daily dose (160 mg) and divide by 6 (q4 h doses) to give size of the IV morphine dose to use for breakthroughs — here 160/6 = ~26 mg).

4. **Could the patient have early cord compression?** Ask: Can you walk? When was the last time you walked? Have you been incontinent of urine and/or faeces? Do a neurological exam including anal tone and sacral sensation, and check for a palpable bladder. Missing spinal cord compression may result in the patient spending their last few weeks or months in a miserable paraplegic state.

Hypercalcaemia

- Rehydrate with 0.9% saline IV (e.g. 4–6 L in 24 h depending on hydration status).
- Once rehydrated consider forced saline diuresis: continue 0.9% saline infusion and give e.g. Furosemide 40 mg bd PO/IV.
- Consider single bisphosphanate infusion (e.g pamidronate) to lower calcium over 2–3 days (max effect at 1 week). Dose varies according to serum calcium level (see below).
- Steroids may help in some conditions e.g. sarcoidosis, malignancy.
- If possible treat the underlying cause.

Disodium pamidronate doses

Corrected calcium	Pamidronate dose
<3 mmol/l	15–30 mg
3–3.5 mmol/l	30–60 mg
3.5–4.0 mmol/l	60–90 mg
>4.0 mmol/l	90 mg

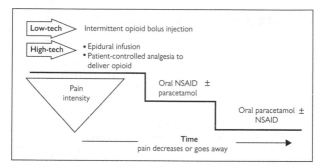

Fig. 18.1 Overview of the management of acute severe pain

Management of acute pain in hospital

1. Effective relief can be achieved with oral non-opioid and NSAIDs. Ibuprofen 400 mg is very effective and is associated with fewer gastrointestinal bleeds than some other NSAIDs. Also effective are paracetamol 1 g and paracetamol combined with codeine.

2. Initial management of moderate pain e.g. in post-surgical patients, should ideally be an oral NSAID such as ibuprofen, supplemented if necessary with paracetamol. In the elderly, paracetamol may be preferred, although it is less effective. There is no evidence that parenteral is more beneficial than oral administration.

3. Opioids are the first-choice treatment for severe acute pain. Additional, often smaller doses can be given if the patient is still in pain and you are sure that all the previous dose has been delivered and absorbed. Repeat doses can be given 5 mins after IV injection, 1 h after IM or SC injection, and 90 mins after an oral dose. The route of administration can be changed to achieve faster control if there is no response to the repeated dose.

4. Titrate opioids against degree of pain relief. Inadequate pain control results from too little drug, too long dosing intervals, too little attention being paid to the patient, or too much reliance on rigid regimens.

5. Morphine is the most appropriate opioid and it is popular amongst pain specialists. Its analgesia lasts a reliable 4 h and is easier to titrate than opioids with a longer half-life. Set up a q4 h regimen which prevents the occurrence of pain (see ⌑ p 676 for an example of a q4 h morphine regimen.)

6. As the pain decreases, the patient can be switched to ibuprofen and paracetamol. Supplementation of morphine with an NSAID allows the morphine dose to be reduced.

Rheumatoid arthritis (RA)

RA is a chronic, systemic inflammatory condition of unknown cause that primarily involves joints. It is associated with disability, accelerated atherosclerosis, and increased mortality. Lack of treatment or poor response to treatment leads to permanent joint destruction and deformity. Onset is usually between the 3rd and 5th decade and RA affects women 2–3 times more frequently than men.

Symptoms: include joint pain, swelling, and stiffness.
Clinical signs: usually chronic symmetrical joint swelling (often PIPs, MCPs, MTPs, wrists, knees); affects the cervical but not the lumbar spine.
Extra-articular disease: anaemia of chronic disease, subcutaneous nodules (usually extensor), fatigue, pleuropericarditis, lymphadenopathy, nerve entrapment (e.g. carpal tunnel syndrome), mononeuritis multiplex, splenomegaly, episcleritis, scleritis, Sjögrens syndrome, and lung fibrosis.

Diagnosis: by history and physical examination — there is no definitive test.
X-rays: affected joints may show typical changes (soft tissue swelling, symmetric joint space narrowing, bone erosions, and deformities).
Immunology: rheumatoid factor is positive in approximately 80% of patients (false positive in 5% of healthy people, more often in old age, chronic infections, liver disease, fibrotic lung disease, and other rheumatic diseases).

Complications: patients with longstanding RA and poor disease control may develop irreversible joint damage and deformity, limited functional capacity and atlanto-axial instability.

Management
- *Non-pharmacologic:* patient education, aerobic and resistance exercise, physical and occupational therapy.
- *Pharmacologic:* disease-modifying anti-rheumatoid drugs (DMARDs) are critical to prevent permanent damage. They should be prescribed as early as possible and are often needed lifelong. Monitoring for drug toxicity is needed (see box). DMARDs are used alone or in combination for disease control. Most widely used are methotrexate, sulfasalazine, and antimalarials — chloroquine and hydroxychloroquine. A common combination is methotrexate + sulfasalazine + hydroxy-chloroquine. Other DMARDs include leflunomide, cyclosporin, and biologic agents. These biologic agents include anti-TNF drugs (infliximab, etanercept, and adalimumab), anti-IL-1 (anakinra), anti CD-20 (rituximab), and CTLA4 Ig (abatacept). All are extremely expensive. Rarely used DMARDs include: gold salts, penicillamine, chlorambucil, cyclophosphamide and azathioprine.
- *Oral NSAIDs* decrease pain and swelling; they only provide symptomatic relief and do not affect other outcomes, and if used, should always be used with DMARDs.
- *Corticosteroids* can be used orally in low-doses (equivalent to <10 mg prednisolone/day) or as intra-articular injections. If steroids are used, it is almost always with a DMARD.
- *Surgery* for deformity/complications.

Differential diagnosis of RA

- Acute viral polyarthritis: caused by hepatitis, rubella.
- Parvovirus: self-limited (weeks); history of rash IgM viral antibodies.
- Connective tissue diseases: symmetric polyarthritis without joint deformities. Look for other multi-systemic features.
- Septic arthritis: usually acute monoarthritis. Immediate joint aspirate (for Gram and ZN stain, crystals, culture) and antibiotics are required to prevent permanent joint damage.
- Fibromyalgia: diffuse pain without inflammation. Insomnia and fatigue.
- Reactive arthritis: asymmetric oligoarthritis, sausage digits. Look for urethritis, conjunctivitis, and history of enteric infection.
- Gout/pseudogout: acute episodic attacks. In gout, monoarthritis of the 1st MTP is common. Definitive diagnosis made by finding crystals in synovial fluid.
- Osteoarthritis (see below).
- Paraneoplastic syndromes.
- HIV-associated arthritis (usually reactive arthritis pattern).

Monitoring of drugs commonly used to treat RA

Drug (usual doses)	Monitoring
NSAIDs	FBC ± yearly LFT and creatinine
Methotrexate (7.5–20 mg weekly)	FBC, AST, albumin, creatinine every 4–8 wks
Chloroquine (150 mg [base] daily*)	Fundoscopy and visual fields every 6–12 months
Hydroxychloroquine (400 mg daily)	Fundoscopy and visual fields every 6–12 months
Sulfasalazine (max 2–3 g daily)	FBC 2–4 weekly for 3 months, then 3 monthly

*Note: Chloroquine base 150 mg = chloroquine sulphate 200 mg = chloroquine phosphate 250 mg

Contraindications to drugs for RA

- NSAIDs: GI bleed, peptic ulcer; if NSAID required combine with a PPI.
- Methotrexate: pregnancy, elevated creatinine, alcohol use, liver disease, abnormal LFTs, HIV, HBV, HCV.
- Sulfasalazine: allergy to sulfas, G6PD deficiency.

Osteoarthritis

OA is a chronic, non-inflammatory arthropathy that can be idiopathic or secondary to trauma or other conditions.

Symptoms: non-inflammatory joint pain (see box). The knees, hips, and DIPs are most commonly affected. If unusual joints are involved (elbows, ankles, MCPs) look for secondary causes: previous trauma, hemochromatosis, Wilson's disease, or reconsider diagnosis (could be RA).

Clinical signs: bony swelling, crepitus.

Diagnosis: by history and physical exam.

X-ray findings: non-uniform joint space narrowing, osteophytes, and juxta-articular osteosclerosis.

Management
- Non-pharmacologic: patient education (weight loss if obese, exercise to strengthen muscles around affected joint), physical and occupational therapy.
- Analgesia: paracetamol ± NSAID.
- Glucosamine sulphate: 500 mg tid (under evaluation).
- Intra-articular hyaluronans.
- Intra-articular glucocorticoids.
- Surgery including prosthetic joint replacement.

Classification of joint pain

Inflammatory e.g. RA
- Improves with activity.
- Worse in the morning.
- Morning stiffness >60 minutes.
- Systemic features: sometimes.
- Soft swelling (effusion).
- Sometimes erythema.
- Sometimes warmth

Non-inflammatory e.g. OA
- Exacerbated by activity.
- Worse at night.
- Morning stiffness <30 minutes.
- Systemic features: absent.
- Hard swelling ('bony').
- No erythema.
- No warmth.

Systemic lupus erythematosus (SLE)

A multi-system chronic inflammatory disease characterized by facial rash, photosensitivity, alopecia, nephritis, serositis, arthritis, CNS involvement, vasculitis, and fever. A etiology is unknown. Women are affected 10 times more often than men; peak incidence is between 15 and 40 years of age. Causes of death include infections and disease activity in early phases of the disease, and atherosclerosis in the long-term.

Clinical features
- *General*: fever, fatigue, weight loss.
- *Joints*: arthralgia/arthritis (may be similar to RA, but usually non-erosive).
- *Skin*: photosensitive rash, purpura, alopecia, livedo reticularis, mouth ulcers.
- Raynaud's phenomenon.
- *Renal*: nephritic or nephrotic syndrome; renal failure.
- *CNS*: depression, psychosis, seizures.
- *Serositis*: pleural and pericardial effusion.
- *Pulmonary*: pneumonitis, fibrosis, bronchiolitis.
- *Cardiovascular*: hypertension, pericarditis, sterile (Libman–Sachs) endocarditis.
- *Blood*: normocytic anaemia, haemolysis (Coombs positive), leukopenia, thrombocytopenia.
- Thrombosis and miscarriage, which may be part of the antiphospholipid antibody syndrome.

Laboratory tests: several auto-antibodies that react with the cell nucleus are a feature of the disease. Anti-nuclear antibodies (ANA) are positive in more than 95% of patients. However, ANA are not specific; patients with other rheumatic conditions or chronic diseases, and 5% of normal subjects have positive ANA. Anti-double-stranded DNA and particularly anti-Smith (anti-Sm) antibodies are more specific but less sensitive.

Diagnosis: American College of Rheumatology diagnostic criteria for SLE are given in the box opposite: 4 or more criteria should be present to make the diagnosis, but some patients meet fewer than 4 criteria.

Management
- *Education*: sun avoidance, sunscreen, hat, long sleeves.
- *NSAIDS*: useful for musculoskeletal symptoms and serositis.
- *Antimalarials* (chloroquine/hydroxychloroquine): effective for skin and musculoskeletal symptoms; may prevent renal and CNS flares.
- *Systemic corticosteroids*: prednisolone <0.5 mg/kg for moderate disease; higher doses (1 mg/kg) for severe or lifethreatening disease, including renal disease, pneumonitis, severe cytopenias, or CNS lupus. Consider high-dose IV methylprednisolone boluses for severely ill patients. Corticosteroids should be tapered early according to response; combine with steroid sparing agents to minimize steroid side-effects.
- *Cyclophosphamide*: used to treat severe disease including proliferative lupus nephritis, vasculitis, CNS involvement, and alveolar hemorrhage.
- *Azathioprine*: as a steroid-sparing agent.

- *Mycophenolate mofetil*: used to treat lupus nephritis; may be as effective as cyclophosphamide with less adverse events.
- *Others*: rituximab, chlorambucil, cyclosporin. For refractory skin involvement: thalidomide.
- *Anticoagulation* for the antiphospholipid syndrome.

American College of Rheumatology diagnostic criteria

4 or more of the following are required to diagnose SLE:

1. Malar rash
2. Discoid rash
3. Photosensitivity
4. Oral ulcers
5. Arthritis
6. Serositis
7. Renal involvement: proteinuria (>0.5 g/day) or cellular casts
8. Neurologic disorders: seizures or psychosis
9. Hematologic disorders: hemolytic anemia, leukopenia, lymphopenia or thrombocytopenia
10. Immunologic disorders: positive LE cell, anti-DNA, anti-Sm
11. Antinuclear antibody

Markers of poor prognosis in patients with SLE

- Diffuse proliferative renal disease.
- Hypertension.
- Male sex.
- Lower socio-economic and education status.
- Black and Hispanic ethnicity.
- Antiphospholipid antibodies.
- Disease activity involving multiple organs.

Typhoid and paratyphoid fevers

These conditions, also called enteric fever, follow infection with Salmonella spp. (*S. typhi* → typhoid; *S. paratyphi* types A, B, C → paratyphoid). They are endemic and important causes of morbidity across the developing world. Typhoid is most severe; paratyphoid B mildest, with types A and C falling somewhere in between. **Early antibiotic treatment** is essential to ↓ mortality — start empirically if clinical suspicion strong. Following 1° multiplication in mesenteric lymph nodes, bacteria infect cells of the reticuloendothelial system where multiplication occurs again. This produces a 2° bacteraemia, infection of multiple organs, and clinical illness. If untreated, 20% die from overwhelming toxaemia or 2° organ involvement, particularly encephalopathy, toxic myocarditis, or GI haemorrhage and peritonitis. Importantly for infection control, chronic asymptomatic gall bladder infection is common — carriers have highly infectious stools.

Transmission: via ingestion of food or water contaminated by infected faeces/urine. Gastric acid is protective so any condition that decreases its production increases an individual's susceptibility to infection.

Clinical features: Incubation period is 10–20 days; untreated illness typically lasts ~4 weeks (may be shorter in severe infections and vice versa).

- *1st week*: non-specific features of malaise, headache, rising remitting fever with mild cough, constipation.
- *2nd week*: patient becomes toxic and apathetic; sustained high temperature with relative bradycardia; rose spots (2–4 mm pink papules on central torso, fading on pressure) may transiently occur; distended abdomen; hepatomegaly and/or splenomegaly.
- *3rd week*: increasing toxicity with persistent high temp; the patient becomes delirious and weak with feeble pulse, tachypnoea ± basal crepitations, profuse 'pea soup' diarrhoea. Look and listen for abdominal distention and bowel sounds. Neurological complications may occur (may rarely be the presenting complaint). Death occurs during week 2, 3, or 4.
- *4th week*: if the patient survives, fever, mental state, and abdominal distension gradually improve. GI complications occur at any time, most commonly in weeks 2–4.

Diagnosis: culture of bone marrow (best), blood, stool, or rectal swab.

Management
- Give antibiotics — see box.
- Give dexamethasone (3 mg/kg IV stat, then 1 mg/kg q6 h for 2 days) to patients with shock or ↓ consciousness — it may reduce mortality.
- Toxic patients must be observed carefully for signs of GI haemorrhage (treat conservatively) or peritonitis (treat with surgery).

Relapse: up to 20% of treated patients relapse after treatment and initial recovery. Relapses are generally milder and shorter than 1° illness; 2nd and 3rd relapses have been reported, therefore follow-up if possible. Co-infection with schistosomes may result in chronic/recurrent fever since the bacteria survive within parasites, protected from antibiotics.

Prevention: improved sanitation, vaccination.

Treatment of typhoid

First-choice antibiotics vary due to local resistance

In Africa and the Americas
Alternatives are:
- chloramphenicol 1 g PO qds for 10–14 days.
- amoxicillin 500 mg PO tds for 10–14 days.
- co-trimoxazole 960 mg PO bd for 10–14 days.

In Asia
Although chloramphenicol, amoxicillin, and co-trimoxazole remain effective in some areas, in many areas MDR strains (resistant to chlorampenicol, amoxicillin, co-trimoxazole) and strains with reduced susceptibility to fluoroquinolones are common. Alternatives are:
- ciprofloxacin 500–750 mg PO bd for 7–14 days.
- ceftriaxone 60 mg/kg IV od for 7–14 days.
- azithromycin 500 mg PO od for 7 days (not in severe disease).

In severe disease
Dosages for each drug can be increased 1.5 × initially and given IV.

Rickettsioses (typhus fevers)

Rickettsioses are zoonoses caused by small intracellular bacilli. Ticks, fleas, or mites act as vectors and/or reservoirs.

Spotted fever group rickettsioses

These are transmitted by the bite of ixodid (hard) ticks. Dogs, rodents, and other animals are the reservoir. After 3–14 days' incubation fever, headache, muscle pain, rash, local lymphadenopathy, and an inoculation eschar (small ulcer with black centre and red areola) typically develop.

- 'Rocky mountain spotted fever' (*Rickettsia rickettsii*, USA) is frequently severe (mortality 13–25% in untreated cases). There is no eschar.
- 'Boutonneuse fever' or 'Mediterranean spotted fever' (*Rickettsia conorii*, Africa, India, Europe, and the Middle East) is usually less severe.
- 'African tick bite fever' (*Rickettsia africae*, sub-Saharan Africa) is milder. Multiple eschars and outbreaks in groups of travellers may occur.
- Other forms include 'Queensland tick typhus', 'North Asian Tick fever'.

Rickettsial pox

Rickettsia akari is transmitted by mites in the Eastern USA and former Soviet Union. The rash is vesicular and may be confused with chickenpox.

Epidemic (louse-borne) typhus fever (*Rickettsia prowazekii*)

Rickettsia prowazekii is transmitted between humans by the human body louse in cold, unhygienic conditions, particularly during war and famine. The disease is endemic in mountainous areas in eastern Africa, Mexico, Central and South America, and Asia.

- Rickettsia are excreted in the faeces of infected lice and inoculated into the abrasions or the bite wound by scratching.
- After 1–2 weeks' incubation there is abrupt onset of fever, headache, prostration, myalgia, conjunctival injection, rales. There is no eschar. A macular rash appears on day 5 or 6. Fatality ranges from 10–40% (untreated) and increases with age.
- Brill–Zinsser disease is a milder recrudescent disease which may occur years later in those who have not been adequately treated.

Endemic (flea-borne) typhus fever (*Rickettsia typhi*)

This is transmitted from rats to humans by fleas. It is found worldwide where rats and humans co-exist. Rickettsia are transmitted in flea faeces during a blood mean. The illness is similar to epidemic typhus but milder.

Cat flea typhus/flea-borne spotted fever (*Rickettsia felis*)

This is a recently recognized illness with a clinical picture similar to the spotted fever group but is transmitted by the cat flea.

Scrub typhus (Orientia tsutsugamushi)

Scrub typhus is transmitted by the bite of trombiculid mites living in sharply delimited areas ('mite islands') in central, east, and southeast Asia, and northern Australia.

- A punched out eschar develops after 6–21 days followed by a severe acute febrile illness resembling typhus. Pneumonitis is common. Case fatality varies widely with infecting strain and increasing age.
- Unlike other rickettsial illnesses, repeat infections may occur, since immunity does not cross-protect against heterologous strains.

Diagnosis and management of rickettsial infection

Diagnosis is often clinical in the right epidemiological setting. It can be verified by serology, PCR, or isolation of rickettsia in cell culture from samples early in infection.

Management: Give antibiotics (in severe cases, drugs can be given IV):

- Doxycycline 100 mg PO bd or 200 mg od for 7–10 days is standard therapy for rickettsial infections. In some situations (e.g. louse-borne typhus) a single 200 mg dose is sufficient.
- Alternative: chloramphenicol 500 mg PO QID for 7–10 days.

PAEDIATRIC NOTE

Doxycycline is favoured for treatment of moderate to severe rickettsial infections in children. Milder infections (e.g. Mediterranean spotted fever) can be treated with newer macrolides e.g. azithromycin 10 mg/kg/day for 3 days.

PUBLIC HEALTH NOTE

- **Lice:** apply residual insecticide powder to clothes and persons in situations favouring infestation; re-apply regularly. Provide facilities for bathing and washing clothes and bedclothes. In epidemic situations, apply residual insecticide to all contacts or the entire community.
- **Ticks:** look for and remove attached or crawling ticks after exposures. De-tick dogs. Use tick repellants and protective clothing to avoid contact.
- **Fleas:** apply residual insecticides to rat burrows or harbourages. Wait until flea populations have been reduced before instituting rodent control measures (to avoid increased human exposure to fleas).

Ehrlichia, Bartonella, and *Coxiella*

Bartonella are intracellular bacteria with tropism for erythrocytes and endothelial cells.

- *B. quintana* is transmitted by the human body louse amongst the homeless, those living in crowded, unhygienic conditions, and during war. It causes **trench fever**, chronic bacteraemia, and endocarditis in the immunocompetent, and **bacillary angiomatosis** (BA) in the immunocompromised.
- *B. henselae* is transmitted amongst cats by the cat flea and to humans by cat scratch or bite. It causes **cat scratch disease** (uncommonly bacteraemia and endocarditis in immunocompetent persons) as well as **bacillary angiomatosis** and **peliosis hepatis**.
- *B. bacilliformis* is transmitted by sandflies in the Andes and causes **Oroya fever** (especially in tourists and transient workers) and **verruga peruana** (especially amongst natives of the Peruvian Andes).

Human ehrlichioses are tick-borne zoonoses caused by intracellular bacilli. The organisms are found in vacuoles within leukocytes where they divide to form a cluster (morula). *Ehrlichia chafeensis* infects monocytes whilst *E. ewingii* and *Anaplasma phagocytophilum* infect neutrophils.

- *Ehrlichia chafeensis* and *E. ewingii* are transmitted from a variety of vertebrates (particularly deer and dogs) to humans by the Amblyomma tick in the southern USA.
- *A. phagocytophilum* is transmitted from vertebrates (particularly ruminants and rodents) to humans by Ixodid ticks in the USA and Europe.

Coxiella burnetii is an intracellular coccobacillus that causes **Q fever**. It infects a wide variety of animals (especially cattle, sheep, and goats), including ticks. Animals shed *C. burnetii* in milk, faeces, urine, and, particularly, birth by-products. Hides and wool may be contaminated with tick faeces containing concentrated organisms. Humans acquire infection through inhalation of infected aerosols (which may be air-borne over considerable distances), ingestion of unpasteurized dairy products, or contact with contaminated clothing. Person-to-person spread is rare.

Clinical features

- **Trench fever** presents with acute onset fever ('5 day fever'), headache, dizziness and shin pain. Most cases are self-limiting. A minority develop chronic infection (attacks of fever, chronic bacteraemia, endocarditis).
- **Cat scratch disease** usually presents as a tender, self-limiting (2–3 months) regional lymphadenopathy without fever. Complications are rare (retinitis, encephalopathy, visceral forms).
- **Bacillary angiomatosis and peliosis hepatis** are due to vascular proliferative lesions in the skin or liver but can involve any organ. They typically occur in immunocompromised (HIV) patients. Skin lesions are nodules or papules which may be red to purple, ulcerate, or bleed.
- **Oroya fever** is life-threatening septicaemia with haemolysis. It is often complicated by bacterial super-infection (especially Salmonella, other Gram-negatives, and *S. aureus*). **Verruga peruana** presents with benign cutaneous vascular lesions.

- **Ehrlichiosis** presents with an acute flu-like illness which may be accompanied by rash, vomiting and meningoencephalitis. Leukopenia, thrombocytopenia, and raised hepatic transaminase levels are common. Illness caused by *E. chafeensis* is generally more severe, with a 3% fatality rate. *E. ewingii* generally causes disease in immuno-compromised patients.
- **Q fever** may be asymptomatic or present as an acute flu-like illness with varying hepatitis and pneumonia. Culture-negative endocarditis is an important chronic presentation. *C. burnetti* can recrudesce in pregnancy causing abortion. There is an association with chronic fatigue syndrome.

Diagnosis

- Serology or PCR.
- Examination of peripheral blood films for morulae within neutrophils or monocytes (ehrlichiosis) or bacilli within or adherent to erythrocytes (Oroya fever).
- For cat scratch disease, large rods can be seen in tissue sections stained with Warthin–Starry silver stain (but not Gram or ZN stains).

Management

- **Trench fever:** doxycycline 200 mg PO od for 4 weeks plus gentamicin 3 mg/kg IV od for the first 2 weeks.
- **Cat scratch disease:** no therapy unless extensive or complicated: azithromycin 500 mg PO on day 1 then 250 mg PO on days 2–5.
- **Bacillary angiomatosis** and **peliosis hepatis:** azithromycin 250 mg PO od or erythromycin 500 mg PO qds for 2–3 months.
- **Oroya fever:** ciprofloxacin 500 mg PO bd for 10 days.
- **Ehrlichiosis:** doxycycline 100 mg BID PO or IV for 7–10 days.
- **Q fever:** doxycycline 100 mg PO BID for 7–10 days. *C. burnetti* endocarditis requires 18 months doxycycline plus hydroxychloroquine.

PUBLIC HEALTH NOTE

Control or avoidance of the vectors: delousing of clothing and body with powder; preventative measures against tick bites. Cat scratches and bites should be thoroughly cleaned and cat fleas controlled to prevent cat scratch disease. Persons at risk of Q fever (abbatoir workers, farmers, researchers) should be educated on sources of infection and safe disposal of infected materials (especially birth products). Milk should be pasteurized. Q fever vaccine is available for those at high risk in some countries.

PAEDIATRIC NOTE

- Rifampicin may be useful for ehrlichiosis in pregnancy or in children.
- Co-trimoxazole or the newer macrolides (e.g. azithromycin) are useful for the treatment of Q fever in children.
- Erythromycin 10–15 mg/kg qds for 7–10 days may also be used to treat Q fever in children.

Relapsing fevers

Relapsing fevers are acute febrile illnesses caused by *Borrelia spirochaetes* which, if untreated, will relapse repeatedly between afebrile intervals of 5–9 days. Epidemic louse-borne relapsing fever, caused by *Borrelia recurrentis*, is transmitted by human body lice (*Pediculus humanus*). It is now confined to the horn of Africa. Endemic tick-borne relapsing fever is caused by more than 15 *Borrelia* species and transmitted by a variety of soft (argasid) ticks (genus *Ornithodoros*). It is widely distributed in tropical and temperate countries except Australasia and Pacific islands. Rarely, these spirochaetes can be transmitted by blood transfusion.

Louse-borne relapsing fever (LBRF)

Transmission: lice are infected by feeding on human blood. They transmit *B. recurrentis* to a new human host not by bites but through contamination of broken skin or intact mucosae by their coelomic fluid when ruptured by scratching. Humans are the sole host and reservoir. Transmission tends to increase in the cold, rainy season when people wear more clothes and crowd together indoors for warmth, conditions that encourage louse infestation. Historically, LBRF has caused massive pandemics in Africa, the Middle East, and Europe (1903–36, 50 million cases with 5 million deaths; 1943–6 10 million cases), exacerbated by wars, crowding, floods, famines, and forced migration.

Clinical features: after an incubation period of 4–17 (average 7) days, there is sudden high fever, chills, headache, confusion, myalgias, arthralgias, fatigue, dizziness, cough, anorexia, nightmares, and prostration. Examination reveals bleeding (epistaxes, subconjunctival haemorrhages, petechiae), tender splenomegaly and hepatomegaly, jaundice, and chest signs. The first attack ends dramatically with a febrile crisis, either spontaneously on about the fifth day if untreated or with a Jarisch–Herxheimer reaction precipitated by antibiotic treatment. Inadequately treated patients may suffer their first relapse about one week later. Subsequent attacks tend to be less severe. Pregnant women are at high risk of abortion. Death is due to myocarditis, liver failure, severe bleeding due to thrombocytopenia, DIC and hepatic dysfunction, ruptured spleen, splenic infarctions, and bacterial superinfection (dysentery, salmonellosis, typhoid, typhus, malaria, tuberculosis). During the J–Hr, patients may die from hyperpyrexia, hypovolaemic shock, or pulmonary oedema. Untreated case fatalities of 40% or higher have been reported during epidemics. Treatment can reduce this to <5%.

Jarisch–Herxheimer reaction (J-Hr): Within a few hours of treatment, the patient becomes restless and then develops rigors with soaring temperature, respiratory and pulse rates, and blood pressure, associated with vomiting, diarrhoea, coughing and delirium. This is followed by the flush phase during which there is profuse sweating and vasodilatation sometimes complicated by hypovolaemic shock or acute pulmonary oedema attributable to myocarditis. The incidence of J–Hr varies from 33–100%.

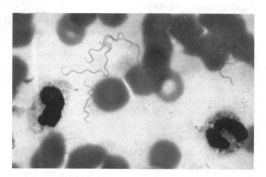

Fig. 18.2 Blood film showing several *Borrelia duttoni* spirochaetes in a patient with untreated TBRF.

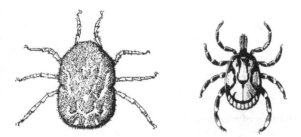

Fig. 18.3 (Left): soft tick (genus *Ornithodoros*) vector of tick-borne relapsing fever; (right): hard tick (genus *Ixodes*). Hard ticks are the vectors of Lyme disease, rickettsial infections, and tick-borne encephalitis.

Tick-borne relapsing fever (TBRF)

Transmission: ticks are infected by feeding on animal or human blood or acquire spirochaetes congenitally (transovarially). They transmit borreliae to a new animal or human host via their saliva while taking a blood meal or by contaminating the bite wound with their coxal gland secretion. They are reservoirs as well as vectors. Peri-domestic rodents are the main vertebrate reservoir. Ecology and species of borreliae and tick vary geographically. Only classic East African TBRF (*B. duttonii* transmitted by *O. moubata* complex) is not a zoonosis. Risk of infection is associated with sleeping in tick and rodent friendly thatched or mud houses or log cabins. Tick bites are painless. They feed for only a few hours at night and then drop off, so exposure is usually unsuspected.

Clinical features: after an incubation period of 2–18 days, presenting symptoms are similar to those in LBRF but are usually milder and less protracted. Epistaxis, abdominal pain, diarrhoea, and cough are described. Splenomegaly and splenic infarction are common but hepatomegaly and jaundice are unusual. Transient neurological problems occur in 5–10% of patients: paraesthesiae, cranial never palsies (especially VII), visual symptoms, hemiparesis or paraparesis, lymphocytic meningitis. Various erythematous and petechial rashes may appear. Fever may recur up to 13 times, separated by gaps of a few days to 3 weeks in untreated patients. Pregnancy is aborted in up to one third of cases.

Diagnosis: diagnosis of LBRF is by finding spirochaetes (sometimes >500,000/mm^3) in Giemsa-stained blood films. In TBRF, spirochaetaemia may be scanty and intermittent. Peripheral neutrophil leucocytosis is followed by leukopenia after the febrile crisis. Serology is not useful. Thrombocytopenia, coagulopathy, and liver dysfunction are common.

Management of relapsing fever

- Single-dose antibiotic therapy is curative for LBRF:
- Adults: tetracycline 500 mg PO (for sick patients, 250 mg IV) stat.
- Pregnant women or children: erythromycin adult 500 mg children 10 mg/kg PO (for sick patients, erythromycin IV) stat *or*
- For mixed infections with louse-borne typhus (adults): doxycycline 100–200 mg PO stat.
- Benzylpenicillin and chloramphenicol are also effective.
- For TBRF, longer courses of the same drugs (e.g. adults: tetracycline 500 mg qds PO for 10 days) are required.
- Consider treating complicating bacterial infections (typhoid etc.)
- For the severe J–Hr precipitated by antibiotics:
- Control pyrexia by physical cooling.
- Prevent hypovolaemia with IV fluids.
- Nurse in bed for 48–72 h to prevent fatal postural hypotension.
- Treat acute pulmonary oedema 2° to myocarditis with digoxin.

Control of relapsing fever   PUBLIC HEALTH NOTE

- *LBRF:* delouse infested clothes (heat, insecticide); bathe patients (soap and 1% Lysol [Cresol]*); decontaminate using 10% DDT, 0.5–1% malathion, 2% temephos, 1% propoxur, or 0.5–1% permethrin. This is essential to control an epidemic.
- *TBRF:* kill or deter ticks with residual insecticides in dwellings, repellents (DEET), improved house contruction, rodent control.

* Cresol requires precautions to prevent absorption through skin

Leptospirosis

Leptospirosis is primarily a disease of wild and domestic mammals, which may asymptomatically pass large numbers of leptospires in their urine. All pathogenic leptospires are spirochaetes belonging to the genus *Leptospira*, the taxonomy of which continues to evolve. They can be divided by phenotyping into 24 serogroups and >250 serovars, and by genotyping into >17 genomospecies. However, there is no relationship between the infecting serovar and clinical manifestations or severity of illness in humans. Leptospirosis in endemic regions is usually related to agricultural exposure and is increasingly recognized in travellers returning from developing countries.

Transmission

Leptospires enter the body through cuts or abrasions of skin or mucous membranes after immersion in contaminated water (pools, canals, rivers), or through close animal contact. Rats are the most common source of human infection in developing countries, and dogs and livestock in industrialized countries. Following infection, leptospiraemia develops and the spirochaetes spread to multiple organs. Clinical manifestations of leptospirosis reflect organ dysfunction resulting from direct effects of leptospires and/or host immune responses to infection.

Clinical features

These vary from subclinical infection, through a self-limiting febrile illness, to a potentially lethal multi-system illness with jaundice, renal failure, and pulmonary haemorrhage (Weil's syndrome):

- Subclinical infection — common in endemic areas where seroprevalence is typically 5–10%.
- Clinical disease — 1–3 weeks post-infection there is sudden onset of fever, headache, severe myalgia, nausea and vomiting, and conjunctival suffusion or haemorrhage. In severe infection, the patient is prostrate with high fever, haemoptysis, dyspnoea, jaundice, and symptoms and signs of respiratory, renal, or multi-organ dysfunction which mimics sepsis syndrome. In mild cases, a 2-day remission occurs after 4–7 days, but this may progress to a second immunopathological phase. If this is severe, the patient's condition worsens with persistent high fever, myocarditis, widespread haemorrhage, renal failure, and shock.
- Death in leptospirosis is due to multi-organ failure. Severe pulmonary haemorrhage (2° to endothelial damage rather than consumption of clotting factors) has been reported as an important cause of death in recent epidemics in Central America and Southeast Asia.

Diagnosis

Early diagnosis is difficult due to the non-specific presentation similar to other infections that present as undifferentiated febrile syndrome (e.g. malaria, dengue, and rickettsial infections). Definitive diagnosis of leptospirosis is made by recovery of leptospires from clinical specimens or detection of leptospiral antibodies. Leptospires can be isolated from blood or CSF during the first 7–10 days of illness, and from urine during the

2nd and 3rd week of illness. Culture is difficult, requires several weeks of incubation, and has low sensitivity. The microagglutination test is the standard for serological diagnosis of leptospirosis. Several rapid serological tests, using whole *Leptospira* antigen preparations, have been developed. All of these have low sensitivity (39–72%) during the acute phase of illness, but serology 10–21 days into the illness is more sensitive.

Management

Management combines supportive treatment with antibiotic therapy; antibiotics should be used at any stage of leptospirosis.

- *Mild disease*: doxycycline 100 mg bd for 7 days, started within 3 days of the onset of symptoms, will hasten recovery.
- *Moderate or severe disease*: benzylpenicillin 1.2–2.4 g IV q6 h for 5–7 days (even if the patient has been ill for several days).
- Alternatives for severe disease: ampicillin 1 g IV q6 h or cefotaxime 1–2 g IV q12 h or ceftriaxone 1–2 g IV od. Chloramphenicol is NOT effective.
- Severe disease may require organ support including haemodialysis in an ICU setting.

The Jarisch–Herxheimer reaction may occur 4–6h after initiation of IV antibiotics in some patients.

Prevention of leptospirosis   PUBLIC HEALTH NOTE

- Education of at-risk groups to reduce exposure.
- Control rodent populations.
- Vaccinate domestic animals.
- Consider chemoprophylaxis in very high-risk groups e.g. sewer workers — the protective efficacy of doxycycline 200 mg weekly is ~95%.

Brucellosis

A chronic granulomatous disease of worldwide distribution caused by the Gram-negative bacillus, *Brucella*. Four species are responsible for almost all human infections, namely *Brucella melitensis* (majority of cases), *B. abortus*, *B. suis*, *B. canis*. The organism lives and multiplies within phagocytes in the reticuloendothelial system. The cellular immune response, in particular the interferon-γ pathway, is important in pathogenesis.

Transmission

Brucellosis is predominately an occupational disease of those working with animals or their products (tissue, blood, urine, vaginal discharges, aborted fetuses and placentas). Entry is through breaks in the skin or inhalation of aerosols (stables, abbatoirs and laboratories). Sporadic cases and outbreaks occur following ingestion of unpasteurized dairy products (particularly soft cheese, milk, butter and ice-cream).

Clinical features

A variable incubation period (usually 2–4 weeks, may be months) is followed by acute or insidious onset of fever (may be rigors), constitutional symptoms, and malodorous perspiration. Lymphadenopathy and hepatosplenomegaly may be present. Complications can affect virtually any organ system, including:

- Osteoarticular (spondylitis, peripheral arthritis, sacroiliitis).
- Reproductive (epididymoorchitis, spontaneous abortion).
- Hepatitis, peritonitis.
- Central nervous system (meningitis, encephalitis, abscess).
- Endocarditis (responsible for most mortality).

Diagnosis

The serum agglutination test is most widely used (single titre >1:160 or rising titre), but cross-reacts with other Gram-negatives. ELISA (IgG, IgM, IgA) has greater sensitivity and specificity. PCR is promising. Culture from blood or tissue is confirmatory, but is relatively insensitive and requires prolonged incubation.

Management

Doxycycline (200 mg PO od for 6 weeks) plus **either** streptomycin (15 mg/kg (max 1 g) IM daily for 2–3 weeks) **or** rifampicin (600–900 mg PO od for 6 weeks). Relapse occurs in ~10% and should be treated with the same regimen. Ciprofloxacin/ofloxacin plus either rifampicin or doxycycline may be an alternative. Rifampicin and co-trimoxazole are useful in pregnancy.

Paediatric doses   PAEDIATRIC NOTE

Use combination regimen of 2 or the following:
- rifampicin 15 mg/kg (max 600 mg) PO od for 6 weeks.
- co-trimoxazole: sulphamethoxazole 20 mg/kg + trimethorpim 4 mg/kg (max 800 mg + 160 mg) PO bd for 6 weeks.
- gentamicin 2.5 mg/kg IV or IM) tds for 2 weeks.

Prevention and Control   PUBLIC HEALTH NOTE

- Pasteurize (or boil) milk products.
- Protective clothing for those at risk.
- Screen livestock by serology or by testing cow's milk and eliminate infected animals.
- Vaccinate animals in high prevalence areas; vaccinate animals using live attenuated vaccine (no human vaccine is available; the vaccine strain may cause disease in humans if accidentally inoculated).
- Identify the source of outbreaks (usually milk or milk products from an infected herd); recall all affected products.

Plague

An acute illness caused by the Gram negative coccobacillus, *Yersinia pestis*, that can be rapidly fatal unless treatment is started early. Empirical antibiotic therapy is thus essential when clinical suspicion is high. It is enzootic among animals (mainly rodents) in many countries in Africa, S.E. Asia, and the Americas (including S.W. USA) and occasionally infects humans.

- The most common clinical form is **bubonic** plague, in which bacteria spread to lymph nodes. Bubonic plague has a 1–15% death rate in treated cases and a 40–60% death rate if not treated.
- Primary **pneumonic** plague occurs after inhalation of bacteria in droplets coughed from a patient with pneumonic plague, resulting in a fulminant pneumonia and sepsis which is uniformly fatal if not treated within 24 h. Pneumonic plague might also occur as a result of biological warfare or terrorism. Secondary pneumonic plague may complicate septicaemic plague.
- **Septicaemic** plague may be primary, or occur as a complication of bubonic or pneumonic plague. Infection may spread to every organ including the lungs, liver, spleen, kidneys, and, rarely, CSF causing meningitis. The mortality is ~40% in treated cases and ~100% in untreated cases.

Transmission

Bubonic plague is transmitted via the bite of infected rodent fleas. Most sporadic human infection comes from sylvatic rodents (e.g. ground squirrels, prairie dogs), occasionally from domestic cats. Outbreaks, however, are associated with urban rats, and spectacular die-offs of rats may herald an outbreak. Pneumonic plague is transmitted from person to person.

Clinical features

Bubonic plague: the first specific sign is usually local lymphadenitis in the nodes draining the site of the flea bite. After 2–7 (always <15) days, a 'bubo' forms in these nodes. There is typically a short prodrome of fever, malaise, headache, and, in some cases, a dull ache in the nodes for up to 24 h before the bubo is apparent. The enlarged nodes are extremely painful and swollen, the overlying skin warm, red, oedematous, and adherent. The mass is non-fluctuant and immobile.

Pneumonic plague: initially intense headache, malaise, fever, vomiting, prostration. Later, cough, dyspnoea, bloodstained sputum with few chest signs, ↓ consciousness. CXR shows multilobar consolidation or broncho-pneumonia — paucity of chest signs compared with the CXR is characteristic. This picture needs to be distinguished from ARDS, which may occur in bubonic and septicaemic forms of plague. Rapid deterioration and death from multi-organ/respiratory failure is common.

Septicaemic plague: presents with fulminant sepsis, multi-organ failure, and skin bleeding.

Diagnosis

Fever plus localized lymphadenopathy in endemic area; aspiration of a bubo for culture and Giemsa/Gram-stained smear (bipolar coccobacillus); blood, sputum, CSF for culture; acute and convalescent serology. Antigen detection directly on clinical samples, if available, may give rapid diagnosis.

Management

For severe disease: antibiotics must be started without delay and continued for 7–10 days:

- Most clinical experience is with streptomycin 15 mg/kg IM bd.
- Alternatives with good activity in vitro, but comparatively little clinical experience include: gentamicin 5 mg/kg IV od; ciprofloxacin 10–15 mg/kg (max 750 mg) IV/PO bd; chloramphenicol 25 mg/kg (max 750 mg) IV/PO qds (treatment of choice for meningitis).
- For milder cases: tetracycline 500–1000 mg PO qds or doxycycline 100 mg PO bd (avoid tetracyclines in children).

Control of plague   PUBLIC HEALTH NOTE

- Control rodents and fleas — fleas must be dealt with before rodents during outbreaks.
- Avoid contact with reservoir species (surveillance, public education)
- Vaccination (currently not generally available).
- Notify suspected cases to both local health authorities and the WHO.
- Isolate pneumonic plague patients until at least 3 days after starting antibiotics and clinically improving — they are highly infectious.
- Consider prophylaxis with tetracycline for close contacts of pneumonic plague (2–3 m) and medical staff.

Melioidosis

A disease caused by the bacterium *Burkholderia pseudomallei* that is endemic in south and southeast Asia (including the Indian subcontinent), northern Australia, the Caribbean, and probably elsewhere in the tropics. It is a major cause of septicaemia in N.E. Thailand. The bacterium is present in mud and surface water (rice paddy); people in regular contact with either are probably infected by inoculation or inhalation.

Clinical features

Clinical presentation may occur acutely following infection or after a latent period of up to several years. Infection is often subclinical; clinical illness commonly presents as septicaemia, or focal infection of the lung (cavitating pneumonia with profound weight loss which may be confused with TB), bone, or (in children) parotid glands (although any organ may be affected). Septicaemia causes rapid deterioration with metastatic abscesses in lung, liver, and spleen. A failure to respond to empirical regimens for sepsis (e.g. penicillin plus aminoglycosides) may suggest this diagnosis in endemic regions.

Glanders is a similar disease of horses caused by *Burkholderia mallei*; although transmission to humans is described as very rare.

Diagnosis

- Culture of clinical specimens (blood, pus, sputum, etc). *Burkholderia pseudomallei* grows on most routine culture media, but an oxidase-positive gram-negative rod may be disregarded as an environmental pseudomonad — therefore be alert to the diagnosis in the right clinical and epidemiological setting. Its identity may be confimed by biochemical tests and characteristic colonies on Ashdown's media.
- Direct immunofluorescence of clinical specimens.
- Serology — problems of specificity and sensitivity, particularly in endemic areas where a large proportion of the population may have serological evidence of previous infection.

Management

- *Treat sepsis with intravenous antibiotics:* ceftazidime 50 mg/kg (max 2 g) tds for at least 14 days or until clinical improvement (alternatives: co-amoxiclav, imipenem, meropenem).
- *Then give oral therapy to prevent relapse: either* co-trimoxazole 960 mg (child 480 mg) bd *plus* doxycycline 100 mg bd for 20 weeks, *plus* chloramphenicol 500 mg qds for the first 4 wks; *or* co-amoxiclav 625 mg tds + amoxicillin 500 mg tds for 20 wks.
- The oral regimen above may be given intravenously for sepsis in beta-lactam allergic patients (or if beta-lactams not available), but it is not as effective as ceftazidime.
- Resistance to these drugs may develop during treatment.

Anthrax

Anthrax is a zoonosis resulting from infection with the spores of the Gram-positive rod *Bacillus anthracis*. Anthrax is a disease of a variety of grazing animals (sheep, cattle, goats) in parts of Asia, Africa, South and Central America, southern Europe, the Caribbean, and the Middle East. The resistant spores may remain viable in soil or animal products for many years.

Transmission

Anthrax is primarily an occupational disease of workers who process hides, hair, bone products, and wool and of those who handle infected animals (veterinarians, wildlife workers). Spores may be dispersed by wind, water, scavengers, or transport of animal products. Outbreaks can occur following ingestion of contaminated meat. Since anthrax spores are resistant and can be aerosolized, they have been used as agents of bioterrorism.

Clinical presentation

- *Cutaneous anthrax* accounts for 95% of naturally occurring cases. Spores are inoculated into the skin through abrasions or cuts. A short incubation period (typically 1–5 days) is followed by an itchy papule which progresses to a vesicle, ulcer, and, finally, a painless black eschar with extensive local oedema and surrounding purple vesicles. This heals spontaneously in 1–3 weeks; however, bacteraemic spread and overwhelming septicaemia may occur. Neck lesions may lead to airway obstruction — consider early tracheostomy.
- *Inhalational anthrax* usually occurs 1–4 days following exposure, but may be delayed for up to 98 days. This biphasic illness presents with symptoms of a viral upper respiratory tract infection followed by sudden onset of haemorrhagic mediastinitis with fever, hypoxia, dyspnoea and shock. Treatment in the late stages is usually unsuccessful, with mortality rates of up to 90%.
- *Gastrointestinal anthrax* follows ingestion of contaminated meat. Severe abdominal pain, bloody diarrhoea, massive ascites, and sepsis occur. Mortality is >50%.
- *Other forms* include meningitis (which may complicate any of the other forms) and oropharyngeal anthrax.

Diagnosis

Rapid diagnosis is by demonstrating bacilli in smears from fluid from under the eschar, or other site-of-disease sample (or using newer methods such as PCR, direct immunofluorescence). Culture blood, lymph node, or CSF.

Management

- Early, aggressive antibiotic therapy is vital: give benzylpenicillin 2.4 g IV 4 hourly for 10 days. Naturally (or genetically modified) penicillin-resistant mutants can occur, so some authorities recommend substitute (or add) ciprofloxacin 400 mg IV bd followed by 500 mg PO bd for 60 days (optimum duration not yet established). Doxycycline is an alternative.
- Surgical debridement of the black, necrotic eschar is contraindicated. The eschar becomes sterile in <2 days.
- Post-exposure prophylaxis should be considered following possible aerosol exposure: ciprofloxacin 500 mg PO bd for 60 days.

Prevention of anthrax   PUBLIC HEALTH NOTE

- *Disinfection:* spores are resistant to dessication, heat, UV light, gamma irradiation, and many disinfectants. For disinfection of discharge from lesions or soiled materials use hypochlorite, hydrogen peroxide, peracetic acid, or gluteraldehyde (or burn or autoclave where possible).
- *Vaccination:* Immunize high-risk persons with cell-free, supernatant-derived vaccine (regular boosters required).
- *Veterinary public health measures:* disposal of infected carcasses (incinerate at site, do not bury or transport if possible); vaccination of all domestic animals at risk (with annual re-immunization).
- *Control occupational exposure:* control dust; ventilate work areas; wear protective clothing; disinfect wool/hides/bone prior to processing.

Paediatric doses   PAEDIATRIC DOSES

- Ciprofloxacin 10–15 mg/kg (max 400 mg) IV bd followed by 10–15 mg/kg (max 500 mg) PO bd.
- If penicillin susceptible, use IV benzylpenicillin 150 mg/kg daily in 4 divided doses.
- For children >12 years, use adult doses (see text).

African trypanosomiasis

Human African trypanosomiasis (HAT), also called 'sleeping sickness', is a protozoan disease caused by *Trypanosoma brucei* spp. that is confined to sub-Saharan Africa. Two forms exist — see Fig.18.4.

Transmission: the disease is transmitted to humans by the bite of tsetse flies, genus *Glossina*. Humans are usually infected by *T.b. gambiense* around waterholes or rivers and by *T.b. rhodesiense* in areas of savanna or recently cleared bush. Humans are the principal reservoir of *T.b. gambiense* but are incidental hosts of *T.b. rhodesiense*, which is a zoonosis that affects game animals and cattle.

Pathogenesis: after inoculation, a local inflammatory reaction results in an itchy, painful chancre (*T.b. rhodesiense*) and regional lymphadenopathy (both *T.b. rhodesiense* and *T.b. gambiense*). Invasion of the bloodstream and lymphoreticular system follows — the haemolymphatic (early) stage. Trypanosomes then invade the CNS, producing the meningoencephalitic (late) stage of the disease. Trypanosomes escape the host immunological response by changing their surface antigens (antigenic variation).

Clinical features: *T.b. gambiense* HAT is a chronic disease that develops insidiously. Evolution towards the late stage of the disease and death generally takes months or years. By contrast, *T.b. rhodesiense* HAT is usually an acute, sometimes fulminant disease. Both forms are almost invariably fatal if left untreated.

Gambian trypanosomiasis

A chancre is rarely seen at the site of inoculation. After an asymptomatic period of months–years, the early stage of infection is characterized by irregular fevers with fatigue, arthralgia, myalgia, pruritus, and headaches. Lymphadenopathy, often in the posterior cervical triangle (Winterbottom's sign), is common; lymph nodes are soft and non-tender; splenomegaly is rare. Trypanosome invasion of the CNS results in headaches, changes in personality, apathy, and forgetfulness; psychosis (abnormal behaviour, agitation, delusions) may also occur. A variety of CNS signs may be seen: pyramidal (focal motor weakness), extra-pyramidal (a resting tremor is common), and cerebellar (ataxia). Late features include daytime somnolence progressing to coma and seizures. Patients ultimately die of starvation, intercurrent bacterial infections, or convulsions.

Rhodesian trypanosomiasis

An area of painful induration — the 1° chancre — often develops at the bite site, subsiding by 2–3 wks. After a 1–3 wk incubation period, trypanosomes enter the blood causing an acute severe illness with high fever, chills, malaise, severe headaches, weight loss, myalgia, and arthralgia. An erythematous rash that may be macular, papular, or circinate sometimes occurs. The disease often runs a fulminant course with multiple-organ failure and early death. CNS involvement produces meningoencephalitis that progresses rapidly and is fatal within 1–3 months if untreated. Myocarditis, resulting in atrial or ventricular dysrhythmia or heart failure, may precede meningoencephalitis.

Epidemiology of human african trypanosomiasis

Two forms of HAT exist with different clinical and epidemiological features: *T.b. gambiense* is present in Central and West Africa, and *T.b. rhodesiense* in East Africa. An estimated 50,000–70,000 people are thought to be currently infected. The incidence of *T.b. gambiense* HAT, which had increased sharply during the past decades in war-torn countries of Africa because of the collapse of disease control measures, has been on the decrease since year 2000. Human infections with *T.b. rhodesiense* are sporadic but outbreaks occur. Travellers to game parks in East Africa have a significant risk of being infected.

In Uganda, Rhodesian HAT is expending north-west towards the Gambian HAT endemic area. This geographical overlap would cause a significant problem in diagnosis and treatment.

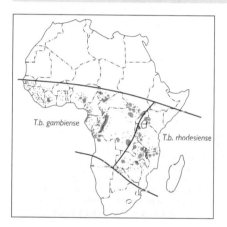

Fig. 18.4 Endemic foci of Gambian and Rhodesian trypanosomiasis. (Reproduced with permission from the WHO)

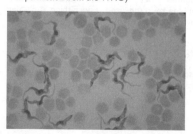

Fig. 18.5 Bloodstream trypomastigote forms of *T. b. rhodesiense* on a peripheral thin blood smear.

Diagnosis: in most Gambian HAT control programmes, initial screening for infection relies on the card agglutination trypanosoma test (CATT), a very sensitive and practical serological test. No such serologic assay exists for Rhodesian HAT. The direct microscopic observation of trypanosomes in lymph node aspirates, blood (Giemsa-stained thick smear, quantitative buffy coat, haematocrit or mini-anion exchange centrifugation techniques) or CSF (double centrifugation) confirms the diagnosis. The sensitivity of blood examination is higher for *T.b. rhodesiense* because circulating trypanosomes are more numerous.

Staging of disease: by lumbar puncture is mandatory before considering the use of the toxic drugs for CNS involvement. CSF findings indicating trypanosomal meningoencephalitis are the presence of:
- Trypanosomes.
- Increased number of leukocytes (>5 per mm^3) *and/or*
- Elevated total or specific (anti-trypanosomal) IgM in the CSF.

Treatment: The choice of treatment depends on the stage of the disease and whether the disease is Gambian or Rhodesian.
Note: following a recent agreement between the pharmaceutical industry and the WHO, drugs for HAT are being donated to the WHO.

Gambian HAT
- *Early stage:* pentamidine isethionate 4 mg/kg IM od for 7 days.
- *Late stage:* (first choice treatment): eflornithine 100 mg/kg IV qds for 14 days, diluted in normal saline and infused over 2 h.
- *Late stage: (alternative only if eflornithine not available)*: melarsoprol by slow IV injection (using a glass syringe, or drawing up and injecting with a plastic syringe as quickly as possible since the drug binds to plastic); very irritant, avoid extravasation; patients should remain supine and fasting for ≥5 h after the injection. Strictly only to be given IV (risk of soft tissue necrosis). Sequential regimen (i.e. 3 cycles of 3 daily injections of 3.6 mg/kg with a resting period of 7–10 days between each cycle) are gradually being replaced by the more practical regimen of 2.2 mg/kg/day for 10 consecutive days that showed a similar efficacy and toxicity profile.

Note: resistance to melarsoprol (up to 30% treatment failure) is present in parts of Angola, Uganda, Central African Republic, DRC, and southern Sudan. In these areas, eflornithine must be used. Eflornithine is a safer treatment than melarsoprol provided that adequate nursing care is given.

Rhodesian HAT
- *Early stage:* suramin 5 mg/kg by slow IV injection on day 1, followed by 20 mg/kg on days 3, 10, 17, 24, and 31.
- *Late stage:* melarsoprol in sequential regimen. The 10-day continuous regimen has not been evaluated for *T. b. rhodesiense*. Eflornithine is thought to be ineffective.

Adverse effects of drugs used for HAT

- *Eflornithine:* leukopenia, anemia, thrombocytopenia, soft tissue infections, and convulsions.
- *Melarsoprol:* encephalopathic syndrome (see below), polyneuropathy, severe (sometimes bloody) diarrhoea, and rash.
- *Pentamidine isethionate:* hypoglycemia (frequent), hypotension, sterile abscess, and pancreatitis (rare).
- *Suramin:* anaphylactic shock, fever, neurological, haematological, and/or renal toxicity.

Melarsoprol-induced encephalopathic syndrome (ES)

Occurs in 5–10% of treated patients, producing status epilepticus and coma. Mortality is ~50%. May be partially prevented by oral prednisolone 1 mg/kg PO od given during melarsoprol treatment. Onset of fever, tachycardia, headache, tremor, and conjunctival suffusion during melarsoprol treatment should be considered as a warning. Melarsoprol treatment should be stopped immediately; it can be restarted once symptoms subside. Some authorities recommend the use of high-dose dexamethasone IV (e.g. 30 mg loading dose followed by 15 mg every 6 h for adults) for treatment of ES or impending ES.

PAEDIATRIC HEALTH NOTE

HAT in neonates and infants can be 2° to mother-to-child transmission or early exposure to tsetse fly bites. Delayed diagnosis is common in young children due to non-specific symptoms and signs. Chronic neurodevelopmental disorders are common sequelae of late stage HAT.

Due to decreased bioavailability of eflornithine in children <12 years, the daily total dose of eflornithine must be increased to 500–600 mg/kg (~150 mg/kg qds) in this age group.

Prevention and control of HAT   PUBLIC HEALTH NOTE

- **Screening:** Gambian HAT control programmes rely on active case finding through systematic screening of communities and treatment of all those infected (human beings are the only significant reservoir). In areas of low prevalence of Gambian HAT, the integration of disease management within existing health structures is a challenge.
- **Vector control** by tsetse fly trapping is cumbersome but effective, particularly in Rhodesian HAT control programmes.
- **In outbreaks** of Rhodesian HAT, a combined programme of vector control, treatment of infected cattle, and active detection and treatment of human cases should be implemented.
- **Challenges:** Better diagnostic tools and drugs are urgently needed.

American trypanosomiasis

A parasitic disease of south and central America, also called Chagas' disease, that is caused by the protozoa *Trypanosoma cruzi*. It may result in fatal cardiomyopathy and GI tract dilatation. The acute infection is often subclinical in adults and children, although potentially severe and fatal in the latter.

Pathogenesis

Parasites invade mesenchymal tissues such as heart muscle and intestinal smooth muscle where they persist in their amastigote form, without necessarily re-entering the blood, making detection and chemotherapy difficult. In ~70% of adults, an adequate immune response controls infection, producing a benign chronic phase ('indeterminate form'). Persistent infection and immune dysregulation causes chronic disease in 30% of cases: destruction of the GI autonomic ganglia leading to chronic dilatation of hollow viscera and, in the case of the heart, arrhythmias.

Transmission

Occurs through contamination of mucous membranes, conjunctivae, and skin by the faeces of nocturnal house-dwelling reduviid bugs. Domestic and wild animals are reservoirs for the infection; however, repeated infection of humans and vector in the absence of natural hosts can occur. Oral infection may occur: sudden outbreaks may occur in association with ingestion of accidentally infected food or drink. Congenital infection occurs, and transmission may also occur via infected blood products or donor transplant organs.

Clinical features

Acute infection: most cases are subclinical with non-specific symptoms. Parasites invading the bite site cause a local swelling, the chagoma, and lymphadenopathy. If close to the eye, unilateral eyelid oedema may occur (Romaña's sign), a characteristic feature that remains for about 2 months (c.f. bacterial conjunctivitis which usually only persists for up to 10 days). 2–4 wks post infection, parasite entry into the blood coincides with the onset of fever. Other features include: a non-pruritic rash of sharply-defined, small macules on the trunk which fades after 7–10 days; swelling, particularly of the face; hepatosplenomegaly; cardiac dysrhythmia or insufficiency; meningoencephalitis (often mild, but fatal in ~10% children).

Chronic infection: (seropositive cases) is clinically different in the cardiac and digestive forms (affecting ~25% of infected cases) and the so-called indeterminate form (~75% of the cases, asymptomatic and with normal resting ECG, colon and chest X-ray).

The cardiac form includes frequent arrhythmias, conduction disorders, ventricular aneurisms, thromboembolic events, and risk of sudden death with progressive dilated cardiomyopathy and cardiac failure ± valvular incompetence in late stages. 5 stages are recognized on clinical and echocardiographic criteria (see p 710).

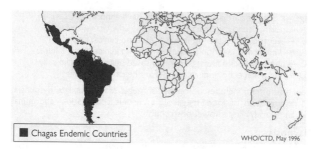

Fig. 18.6 Distribution of American trypanosomiasis.

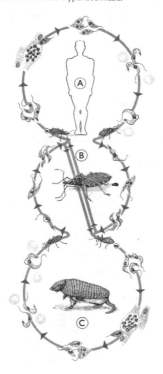

Fig. 18.7 Life cycle of *T. cruzi*: The reduviid bug (B) transmits infection via its faeces when taking blood meals from animal reservoirs such as the armadillo (C) or humans (A). (Adapted from G.Piekarski, *Medical parasitology in plates*,1962, with kind permission of Bayer Pharmaceuticals.)

Stages of chronic cardiac involvement (all have abnormal ECGs):
- A — normal echo, no heart failure.
- B1 — ventricular ejection fraction > 45%, no clinical heart failure.
- B2 — ventricular ejection fraction < 45%, no clinical heart failure.
- C — abnormal echo findings, compensated heart failure clinically.
- D — abnormal echo findings, refractory heart failure clinically.

The digestive form includes oesophagitis, megaoesophagus, late dysphagia, and regurgitation of food; megacolon, chronic constipation, abdominal pain, and (rarely) large bowel obstruction.

Diagnosis

Serology for anti-*T. cruzi* IgG is the main diagnostic tool. Parasites may also be detected directly in wet mount or Giemsa-stained blood films or CSF precipitate; parasite DNA may be detected by PCR. *T. rangeli*, which is not a cause of human disease, may be mistaken for *T. cruzi*.

Management

- *Acute phase*: current treatment is effective at this point. Give *either*:
  - Benznidazole 5–7 mg/kg/day (children 10 mg/kg/day) PO in two divided doses for 60 days *or*
  - Nifurtimox 8–10 mg/kg PO in three divided doses (children 15 mg/kg PO in four divided doses) for 90 days.
- *Chronic phase*: benznidazole is also indicated in this phase but it may be not so effective.
- *Symptomatic treatment*: is often necessary for later complications: CCF, arrhythmias (see 📖 pp 344–346), AV block, and sick-sinus syndrome.
- *Pacemakers* are implanted in patients with severe bradyarrhythmias.
- *Surgery*: may be required for megaoesophagus or megacolon.

Congenital infection

Transmission from infected mother to newborn children varies from 1% to 12% in different Latin American countries and should be evaluated in seropositive mothers. Congenital infection is confirmed by identification of parasites in the infant's blood and/or detection of infant anti-*T. cruzi* IgG 6–9 months after birth (assuming vector and other modes of transmission have been excluded). Congenital Chagas' disease is considered acute and requires trypanocide treatment. Notification is mandatory.

Prevention and control of Chagas' disease

- Limit exposure to the vector: improved housing, chemical disinfection of houses.
- Promote the use of mosquito nets.
- Screen blood for transfusion.

Chagas' disease is a clear example of public policy success, with 5 separate large-scale vector control programmes with modern pyrethroid insecticides being implemented in the last few decades in different Latin American countries. There is now mandatory notification of acute cases for intense epidemiological surveillance. Microepidemics of acute cases due to oral transmission through contaminated food such as meat, sugar cane juice, or açai (*Euterpe oleracea*) fruit juice, have been described, especially in the Amazon Region and in the south of Brazil.

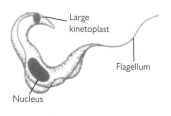
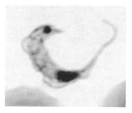

Large
kinetoplast

Flagellum

Nucleus

Fig. 18.8 *T. cruzi* as seen in a blood film.

Visceral leishmaniasis (kala-azar)

A severe systemic protozoal disease, caused by *Leishmania donovani* or *L. infantum* (called *L. chagasi* in S America). VL is increasing in incidence and causes major epidemics with high mortality. The disease is seasonal and geographically focal.

Pathogenesis: at infection, promastigotes (flagellate form) invade macrophages, becoming amastigotes (rounded form) which spread within spleen, bone marrow, liver, lymph nodes, and other tissues. Infection may be subclinical, controlled by an efficient cell-mediated immune response. Latent infections are reactivated during immunosuppression, especially HIV. In clinical disease, the immune response is ineffective and the parasite continues to multiply, producing pancytopenia and profound immunosuppression.

Transmission: is by the nocturnal bite of female *Phlebotomus* and *Lutzomyia* sandflies. In southern Europe, Brazil, etc. dogs are the major reservoirs of *L. infantum*/*L. chagasi,* a zoonotic form of VL which affects humans rarely (mainly infants and those with HIV). Humans are the hosts of highly endemic Indian and E. African *L. donovani* parasites, sandflies spreading infection human to human. Patients with post kalar dermal leishmaniasis (PKDL) can be long-term reservoirs of infection.

Clinical features: ~2–6 months' incubation period (asymptomatic) and ~1–4 months symptoms have elapsed by the time the patient presents. Initially, the patient may appear relatively well, is ambulant, and has a good appetite. Afternoon fevers (without rigors) and night sweats develop, lasting weeks–months. Dry cough and epistaxis are common. The patient notices wasting, weakness, and abdominal distension or pain due to the splenomegaly. The spleen enlarges and can reach the RIF, though a modest splenomegaly is more common. Anaemia causes fatigue. Diarrhoea, moderate hepatomegaly, ~1–2 cm lymphadenopathy (in Africa), pedal oedema, darkened skin, and zoster are also seen, as well as neurologic signs (confusion, ataxia, convulsions, deafness) in some. Dysentery, pneumonia, and TB may develop due to immunosuppression; malaria, measles, or influenza can be severe or fatal. Death is almost inevitable if untreated; it may follow sepsis, epistaxis, or anaemic heart failure.

During treatment: 3–10% of patients will succumb to the complications above, or die suddenly from antimonial-induced arrhythmias. The risk of death during treatment is much higher in those aged >45 yrs or <4 yrs, or with the following: severe anaemia (Hb<8 g/dL), severe malnutrition (BMI <13 kg/m^2), inability to walk unaided, and symptoms for >5 months.

Diagnosis: serology — most patients (>90%) have very high anti-*Leishmania* antibody titres on the direct agglutination test or a positive rapid dipstick test (rK39) using recombinant *Leishmania* antigen. Diagnosis is confirmed by finding parasites in Giemsa-stained smears of spleen aspirates (95% sensitive, but requires training) or lymph node/bone marrow aspirates (60–80% sensitive). Culture of aspirate improves diagnostic yield; cultures on other media can eliminate differential diagnoses (e.g. typhoid, brucellosis, miliary TB). In HIV co-infected patients, parasites are often numerous in skin, gut, liver, and on bronchoalveolar lavage.

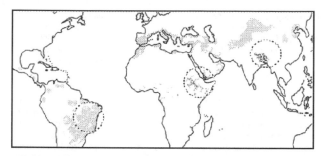

Fig. 18.9 The global distribution of viceral leishmaniasis (kala-azar). The species are *L infantum/L. chagasi* (dotted area) and *L donovani* (hatched area). 90% of all VL cases occur in Bangladesh, Brazil, India, Nepal, and Sudan. Up to 500,000 cases of kala-azar occur during an epidemic year.

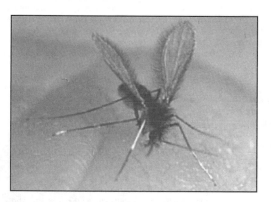

Fig. 18.10 The female phlebotomine sandfly is about half the size of a mosquito and feeds nocturnally. Several species transmit visceral or cutaneous leishmaniasis (Courtesy WHO/TDR).

Prevention: spraying to reduce sandfly vectors (in urban areas) and culling canine/rodent reservoirs. Insecticide-treated bednets reduce risk of VL by ~50%. Deltamethrin-impregnated dog collars reduce transmission of *L. infantum/L. chagasi*. In areas of human to human spread, case identification and treatment of visceral leishmaniasis and PKDL cases reduces transmission.

Management

VL is usually responsive to IM or IV pentavalent antimony (Sb^v) — 20 mg/kg IM od for 30 days. Meglumine antimoniate (85 mg Sb^v/ml) or sodium stibogluconate (100 mg Sb^v/ml) are equivalent; good-quality generic stibogluconate is as effective as brand-name preparations. There is no upper limit on the daily dose. 1° Sb^v resistance is a major problem in India; 2° resistance occurs in relapsed patients. Cardiac arrhythmias (may be fatal), pancreatitis, and other side-effects are well-recognised with antimonials, especially in HIV co-infected patients.

Patients who relapse following the 1st course can be retreated with the same daily dosage of Sb^v for a longer course, ensuring that at least 2 test-of-cure aspirates are parasite-free before the patient is discharged. Alternative: give infusions of amphotericin B 0.5 mg/kg/day (or 1 mg/kg on alternate days) to a total dose of 15 mg/kg, or liposomal amphotericin B 2–4 mg/kg/day to a total of >20 mg/kg over 7–10 days.

Second-choice drugs include paromomycin (also called aminosidine) 15 mg/kg/day IV/IM for 21 days. Miltefosine 2.5 mg/kg/day (for patients weighing 8–20 kg); 50 mg/day (20–25 kg); or 100 mg/day (>25 kg), for 28 days. It might be teratogenic; do not give to women of childbearing age unless pregnancy can be prevented during treatment and for 2 mths thereafter; unsafe in lactating mothers.

Drug combinations are logical developments for the future, to prevent resistance. Sb^v 20 mg/kg/day plus paromomycin 15 mg/kg/day, both for 17 days, is a safe combination.

Clinical improvement should be evident in 7–10 days. Response can be monitored by fever, haemoglobin, and spleen size. A parasitological response is shown by a negative splenic aspirate (bone marrow or lymph node if spleen impalpable) at the end of treatment. Clinical follow-up is important during next 6 months to detect relapse; by 12 months, the person can be considered cured. Relapse rates should be <5%, except in HIV +ve patients, most of whom will relapse unless antiretroviral treatment started early; even on ART, many will have repeated relapses and the VL becomes drug-resistant.

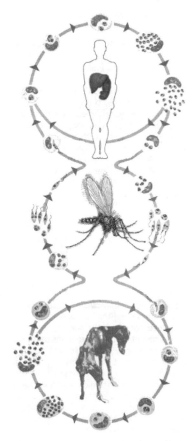

Fig. 18.11 Leishmaniasis (kala-azar) life cycle. The female sandfly inoculates flagellate forms (promastigotes) into man or animals whilst feeding. L infantum/L. chagasi are zoonotic, with a canine reservoir — L donovani has no known animal reservoir in India and several (unproven) animal hosts in Sudan. (Adapted from G.Piekarski, Medical parasitology in plates, 1962,with kind permission from Bayer Pharmaceuticals.)

Influenza

Influenza viruses serogroups A, B, and C are RNA viruses that cause respiratory tract infections in humans. Influenza A can cause epidemic disease and, rarely, can lead to a global pandemic. Human Influenza is spread from person to person in respiratory secretions. The virus evolves through small mutations ('drift') and, infrequently, reassortment of its segmented genome ('shift'), thereby evading existing population immunity. Over the last few years, there has been a global pandemic among poultry and birds of an avian influenza caused by influenza A (H5N1). This has been associated with a very worrying but, to date, relatively small number of infections in humans, usually associated with close exposure to infected poultry. Human infection with this influenza A (H5N1) virus leads to a severe disease with very high mortality (approximately 60%) and major concerns that if the virus adapted to humans it could lead to a global pandemic in humans akin to the devastating pandemic of 'Spanish flu' in 1918. As yet, there is no evidence of efficient transmission between humans of the influenza A (H5N1) virus, although there have been a number of incidents of clustering of cases within families with some evidence of very limited, inefficient human to human transmission.

Clinical features

The illness starts abruptly. Characteristic features are fever, chills, headache, coryza, dry cough, and myalgia. The symptoms are worst in the first 24–48 h and, thereafter, usually improve. In most cases, the patient recovers fully. The most common and important complication of human influenza is 2° bacterial pneumonia, usually due to pneumococcus or *Staphylococcus aureus*. This accounts for the significant mortality associated with influenza infection in the elderly and those with underlying lung disease. Infection with an influenza virus to which humans have no prior immunity (such as with influenza A (H5N1) or in primary influenza infection with a human virus) leads to a severe systemic infection associated with intense viral invasion of the lungs and other organs. In these cases, patients can deteriorate very rapidly with progressive severe bilateral multifocal consolidation and bulla formation. The viral loads (particularly in pharyngeal secretions) are very much higher in influenza A (H5N1) or in primary influenza infection and this can lead to an intense inflammatory response with associated tissue damage.

Diagnosis

Is usually clinical, but can be confirmed by rapid antigen detection from nose or throat swabs or from samples of respiratory secretions using PCR and viral culture.

Management

In uncomplicated cases, is supportive. Early treatment with antibiotics that are active against pneumococcus and *Staph aureus* (e.g. amoxicillin plus flucloxacillin) is indicated if there is any clinical suggestion of 2° pneumonia (e.g. breathlessness, discoloured sputum, or clinical signs of pneumonia). There has been little evidence so far of 2° bacterial infection complicating influenza A (H5N1) disease. Failure to improve as expected after the first 24–48 h of the illness is a warning sign of the development of potential complications. In these cases, the patient needs careful clinical, diagnostic, radiological, and therapeutic reassessment.

Antiviral agents

The neuroaminidase inhibitors (oral oseltamivir and inhaled zanamivir) or inhibitors of the M2 membrane protein (amantadine and rimantadine) have been shown to reduce the duration of illness in patients with influenza and are recommended in more severe disease. The maximum benefit is probably gained by early treatment within 48 h of onset of symptoms but there is theoretical benefit for as long as there is active viral replication. The influenza A (H5N1) outbreaks have generated a great deal of interest in the development of new parenteral antiviral agents and combination therapy. It is likely that in the next few years these will become available. Treatment of close household contacts of proven cases can reduce 2° transmission and would be of particular importance in an epidemic or pandemic. There is increasing resistance to all these drugs and treatment recommendations would ideally be based on knowledge of the sensitivity patterns of the circulating strains. There have been a series of excellent clinical and epidemiological guidelines released relevant to influenza A (H5N1). See:

www.who.int/csr/disease/avian_influenza/en/index.html

| **Prevention** | **PUBLIC HEALTH NOTE** |

- Immunization against known circulating strains is recommended annually for individuals at high risk of developing complications.
- Prophylaxis of health care workers and other high-risk staff is possible with oral oseltamivir and inhaled zanamivir, although data on their use long term (greater than 8 weeks) is not yet available.

Infectious mononucleosis

The clinical syndrome of infectious mononucleosis (IM) classically results from infection with the ubiquitous gammaherpes virus Epstein–Barr virus (EBV). An IM-like illness can also be caused by other organisms including cytomegalovirus, human immunodeficiency virus, and toxoplasma.

Transmission

EBV is transmitted orally via saliva and establishes infection within the oropharynx and circulating B cells. Individuals are usually infected by family members in childhood. If not exposed at this stage, they may acquire EBV during adolescence ('kissing disease') or adult life. EBV persists within the host for life and is intermittently shed in saliva.

Clinical features

Primary EBV infection is usually asymptomatic but causes IM in a very small proportion of children and in 25–50% adolescents/adults. A 4–7 weeks' incubation period is followed by development of fevers, malaise, pharyngitis, lymphadenopathy, and splenomegaly. Hepatitis, thrombocytopena, palatal petechiae, and a morbilliform rash may occur. Less commonly, myocarditis, pericarditis, pneumonitis haemolytic anaemia, or nephritis develops. Symptoms persist for 3–6 weeks and resolve spontaneously. An atypical form of disease in which neurological features such as meningitis, encephalitis, neuritis, or transverse myelitis predominate is recognized. IM is rarely fatal, although deaths have occurred 2° to splenic rupture, upper airway obstruction, encephalitis, hepatitis, and haemophagocytosis. Very rarely, a persistent form of disease known as chronic active EBV infection develops. This is characterized by a high viral load, failure of maturation of specific humoral immunity, and virus infection of NK or T cells, and has a 50% mortality rate. Primary EBV infection may also be fatal in those who are immunosuppressed or suffer from the X-linked lymphoproliferative syndrome.

The life-long persistent phase of EBV infection is almost always clinically silent. In a small proportion of individuals, EBV is implicated in the development of malignancies including nasopharyngeal carcinoma, endemic Burkitt's lymphoma, and Hodgkin's lymphoma. Persistent virus infection can cause B cell lymphoproliferative disease in the immunocompromised and hairy oral leukoplakia in those with HIV infection.

Diagnosis

A lymphocytosis with atypical cells is characteristic of IM. Mild thrombocytopenia and elevated transaminases may occur. IgM heterophile antibodies reactive with antigens found on sheep/horse red cells are usually present and are detected by Paul Bunnell/Monospot tests. IgM antibodies against EBV viral capsid antigens (VCA) confirm the diagnosis of IM. IgG antibodies specific for EBV VCA and the EBV nuclear antigen EBNA1 are detectable during lifelong persistent infection.

Management

The disease is normally self-limiting, requiring only supportive measures such as hydration, analgesics, or mild non-steroidal agents. Contact sports should be avoided in view of splenic enlargement. Prednisolone 0.7 mg/kg for 5–7 days, reducing over next 7 days, may be used in neurological disease, developing respiratory obstruction, or where splenic enlargement causes concern. Amoxicillin should be avoided if treating concomitant bacterial infection as it causes a rash in 90% patients. High-dose acyclovir reversibly reduces levels of replicating virus but has not been shown to clearly alter the clinical course of disease.

Measles

Overall global mortality from measles decreased from ~871,000 in 1999 to ~454,000 in 2004. However, measles still remains a substantial cause of global childhood mortality. Most of the deaths occur in developing countries where measles vaccine coverage is low.

Transmission

Measles is a paramyxovirus. It causes a highly contagious illness with >90% of non-immune people becoming infected if exposed. Transmission follows inhalation of airborne respiratory droplets from an infected person's coughing or sneezing. A child is infectious from 1 day before the onset of symptoms until around 5 days after the start of the rash. The virus can remain infectious in the environment for several hours. There is no animal reservoir. Infection confers lifelong immunity.

Risk factors

Unvaccinated or immunocompromised children (e.g. AIDS or corticosteroid therapy), children living in overcrowded conditions or visiting health facilities are at increased risk of measles. Previously uninfected and unvaccinated adolescents are also at increased risk.

Clinical features

Incubation period: Ranges from 7–14 days.

Prodrome: Generally occurs around 10–12 days from exposure; begins with mild to moderate fever and loss of appetite, followed by conjunctivitis, cough, and coryza. Koplik spots (greyish white spots the size of grains of sand on the inside of the mouth) appear on the 2nd/3rd day, 24–48 h before the rash stage. The prodrome usually lasts 2–5 days.

Rash: The distinctive maculopapular rash appears on the 4th/5th day following the start of symptoms, usually accompanied by high fever. The rash is non-pruritic, begins on face and behind the ears, and within 24–36 h spreads to the entire trunk and extremities (palms and soles rarely involved). It begins to fade 3–5 days after it first appears, initially to a purplish hue and then to brown/black lesions with fine scales.

Recovery: Cough may persist for 1–3 weeks. Measles-associated complications may cause persisting fever beyond the 3rd day of the rash.

Diagnosis

Diagnosis is usually clinical. The WHO defines measles as an illness with generalized maculopapular rash and fever with at least one of the following: cough, coryza, or conjunctivitis. In presence of distinctive clinical symptoms and a history of exposure, laboratory diagnosis is seldom required but, if needed, the following can be used:

- *Serology*: measles-specific IgM or 4-fold rise in measles IgG antibody titres between the acute and the convalescent phase.
- *Microscopy*: detection of multinucleate giant cells with inclusion bodies in nasopharyngeal secretions during the prodrome.

- *Immunofluorescence* can be used to demonstrate measles virus antigens in cells from nasopharyngeal specimens and urine.
- *Virus isolation*: measles virus can be isolated from throat or conjunctival washings, sputum, urine, and lymphocytes.

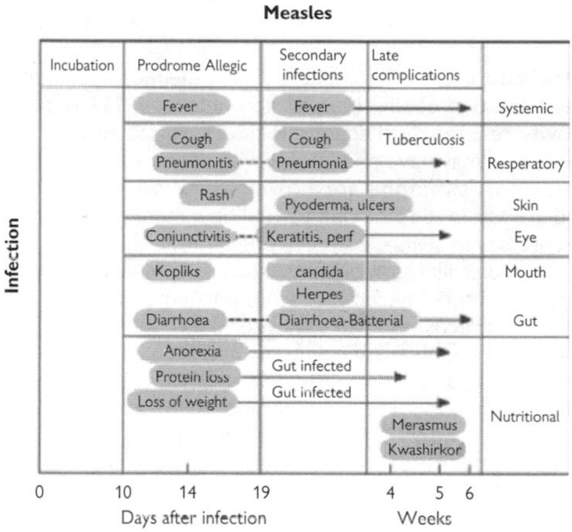

Fig. 18.12 Time course of measles infection.

Complications of measles

Severe measles is more common among unvaccinated young children and adults; immunocompromised, malnourished, or vitamin A-deficient children; or children living in overcrowded conditions. Vaccinated children usually have milder measles. In developing countries, at least one complication is expected in a large proportion of measles cases and one child may have several complications.

- **Pneumonia** is the most common complication and the most common cause of measles-associated deaths. Measles accounts for 6–21% of all cases of acute lower respiratory infections. In developing countries, 8–66% of measles cases may have pneumonia with widely varying case-fatality rates. Respiratory symptoms are a characteristic part of measles presentation and are assumed to be due to viral pneumonitis. In a minority, this progresses to severe giant cell pneumonia, which is characteristically a chronic illness in patients who are immunocompromised. Secondary respiratory infection is usually encountered when a patient is on the way to recovery 7–10 days after the onset of rash. The predominant bacteria are *S. aureus*, *E.coli*, *Pseudomonas*, *S. pneumoniae*, and other *Streptococcus* spp.
- **Diarrhoea** is the 2nd most common complication of measles. 1–7% of all diarrhoea episodes and 9–77% of all diarrhoea deaths in under-5-yr-olds in developing countries are measles-associated. From 8–80% of measles cases may have diarrhoea, with variable case-fatality rates. Most measles-associated diarrhoea occurs within 4 days of rash onset. Limited data shows that the distribution of diarrhoeal pathogens is similar in diarrhoeal patients with or without measles.
- **Other serious complications** include blindness, acute encephalitis, and subacute sclerosing panencephalitis (SSPE). Incidence of blindness has decreased due to vitamin A supplementation programmes and administration of vitamin A during measles. Acute encephalitis occurs in ~1/10,00 cases. SSPE occurs years after the primary illness in ~1/100,000 cases.
- **Other common complications** include acute malnutrition, mouth ulceration, and otitis media. Immune suppression and increased incidence of pneumonia, diarrhoea, and malnutrition persist after the acute illness, lasting ~6–8 weeks from rash onset.

Management

In most patients, measles is an acute self-limiting disease.
- Ensure adequate nutrition, hydration, and support, including education of mother about complications.
- Give vitamin A (dose and regimen, 📖 p 649). This corrects vitamin A deficiency, decreases severity of illness and case-fatality.

If specific symptoms/signs or conditions are present:
- Give paracetamol for high fever (>38.5°C).
- Treat mouth ulcers with gentian violet 0.25%.
- Give topical antibiotics if cornea cloudy or pus draining from the eyes.
- Manage diarrhoea/dysentery and dehydration as outlined on 📖 p 248.
- Give broad-spectrum antibiotics for treatment of acute otitis media or 2° pneumonia.

- The role of antibiotic prophylaxis for 2° bacterial pneumonia has not been established.

Control of measles

All children should be immunized: Give 1st dose of measles vaccine at the age of 9 months or shortly thereafter. At least 90% of children should be immunized. A 'second opportunity' for measles immunization is provided to all children. This assures measles immunity in children who failed to receive a previous dose of measles vaccine, as well as in those who were vaccinated but failed to develop immunity (10–15% of children vaccinated at 9 months of age). Providing measles vaccine to displaced persons living in camp settings within a week of entry should be a public health priority. (Measles vaccine is covered further on 🕮 p 821). Measles surveillance enables prompt recognition and investigation of outbreaks, and provides information on programme impact.

Hospital admission triage during an epidemic

During a measles epidemic, decide which clinical signs should determine whether a patient is ill enough to warrant admission to hospital. The following criteria were used to grade illness severity in one epidemic.

	Degree of severity			
	Severe	Mod/Sev	Moderate	Mild
Oral lesions				
Buccal mucosa	+	+	+	+
Gingiva	+	+	±	−
Tongue/palate	+	+	−	−
Haemorrhagic	+	−	−	−
Rash				
Haemorrhagic	+	−	−	−
Confluent	+	+	−	−
Desquamating	+	±	−	−
Widespread	−	−	+	−
Scattered	−	−	−	+
Systemic upset				
Bronchopneumonia	+	+	−	−
Cough	+	+	+	−
Coryza	+	+	+	+
Diarrhoea	+	+	+	−
Bloody diarrhoea	+	−	−	−

Other signs that may warrant admission include: severe mouth or skin ulceration, corneal ulceration, convulsions/LOC, laryngeal obstruction, and marked dehydration. If the child is malnourished or underweight, these signs should be considered with greater seriousness.

Arboviruses

Arboviruses are transmitted to man by arthropod vectors — insects (mosquitoes, sandflies) and ticks. A large number cause clinical disease. They occur throughout the world (although the geographical range of individual viruses is limited) and most are zoonoses (infection in man is incidental) but may become epidemic. The illnesses caused by arbovirus infections can be broadly classified into four overlapping syndromes:

1. Acute benign fever, with or without rash
2. Acute encephalitis
3. Haemorrhagic fever (see later)
4. Polyarthritis and rash

Overall, dengue causes more illness and death than any other arboviral infection. Locally, other viruses may be more important. Yellow fever has the potential to cause disastrous epidemics. Japanese encephalitis — a common and important arboviral infection in parts of Asia — is considered on 📖 p 413.

Dengue and dengue haemorrhagic fever

Dengue is transmitted from infected to susceptible humans by day-biting *Aedes* mosquitoes — domestic mosquitoes that breed in human-made containers. There are four viral serotypes (1, 2, 3, and 4). Infection with one serotype does not induce solid immunity to the other serotypes, and so an individual may be infected with dengue more than once. Dengue is not transmitted directly from one person to another and, therefore, no special infection control measures are required for suspected cases in hospital.

The most intense transmission occurs in South-east Asia, but in recent years there have been dramatic increases in dengue transmission in the Indian subcontinent and the Western hemisphere. An estimated 50–100 million people are infected with dengue each year. In established areas of intense dengue transmission (such as S.E. Asia), almost all infections occur in children, and adults are immune to locally circulating serotypes of dengue virus. In contrast, if a particular serotype of dengue is newly transmitted in a geographical area, both adults and children will become infected.

Clinical features and classification: Dengue virus infection may be subclinical, may present as an undifferentiated febrile disease with maculopapular rash (particularly in infants and young children), or may result in a typical febrile illness with or without bleeding and/or shock. Conventionally, typical dengue syndromes have been classified into two groups, classical dengue fever (DF) and dengue haemorrhagic fever (DHF). Current diagnostic criteria for DHF are based on clinical observation and simple laboratory tests — see box 📖 p 725. The presence of vascular leak is the key feature that distinguishes DHF from DF. Individual patients may have varying degrees of bleeding and/or shock (and sometimes other serious complications, such as encephalitis) and, therefore, the clinical utility and specificity of the current classification is limited.

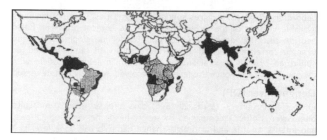

Fig. 18.13 Distribution of dengue fever. The black areas indicate recent dengue activity and the grey areas are those at risk in the future. (Reproduced from the *WHO Report on Global Surveillance of Epidemic–prone Infectious Diseases* with permission of the WHO.)

WHO case definition of DHF

The following must all be present:
1. Fever, or history of acute fever
2. Haemorrhagic tendencies, evidenced by at least one of:
- Positive tourniquet test.
- Petechiae, ecchymoses, or purpura.
- Bleeding.
3. Thrombocytopaenia
4. Evidence of plasma leakage
- Haematocrit >20% above average.
- Drop in haematocrit >20% after volume replacement.
- Clinical signs (e.g. pleural effusion, ascites).

WHO case definition of DSS

All of the above, plus evidence of circulatory failure including:
- Rapid and weak pulse.
- Narrow pulse pressure (<20 mmHg).
or
- Hypotension.
- Cold, clammy skin and restlessness.

Laboratory diagnosis: requires specialist laboratories, so is not routinely available in parts of the world where dengue is most prevalent. Rapid bedside tests for dengue are currently under development. Dengue viraemia correlates well with temperature, thus virus can be isolated (or confirmed by PCR or viral antigen detection) in a febrile patient with dengue. Conversely, once the fever has resolved, serology is more useful.

Dengue fever (DF)

DF begins abruptly 3–15 (usually 5–8) days after an infected mosquito bite. Fever is often accompanied by severe headache, retro-orbital pain, and intense myalgia and arthralgia (hence name 'break bone fever'). A blanching rash typically appears after a few days; it is a useful clue to diagnosis, if present. DF usually lasts for 4–7 days, followed by complete recovery. Severe complications are uncommon and include: bleeding without evidence of vascular leak (therefore not fulfilling case definition of DHF), in particular of GI tract and menorrhagia; encephalopathy; encephalitis.

Management: is symptomatic. Avoid aspirin because of bleeding risk.

Dengue haemorrhagic fever (DHF)

DHF usually begins in the same way as DF, but after 2–7 days, signs of bleeding and increased vascular permeability become apparent. The most severely ill patients have evidence of circulatory failure known as dengue shock syndrome (DSS) — see box 📖 p 725. Without treatment, mortality is high in patients with DSS, but this is reduced to 1–5% by careful supportive care.

Treatment: Prompt restoration of the volume of circulating plasma is the cornerstone of therapy. Initial resuscitation with Ringer's lactate is indicated for children with moderately severe DSS (pulse pressure 10–20 mmHg); for those with severe shock (pulse pressure <10 mmHg), colloid is used if available e.g. 6% hydroxyethyl starch. The vascular leak syndrome typically resolves within 24–48 h, and careful monitoring is required to avoid fluid overload during the recovery phase. Pulmonary oedema secondary to fluid overload can contribute to mortality.

Prevention: There is currently no vaccine. Vector control is effective but difficult to sustain.

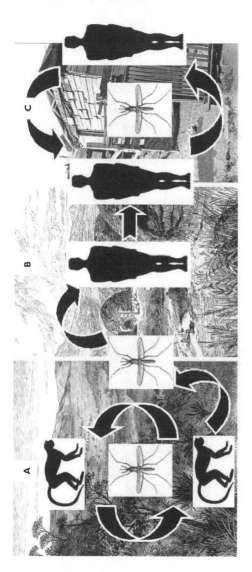

Fig.18.14 Transmission cycles of yellow fever in Africa. (A) Jungle yellow fever is enzootic (but usually asymptomatic) among monkeys and baboons, transmitted by *Aedes africanus*. (B) Savannah yellow fever occurs when *Aedes simpsoni* mosquitoes leave the forest to feed on humans living in villages nearby. (C) Urban yellow fever occurs when the viraemic patient travels to the town and *Aedes aegypti* mosquitoes become infected. This can lead to large epidemics in unvaccinated populations.

Yellow fever

Yellow fever (YF) is a flavivirus that is transmitted by several different culicine mosquitoes. Accurate YF incidence data are lacking — there are ~200,000 cases/year and >30,000 deaths. YF occurs mainly in sub-Saharan Africa; there are far fewer cases in tropical South America and YF does not occur in Asia.

Transmission: (see Fig.18.14): the primary transmission cycle involves non-human primates, but humans may be 'accidentally' infected when they are bitten by an infected mosquito. The disease may then be spread by mosquitoes from infected human to susceptible human, causing explosive epidemics in urban environments.

Clinical features: illness begins abruptly 3–6 days after the bite of an infected mosquito. Characteristic features are fever, chills, headache, widespread myalgia, conjunctival congestion, and relative bradycardia (Faget's sign). After several days, the majority of patients recover. Others deveop a life-threatening illness with increasing fever, jaundice, renal failure, and bleeding (due to thrombocytopaenia and coagulopathy). Death is preceded by shock, agitated delirium, stupor, and coma.

Diagnosis: can be confirmed by virus isolation from blood in the first 4 days of illness or by detection of specific IgM. The WHO will advise on availability of laboratory diagnostic services.

Management: there is no specific anti-viral therapy and treatment is supportive. Direct human to human transmission, without the agency of a mosquito vector, has not been reported. The case fatality rate is not accurately known — perhaps 20% of patients with jaundice will die.

Prevention: Immunization is the cornerstone of prevention — protective immunity is probably lifelong after a single dose of live-attenuated vaccine. Universal immunization in endemic areas would be effective but has not been achieved. The disease is statutorily notifiable to the WHO. In the event of human infection, measures should be taken to prevent or control an outbreak in order to protect public health — see box.

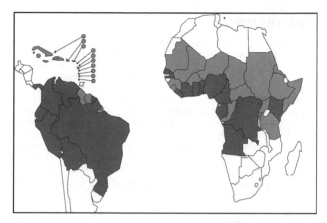

Fig.18.15 Distribution of yellow fever (the WHO). The dark grey areas indicate countries that have reported at least one outbreak of YF 1985–99 and the light grey countries are at risk of YF in the future. (Reproduced from the *WHO Report on Global Surveillance of Epidemic–prone Infectious Diseases* with permission of the WHO.)

**Prevention and control of a   Public health note
yellow fever outbreak**

Management of human cases
1. Notify the WHO (required under international health regulations).
2. Prevent access of mosquitoes to patient for at least 5 days by screening room, spraying with permethrin, lambda cyalothrin or DDT, and using insecticide-treated bednets.
3. Spray patient's home and all nearby houses with insecticide.
4. Identify areas visited by patient 3–6 days before onset (e.g. place of work) and spray with insecticide as appropriate.
5. Immunize family, contacts, and neighbours (if not previously immunized).

Epidemic measures
Urban yellow fever
1. Mass immunization.
2. Eliminate and/or treat *Aedes* breeding sites.
3. Widespread insecticide spraying inside houses should be considered.

Jungle yellow fever
1. Immunize all people living near or entering forested area that is presumed focus.
2. Ensure non-immunized or just immunized (within 1 week) individuals avoid tracts of forest where infection has been localized.

Chikungunya

Chikungunya is a mosquito-borne alphavirus that has a wide geographical range — sub-Saharan Africa, India, Indian Ocean islands, much of S.E. Asia — and can cause explosive outbreaks of disease. The illness begins abruptly 4–7 days after the bite of an infected *Aedes* mosquito. *Common features* are fever, chills, headache, photophobia, vomiting, lymphadenopathy, and a predominantly truncal rash that appears on the 2nd to 5th day of onset. Minor haemorrhagic phenomena can oocur. A striking feature is myalgia and severe arthralgia/arthritis affecting single or multiple joints. The strain responsible for the recent Indian Ocean islands outbreak may be more virulent — there have been confirmed cases of meningo-encephalitis in neonates and the elderly, and Chikungunya infection was associated with death in elderly patients with co-morbidity.

Diagnosis: is made by IgM-capture ELISA. PCR is useful for diagnosis with acute samples.

Treatment: is symptomatic. Recovery in 5–7 days without serious complications is usual. Prolonged joint pain and stiffness may occur — 12% of patients have chronic arthralgia 3 years after onset of illness.

Viral haemorrhagic fevers (VHF)

Overview: Infections that cause haemorrhagic fever (HF) evoke great fear. The term defines a clinical syndrome, not a specific cause. Viral haemorrhagic fevers (VHF) occur in most parts of the world — see box. Knowledge of local HF viruses is essential in assessing the risk to an individual patient. Acute bacterial infections (especially meningococcal disease, leptospirosis, rickettsial infection) and falciparum malaria may produce a similar clinical picture and require specific treatment.

The management of HF always includes general support. Infection control measures to protect medical, nursing, and laboratory personnel should be instituted until more information becomes available. If a VHF that can be spread from person to person (in particular, Ebola, Marburg, Crimean–Congo HF, but also Lassa fever, Bolivian HF, and Argentine HF) is plausible, based on time and place of exposure, then local experts, the WHO, or CDC should be consulted immediately to advise on infection control and to help expedite diagnosis.

Viruses belonging to four different families of RNA viruses cause HF.

Clinical features: VHF typically begins with a non-specific illness — fever, myalgia, and malaise. Within a few days, the illness progresses with increasing prostration, specific organ involvement, and evidence of vascular damage (injected conjunctivae, oedema, organ dysfunction, haemorrhage). Severe cases develop shock, CNS involvement, or extensive bleeding.

Diagnosis: The particular clinical features associated with different viruses are listed on 📖 p 735. but, in general, accurate diagnosis requires virological confirmation in a specialist laboratory.

Management: In addition to supportive therapy, antiviral therapy with ribavirin has been shown to be effective in reducing mortality in severe cases of Lassa fever. Ribavirin is probably also effective in other arenavirus infections, Crimean–Congo HF, and HF with renal syndrome, if administered early in the course of infection. If available, ribavirin could also be considered for treatment of severe Rift Valley fever.

Classification of HF viruses and modes of transmission

	Important examples	Modes of transmission
Arenaviruses	Guanarito **Junin** **Machupo** **Lassa**	All have rodent reservoir Humans infected by aerosols of rodent excreta or other close contacts with rodents
Bunyaviruses	Rift Valley Fever **Crimean–Congo** Hantaan	Mosquito bite; aerosol or contact with blood of domestic animals Tick bite; aerosol or contact with slaughtered cattle or sheep Aerosols of rodent excreta or other close contacts with rodents
Filoviruses	**Ebola** **Marburg**	Index case probably infected from non-human primates Person to person spread by contact with body fluids (? aerosol) is most important route of transmission to humans
Flaviviruses	Yellow fever Dengue Kyanasur forest disease	Mosquito bite Mosquito bite Tick bite

Viruses listed in bold may spread from person to person and necessitate special attention to infection control

Important HF viruses and their distribution in tropical and subtropical regions

Africa
- Crimean–Congo HF.
- Dengue.
- Ebola.
- Lassa.
- Marburg.
- Rift Valley fever.
- Yellow fever.

Asia
- Crimean–Congo HF.
- Dengue.
- Kyanasur forest disease.
- HF with renal syndrome (Hantavirus).

Americas
- Argentine (Junin) HF.
- Bolivian HF (Machupo virus).
- Dengue.
- HF with renal syndrome (Hantavirus).
- Venezualan HF (Guanarito virus).
- Yellow fever.

Management of VHF contacts and isolation precautions

- Determine index case's places of residence and activities over last 3 weeks, and search for unreported or undiagnosed cases.
- Establish surveillance for individuals at risk — all close contacts within 3 weeks of onset of illness and laboratory staff handling specimens. Surveillance comprises body temperature measurement twice daily until 3 weeks after last possible exposure. If oral temperature exceeds 38.3°C, the contact should be hospitalized immediately in strict isolation.
- Reinforce and ensure the use of universal precautions in non-isolation areas of the health facility.
- Isolate the VHF patient.
- Wear protective clothing (enhanced by use of two sets of gloves, two sets of clothing, plastic apron, boots, eyewear, bonnet, and mask) in the isolation area, cleaning and laundry area, laboratory, or when in contact with the patient. (Because of experimental infection of primates by aerosols, the observed high mortality among health care workers, and the desire to provide the maximum protection, masks which meet the US HEPA or N series standards are recommended.)
- Handle needles and other sharp instruments safely. Do not recap needles. Dispose of non-reusable needles, syringes, and other sharp patient-care instruments in puncture-resistant containers.
- Avoid sharing equipment between patients. Designate equipment for each patient, if supplies allow. If sharing equipment is unavoidable, make sure it is not reused by another patient until it has been cleaned, disinfected, and sterilized properly.
- Disinfect all spills, equipment, and supplies safely. (This is enhanced by using disinfectant sprayers and 0.05% hypochlorite solutions.)
- Dispose of all contaminated waste by incineration or burial (including safe disposal of corpse).
- Provide appropriate information to the families and community about the prevention of VHF and the care of infected patients.

Table 18.1 Clinical features of VHFs*

Disease	Incubation period (days)	Case infection ratio	Case fatality rate	Features of severe disease
Arenaviridae				
South American HFs	7–14	>50%	15–30%	Overt bleeding and shock; CNS involvement (dysarthria, intention tremor) common
Lassa fever	5–16	Mild infection common	2–15%	Prostration and shock; fewer haemorrhagic or neurological manifestations cf. South American HF
Bunyaviridae				
Rift Valley fever	2–5	1%	50%	Bleeding, shock, anuria, jaundice; encephalitis and retinal vasculitis occur but are distinct from HF syndrome
Crimean–Congo HF	3–12	20–100%	15–30%	Most severe bleeding and bruising of all the HFs
HF with renal syndrome (Hantavirus)	9–35	>75%	5–15%	Febrile stage followed by shock and renal failure; bleeding at all stages
Filoviridae				
Marburg or Ebola	3–16	High	25–90%	Most severe of HFs; marked prostration; maculopapular rash common
Flaviviridae				
Dengue	See 📖 p 724			
Yellow fever	See 📖 p 728			
Kyasanur Forest disease	3–8	Variable	0.5–9%	Typical biphasic illness — fever and haemorrhage followed by CNS involvement

*Adapted from Peters and Zaki, in *Tropical Infectious Diseases* (eds. Guerrant, Walker, and Weller)

Prevention of infection in the health care setting

Hospitals concentrate in one-place infectious patients, vulnerable patients, invasive procedures, surgery, and resistant microbial flora. Nosocomial infections are a large, under-recognized and preventable problem in tropical hospitals and clinics, and risk of health care-associated infection in tropical and low-income countries is high:

- In one Thai hospital studied 36% deaths were from nosocomial infection.
- Nosocomial infections were the 3rd most common infectious cause of death in Mexico (after pneumonia and gastroenteritis).
- In Ebola outbreaks, hospitals became foci of transmission to the community at large.

There is a substantial risk of infection to both patients and health care workers (HCWs) in these settings. Risk of nosocomial transmission of certain infections is especially high in low-income settings e.g. measles, gastrointestinal infections incl. typhoid and cholera, and TB. Basic elements of hygiene and infection control are commonly overlooked.

Minimum requirements

Gloves, disposable needles, and hand hygiene are absolute necessities for any health service. Resources should not be wasted on ineffective measures such as disinfecting floors or wearing of surgical masks by HCWs on the wards.

Hand hygiene

Health care workers' hands are the main route of transmission for many gastrointestinal, wound, and respiratory pathogens. This is largely preventable by consistent hand cleansing. Provision of soap and water near the bedside in every health facility is ideal, but not always feasible. Re-use of towels decreases the efficacy of hand washing.

Alcohol-based hand cleansers are as effective as hand washing against most pathogens, more convenient, and quicker to use and less irritating to the hands. The basic ingredients (980 ml isopropyl alcohol and 20 ml glycerine) are inexpensive. Routine hand cleansing between patients should be practised — particularly by doctors, who often have poor compliance with hand hygiene.

Mechanical barriers: gloves, etc.

Gloves are essential for all invasive procedures and any examination involving exposure to body fluids. A face shield or goggles should be used for procedures that may involve direct spraying (e.g. an arterial spurter in surgery) or aerosolization of body fluids.

Enteric precautions and isolation

Patients who are incontinent with diarrhoea or who may have an epidemic pathogen such as cholera, should be in a single room, if at all possible. Gloves should be worn when examining the patient or handling contaminated materials. Contaminated areas should be cleaned with hot soapy water and equipment, with a disinfectant.

Respiratory isolation (includes TB, measles, varicella)

Many respiratory pathogens, from respiratory syncytial virus (RSV) to SARS, are present in large droplets which are transmitted over short distances or by hand contact. TB, measles, and varicella are transmitted by small aerosolized particles which travel much farther.

HCWs and patients are exposed to a significant risk of nosocomial TB infection; especially vulnerable are HIV-infected individuals. Much of the risk occurs before the diagnosis is made and treatment initiated i.e. in casualty and medical wards. Ideally, TB suspects should be identified and isolated when first seen; however, TB is in the differential diagnosis of at least half of new medical admissions, which may make it impossible to isolate all TB suspects.

- Priority should be given to patients with possible drug resistant TB (e.g. treatment failures).
- Separate immune suppressed patients and small children from those with suspected TB.
- Ventilation and sunlight should be high priorities in the design and operation of all health facilities in low-income countries.
- Standard surgical masks worn by HCWs provide little if any protection against TB. When worn by infectious patients e.g. going down to the X-ray suite, they may ↓ dissemination of aerosolized organisms. High-efficiency masks are expensive and require a good fit to be effective.
- TB culture laboratories, but not those doing smear microscopy, carry an increased risk of TB exposure and should be equipped with protective hoods and adequate ventilation.
- HIV-infected HCWs should be encouraged to work in settings where the risk of TB transmission is less e.g. non-clinical roles or paediatrics.

Sterilization and disposal

- The highest priority is to ensure that needles cannot be re-used in the community.
- Standard sterilization equipment should be used for surgical and other hospital equipment and protocols for their use and maintenance followed strictly.
- Every health care facility should have a provision for the disposal or incineration of medical waste.

Needle and sharps risk

In the tropics, the risk of nosocomial blood-borne infection is high. Injections are often given under risky conditions, by 'informal' or 'alternative' health care providers in many communities. Both HCWs and patients are at risk. Agents transmissible by this route include HIV, hepatitis B, hepatitis C, HTLV 1, syphilis, malaria, and dengue. Most patients with blood-borne infections cannot be identified by history or clinical findings. Routine testing of patients for HIV and other blood-borne infections has many benefits but contributes little to the protection of HCWs. The best preventative strategy is the **routine** application of 'universal' 'or 'standard' precautions to all patients, in all settings. This applies particularly to handling of needles and other sharps, but also to the use of gloves when there is any possibility of exposure to blood or body fluids. Consistent application of these principles dramatically reduces the risk of occupational infection among HCWs.

- Every HCW using a needle for any procedure should have a puncture-proof container at the bedside before starting the procedure, and use it for disposal rather than recapping the needle.
- Non-reusable needle systems are a more costly alternative.
- Every HCW in contact with patients or specimens should be vaccinated against hepatitis B (unless shown to have hepatitis B surface antigen or antibody).

Only use injectable drugs when there is a clear therapeutic advantage — ignore the preference for injections among some patients.

Post-exposure prophylaxis (PEP)

When sharps injuries occur, post-exposure prophylaxis can reduce the risk of HIV infection by over 80%. Every health care facility should have: a) a protocol for sharps injuries and b) rapid access to initial doses of antiretroviral drugs for PEP.

Action in sharps injury or blood exposures:

- 'First aid' — cleaning and irrigation of the wound or exposed area.
- Assessment of the level of risk involved e.g. penetrating injury, hollow bore or solid needle (the former is much higher risk), exposure of mucous membranes or non-intact skin to blood or body fluids.
- Determine the HIV status of the source patient. This commonly involves some delay if the patient's HIV status is not already known, and it is often necessary to start PEP while waiting for the result. Although there may be local differences of approach, source patients should be informed and agree to HIV testing.
- If a potentially risky exposure is thought to have occurred from an HIV-infected source patient (or while awaiting source patient results), PEP should be initiated immediately (within 1–2 h). Animal models suggest that PEP efficacy correlates with the speed of administration after the exposure.
- If it proves impossible to determine the HIV status of the source patient, a decision regarding PEP must be made on the likelihood of the source patient having HIV.

Suggested PEP regimens vary, typically including at least two drugs such as zidovudine and lamivudine. The standard duration is 28 days. Nelfinavir or lopinavir/ritonavir (Kaletra) is often used when three-drug therapy is recommended. Nevirapine should not be used in this setting because of its high risk of serious reactions.

PEP recipients should be informed about possible adverse effects. If the regimen involves zidovudine, a haemoglobin and white blood cell count should be checked at about two weeks after PEP initiation, if possible. HIV testing should be offered, usually at 0, 3, and 6 months post exposure and safer sex practices recommended until a final negative result is received. Follow-up for hepatitis B and C should be carried out depending on source patient status, if local resources permit.

Isolation for known or suspected viral haemorrhagic fevers (VHF)

The critical element in the prevention of transmission from patients to HCWs or other patients is the rigorous and consistent implementation of 'standard precautions' as indicated above. External agencies such as the CDC commonly become involved and may provide additional resources and equipment such as high-efficiency masks which should be worn if available. An infection control manual for VHFs in the African health care setting is available at:

http://www.cdc.gov/ncidod/dvrd/spb/mnpages/vhfmanual.htm

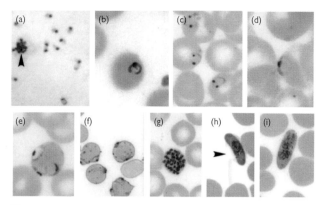

Plate 1 *Plasmodium falciparum:* (a) thick film showing ring trophozoites + schizont (arrow); and thin films showing: ring trophozoites [(b) to (f)] — note the single and double chromatin dots, multiply infected erythrocytes, accolé form (d) and Maurer's clefts (f); schizont (g); macrogametocyte (h); and microgametocyte (i). (Reproduced with permission from the *WHO Bench Aids for the Diagnosis of Malaria Infections,* 2nd edn.)

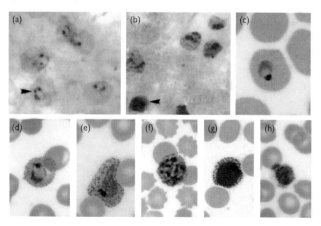

Plate 2 *Plasmodium vivax:* thick films (a) and (b) showing ring forms; and thin films showing: ring trophozoites of varying size and shape [(c) to (e)], schizont (f), microgametocyte (g), and macrogametocyte (h). Note Schuffner's dots seen as stippling in the surface of the erythrocyte. (Reproduced with permission from the *WHO Bench Aids for the Diagnosis of Malaria Infections,* 2nd edn.)

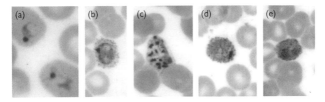

Plate 3 *Plasmodium ovale:* thin films showing trophozoites [(a) and (b)]; schizont (c); microgametocyte (d); and macrogametocyte (e). (Reproduced with permission from the *WHO Bench Aids for the Diagnosis of Malaria Infections*, 2nd edn.)

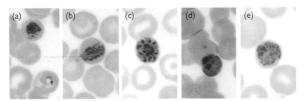

Plate 4 *Plasmodium malariae:* thin films showing trophozoites (a), including band form (b); schizont (c); macrogametocyte (d); and microgametocyte (e). (Reproduced with permission from the *WHO Bench Aids for the Diagnosis of Malaria Infections*, 2nd edn.)

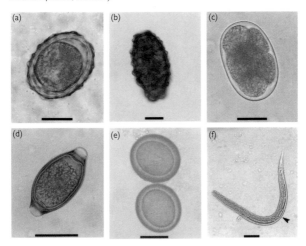

Plate 5 Faecal parasites 1: (a) Ascaris egg (fertile); (b) Ascaris egg (infertile); (c) Hookworm egg; (d) Trichuris egg; (e) Taenia eggs; (f) Rhabtidiform larva of *Strongyloides stercoralis*. [Scale: bar = 25 μm] (Reproduced with permission from the *WHO Bench Aids for the Diagnosis of Faecal parasites*)

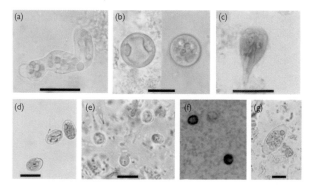

Plate 6 Faecal parasites 2: (a) *Entamoeba histolytica* trophozoite (note phago-cytosed erythrocytes); (b) *E. histolytica* cysts; (c) *Giardia lamblia* trophozoites; (d) *G. lamblia* cysts; (e) *Cryptosporidium parvum* oocysts (wet prep); (f) *Cryptosporidium parvum* oocysts (Ziehl–Neelsen stain); (g) *Isospora belli* cyst. [Scale: bar = 10 μm] (Reproduced with permission from the *WHO Bench Aids for the Diagnosis of Faecal parasites*.)

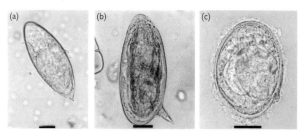

Plate 7 **Schistosomiasis eggs:** (a) *S. haematobium* (in urine); (b) *S. mansoni* (in stool); (c) *S. japonicum* (in stool). [Scale: bar = 25 μm] (Reproduced with permission from the *WHO Bench Aids for the Diagnosis of Faecal parasites*.)

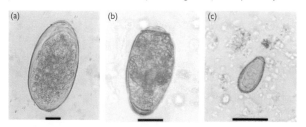

Plate 8 **Other trematodes**: (a) *Fasciola hepatica* egg; (b) *Paragonimus westermani* egg; (c) *Clonorchis sinensis* egg. [Scale: bar = 25 μm] (Reproduced with permission from the *WHO Bench Aids for the Diagnosis of Faecal parasites*.)

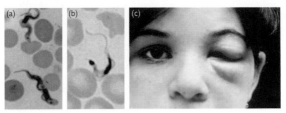

Plate 9 Trypanosomes: (a) *Trypanosoma b. rhodesiense* (Giemsa); (b) *Trypanosoma cruzi* (Leishman stain); (c) Romaña's sign (unilateral oedema and conjunctivitis at the portal of entry in acute Chagas' disease) ((c) Reproduced with permission from the WHO).

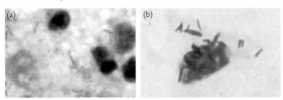

Plate 10 Mycobacteria: (a) *M. tuberculosis* in sputum smear; (b) *M. leprae* in skin smear — note acid-fast bacilli in and around macrophage (both Ziehl–Neelson stain). Reproduced with Permission of Tropical Health Technology.

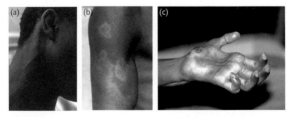

Plate 11 Leprosy: (a) great auricular nerve, and (b) hypopigmentation in tuberculoid leprosy; (c) typical deformity and neuropathic ulcer in lepromatoous leprosy. ((b) Reproduced with kind permission from Anthony Bryceson; (c) reproduced with permission from the WHO.)

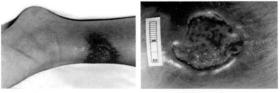

Plate 12 Buruli ulcer — note the undermined edges of the ulcer. (Reproduced with permission from Johnson *et al.* (2005) Buruli ulcer: New Insights, New Hope for Disease Control, *PLOS Med*, 2(4) e108.)

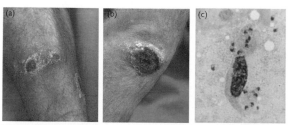

Plate 13 Leishmaniasis: (a) leg and (b) elbow with cutaneous leishmaniasis from Belize due to *Leishmania braziliensis*; (c) *Leishmania* amastigotes in slit skin smear.

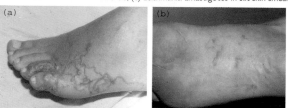

Plate 14 Cutaneous larva migrans. (Reproduced with kind permission from (a) Anthony Bryceson and (b) Terence Ryan.)

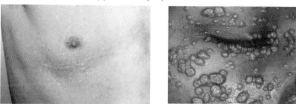

Plate 15 Larva currens.   **Plate 16 Moluscum contagiosum.**

Plate 15 reproduced with the kind permission of Anthony Bryceson; plate 16 reproduced with permission from Cotell and Roholt (1998) Images in clinical medicine. Molluscum contagiosum in a patient with the acquired immuno deficiency syndrome. *N Engl J Med*, 338:888).

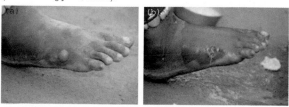

Plate 17 Dracunculiasis: the female guinea worm induces a painful blister (a), through which she protrudes (b) to lay her eggs.

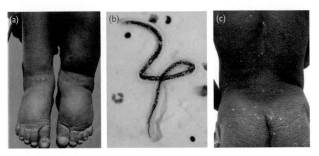

Plate 18 Filaria: (a) lymphoedoema (elephantiasis), due to (b) *Wuchereria bancrofti* (blood smear, haematoxylin); (c) onchocerciasis — chronic papular onchodermatitis. ((a) and (c) reproduced with kind permission from Anthony Bryceson).

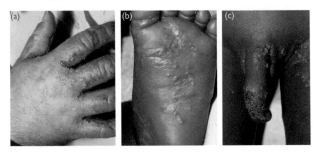

Plate 19 Scabies: (a) hand (note predilection for web spaces), (b) foot, (c) groin. (Reproduced with permission from TALC).

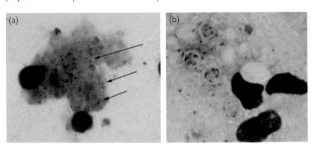

Plate 20 Pneumocystis pneumonia (PCP): (a) *Pneumocystis jirovecii* trophozoites in bronchoalveolar lavage (BAL) from patient with HIV (Giemsa). The trophozoites are small (1–5 μm), and only their nuclei, stained purple, are visible (arrows). (b) 3 *Pneumocystis jirovecii* cysts in BAL (Giemsa stain). The rounded cysts (4–7 μm) contain 6 to 8 intracystic bodies, whose nuclei are stained by Giemsa; the walls of the cysts are not stained; note the presence of several smaller, isolated trophozoites.

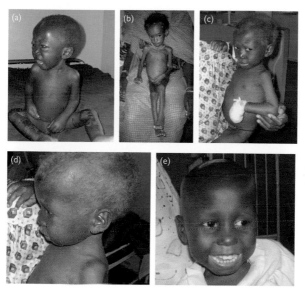

Plate 21 Malnutrition: (a) kwashiorkor — miserable affect, periorbital and limb oedema, protuberant belly, skin and hair changes; (b) marasmus — severe wasting; (c) & (d) marasmus-kwashiorkor — wasting, hair changes, and early skin changes in axilla and groin; (e) is the same child one month later after nutritional rehabilitation

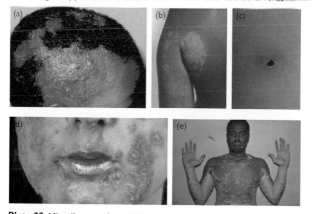

Plate 22 Miscellaneous dermatology: (a) tinea capitis; (b) tinea corporis; (c) Rickettsial eschar (African tick bite fever); (d) impetigo; (e) vitiligo. (Reproduced with permission from (a) TALC; (b), (d), (e) Terence Ryan.)

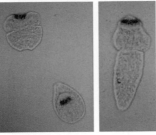

Plate 23 Hydatid sand: *Echinococcus granulosus* protoscolices in hydatid cyst fluid.

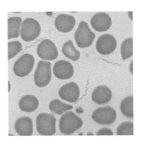

Plate 24 *Borrelia recurrentis* spirochaetes in blood film.

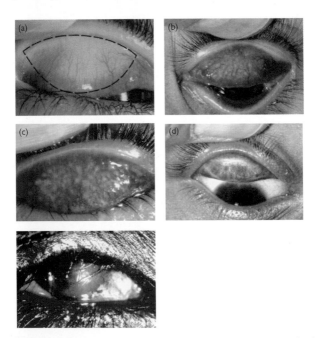

Plate 25 Trachoma: (a) normal tarsal conjunctiva (area to be examined outlined by dotted line); (b) follicular trachomatous inflammation (>5 follicles in the upper tarsal conjunctiva); (c) intense trachomatous inflammation (inflammatory thickening partially obscures numerous follicles); (d) trachomatous scarring (white bands or sheets in the tarsal conjunctiva); (e) trachomatous trichiasis and corneal opacity (eyelashes rub on cornea which eventually clouds).

Mental health

Section editor   **Vikram Patel**

Introduction

Mental illnesses are a major public health problem, accounting for 12.7% of the global burden of disease. Projections indicate this will increase. Common mental disorders (depression and anxiety), alcohol use, and psychoses (schizophrenia and bipolar disorder) are the leading psychiatric causes of disability.

In most communities, mental illnesses are equated with psychoses. Depression and anxiety and substance abuse, which account for most mental morbidity, are seen as being social problems with physical symptoms being the typical clinical presentations. Try to use locally useful labels of illness, rather than emphasis on psychiatric diagnoses, to improve the recognition of mental disorders and improve patient compliance. Mental illnesses are more common in people with physical illnesses, particularly chronic conditions, and may complicate the treatment of physical disorders: e.g. mothers with depression are more likely to have low birth weight babies and their infants are more likely to be malnourished. People with HIV/AIDS have a higher rate of mental disorders, which may interfere with their HIV care. Mental disorders are associated with higher mortality, through suicide, physical disease (e.g. liver damage from alcohol abuse), and worsening of the outcome of co-morbid physical health problems.

Most mental disorders can be treated effectively using cheap and relatively simple interventions, delivered by 1° or community health care workers. Yet most mental disorders are not recognized by health workers and treated inappropriately or not treated at all. Lack of knowledge, fear about not being skilled to provide treatment, not having enough time, and the stigma attached to mental disorders (particularly psychoses) are major obstacles to meeting the mental health needs of people.

Terms for mental illness

The terms used to detect mental disorders are heavily influenced by language. For example, if very few patients complain of 'depression', then the term 'depression' as a diagnosis has limited meaning for doctors or patients. However, in all languages, one can find locally meaningful words to describe emotional and behavioural states that doctors may diagnose as a mental disorder. Find out what the most appropriate words are for the descriptions in the box opposite and use these to help communicate with your patients and other health workers more effectively.

Terms for mental illness — making sense of mental illness

- An illness where the person thinks too much, cannot sleep, and is tired all the time (probable diagnosis: common mental disorders = anxiety and depression).
- An illness where the person gets very scared or frightened for no reason (probable diagnosis: panic disorder or PTSD).
- An illness where the person behaves in a strange way, says strange things, holds strange beliefs (diagnosis: severe mental disorders = psychoses).
- An illness where the person drinks too much alcohol or uses drugs.
- An illnesses in which a child does not learn as well as others in school.

Suicide and deliberate self-harm

Deliberate self-harm may take many forms e.g. deliberate overdosing with medication, self-poisoning with pesticides, self-cutting, hanging, or burning. The motivations can vary widely and several may play a role simultaneously. There are large variations between countries in the rates and methods used depending on socio-cultural, economic, and political conditions. In many cases, the patient may be suffering from a mental illness, typically depression or alcohol use, or a chronic physical illness (such as HIV/AIDS). Major risk factors are: social factors, particularly financial difficulties and gender-based violence, and, in young people, educational pressures and conflict with parents or partners. The lethality of suicide attempts varies considerably between sexes and populations, both due to the method used and the availability and access to emergency medical care.

Consider suicide risk in all patients with mental illnesses. Patients are rarely embarrassed, and often very relieved, to be tactfully asked about suicide. Asking about suicidal thoughts does not ↑ risk for suicide. Simple questions you might ask are:
- 'Feeling as you've described recently, have you felt that life was a struggle? Have you felt as if there was no point in living anymore?'
- 'Patients with similar difficulties to you sometimes tell me they feel like ending their life. Have you felt like that?'

Management
- Ensure that the patient is out of immediate danger. 1st treat the medical consequences of the suicide attempt.
- Suicide is a sensitive and personal matter. Talk to the patient in private. Give the patient enough time to feel comfortable and share their reasons frankly.
- Do not make judgements about the patient's character; do not make reassuring statements without fully understanding the patient's situation because this may make the patient feel even more hopeless.
- Talk to family or friends for their version of the patient's recent life situation and health.
- Assess mental state (common mental disorders, alcohol or drug dependency, and psychotic disorders) and offer appropriate treatment.
- Help the patient address the main problems. These may be psychological, social (e.g. financial problems, relationship difficulties), or physical (e.g. chronic illness); see box on 📖 p 745.
- Enlist the help of others (e.g. relatives or friends, social workers, counsellors), with the consent of the patient.
- Ensure you give a follow-up appointment within 2 weeks.
- Assess future suicide risk. It may be necessary to agree to remove dangerous/sharp objects from the patient's home, and even to ensure constant supervision by relatives if you feel the risk for suicide is high.

Assessment of future suicide risk

- *Intention of act*: what was their motivation? Ask about associated actions and thoughts; go through what led up to the act and afterwards. Was there planning/preparation?
- *Method chosen*: how lethal or dangerous was the method chosen? Why did they choose this method, and did they consider alternatives? Did they make any 'final acts' (e.g. writing a suicide note)? Did they take precautions to avoid discovery?
- *What did the act represent*: a wish to die/for help/something else? Did they seek help or tell anyone? Was medical attention willingly sought or were they coerced?
- *Present feelings and intentions*: do they regret or feel guilty about the act or being discovered? Have they changed how they feel? If they go home, will they cope? What do they want now: to die or get help? Will they accept treatment?
- *Precipitation*: what problems led to the act? Are these likely to recur or persist? What can be done about them?
- *Resources*: what resources are available (self/friends/family/community/health services)? Is the patient isolated? How can this be addressed?
- *Mental disorder*: is the patient severely depressed or psychotic? Will she/he take treatment?
- *Protective factors*: do they have hope for future improvement? Do they have supportive children/partner/family/friends or strong convictions or religious beliefs that would prevent them from committing suicide?
- *Personal history*: previous attempts, chronic pain or illness, social isolation, unemployment, and older age (all ↑ risk of eventual suicide).

Common mental disorders

Common mental disorders are depressive and anxiety disorders, most often seen in 1° care. Though psychiatric classifications deal with depressive disorders and anxiety disorders separately, many patients have symptoms of both disorders, both have similar risk factors, and both respond to the similar treatments. Hence the broader term of 'common mental disorders' is often used when describing the practical, clinical approach to these disorders.

Common mental disorders are amongst the most important causes of morbidity and are the leading mental health cause of disability worldwide. However, these disorders are often missed, because few patients complain of psychological symptoms. Moreover, there is a tendency to prescribe benzodiazepines or placebo treatments when specific and efficacious treatments exist: antidepressants and brief psychological treatment.

Clinical features

Although the terms 'depression' and 'anxiety' imply a sad mood or feeling fearful, few patients complain of emotional or cognitive (thinking) symptoms. Patients classically have physical complaints. On inquiry, you can readily elicit emotional and cognitive symptoms. Sometimes, relatives may misinterpret these symptoms as signs of laziness. In some individuals, severe symptoms of anxiety may dominate in the form of panic attacks and phobias (see below). Panic attacks may present as an emergency e.g. with acute chest pain.

Diagnosis

Anxiety and depression are normal human experiences in certain situations e.g. to feel miserable when a relative dies, or a medical student before an examination will feel anxious and tense. Depression and anxiety become an illness if lasting >2 weeks, interfering with daily life, or causing severe symptoms. Suspect a common mental disorder when physical complaints do not fit into the pattern of common physical illnesses. Remember that common mental disorders are more frequent in persons with chronic physical health problems; always assess depression and anxiety in such patients. Other risk groups are persons using drugs or alcohol, tobacco users, women, and people facing severe economic or social difficulties.

In all patients, inquire about drug and alcohol misuse (alcohol/drugs may be used to self-treat anxiety, or anxiety and depression may be the consequence of dependence). Rarely, anxiety and depression may be the presenting symptoms of another medical disorder e.g. hypothyroidism, thyrotoxicosis, Cushing' syndrome.

Clinical features of depression

Presenting complaints
- tiredness, fatigue, and weakness.
- vague aches and pains all over the body.
- disturbed sleep (usually worse, but occasionally too much sleep).
- poor appetite (sometimes ↑ appetite).

Complaints on inquiry
- feeling sad and miserable.
- feeling a loss of interest in life, social interactions, work, etc.
- feeling guilty.
- feeling hopeless about the future.
- difficulty making decisions.
- thoughts that one is not as good as others (low self-esteem).
- thoughts that it would be better if one was not alive.
- suicidal ideas and plans.
- difficulty in concentrating.

Clinical features of anxiety

Presenting complaints
- palpitations.
- a feeling of suffocation.
- chest pain.
- dizziness.
- trembling, shaking all over.
- headaches.
- pins and needles (or sensation of ants crawling) on limbs or face.
- poor sleep.

Complaints on inquiry
- feeling as if something terrible is going to happen.
- feeling scared.
- worrying too much about one's problems or one's health.
- thoughts that one is going to die, lose control, or go mad.

Common management principles

- Use a stepped care approach i.e. give advice to all patients and reserve medication or psychological treatment for those who do not recover or are extremely depressed (e.g. actively suicidal). Advice should emphasize the link between thoughts, feelings, and physical responses e.g. reminding the patient about physical sensations when they are very scared. Explain how stress can lead to health problems, including physical complaints.
- After confirming diagnosis, assess suicide risk (see 📖 p 745): there is no evidence that asking about suicide 'puts ideas into their head'.
- Reassure families and the patient that simply because there are no physical signs or diagnoses, this does not mean the patient is 'making it up'.
- Avoid unnecessary medical investigations and placebo treatments.
- Identify and ↓ stimulants that predispose to anxiety (e.g. cigarettes, steroids, chewing khat (*Catha edulis*), alcohol).
- Identify and discuss ways of ↓ work pressures, disabilities, or conflict at home. Speak with the spouse or relatives.
- Encourage the patient to stop concentrating on negative ideas or acting on them (e.g. leaving work).
- Avoid the 'pull yourself together' or 'there is nothing wrong with you' approach — the patients are caught up in guilt and feelings of failure and do not need outside blame.
- A problem-solving approach may be useful, focusing on small, defined steps (see box).
- Medication is useful for moderate and severe depressive episodes with 70–80% patients showing an improvement. (see box).
- If patient does not respond: review diagnosis, ensure complaince with medication, ↑ dose to the maximum permitted dose, consider referral to other agencies for social issues, and consider changing medication to an alternative class.

Psychological treatments for common mental disorders

Anxiety reduction techniques

These techniques need to be practised, ideally daily, to develop the ability to relax before and during stressful situations.

- *Progressive muscle relaxation*: in a quiet environment, close eyes, tensing then relaxing muscles, starting from feet, then legs, then thighs, etc, up to the head. Concentrate on the relaxed feelings.
- *Controlled breathing*: close eyes; breathe in and out to a slow count of 4 or 5. Continue for 5 mins. The patient can chant in his mind a religious or calming word while exhaling.
- *Imagery*: visualize a scene that is calm, safe, and relaxing. Concentrate on the details — smells, sounds, and feel of the place.
- *Distraction*: focus attention away from anxious thoughts and sensations and on to something relaxing and absorbing.

Problem solving

Common mental disorders are often the consequence of practical problems the patient is facing in their daily lives. Unfortunately, the disorders impair the ability of the patient to take the steps necessary to overcome their problems. Problem solving aims to empower the patient to regain control over their lives.

- Explain the treatment.
- Define the problems (what are the different problems faced by the patient).
- Summarize the problems (how are these problems related to the patient's symptoms).
- Select one problem and choose the goals (why should the patient overcome the problem).
- Define solutions (the action to be taken to overcome the problem).
- Review the outcome of the actions taken (did it make the problem less; did it help improve the patient's mood).

Group therapy

In many places, people are accustomed to meet in groups to discuss personal problems. For example, women may meet regularly to discuss their health or social condition. Similar groups may be used for patients with common mental disorders. Discussion about symptoms, their causes, and how individuals cope with their problems, helps each group member in their recovery.

Specific presentations of common mental disorders

Recurrent depression

Some patients suffer from repeated episodes of depression. Consider long-term follow up, (e.g. once a month) to discuss personal and social issues, and continue antidepressants for 2 yrs or more. Consider a long-term prophylactic medication (e.g. lithium or sodium valproate).

Phobic disorder

A phobia is a fear of a specific situation that is out of proportion to the objective risks, beyond voluntary control, and not responsive to reasoning. It results in avoidance of situations in which the trigger might occur (e.g. crowds, open spaces, travelling, social events). Patients may become confined to their house. Phobias can be managed by anxiety reduction techniques (see box). Use graded exposure (e.g. to feared situation such as crowds) to ↓ avoidance and escape the cycle of reinforcement. Antidepressants may also be effective.

Panic disorder

Recurrent, frequent, unexpected panic attacks in which the patient experiences severe, acute anxiety accompanied by chest pain, breathlessness, or dizziness that are typically the result of hyperventilation. Panic attacks are best managed using anxiety reduction techniques. Antidepressants are also effective and anxiolytics can be used for short-term relief.

Obsessive-compulsive disorder

Obsessional thoughts are recurrent thoughts, ideas, or images that are distressing to the patient who makes efforts (often unsuccessful) to get rid of them e.g. thoughts of being dirty or blasphemous or ugly. Compulsions are behaviours that are repeated (e.g. cleaning or counting rituals) even though the patient recognizes that this is irrational, but is unable to resist the urge to carry them out. This disorder is managed using psychological treatments (e.g. cognitive behavioural techniques) or antidepressants (e.g. fluoxetine, clomipramine).

Medicines for common mental disorders

Antidepressants

Antidepressants are the most effective medications, irrespective of the types of symptoms the patient presents with. There are two major classes of antidepressants.

- *Tricyclic antidepressants* e.g. imipramine or amitryptiline initially 25 to 50 mg PO at night. Minimum effective dose is 75 mg; max daily dose 150 mg, given as a single night-time dose.
- *Selective serotonin reuptake inhibitors* e.g. fluoxetine, initially 20 mg PO od (also the minimum effective dose), max daily dose 60 mg given as a single dose in the morning.

Choice of antidepressant is influenced by:

- Toxicity (if risk of overdose is high, avoid tricyclics).
- Side-effect profile (avoid amitryptiline and imipramine in patients with heart disease).
- Symptoms: consider more sedative medication (e.g. amitryptiline, imipramine) in anxious or sleep-deprived patients.

Regimen is as follows:

- Start at a low dose and ↑gradually over a few weeks to the minimum effective dose, with regular reviews to assess side-effects, compliance, and suicidal ideation.
- Explain that side-effects generally fade after 2–3 weeks and that maximum benefit builds up over 3–6 weeks, provided medication is taken every day.
- Once improved, continue the antidepressant for >6 mths, to minimize the risk of relapse.
- Withdraw medication gradually to avoid discontinuation syndromes.

Benzodiazepines or other medicines

- Anxiolytics (e.g. diazepam 2 mg PO tds, ↑as necessary to 5–10 mg tds) are effective for short-term (<2 weeks) acute relief of severe anxiety symptoms. Dependence and reinforcement of anxiety may occur with longer use.
- Beta-blockers (e.g. propranolol 40 mg PO bd or tds) are effective in ↓ autonomic symptoms (e.g. palpitations and tremor).

Severe mental disorders (psychoses)

This group consists of schizophrenia, manic-depressive psychoses (also called bipolar disorder), and brief or acute psychoses. These illnesses are relatively rare. They are characterized by marked behavioural problems and strange or unusual thinking. The majority of patients of all cultures in psychiatric hospitals suffer from psychoses.

Clinical features

- *Delusions:* false beliefs, not in keeping with the patient's cultural or educational background: e.g. the body or mind are under external control, or that thoughts are being inserted, withdrawn, or broadcast from their mind, or persecutory or grandiose delusions, or other very bizarre beliefs.
- *Hallucinations:* the experience of their thoughts being spoken aloud, or other persistent auditory, visual, olfactory, or somatic hallucinations.
- *Thought disorder:* inability to communicate coherently, with thinking and speech becoming illogical and irrelevant.
- *Disturbed behaviour:* both aggressive or agitated; withdrawn or apathetic behaviour may be seen.
- *Insight* (the awareness of being ill and needing treatment) is often seriously impaired.
  The three psychoses are distinguished through the following criteria:
- *Duration of symptoms:* if symptoms have occurred for the 1st time <1 mo before, then the most likely diagnosis is acute or brief psychosis.
- *Affective/mood symptoms:* if there are marked depressive or manic features, the most likely diagnosis is bipolar disorder.
- *Cognitive impairment e.g. disorientation:* indicates the probability of acute psychoses (e.g. organic psychosis or delirium).
- *Chronicity:* if symptoms have been continually evident for >6 mths, the likely diagnosis is schizophrenia.
- *Episodic course:* with periods of relatively normal health in between, is typical of bipolar disorder.
- *Presence of a trigger:* although any of the psychoses may be precipitated by a trigger, these are the hallmark of acute or brief psychoses.

Schizophrenia

A severe mental disorder which usually begins before the age of 30. Apart from the usual symptoms of psychoses, patients may also show catatonic behaviour (stupor, mutism, posturing), negative symptoms (unexplained apathy, not speaking, incongruous affect), and marked social withdrawal. Schizophrenia is often a long-term illness which may last months — years and may require long-term treatment. There is often a family history of mental illness.

Manic depressive illness or bipolar disorder

A chronic psychosis characterized by episodes of 'high' mood or mania and 'low' mood or depression. Usually begins in adulthood and generally is diagnosed because of the manic phase, characterized by agitation, inappropriate behaviour (e.g. spending money excessively or sexually inappropriate behaviour), ↓sleep, ↑levels of energy, irritability, suspiciousness, rapid thinking and speech, and grandiose delusions (e.g. believing one has special powers). The depressed phase is similar to depression in common mental disorders except that it is usually more serious. A typical feature of this condition is that it is episodic. There are periods, from months — years, when the person is completely well, even if they are not taking treatment. There is often a family history of mental illness. Bipolar disorder diagnosis requires ≥1 manic episode. Differential diagnosis of manic episodes includes alcohol or drug misuse and acute psychoses.

Acute or brief psychoses

Usually start suddenly and are characterized by florid or marked psychotic symptoms. Most patients recover completely within a month and do not need long-term treatment. Typically caused by a sudden severe stressful event e.g. the death of a loved person, or may be induced by amphetamines or cannabis or by a severe medical or brain illness; when this happens, the condition is also called a 'delirium'. Delirium needs urgent medical treatment. The presence of fever, other signs of a physical illness, disorientation and altered consciousness, and history of head injury should raise the suspicion of delirium. Sometimes, an acute psychotic episode may be the presenting event heralding a schizophrenic illness.

Management of severe mental disorders

- Treatment should be started as soon as possible since untreated psychosis is linked with ↑disability.
- Acutely disturbed patients, especially those with acute manic episodes, may need to be admitted to hospital and require intensive nursing. If this is not available, try to arrange a safe environment.
- Respect the patient's rights and dignity, irrespective of how disturbed she/he may be. Avoid confrontation/argument and where it is necessary to intervene, do it calmly and firmly.
- Minimize the risk of harm to the patient with behavioural disturbance and others. Promote a calm, relaxed atmosphere and minimize stress.
- Agitation and/or psychotic symptoms should be treated with an antipsychotic medication; if these are not sufficient, then sedative medication (benzodiazepines) may be required for short periods.
- Treat with antipsychotic medication — see box, ⬚ p 756.
- If there is no or incomplete response: ↑dose.
- Assess compliance; discuss reasons for non-compliance (e.g. poor insight, intolerable side-effects) and address these reasons (e.g. switch antipsychotic drug to an alternative with fewer side-effects).
- Family intervention: discuss the illness with supportive family members, and counsel them to ↓levels of stress and hostility in the family. A sympathetic explanation that the patient is suffering from an illness that can be treated may help allay fears about the cause and implications of the illness. In particular, advise that schizophrenia and bipolar disorder need long-term treatment.
- Once the patient has recovered from acute symptoms, offer sheltered work or appropriate training to help develop occupational and self-care skills.
- Activity or distraction may ↓ severity or burden of symptoms, such as hallucinations.
- Counsel the patient regarding cessation of substance abuse, especially cannabis which can exacerbate psychoses.
- Mood stabilizers are indicated for patients with chronic affective disorders (bipolar disorder). They are only effective if patient complies for >6 mths — these must be taken for >2 yrs (see box).
- Develop a therapeutic relationship with the patient and invite the patient for regular reviews to assess mental health and provide medication.

Antipsychotic drugs for severe mental disorders

Antipsychotic drugs can be conveniently grouped into:
- *Conventional drugs* including chlorpromazine, trifluoperazine, and haloperidol. These drugs are older and generic (and thus cheap), but are associated with more extrapyramidal and anticholinergic side-effects.
- *Atypical drugs*: these include risperidone, olanzapine, and clozapine. These are newer, more expensive (while still patented), and associated with less extrapyramidal and anticholinergic side-effects (although clozapine is associated with potentially serious bone-marrow suppressive side-effects).
- *Depot medication*: these are long-acting, injectable formulations of drugs (conventional or atypical) e.g. flupenthixol decanoate and haloperidol decanoate.

Starting dose

Drug-naïve patients should be started on a low dose and this dose increased based on clinical response (e.g. haloperidol 1.5–3 mg PO bd (3–5 mg bd if severe), increased up to a maximum of 15 mg bd; or risperidone 2 mg nocte (4 mg nocte if severe), increased if necessary up to a maximum of 8 mg nocte). Benefit should become apparent within 2 weeks and continued improvement occurs for 3–6 months.

Length of treatment

For acute psychoses and affective psychoses, antipsychotic drugs may be gradually reduced after the patient has been well for >3 mths. For schizophrenia, the medication may need to be continued for longer periods, sometimes for many years. Depot medication may be especially useful for these patients; a test dose of a depot must always be administered the first time these drugs are being used.

Issues with treatment of schizophrenia

Most patients with schizophrenia will respond to an antipsychotic; however, the majority will relapse within 2 yrs if they stop medication. ~25% of patients do not respond adequately, despite being compliant. They should be switched to an alternative drug, ideally from a different class. Patients who remain psychotic despite adequate trials of antipsychotics are often termed 'treatment resistant'. The diagnosis should be reviewed. Where the diagnosis is schizophrenia, a trial of clozapine is warranted (2/3 will respond to clozapine). Withdraw other antipsychotics and commence clozapine 12.5 mg PO od or bd initially, gradually titrated up to 300 mg (max 900 mg) over 2–3 weeks in 25–50 mg increments. Monitor FBC weekly for 4 months initially, and monthly thereafter (causes agranulocytosis).

Side-effects of antipsychotic medication

Warn the patient about likely side-effects: acute and chronic movement disorders and anticholinergic effects for conventional drugs, ↑appetite and weight, sedation, and hyperprolactinaemia (gynaecomastia, galactorrhoea, dysmennorrhea, and sexual dysfunction).

Movement disorders include:
- Acute dystonia (e.g. painful ocular deviation, neck twisting, or muscle spasms) may occur within hours.
- Parkinsonism: tremors and rigidity.
- Akathisia: severe motor restlessness.

Movement disorders should be managed by:
- ↓ dose.
- Switching from a conventional to atypical antipsychotic.
- Acute dystonias should be treated with an anticholinergic such as procyclidine 5–10 mg IM, which can be repeated after 20 mins.
- Parkinsonism may be treated with an anticholinergic (e.g. procyclidine. 2.5 mg PO tds, increasing gradually up to max 30 mg in divided doses).
- Akathisia can be managed with a benzodiazepine.

Mood stabilizers

These are drugs used to prevent episodes of mania or depression in people with recurrent depressive disorder or bipolar disorder. The most effective are lithium and sodium valproate. Both must be taken regularly and require monitoring, especially lithium
- *Lithium carbonate* — start with 400 mg od. Adjust dose (sometimes to >1 g/day) to achieve a serum lithium concentration of 0.4–1 mmol/L 12 h after a dose 4–7 days after starting treatment. Warn patients about signs of toxicity: coarse tremor, nausea, diarrhoea, confusion, fits. Blood levels should be measured weekly until stable, and then at least 6 monthly.
- *Sodium valproate* is an effective mood stabilizer and has the advantage of being effective for epilepsy, being less toxic in overdose, and requiring less blood monitoring. Start with 750 mg daily in 2–3 divided doses and ↑ according to clinical response (or blood levels of 50–75 mg/L) up to 1–2 g/day in divided doses.

Mental retardation (learning disability)

Mental retardation (MR) is not a mental illness in the strict sense of the word. The mental abilities of the child are slower or delayed compared to other children. There is impairment in cognitive, social, language, and motor development, with onset during childhood. The prevalence of moderate to severe retardation varies from 1–20/1000 worldwide. Persons with mental retardation are often brought to health workers by concerned family members for many reasons such as self-care, school difficulties, and behavioural problems such as aggression.

Clinical features

- Delays in achieving milestones e.g. sitting, walking, speaking.
- Difficulties in school e.g. coping with studies and repeated failure.
- Difficulties in relating to others, especially other children of same age.
- In adolescents, inappropriate sexual behaviour.
- In adults, problems in everyday activities e.g. cooking, managing money, finding and staying on in a job.

There are degrees of mental retardation:

- Mild retardation may lead only to difficulty in schooling but no other problems.
- Moderate retardation may lead to failure to stay in the school system and difficulties in self-care such as bathing.
- Severe retardation often means the person needs help even for simple activities such as feeding.

Whereas persons with mild retardation may spend their entire lives without being 'detected', those at the severe end are diagnosed in early childhood because of the obvious severity of the disability. People with mild retardation may be able to live alone and work in certain jobs; however, severe affected people will almost always need close supervision and care.

Assessment

- An informant such as a parent is essential.
- Record nature and extent of mental retardation — take a developmental history and consider delay in communication and social interaction; motor function and self-care; and functional academic skills.
- Identify additional problems — such as self-harm or harm to others; impulsive or dangerous behaviour.
- Determine aetiology — see box opposite. In most cases, however, no definite aetiology will be identifiable.
- Identify co-existing psychiatric diagnoses — prevalence is 2–4-fold higher in people with mental retardation than the general population.

Causes of moderate to severe mental retardation

Prenatal (50–70%)
- Genetic e.g. Fragile X; Down's syndrome.
- Congenital infections with HSV 2, rubella, HIV, toxoplasmosis, syphilis, CMV.
- Exposure to toxins such as alcohol.
- Maternal disorder such as pre-eclampsia.

Perinatal (10–20%) — low birth weight, extreme prematurity, delivery problems resulting in asphyxia or brain trauma, neonatal sepsis, encephalitis, kernicterus.

Postnatal (5–10%) — brain damage due to trauma, infections, toxic agents (e.g. lead poisoning), iodine deficiency, malnutrition.

Management
- 1st be certain that the child has MR. MR implies that the child has a an incurable problem. It is a label which can cause great unhappiness, so use it with care. If in doubt, get a 2nd opinion from a child or mental health specialist.
- Once you are confident that the child has MR, determine its severity. The abilities a child has will be an important indicator of how much progress the child is likely to make in the years ahead.
- If the child has a specific medical problem e.g. low thyroid function, sensory impairment, or seizures, treat these. Other than these rare situations, there are no indications for using medicines to treat MR. Do not use 'brain tonics' and other medicines supposed to help 'mental function'. Use antipsychotics or antidepressants to treat psychoses or common mental disorders in people with MR.
- Reassure the family that, even though the child has limited mental abilities, he will achieve many milestones in life. They must be prepared to accept a delay in these milestones and be realistic in what they expect their child to achieve. Explain that there is no cure and that they should not waste money on false claims of cures.
- Teach the parents how to help the child in daily activities e.g. in toileting and feeding, by breaking down activities into smaller bits.
- Use reward and praise whenever the child succeeds in any activity, however small. Find activities which can help the parent spend time with the child and yet allow other household activities to be done e.g. the child could learn to help the mother in daily chores in the house.
- Never ignore the child's educational needs. Some parents feel like giving up on the child's education when they discover that the child has MR. Stress to the parents their child needs education just as any other child. Refer the family to local schools for children with special needs.
- Provide information about any special schemes to help families with children with MR either through financial or educational help.
- Stay in regular touch with the family. Some families go through a lot of stress because of caring for a child with MR, especially when the MR is severe. Caring can itself be a cause of stress and mental health problems. Refer parents to support groups.

Disorders due to substance abuse

The most common substances of abuse/dependence are alcohol and tobacco. Others include: glue or benzene (which is inhaled); heroin; cocaine; amphetamines; cannabis; benzodiazepines. The origin of benzodiazepine abuse is often iatrogenic.

Alcohol and drug abuse is rarely the main reason for seeking health care. Instead, the health worker has to be alert to the possibility of substance abuse (e.g. repeated unexplained injuries or absence from work). Many patients with substance abuse problems also develop other mental disorders, particularly, common mental disorders. Suicide is more common, and psychoses can occur both during intoxicated and withdrawal states.

Dependence

A person is said to be dependent on alcohol or drugs when their use harms the person's physical, mental, or social health. The diagnosis of a dependence syndrome should be made if ≥3 of the following are present:

- Strong desire/compulsion to take the substance.
- Difficulties controlling substance-taking behaviour in terms of onset, termination, or levels of use.
- Withdrawal: a physiological state when use of the substance has been stopped or reduced. The patient may use the substance to relieve or avoid withdrawal symptoms.
- Tolerance: ↑ doses are required to achieve a given effect.
- Neglect of alternative interests: obtaining and taking the substance gradually grows to dominate the individual's life.
- Continued use despite evidence of harmful consequences: the user must be aware of these consequences.

Dependence problems lead to great damage to individuals, their families, and to the community. For example, alcohol not only harms the drinker due to its physical effects, but also is associated with high suicide rates, marriage problems and domestic violence, road traffic crashes, and poverty.

Harmful use is substance abuse not fulfilling the above criteria but causing significant damage to mental or physical health. There are often major social consequences.

Management of dependence

There is increasing evidence that dependent patients have ↓ ability to control substance use — it is not just 'a lack of willpower'. Ask 'open' questions and use 'reflective listening', clarify concerns, convey empathy and collaboration, and motivate patients to reach their own conclusions about the effects of substance misuse.

Advise the patient that dependence is an illness with serious health effects, and stopping or ↓ use will bring mental and physical health, social and economic benefits. Explain the symptoms of withdrawal. Abstinence should be the goal in the majority of cases, although ↓ levels of use are sometimes appropriate.

Questions to assess alcohol abuse: the CAGE questionnaire

Alcohol dependence is likely with 2 or more positive answers:
- have you ever felt you should **CUT** down your drinking?
- have people **ANNOYED** you by criticising your drinking?
- have you ever felt bad or **GUILTY** about your drinking?
- have you ever had a drink first think in the morning to steady your nerves or get rid of a hangover (**EYE**-opener)?

For patients willing to stop now or control their use, help them:
- Set a definite day to quit/begin controlled use.
- Enlist the help of a friend or relative who is not using the substance to be a buddy and help the person.
- If ↓ use, agree a clear and specific goal for reduction (e.g. no more than 4 units of alcohol/day and 2 alcohol-free days/week).
- Agree strategies to control use (e.g. slow down drinking to <1 unit/hr, introduce alternative behaviour such as drinking fruit juice, chewing gum, exercise).
- Identify high-risk situations (social or stressful occasions) and strategies to avoid or cope with these.
- Make plans to avoid substances (e.g. develop assertiveness skills to respond to friends who are using substances).
- Discuss symptoms and management of withdrawal (see later).
- Medicines may be available for withdrawal from opiates (e.g. methadone) — these need specialist assessment and monitoring.
- Minimize risk of harm due to substance abuse e.g. advise not to drive after drinking, never to share needles, regarding safe sexual practice.
- Prevent iatrogenic abuse by using benzodiazepines cautiously, and never for more than four weeks running.

If the attempt is unsuccessful:
- Identify areas of success (e.g. cut down use for a period).
- Discuss situations/triggers for relapse; can changes be made?
- Try again.

If the attempt is successful
- Consider the use of medicines used to ↓ risk of relapse (e.g. disulfiram or acamprosate for alcohol dependence).
- Relapse is common and often occurs because the person is not able to deal with life difficulties. Once drug use is stopped, discuss ways in which the person could cope. Identify different things a person can do to ↓ risk of taking drugs such as: giving up friends who also use drugs; getting back to work, school, other enjoyable activities; learning relaxation and problem-solving; joining community groups which help substance abusers (e.g. Alcoholics Anonymous).

Withdrawal states

Many states show these general effects:

- anxiety.
- tremor.
- fever.
- sleep disturbance.
- tachycardia.
- gastro-intestinal disturbance.

In addition, the following symptoms may occur during withdrawal from specific substances:

- *Opiate:* hypertension, tachycardia, dysphoria, agitation, insomnia, diarrhoea and vomiting, shivering, sweating, lacrimation, rhinorrhoea, dilated pupils, piloerection ('gooseflesh'), muscle aches.
- *Alcohol:* fits, confusional states including delirium tremens (severe confusional state with visual and auditory hallucinations and paranoid ideation); risk of Wernicke's encephalopathy (ophthalmoplegia, nystagmus, and ataxia with confusion due to thiamine deficiency).
- *Benzodiazepines/barbiturates:* weight loss, vivid dreams (REM sleep rebound), tinnitus, irritability, impaired memory and concentration, perceptual disturbance (hypersensitivity to sound, light and touch, derealization and depersonalization), confusional states, and fits.

Timing

Withdrawal states usually begin 4–12 h after the last dose, peak at 48–72 h, and last 7–10 days. Benzodiazepine withdrawal begins later, usually 1–14 days after the last dose and may last many months. The confusional states and fits associated with alcohol, benzodiazepine, and barbiturate withdrawal are potentially life-threatening. Withdrawal states should be avoided as much as possible by using a gradual reducing regime and being treated rapidly when identified.

Management

Opiate withdrawal

If there are clinical features of withdrawal, prescribe a single dose of dihydrocodeine (e.g. 120 mg; alternative codeine). Reassess after 4 h, and prescribe another 120 mg. This can be repeated once more. The patient should not receive more than 360 mg dihydrocodeine in the first 12 h. After the initial 12 h, the dose can be increased to 480 mg over the next 24 h. Gradually d dose over 5–10 days.

Do not prescribe dihydrocodeine on an 'as required' basis. The patient must be assessed before each dose in the early stages. Write on the prescription — 'do not give if drowsy, sedated, ataxic, with slurred speech or asleep'. Do not give if the patient has been away from the ward and you suspect illicit drug use; do not allow the patient to leave the ward for 4 h after increasing the dose. Do not give dihydrocodeine to patients on discharge.

Alcohol withdrawal

Admission may be advisable, particularly if there is a Hx of previous severe withdrawals (e.g. confusion, fits), poor physical health (e.g. liver failure), or mental health (e.g. suicidal ideation). A reducing dose of a substitute benzodiazepine is given over 7–14 days e.g. initial dose of chlordiazepoxide 10–50 mg PO qds.

- Higher doses may be required. As an in-patient, this judgement can be based on symptoms of withdrawal, with more frequent dosing.
- A short-acting drug (e.g. lorazepam 1 mg od or bd) may be used instead for patients with significant liver failure.
- B-complex vitamins should be given parenterally to prevent or treat Wernicke's encephalopathy.

Benzodiazepine withdrawal

Most common with short-acting agents e.g. lorazepam. Change to an equivalent dose of a long-acting benzodiazepine such as diazepam (lorazepam 0.5 mg is equivalent to diazepam 5 mg). Then gradually ↓ dose every 2–3 weeks in steps of diazepam 2–2.5 mg. If withdrawal symptoms occur, maintain the dose until symptoms improve. Thereafter, ↓dose further, in smaller steps if necessary. If dependency is chronic, this may take up to 12 weeks.

Adjustment disorders and bereavement

An adjustment disorder is a state of emotional disturbance and impaired social functioning that develops shortly after (<3 months) or during a stressor. There may be affective, cognitive, and behavioural symptoms. Stressors may take many forms (e.g. bereavement, diagnosis of a major illness such as HIV/AIDS, migration). Adjustment disorders are common in people with physical disorders, and should be considered if rehabilitation is slower or poorer than expected.

Bereavement: may be abnormal in form and/or severity compared to cultural norms. Four stages have been described:
- Shock and numbness.
- Preoccupation (yearning or anger, etc.).
- Disorganization (loss is reluctantly accepted).
- Resolution.

These may not necessarily occur in this order. Bereavement is considered abnormal when symptoms are not related to the loss — such as feelings of worthlessness or inappropriate guilt. Abnormal perceptions involving the lost person (e.g. hearing them whispering) can be a feature of normal bereavement, but hallucinatory phenomena not involving the lost person are indications of abnormal (or pathological) bereavement.

Management
- Allow the individual to talk about the loss and its circumstances, and to discuss the feelings that are provoked, particularly guilt and anger.
- Involve the others in the family, and aim to ↑ social support.
- Identify steps that can be taken to modify causes of stress.
- Medication should be avoided unless there is depression or psychosis. If there is severe insomnia, hypnotics may be used — but only for <2 weeks.

Post-traumatic stress disorder

An incident which makes a person fear for their life or causes extreme distress is a traumatic event e.g. rape; war; major disasters. Many persons affected by trauma will experience some emotional reaction. These include a feeling of being numb or in a daze, scared, sleep difficulties, repeated thoughts of the event, irritability, nightmares, and poor concentration. This is a normal response to a traumatic incident and lasts for a short period (~2–4 weeks). In a few people, however, these experiences continue for months (even years) after the trauma. They begin to interfere with the person's daily life and may lead to new problems such as alcohol abuse or problems in relationships with other people. This called post-traumatic stress disorder (PTSD).

Clinical features

Clinical features of PTSD include:
- Experiencing the trauma again and again through visions of the incident, nightmares, and 'flashbacks'.
- Avoiding things: the person avoids situations which remind her of the traumatic incident; she is unable to remember things related to the trauma and feels emotionally distant from people.
- ↑ arousal: sleep is disturbed, the person feels irritable, has difficulty concentrating and is easily startled or scared. Panic attacks may occur.
- Many patients with PTSD feel depressed and lose interest in daily life, feel tired or suffer aches and pains, and have suicidal feelings.

Management

- Encourage the person to talk about what happened. Group discussions are helpful, especially when the traumatic event has affected many persons, such as refugees.
- Reassure that emotional reactions are normal and not a sign of madness.
- Encourage person not to avoid situations that remind them of the event.
- The victim should not be left alone for some days. Make sure that they are staying with caring relatives or friends.
- For panic attacks, follow the steps suggested earlier.
- For acute severe symptoms, use benzodiazepines for up to 4 weeks.
- A course of antidepressants may help some patients.

Mental disorders in children and adolescents

In younger children, the most common and disabling disorders are developmental; whilst in adolescents, emotional and behavioural disorders linked to difficulties in school or at home are most common. Mental retardation is a commonly recognized type of developmental disorder.

Other developmental and mental disorders in children include:

- Autism and other pervasive developmental disorders, characterized by delays or loss of language abilities and marked impairment in social relationships; typically presents in early to mid-childhood.
- Attention deficit and hyperactivity, marked by impulsivity, hyperactivity, and poor concentration; typically presents while the child is in primary school.
- Learning disabilities (specific) marked by specific impairments in learning and cognitive abilities such as reading and writing; typically presents when the child is in secondary school.

In adolescence, the most common mental disorders are depression, substance abuse, psychoses, and conduct disorders (characterized by antisocial behaviours). Mental health problems in adolescents may be managed in a similar way to the way described earlier in the chapter. Developmental disorders may require a specialist approach to diagnosis and management. In general, if a child is brought to you with the complaint of behaviour problems or difficulties in school, take a developmental history first to rule out MR. Once MR has been ruled out, consider the possibility of these conditions.

Child abuse

Children can be abused physically, emotionally, or sexually, affecting their health and development. Both boys and girls can be abused, most often by someone they know well. Abused children may have problems with:

- *Physical health:* bruises or cuts, fractures, cigarette burns; severe cases can lead to death.
- *Sexual health:* injuries to the sexual organs, pregnancy, and STIs.
- *Mental health:* fear, aggression, poor concentration, bed-wetting having previously gained control, depression, antisocial behaviour, self-harm.
- *School performance:* ↓in school performance.

Diagnosis
- Ask the family; few adults will openly report that they feel a child they know is being abused. It is essential that, if you suspect child abuse, you ask the adult in a frank and open way about whether they think the child is being physically, emotionally, or sexually hurt.
- Ask the child: interview the child with her mother, or with another adult who is definitely not a suspected abuser and whom the child trusts. Do not ask questions about abuse until you have established rapport with the child. If this means spending more time, then do so. Ask: 'Sometimes, children can get hurt by a grown-up person. Has anyone grown-up hurt you recently?' Do not force the child.
- Examine the child: a child who has been abused is likely to be very sensitive to being examined physically. Respect the child's privacy. Explain what you are doing and why. Have a trusted family member present during the examination. Document the findings in detail. These may be needed in a police investigation. A thorough examination of the child should include weight and height, injuries on the body, and injuries or inflammation of the sexual organs, including the anus.

Management
- Your priority is the health and safety of the child. If you suspect the child's life is in danger, refer the child immediately to a place of safety.
- Talk to the family members. Explain why you suspect abuse. Many parents are not aware that their actions can be so damaging to the child's health. Just telling them about the dangers of beating a child or neglecting emotional needs may bring about change in their behaviour.
- If you suspect sexual abuse, then it is unlikely that the family will accept it easily, particularly if the abuser is someone close to the family. Do not accuse anyone. Instead, share your concerns openly with the family and stress that if the abuse continues, the child's health will be even more seriously affected.
- Teach the child how to ensure his safety. Explain that the abuse is not his fault and he should not feel guilty for having spoken out about the abuse. It is important to make sure this never happened again. Some suggestions on how to prevent abuse from recurring are: to tell the abuser not to touch him in a firm manner; to run away from the abuser to be with another adult who can protect you.
- Put the family in touch with community supports. This might include child support groups, family violence groups, legal support, child protection agencies, the police, or specialist health professionals.
- If the child abuse persists or is very serious, refer to a specialist team.
- Keep in close touch with the child and the family at regular intervals for at least 6 months. Very often, the abuse stops once it has been openly discussed. If it does not, you may need to encourage the family to take action to stop it. Talk to the child each time; many children do recover from the trauma, but some children will develop mental health problems.

Trauma and obstetric emergencies

Section editors **Douglas Allan Wilkinson**
Jenny Thompson

ABCDE of trauma assessment

Initial assessment (the primary survey) of multiply-injured patient must identify and treat life-threatening injuries. Multiple casualties require prioritization (triage) according to need and available resources.

The ABCDE system allows rapid systematic assessment and simultaneous treatment of life threatening injuries. Do not move onto the next system until the current problem is treated. If the patient deteriorates, go back to the beginning and assess again.

- Airway — can the patient talk to you and breathe freely?
  — give supplemental oxygen if available
- Breathing — is the patient breathing (look, listen, and feel)?
  — is breathing adequate?
- Circulation — can peripheral or central pulses be felt?
  — is capillary refill <3 seconds?
- Disability — use AVPU for rapid neurological assessment
  - **A**lert/Awake.
  - **V**erbal response.
  - **P**ainful response.
  - **U**nresponsive.
- Exposure — undress the patient and look for injury.

Airway management

If the patient can speak clearly, they have a patent airway and are breathing. Signs of airway obstruction include:
- snoring or gurgling.
- stridor.
- using accessory muscles of respiration.
- cyanosis agitation.

Treatment
1. Simple airway management
- chin lift/jaw thrust.
- suction.
- insert an adjunct oral or nasopharyngeal airway.

If these manoeuvres do not help or the patient is apnoeic, hypoxic, unconscious, or has severe head chest or neck trauma, move onto:

2. Advanced airway management
- tracheal intubation (with neck immobilization).
- surgical access — cricothyroid puncture or tracheostomy depending on equipment, skill, and resources.

Breathing (ventilation) management

Once the airway is patent, the next priority is adequate ventilation.
Inspect (look) for the following:
- respiratory rate and pattern.
- cyanosis.
- chest injury e.g. penetrating injury, flail chest, or a sucking injury.
- use of accessory muscles or respiration i.e. breathing is hard work.
Palpate (feel) for:
- tracheal shift.
- broken ribs.
- subcutaneo.us emphysema.
- percuss for hyperresonanace or dullness.
Auscultate (listen) for:
- pneumothorax (decreased breath sounds on side injury).
- abnormal sounds in chest.

Management
- **Pneumothorax:** if under tension, immediately insert a large bore needle (e.g. 16 g venflon) into the second intercostal space in the midclavicular line. Insert an intercostals drain once decompressed.
- **Penetrating injury:** may require surgical exploration.
- **Flail chest:** will require analgesia, O2, chest drain ± ventilation.
- **Sucking chest wound** (open pneumothorax): apply waterproof patch secured on three sides, a chest drain, and give analgesia.
- **Massive haemothorax:** obtain iv access, give fluid resuscitation, and insert a chest drain. Start surgical exploration if >1500–2000 ml blood initially or >200–300 ml/hr.

Circulatory management

The goal is to stop bleeding and restore oxygen delivery to the tissues.
Fluid resuscitation is essential, as the usual problem is blood loss.
- Insert two large bore (14–16 G) cannulae. A peripheral cut down may be necessary.
- Take blood specimens for the laboratory e.g. crossmatch.
- Start warmed (in a bucket of warm water) crystalloid infusion.

Stop bleeding

- **Limb injuries:** do not use tourniquets. Place gauze packs under the fascia, plus manual compression of proximal artery, plus compressive dressing of the entire injured limb.
- **Chest injuries:** chest wall arteries are the most common source of bleeding. Place an intercostal chest drain and give iv ketamine (see Table 20.1) for pain relief. The expanded lung should tamponade bleeding.
- **Abdominal injuries:** a damage control laparotomy (DCL) is required as soon as possible if fluid resuscitation fails to achieve a systolic BP of 80–90 mm Hg. DCL is not a surgical procedure but a resuscitative one, involving gauze packing of bleeding abdominal quadrants and temporary closure of the abdominal wound with towel clamps. The procedure should be observed before being done, but should be within the capabilities of any trained doctor or nurse and is carried out under ketamine anaesthesia. DCL can save lives.
- **Pelvic fractures:** stabilize the pelvis — by tying a sheet around pelvis.

Volume replacement and warming

- **Warm fluid replacement:** hypothermic patients do not clot so well! Even in hot climates, trauma patients quickly become hypothermic, especially when being treated outside. IV and per-oral fluids should have a temperature of 40–42°C.
- **Hypotensive fluid resuscitation:** if haemostasis is not complete, control blood loss by maintaining systolic BP at 80–90 mmHg until definitive haemostasis can be achieved.
- **Blood transfusion:** consider transfusion when there is persistent haemodynamic instability despite fluid resuscitation or when Hb is <7 g/dl with ongoing bleeding. Use type O negative packed cells if cross-matched or type-specific blood is not available. Remember the patients' family or friends may be able to donate blood for them but beware of incompatibility and blood-borne infections.
- **Per-oral fluid resuscitation:** is safe and efficient if the patient has a gag reflex and is without abdominal injury. Oral fluids should contain low concentrations of sugar and salt to avoid 'osmotic pull' into the intestines. Diluted cereal porridges based on local foodstuffs are ideal.

Analgesia

Ketamine 0.2 mg/kg in repeated doses is the drug of choice as it has positive ionotropic effects and does not depress gag reflex.

Shock

Defined as inadequate organ perfusion leading to inadequate tissue oxygenation. In the trauma patient, often due to haemorrhage and hypovolaemia but can occur from other causes.

1. **Haemorrhagic (hypovolaemic shock):** due to acute loss of blood or fluids. It is easy to underestimate blood loss. Remember that large volumes may be hidden in abdomen, pleura, femoral, or pelvic fracture (latter may lose >2 L). In young fit patients, signs of blood loss may not be obvious until >1 L has been lost.

Table 20.1 Cardiovascular parameters associated with blood loss in an adult

Blood loss	Up to 750 ml	750–1500 ml	1500–2000 ml	>2000 ml
Heart rate	<100	>100	>120	>140
Blood pressure	↔	Systolic, normal	↓	↓
Capillary refill	↔ (<3 secs)	Prolonged	Prolonged	Prolonged
Respiratory rate	↔	20–30 per min	30–40 per min	>40 per minute
Urine volume	> 30 ml/hr	20–30 ml/hr	5–15 ml/hr	<10 ml/hr
Mental state	Normal	Mild concern	Anxious/confused	Coma

2. *Cardiogenic shock:* due to inadequate cardiac function. May be due to:
- myocardial contusion.
- cardiac tamponade.
- tension pneumothorax (preventing venous return).
- penetrating wound to heart.
- myocardial infarction.

Assessment of JVP and ECG may be helpful. *Treat:* the cause.

3. *Neurogenic shock:* classically presents as hypotension with no reflex tachycardia or skin vasoconstriction. Cause is loss of sympathetic tone secondary to spinal cord injury. *Treatment:* fluids, vasoconstrictors, stabilization ± surgery to spine. Exclude other causes of shock.

4. *Septic shock:* rare in early phase of trauma, but common in weeks following injury. Most commonly seen in penetrating abdominal injuries and burns patients. Common cause of late death in trauma patient. *Treatment:* treat cause of sepsis early (see 🕮 p 670), support organs.

Urine output: useful marker of intravascular volume status and response to resuscitation. Expect an output of >0.5 ml/kg/h if resuscitation is adequate.

Secondary survey

A secondary survey is only done when the patient's ABCs are stable. If any deterioration occurs during this phase, a second primary survey (ABCDE) must be performed to find and treat the problem. Documentation is required for all procedures undertaken.

Head-to-toe examination is now undertaken, noting particularly:

1. Head examination
- scalp and ocular abnormalities.
- external ear and tympanic membrane injury.
- periorbital soft tissue injuries.

2. Neck examination
- penetrating wounds.
- subcutaneous emphysema.
- tracheal deviation.
- neck vein appearance.

3. Neurological examination
- brain function — assess using the Glasgow Coma Scale (📖 p 399).
- spinal cord motor activity.
- sensation and reflex.

4. Chest examination
- clavicles and all ribs.
- breath sounds and heart sounds.
- ECG monitoring (if available).

5. Abdominal examination
- surgical exploration is required for a penetrating wound.
- blunt trauma — insert a nasogastric tube (not in the presence of facial trauma).
- rectal examination.
- insert urinary catheter (check for meatal blood before insertion).

6. Pelvis and limbs
- fractures.
- peripheral pulses.
- cuts, bruises, and other minor injuries.

7. X-rays (if possible, and where indicated)
- NB chest, lateral neck, and pelvis X-rays may be needed during primary survey.
- cervical spine films (important to see all 7 vertebrae).
- pelvic and long bone X-rays.
- skull X-rays may be useful to search for fractures when head injury is present without focal neurological deficit, but is seldom indicated.

Chest trauma

About 25% of trauma deaths are due to thoracic injury. However, most patients with thoracic trauma can be effectively managed by simple manoeuvres. Respiratory distress may be caused by: rib fractures/flail chest, pneumothorax, tension pneumothorax, haemothorax, pulmonary contusion (bruising), open pneumothorax, aspiration. Haemorrhagic shock may be due to: haemothorax, haemomediastinum.

- **Rib fractures:** may damage underlying lung and produce lung bruising or puncture. The ribs usually become fairly stable within 10 days to two weeks. Firm healing with callus formation is seen after about six weeks.
- **Flail chest:** the unstable segment moves separately and in an opposite direction from the rest of the thoracic cage during the respiration cycle, causing severe respiratory distress. This is a medical emergency and can be treated with positive pressure ventilation and analgesia.
- **Tension pneumothorax:** develops when air enters the pleural space but cannot leave. The consequence is progressively increasing intrathoracic pressure in the affected side, resulting in mediastinal shift. Urgent needle decompression is required prior to the insertion of an intercostal drain. The trachea may be displaced (a late sign).
- **Haemothorax:** is more common in penetrating than non-penetrating injuries to the chest. Continuing haemorrhage will cause severe hypovolaemic shock and respiratory distress due to compression of lung on the involved side. Therapy consists of the placement of a large chest tube.
  - A haemothorax of 500–1500 ml that stops bleeding after insertion of an intercostal catheter can generally be treated by closed drainage alone.
  - A haemothorax of greater than 1500–2000 ml or with continued bleeding of more than 200–300 ml per hour may be an indication for further investigation e.g. thoracotomy.
- **Pulmonary contusion (bruising):** is common after chest trauma and may be a life-threatening condition. The onset of symptoms can be slow. It is likely to occur in cases of high-speed crashes or falls from a great height. Clinical features include: shortness of breath, hypoxaemia, tachycardia, absent breath sounds, rib fractures, and cyanosis.
- **Open or 'sucking' chest wounds of the chest wall:** the lung on the affected side is exposed to atmospheric pressure causing it to collapse and a shift of the mediastinum to the uninvolved side. Rapid treatment is required. A seal (e.g. a plastic packet) is sufficient to stop the sucking. Care must be taken to ensure an open chest wound does not tension the lung, and leaving one side of the seal open will allow venting of any tension. In compromised patients, intercostal drains, intubation, and positive pressure are required.
- **Other thoracic injuries** carry a high mortality even in regional centres. They include myocardial contusion, pericardial tamponade, thoracic great vessel injuries, rupture of trachea or major bronchi, trauma to oesophagus, and diaphragmatic injuries.

Abdominal trauma

The abdomen is commonly injured in multiple trauma. The most common organ injured in penetrating trauma is the liver and, in blunt trauma, the spleen is often torn and ruptured. The first priority is to undertake the primary survey with evaluation of ABCDE.

Any patient involved in any serious accident should be considered to have an abdominal injury until proven otherwise. Unrecognized abdominal injury remains a frequent cause of preventable death after trauma.

There are two basic categories of abdominal trauma:
- **penetrating trauma** where surgical consultation is important e.g. gunshot, stabbing.
- **non-penetrating trauma** e.g. compression, crush, seat belt, acceleration/deceleration injuries.

About 20% of trauma patients with acute haemoperitoneum (blood in abdomen) have no signs of peritoneal irritation at the first examination and the value of repeated primary survey cannot be overstated. Blunt trauma can be very difficult to evaluate, especially in unconscious patients.

Complete physical examination of the abdomen includes rectal examination, assessing sphincter tone, integrity of rectal wall, blood in the rectum, prostate position. Check for blood at the external urethral meatus. Urinary catheterization (with caution in pelvic injury) is important. Women should be considered pregnant until proven otherwise. The foetus may be salvageable and the best treatment of the foetus is resuscitation of the mother. A pregnant mother at term, however, can usually only be resuscitated properly after delivery of the baby.

Diagnostic peritoneal lavage (DPL)

May be helpful in determining the presence of blood or enteric fluid in abdomen. If there is any doubt, a laparotomy is still the gold standard. The indications for DPL include: unexplained abdominal pain, trauma of the lower part of the chest, hypo-tension/haematocrit fall with no obvious explanation, abdominal trauma in a patient with altered mental state (drugs, alcohol, brain injury), patient with abdominal trauma and spinal cord injuries, and pelvic fractures. The relative contraindications for the DPL are: pregnancy; previous abdominal surgery; operator inexperience; the result will not change management.

Pelvic fractures

Often complicated by massive haemorrhage and urology injury. Examine the rectum for the position of the prostate, the presence of blood, and rectal/perineal laceration. The management of pelvic fractures includes: resuscitation and immobilization, analgesia, transfusion, and consideration of surgery.

Head trauma

Early assessment and treatment of head-injured patients is essential to improve survival and outcome. Hypoxia and hypotension double the mortality of head-injured patients. The following conditions are potentially life-threatening; triage casualties carefully and treat what you can with available expertise and resources:

- **Acute extradural haematoma** — classically, a rapid deterioration in conscious level following a lucid interval. A middle meningeal artery bleed causes an acute increase in intracranial pressure and development of contralateral hemiparesis and ipsilateral dilated pupil.
- **Acute subdural haematoma** — tearing of a bridging vein between cortex and dura results in clotted blood in the subdural space ± severe contusion of the underlying brain.

Management of the above conditions is surgical and every effort should be made to do burr-hole decompressions (see 🕮 p 430). The diagnosis can be made on history and examination.

The conditions below should be treated with more conservative medical management, as neurosurgery usually does not improve outcome:

- Base-of-skull fractures — suggested by bruising of the eyelids (Raccoon eyes) or over the mastoid process (Battle's sign), or a cerebrospinal fluid leak from ears and/or nose.
- Cerebral concussion — producing temporary altered consciousness
- Depressed skull fracture — an impaction of fragmented skull that may penetrate the underlying dura and brain.
- Intracerebral haematoma — may result from acute injury or progressive damage secondary to contusion.

Management

Basic medical management for severe head injuries includes:

- ADCDE primary survey with C-spine control.
- Intubation and moderate hyperventilation, producing low normal PCO_2 (to 4.5–5 Kpa). This temporarily reduces intracranial blood volume and intracranial pressure. Hypoxia and hypoventilation may kill patients.
- Sedation with paralysis as necessary.
- Moderate IV fluid input with diuresis i.e. do not overload.
- Nursing head up 20%.
- Prevent hyperthermia.

Record the GCS (🕮 p 399): severe head injury is when GCS is 8 or less; moderate head injury, GCS 9 to 12; and minor head injury, GCS 13 to 15.

Deterioration may occur due to bleeding

Unequal or dilated pupils may indicate an increase in intracranial pressure. Brain injury is never the cause of hypotension in the adult trauma patient. The Cushing reflex is a specific response to a lethal rise in intracranial pressure. This is a late and poor prognostic sign. The hallmarks are: bradycardia, hypertension, decreased respiratory rate.

Spinal trauma

The incidence of nerve injury in multiple trauma is high. Injuries to the C-spine and the thoraco-lumbar junction T12–L1 are common. Other common injuries include brachial plexus injury and nerve damage to legs and fingers.

First priority = primary survey with evaluation of ABCDE

Examination of spine-injured patients must be carried out with patients in the neutral position (i.e. without flexion, extension, or rotation) and with-out any movement of the spine. The patient should be log-rolled (i.e. moved by several people, working together to keep neck and spine immobilized); their neck immobilized with a stiff cervical neck collar or sandbags; and transported in a neutral position (i.e. supine).

- **Vertebral injury** (which may cause spinal cord injury): search for local tenderness, deformities for a posterior 'step-off' injury, and swelling.
- **Cervical spine injury:** look for
  - difficulties in respiration (diaphragmatic/paradoxical breathing)
  - flaccid muscle tone absent reflexes (check rectal sphincter)
  - hypotension with bradycardia (without hypovolaemia).

C-spine X-ray: AP and a lateral X-ray (showing all seven C vertebrae) with a view of the atlas-axis joint.

Neurological assessment

Assessment of the level of injury guides immediate treatment, assesses progression, and gives an idea of prognosis. Ask the patient questions relevant to her/his sensation and try to ask her/him to do minor movements to assess motor function in the limbs.

Motor response	Level	Sensory response	Level
Diaphragm intact	C3, C4, C5	Anterior thigh	L2
Shrug shoulders	C4	Anterior knee	L3
Biceps (flex elbows)	C5	Anterolateral ankle	L4
Extension of wrist	C6	Dorsum big+2nd toe	L5
Extension of elbow	C7	Lateral side of foot	S1
Flexion of wrist	C7	Posterior calf	S2
Abduction of fingers	C8	Perianal sensation	S2–5
Active chest expansion	T1–T12		
Hip flexion	L2		
Knee extension	L3–L4		
Ankle dorsiflexion	L5–S 1		
Ankle plantarflexion	L1–S2		

NB If no sensory or motor function is exhibited with a complete spinal cord lesion, the chance of recovery is small.

Limb trauma

Examination
Must include:
- skin colour and temperature.
- distal pulse assessment.
- grazes and bleeding sites.
- limb alignment and deformities.
- active and passive movements.
- unusual movements and crepitation.
- level of pain caused injury.

Management of extremity injuries should aim to:
- keep blood flowing to peripheral tissues.
- prevent infection and skin necrosis.
- prevent damage to peripheral nerves.

Special issues relating to limb trauma
1. Stop active bleeding by direct pressure, rather than by tourniquet, as a tourniquet can be left on by mistake, resulting in ischaemic damage.
2. *Compartment syndrome:* is caused by increasing pressure inside fascial compartments. Common in injuries with intramuscular haematomas, crush injuries, fractures, or amputations. Increasing pressure results in local circulatory collapse by compression of local vessels and peripheral nerves. Tissue perfusion becomes limited and ischaemic; necrotic muscles with restricted function can even result if the perfusion pressure (systolic BP) is low. Clinical features of compartment syndrome:
- pain out of keeping with injury.
- parasthesia.
- tense compartments.
- pulse lost — but this is a late sign.
- passive stretch test — painful on moving foot or lower limb.

Damage on reperfusion is often serious. If there is local hypoxaemia (high IM pressure, low BP) for more than 2 h, reperfusion can cause extensive vascular damage. Decompression by fasciotomy should be done early. The forearm and lower leg compartments are at particular risk.
3. Traumatically amputated body parts should be covered with moist-ened sterile gauze towels and put into a sterile plastic bag. A non-cooled amputated part may be used within 6 h after injury; a cooled one as late as 18 to 20 h.

Paediatric trauma

Trauma is a leading cause of death in children. Survival of children who sustain major trauma depends on early resuscitation. The initial assessment of the paediatric trauma patient is identical to that for the adult, following ABCD, and finally exposing the child, without losing heat.

- **Blood volume** is proportionately greater in children and is calculated at 80 ml/kg in a child and 85–90 ml/kg in the neonate. A height/weight chart is the easiest method of approximating weight of a seriously ill child.

- **Venous access** in children who are hypovolaemic can be difficult. Useful sites for cannulation include: long saphenous vein over the ankle, external jugular vein, and femoral veins. The intraosseous route can provide the quickest access to the circulation in a shocked child.

- **Recognition of hypovolaemia** can be difficult. The increased physiological reserves of the child may result in the vital signs being only slightly abnormal despite up to 25% of blood volume being lost. Tachycardia is often the earliest response, but this can also be caused by fear or pain.

Table 20.2 Classification of hypovolaemia in children

	Class 1	Class 2	Class 3	Class 4
Blood lost	<15%	15–25%	25–40%	>40%
Pulse rate	↑	>150	>150	↑ or ↓
Pulse press	↔	↓	↓↓	absent
Systolic BP	↔	↓	↓↓	unrecord
Capillary refill	↔	↑	↑↑	absent
Resp rate	↔	↑	↑	↓sighing
Mental state	↔	irritable	lethargic	coma
Urine ml/kg/hr	<1	<1	<1	<1

- **Fluid management:** give 20 ml/kg of crystalloid fluid initially to a child showing signs of Class 2 hypovolaemia or worse, repeated up to 2x (up to 60 ml/kg) depending on the response. Children with little or no response to the initial fluid challenge require further crystalloid fluids and blood transfusion: 20 ml/kg of whole blood or 10 ml/kg of packed red cells should be initially transfused in these circumstances.

- **Heat loss** occurs rapidly due to the high surface-to-mass ratio in a child. A child who is hypothermic may become refractory to treatment.

- **Acute gastric dilatation** is commonly seen in the seriously ill or injured child. Gastric decompression, via a nasogastric tube, is essential.

- **Analgesia** should not be withheld. A recommended regime is a 50 mcg/kg IV bolus of morphine, followed by 10–20 mcg/kg increments at 10 minute intervals until an adequate response is achieved.

Burns

The source of the burn is important e.g. fire, hot water, paraffin, kerosene, electric shock, as this may point towards associated problems e.g. inhalational injury. Electrical burns are often more serious than they appear. Damaged skin and muscle can result in acute renal failure.

Management
- stop the burning (remove source and cool).
- ABCDE, then determine depth and area of burn (Rule of 9's).
- obtain good IV access and give early fluid replacement.

Burned surface area: morbidity and mortality increase with area burned and age, so that even small burns can be fatal in elderly people. Burns >15% in an adult, >10% in a child, or any occurring in the very young or elderly are considered serious.
- Rule of 9's is commonly used to estimate the burned surface area:
Adults: head 9%, torso 18%, arms 9% each, legs 18% each, genitalia 1%.
Children: use the palm of the child's' hand to represent 1% surface area.

Depth of burn
- first degree — red, pain, no blisters.
- second degree — red or mottled, pain blisters.
- third degree — dark and leathery, no pain, dry.
It is common to find all three depths within the same burn.

Fluid resuscitation: in the first 24 h from time of burn, give 2–4 mls/kg/ % surface area burned. Give half in first 8 h and half in next 16 h. e.g. an 80 kg adult with 25% burns would require:

> 80x25x2–4 ml in 24 h = 4000–8000 ml over 24 hour period; 2000–4000 over first 8 hour, then 2000–4000 over the subsequent 16 h.

Other considerations
- The site of the burn determines its severity. Burns to the face, neck, hands, feet, perineum, and circumferential burns (those encircling a limb, neck, etc.) are classified as serious.
- Beware inhalation injury in patient with facial burns, singed facial or nasal hair, hoarseness, and circumferential full thickness burns of the chest or neck. These patients need early intubation or tracheostomy before laryngeal oedema makes it impossible!
- Associated trauma or pre-burn illness.

Serious burns requiring hospitalization
>10% in child, >15% in adult; any in very young, elderly, infirm; full thickness or circumferential; with inhalation; burns of face, hands, feet, perineum. See also: *http://www.bmj.com/cgi/content/full/329/7458/158*

Pregnant trauma patients

The ABCDE priorities of trauma management in pregnant patients are the same as those in non-pregnant patients. However, anatomical and physiological changes occur in pregnancy that are extremely important in the assessment of the pregnant trauma patient.

Anatomical changes

The size of the uterus gradually increases and becomes more vulnerable to damage by both blunt and penetrating injury

- 12 weeks of gestation, the fundus is at the symphysis pubis.
- 20 weeks, it is at the umbilicus.
- 36 weeks, it is at the xiphoid.

The foetus in the first trimester is well protected by the thick walled uterus, pelvis, and large amounts of amniotic fluid.

Physiological changes

- increased tidal volume and respiratory alkalosis.
- increased heart rate.
- 30% increased cardiac output.
- usually lower BP, by 15 mmHg.
- aortocaval compression in the second and third trimester when the woman is lying flat, leading to hypotension.

Special issues in the traumatized pregnant female

- blunt trauma may lead to uterine irritability and premature labour.
- beware partial/complete rupture of the uterus.
- beware partial/complete placental separation (up to 48 h later).
- beware severe blood loss after pelvic fracture.

Management

1. Assess mother according to the ABCDE.
2. Resuscitate in left lateral position to avoid aortocaval compression.
3. Perform vaginal examination with a speculum to look for vaginal bleeding and cervical dilatation.
4. Mark the fundal height and assess tenderness.
5. Monitor the foetal heart rate as appropriate.

Resuscitation of mother may save the baby. However, there are times when the only option to save the mother is to deliver the baby by Caesarian section. **Remember:** aortocaval compression must be prevented in resuscitation of the traumatized pregnant woman.

Obstetric emergencies

More than 99% of all maternal deaths occur in the developing world. Around 50% of women worldwide give birth without a skilled attendant and with no antenatal care. Prevention is the key. The WHO in its Standards for Maternal and Neonatal Care sets out strategies for reducing maternal mortality:

- Family planning.
- Antenatal care.
- Clean/safe delivery.
- Essential obstetric care.

Management

- Assess using ABCDE in the lateral position and resuscitate.
- Be aware that the mother will probably deliver without medical intervention in her next pregnancy, so a uterine scar (from Caesarean section) is best avoided if possible.
- If the baby is alive, Consider Caesarean section or symphysiotomy (division of symphysis pubis).
- If the baby is dead, consider, with the mother's consent, symphysiotomy or destructive procedure (e.g. craniotomy) for baby.
- **Sepsis** may require evacuation of products of conception as well as antibiotics and resuscitation.
- **Eclampsia** (seizures associated with hypertension in pregnancy) is best treated with magnesium sulphate 4 g iv over 10–15 mins.
- **Haemorrhage:** all women need oxygen, 2 large bore venous cannulae, crystalloid, colloid, and blood resuscitation. Treat in left lateral position or manual uterine displacement. Assess for and treat coagulopathy.

Common causes of haemorrhage

- **Uterine atony** — treat with oxytocics/ergometrin/prostaglandin, massage + bimanual compression. Empty the uterus of foetus ± products of conception, repair lacerations, pack the uterus or use Rusch balloon to tamponade bleeding. Manual compression of aorta gives temporary control to allow resuscitation. A B-lynch suture may help at Caesarean. Perform a hysterectomy if necessary.
- **Placenta praevia** — deliver by Caesarean. There is risk of postpartum haemorrhage.
- **Uterine rupture** — perform laparotomy and repair the rupture.
- **Genital tract trauma** — find and repair injury.
- **Uterine inversion** — replace the uterus manually or with water pressure.
- **Ectopic pregnancy** — diagnose and operate.

The following are often associated with coagulopathy as well as haemorrhage: placental abruption, sepsis, dead foetus retained for some time, and amniotic fluid embolus.

For more information on childbirth and its variations, see *www.obgyn-101.org* (select 'procedures') or *www.wikipedia.org*

Poisoning and envenoming

Section editors **Andrew Dawson**
David Warrell

Acute poisoning

Most deaths from acute poisoning are due to deliberate self-poisoning. Although drug poisoning is common in urban areas of the developing world, the majority of deaths occur in rural areas after ingestion of pesticides. Whilst outcome seems to be determined purely by the amount ingested for some pesticides, good management for poisoning by other agents can reduce the death rate.

General management

- Resuscitate and stabilize (see life support algorithms inside front cover). In particular, take care of the airway, intubating any patient unable to protect their own airway (check cough and gag intact).
- Give high-flow oxygen — except for paraquat poisoned patients.
- Place the patient on their left side to reduce risk of aspiration and the passage of poison from stomach; it will also keep the airway open.
- If the patient has taken a pesticide, determine whether he/she needs atropine (see 📖 p 792).
- Suck out secretions as necessary (however, in organophosphate poisoning, patients will require atropine to control secretions).
- Get a history. What has been taken? How much and when? Have a handbook available that lists pesticides by both their chemical class and trade name since many people will only know the latter.
- Calm the patient. An agitated poisoned patient makes management difficult and increases risk of aspiration — consider giving diazepam.
- Watch out for and control convulsions. First-line therapy is diazepam; second-line is phenobarbital (see 📖 p 792).
- Give antidotes according to the poison ingested — poison identity can come from history or recognition of a 'toxidrome' (see box).
- Finally, consider the value of performing gastric emptying or decontamination once everything else is done.
- *Gastric lavage and induced emesis:* are no longer recommended in the routine management of a poisoned patient. Studies have shown little return of poison even when performed in ideal circumstances. Gastric lavage is associated with increased rate of ICU admission and aspiration pneumonia. It should only be considered within an hour of the poisoning and only if it can be done safely in a consenting or intubated patient. Gastric lavage performed in a non-consenting struggling patient has a high risk of aspiration and death.
- *Activated charcoal:* administered orally, is the recommended form of GI decontamination. Activated charcoal offers a large surface area for the poison to bind to, reducing absorption into the body. Give 50–100 g (1 g/kg for children) dissolved in 200–300 ml of water.
- *Multiple doses of activated charcoal:* some poisons are excreted in the bile or diffuse across the intestinal wall into the lumen. In this situation regular repeated administration of activated charcoal q4 h may enhance elimination.
- *Osmotic cathartics:* are no longer recommended. They increase the risk of electrolyte abnormalities with no evidence of benefit.

Toxidromes

Patients are often unable or sometimes unwilling to state the exact poison ingested. Treatment in these situations is based on clinical signs and the locally most likely poison ingested. Toxidromes are collections of signs which may assist in diagnosis (such as the cholinergic or anticholinergic syndromes).

Classification of common pesticides

1. Insecticides

- *Organophosphates (OP):* poisoning is often serious, requiring treatment with atropine, pralidoxime, ± diazepam.
- *Carbamates:* similar to OPs but AChE inhibition is briefer; however, poisoning may still last 2–4 days and patients require ventilation.
- *Organochlorines:* being restricted globally due to environmental persistence. Major problem with significant overdose is status epilepticus.
- *Pyrethroids:* low toxicity but may cause anaphylaxis.

2. Herbicides

- *Chlorphenoxy compounds:* in large overdoses, cause decreased consciousness and rhabdomyolysis resulting in renal failure.
- *Paraquat:* no proven treatment is available. Management appears not to alter clinical course.
- *Propanil:* causes methaemoglobinaemia; few other signs.
- *Glyphosate:* low toxicity unless pesticide and solvent is aspirated.

3. Rodenticides

- *Aluminium phosphide:* very toxic. Consider giving severely poisoned patients magnesium 1 g IV stat, then 1 g q1 h for 3 h, then 1 g q6 h.
- *Zinc phosphide:* less toxic. Treat supportively.
- *Coumarin derivatives:* long-acting warfarin-like compounds. INR >2 or active bleeding requires vitamin K 1 mg (sometimes for prolonged periods).
- *Thallium:* highly toxic. Banned in many countries.
- *Carbamates:* the highly toxic carbamate, aldicarb, is widely used as a rodenticide.

There are many other, often newer, pesticides. None have specific antidotes; conservative management with airway support and diazepam for seizures is probably best.

Acute pesticide poisoning

Early careful resuscitation and supportive care of pesticide-poisoned patients, with correct use of antidotes, will reduce deaths. Most pesticides are dissolved in organic solvents which can cause fatal pneumonia if aspirated; other additives, such as methanol, can cause additional toxicity. After 1 hour, gastric lavage and forced emesis is futile because of a high risk of complications. Activated charcoal should be adminstered orally or by NG tube.

Organophosphates/carbamates: see 📖 p 792.

Organochlorine poisoning: pesticides such as endosulfan, endrin, and the less toxic lindane, cause status epilepticus after large ingestions. *Manage:* with diazepam; give phenobarbital and then general anaesthetic if no response (📖 p 438). Many organochlorines are banned worldwide.

Pyrethroids: synthetic derivatives of the plant-derived pyrethrin. Low toxicity but may cause anaphylaxis. *Manage:* conservatively.

Chlorphenoxy herbicides: include MCPA; 2,4-D; 2,4,5-T (latter two are more toxic). Cause coma and rhabdomyolysis after large overdose. Observe for black urine (indicates myoglobinuria) and muscle pain. *Manage:* keep high urine output with IV fluids. Give sodium bicarbonate 3 mMol/kg if urine is black. Normally has a good outcome if renal failure can be averted.

Paraquat: uniformly fatal if taken in large amounts due to multi-organ failure. Smaller doses may result in fatal lung fibrosis. Patients often have marked ulceration of the mouth since they may just take it into their mouth and then spit it out; oesophageal damage is a poor prognostic sign, implying that the paraquat was swallowed. Intensive haemofiltration may offer some slight benefit; high-dose immunosuppression (cyclophosphamide 15 mg/kg IV od for 2 d; methylprednisolone 1 g IV od for 3 d, followed by PO dexamethasone) may prevent lung fibrosis, but definite evidence is not available. *Manage:* conservatively. Activated charcoal should be given early. Gastric lavage could be considered <1 hour after poisoning but if performed later there is a risk of oesophageal perforation. Oxygen may exacerbate lung fibrosis.

Propanil: causes methaemoglobinaemia. The patient looks cyanosed but is asymptomatic if metHb levels <20%; headaches and low GCS occur as metHb level rises. Death occurs with metHb >70%. *Manage:* give methylthioninium chloride (methylene blue) 1–2 mg/kg IV over 5 mins, repeated after 30–60 mins as necessary, and/or exchange transfusion.

Glyphosate: causes ulcerative damage to the oesophagus but little else. Do not perform lavage since complications may occur after aspiration.

Gastric lavage for pesticide poisoning

- Lavage must not be performed in combative, conscious patients or in patients with reduced GCS unless intubated.
- Lavage should only be considered when patients present <1 h after ingestion of a potentially life-threatening amount of pesticide (organophosphorus, organochlorine, carbamate, or paraquat).
- Use an 18-gauge NG tube for pesticides — a larger bore tube has a higher rate of complications.

Poisoning with corrosives

Acids cause an immediate mucosal burn that scabs over, limiting damage. In contrast, alkalis produce a liquifactive necrosis that produces much deeper tissue damage.

Clinical features: pain in mouth, throat, and abdomen; dysphagia; drooling. Complications include perforation, haemorrhage, and systemic complications of particular corrosives. Patients with significant poisoning are at high risk of strictures in oesophagus or stomach.

Management: give O_2 and obtain IV access for fluid resuscitation. Watch for signs of airway obstruction or GI perforation. GI decontamination is generally not indicated. Careful endoscopy is recommended soon after admission to assess damage to GI tract and manage strictures. Patients with alkali ingestions and circumferential oesophageal burns may benefit from early steroids (hydrocortisone 100 mg BD).

Poisoning with hydrocarbons

- Hydrocarbon toxicity occurs after pulmonary aspiration or after systemic absorption.
- Hydrocarbons can be grouped by volatility/viscosity and systemic toxicity.
- Poisoning with non-volatile, non-absorbed hydrocarbons such as motor oil does not require treatment. The risk of aspiration is low.
- Poisoning with more volatile but non-toxic hydrocarbons, such as kerosene, is very common. Aspiration pneumonia is the main complication so treat conservatively without induction of vomiting or lavage.
  - The management of volatile and toxic hydrocarbons such as phenol is difficult. Lavage may be indicated in hope of preventing systemic toxicity if the patients have taken a significant dose and been admitted <1 h after ingestion. Beware of causing aspiration pneumonia.
  - There is no general antidote; steroids are not indicated.

Organophosphates/carbamates

These pesticides inhibit acetylcholinesterase (AChE) at autonomic, neuro-muscular, and central synapses, causing acetylcholine (ACh) to accumulate and overstimulate receptors. AChE reactivates quickly in carbamate poisoning; the process is much slower in OP poisoning. Atropine competes with and antagonizes ACh at muscarinic receptors; oximes such as pralidoxime reactivate inhibited AChE. If oxime treatment is delayed, the inhibited AChE may become 'aged' and resist reactivation.

Clinical features:

Result from accumulation of ACh at muscarinic synapses (salivation, bronchorrhoea, urination, diarrhoea, bradycardia, small pupils); nicotinic synapses (muscle fasciculation and weakness, tachycardia, large pupils); and CNS synapses (agitation, confusion, drowsiness → coma). Inhibition of AChE over several days may result in failure of the neuromuscular junction: the intermediate syndrome (initially neck flexion weakness — ask patient to lift head from the pillow; sometimes cranial nerve palsies → respiratory muscle weakness and sudden respiratory arrest). Some OPs cause a peripheral motor neuropathy after several weeks.

Diagnosis:

Is normally clinical, based on the typical features. Plasma butyrylcholi-nesterase levels may support the diagnosis.

Management

- Resuscitation and supportive care are the major initial priority. Any decontamination should only be considered after patient stabilization.
- Give oxygen. Intubate early — as soon as the patient's GCS drops <12–13. Give diazepam 10 mg IV slowly over 2–3 mins as required.
- Simultaneously, give atropine 1.2–2.4 mg rapidly as a bolus.
- Watch for a response in the markers of atropinization (see box).
- If no response at 5 mins, double the dose of atropine.
- Continue giving doubling doses of atropine until the chest is clear of wheeze or crackles (beware sounds of aspiration) and pulse is above 80/minute. Tens or, rarely, hundreds of mg may be required.
- Once the patient is atropinized (see opposite), set up an infusion giving 20–40% per hour of the total bolus dose of atropine required.
- For OPs and where the agent is unknown, give pralidoxime 2 g IV slowly over 5–30 mins (a fast injection → emesis and tachycardia), followed by an infusion of 500 mg/hr.
- Treat convulsions with diazepam 10 mg IV slowly over 2–3 mins; repeated as necessary. Intubate and ventilate if required.
- Observe carefully to ensure that (i) the required amount of atropine is being given — increase or decrease as required, and (ii) detect neck weakness (= early intermediate syndrome) early so that a patient can be intubated and ventilated before a respiratory arrest. Also monitor tidal volume regularly.

Markers of atropinization

Sufficient atropine has been given when all of the following are attained:
- Chest clear (no wheeze or crackles).
- Pulse >80 bpm.
- Systolic BP >80 mmHg with urine output >0.5 ml/kg/hr.

Other signs of atropinization include:
- Pupils no longer pinpoint.
- Axilla (or oral mucosa) are dry.

Notes
- Aspiration may complicate the chest criteria. Try to differentiate between local creps of aspiration and generalized creps/wheeze of OP poisoning.
- The pupils may dilate late — after 30 mins or so.
- There is no need to continue to give atropine until the heart rate is 120–140 or the pupils widely dilated. The aim is to reverse the poisoning, not induce atropine toxicity.

Markers of over-atropinization

Too much atropine is being given if:
- Bowel sounds are absent.
- Patient is in urinary retention.
- Patient is confused (not alcohol-related).
- Patient is febrile due to atropine.

Atropine-induced fevers: particularly in patients agitated by alcohol withdrawal and in hot environments — risk causing cardiac arrest.

Agitation: can be decreased with oral or IV benzodiazepines. Reduce temperature by sponging the patient and using a fan.

Acute poisoning with pharmaceuticals/chemicals

Relatively few pharmaceuticals have specific antidotes — the main aim of management for most patients will be supportive care. There is no evidence for any benefit from lavage, forced emesis, or activated charcoal.

- **Benzodiazepines:** patients present with drowsiness, slurred speech, ataxia, rarely coma (small pupils/hyporeflexia), or respiratory failure, due to the drugs' inhibitory effect on the CNS. Most patients can simply be observed. In case of respiratory failure (often with newer, short-acting drugs), intubate/ventilate. Severe poisoning can be briefly reversed with flumazenil 0.2 mg IV over 15 secs repeated with doses of 0.1 mg at 60 sec intervals if required, up to a maximum of 1 mg. This drug must not be used if there are signs of tricyclic antidepressant toxicity.

- **Cardiac glycosides:** can be due to overdose of digoxin medication or ingestion of a source of natural glycoside (e.g. oleander seeds). Main effects are on the heart: dysrhythmias and conduction block. Atropine 0.5 mg IV for bradycardia is frequently used but is unlikely to prevent severe dysrhythmia. Temporary cardiac pacing can tide the patient through 3rd degree AV heart block. Anti-digoxin antibodies can reverse DC-shock resistant VF or cardiogenic shock in severe poisoning.

- **Isoniazid:** may cause decreased consciousness, convulsions, coma, respiratory arrest, metabolic acidosis. If severe, give pyridoxine by slow IV injection (quantity equal to the quantity of isoniazid taken; if quantity unknown, give 5 g). Repeat at 5–20 min intervals if there is no response.

- **Lithium carbonate:** affects CNS, heart, and kidney. Acute lithium poisoning with normal renal function generally requires only supportive care. In patients with poor renal function and severe poisoning, haemodialysis is the best method to remove lithium. Check serum electrolytes q6–12 h; if hypernatraemia is present, give 5% dextrose until plasma Na^+ returns to normal. Since most patients will be on chronic lithium therapy and have nephrogenic diabetes insipidus, they will require high fluid maintenance rates.

- **Opiates:** are found in analgesics and recreational drugs. Features include respiratory depression, decreased consciousness, and pinpoint pupils. Give repeated bolus of naloxone 0.4 mg (up to 2 mg) IV. After the initial response, an infusion may be needed in long-acting or sustained-release opioids; the starting dose is 50% of the total initial bolus each hour. The major indicator of naloxone response is reversal of respiratory depression. The response time is 9 ± 4 mins to increase respiratory rate to >10/min. If more than 2 mg naloxone is required review the diagnosis — has more than one drug been taken?

- **Paracetamol:** for ingestions of >150 mg/kg, give N-acetylcysteine IV unless paracetamol blood levels can be measured and shown to be safe. Dose = 150 mg/kg in 200 ml of 5% dextrose over 15 mins, followed by 50 mg/kg in 500 ml of 5% dextrose over 4 h, and then 100 mg/kg in 1 litre over 16 h. If liver failure develops, continue since it may improve outcome. If unavailable, give methionine 2.5 g PO repeated q4 h for a total of 4 doses. Check liver and kidney function. Closely monitor blood glucose levels, watching for hypoglycaemia.

- **Salicylates:** severe aspirin poisoning may present with CNS depression, haematemesis, hyperthermia. However, lethal doses may not affect consciousness. Lesser poisoning produces GI pain, N&V, tinnitus. A mixed metabolic acidosis/respiratory alkalosis is common. Metabolic acidosis occurs in young children; respiratory alkalosis more commonly in older patients. Give charcoal and correct electrolyte imbalances. If there are neurological signs, give 50 ml of 50% dextrose IV; repeat if necessary. Any metabolic acidoisis should be corrected (even if there is respiratory compensation) with sodium bicarbonate infusion; patients commonly require potassium supplementation. Goal of bicarbonate treatment = restore normal systemic pH and make the urine alkaline.

- **Tricyclic antidepressants:** may present with signs of CNS toxicity (convulsions, ophthalmoplegia, muscle twitching, delirium, coma, respiratory depression), anticholinergic effects (dry mouth, blurred vision, mydriasis), cardiotoxicity (QRS duration & QT prolongation), hypothermia, pyrexia. Control convulsions; monitor heart and correct arrhythmias; control acidosis. Give IV sodium bicarbonate for cardio-toxicity or for seizures with an initial dose of 3 mmol/kg. This dose can be repeated and titrated against clinical response. The pH should be assessed, if possible, after a total dose of 6 mmol/kg and should not exceed pH 7.55.

- **Cyanide:** late presentations include dyspnoea, cyanosis, or uncon-sciousness. Altered mental status, tachypnoea (in absence of cyanosis), unexplained anion gap metabolic acidosis, and bright red blood are earlier signs. Administer O_2; correct acidosis; give amylnitrite by inhala-tion over 30 secs each minute until other drugs are prepared. Then give: sodium nitrite 300 mg by IV injection over 5–20 mins followed by sodium thiosulfate 12.5 g IV over 10 mins (alternative: dicobalt edetate 300 mg IV over 1 min followed by 50 mls of 50% dextrose. Repeat ×2 if required. Do not use if the diagnosis is uncertain).

- **Metal ions (e.g. gold, mercury, zinc, lead, copper):** acute poisoning can cause coma, convulsions, and death, or affect multiple organ systems. Anticipate and treat shock, renal or hepatic failure. Give penicillamine 1–2 g PO od in 3 divided doses (2 h before meals, if possible) for 2–4 weeks. Get a senior opinion. An alternative option (preferred in mercury poisoning) is dimercaprol (BAL; British anti-Lewisite) 2.5–3 mg/kg q4 h for 2 days; then q6 h on the 3rd day; and bd for days 4–10 or until recovery.

Mushroom poisoning

Mushrooms cause a variety of toxicological syndromes affecting the CNS, kidney, liver, muscle, and GI tract. Clinical features are separated into those appearing early (<6 h) or late (around 6 h or later).

Clinical features

1. Early symptoms starting within a few hrs: gastroenteritis, cholinergic (muscarinic) effects, confusion, visual hallucinations, or antabuse-like reactions to drinking alcohol, according to the species ingested.

2. Delayed symptoms starting 6 h to many days later suggest more dangerous poisoning:

- Gastroenteritis with hepato- and nephro-toxicity (amatoxin poisoning) is caused by the death cap mushroom (*Amanita phalloides*) and others from the *Amanita*, *Galerina*, and *Lepiota* genera. Abdominal pain, vomiting, and watery diarrhoea start after 6–24 (usually 12) hours resulting in dehydration. Hepatic and renal failure evolve over the next few days or weeks.
- Gastroenteritis with neurological symptoms (gyromitrin poisoning) caused by false morel (*Gyromitra esculenta*). Gastroenteritis, bloating, severe headache, vertigo, pyrexia, sweating, diplopia, nystagmus, ataxia, and cramps are followed by delirium, coma, hepatic and renal damage, hypoglycaemia, and haemolysis.
- Renal damage may develop 2–17 days after eating *Cortinarius* species (orellanine poisoning). Fatigue, intense thirst, headache, chills, paraesthesiae, tinnitus and abdominal, lumbar, and flank pain are the prelude to polyuria, oliguria, and anuria.
- Rhabdomyolysis occurs after ingestion of *Tricholoma* species due to a myotoxin.

Management

Give activated charcoal 50 g q2 h for at least 48 h.

- Correct hypovolaemia, acid-base disturbances, hypoglycaemia, and renal failure.
- Give atropine (adult 0.6–1.8 mg IV) for cholinergic features.
- Give physostigmine (adult 1–2 mg IV) or diazepam (adults 5–10 mg IV) for anticholinergic hallucinations.
- For amatoxic fungal poisoning, give large doses of benzylpenicillin (2.4 g q6 h; N-acetylcysteine may have benefit). Liver transplantation may be necessary.
- Gyromitrin fungal poisoning is treated with pyridoxine 25 mg/kg over 30 min, 5% dextrose IV, and diuresis.

Prevention

Discourage the ingestion of any wild fungi, especially those with white gills. Cooking does not destroy their poisons.

Fish and shellfish poisoning

Ciguatera fish poisoning: >50,000 cases occur each year. In some Pacific islands ~1% are affected/year, case fatality 0.1%. Due to accumulation of toxins from the flagellate *Gambierdiscus toxicus* in muscles of carnivorous fish at the top of the food chain. The toxins activate sodium channels. Gastroenteritis develops 1–6 h after eating warm-water shore or reef fish (groupers, snappers, parrot fish, mackerel, moray eels, barracudas, jacks). Gastrointestinal symptoms resolve within a few hours, but paraesthesiae, pruritis, and myalgia may persist for a week to months.

Tetrodoxin poisoning: scaleless porcupine, sun, puffer, and toad fish (order: *Tetraodonitiformes*) become poisonous seasonally. Puffer fish ('fugu') is relished in Japan. Neurotoxic symptoms develop 10–45 min after eating the fish and death from respiratory paralysis 2–6 h later.

Scombroid poisoning (histamine-like syndrome): bacterial contamination and decomposition of e.g. dark-fleshed tuna, mackerel, bonito, and skipjack, and of canned fish releases histamine. Buccal tingling or smarting is followed by flushing, burning, sweating, urticaria, pruritis, headache, abdominal colic, nausea, vomiting, diarrhoea, asthma, giddiness and hypotension.

Paralytic shellfish poisoning: bivalve mollusks (mussels, clams, oysters, cockles, and scallops) become toxic when there is a 'red tide' of algal blooms. Within 30 min of ingestion, paralysis begins and, in 8% of cases, progresses to fatal respiratory paralysis within 12 h.

Management (of all types of fish/shellfish poisoning)
- Promote vomiting and diarrhoea with emetics and purges.
- Scombroid poisoning responds to antihistamines, bronchodilators, and adrenaline.
- Assisted ventilation is required in severe paralytic poisoning.

Prevention: marine poisons are not destroyed by cooking or boiling.
- local advice should be sought about what is safe to eat.
- prevent ingestion of shellfish when there is a 'red tide'.
- very large reef fish (ciguatera poisoning) and any parts of the fish other than muscle should not be eaten.
- notorious species such as Moray eels (ciguatera poisoning) or puffer fish (tetrodotoxin poisoning) should never be eaten.

Leech bite

Land leeches infest the rainforest floor, attaching to legs or ankles. After a painless bite, they ingest blood and then drop off, but the wound continues to bleed and the clot is fragile. Aquatic leeches are swallowed in river or pond water, or they attack bathers, entering the mouth, nostrils, eyes, vulva, vagina, urethra, or anus.

Clinical features

The main effect is blood loss. Other symptoms include secondary infection (by *Aeromonas hydrophila* with medicinal leeches), itching, and phobia. Ingested aquatic leeches attach to the pharynx, producing a sensation of movement at the back of the throat, cough, hoarseness, stridor, breathlessness, epistaxis, haemoptysis, haematemesis, or upper airway obstruction, or they penetrate bronchi or oesophagus. Via the anus, they may reach the rectosigmoid junction, causing perforation and peritonitis.

Treatment

Apply salt, a flame, alcohol, turpentine, or vinegar to the leech to encourage detachment. Control local bleeding with a styptic, such as silver nitrate, or a firm dressing. Penetrating aquatic leeches must be removed endoscopically. Spray with 10% tartaric acid or 1:10,000 adrenaline (nasopharynx, larynx, trachea, or oesophagus) or irrigate with concentrated saline (GU tract and rectum).

Prevention

Trousers, socks, and footwear should be impregnated and skin anointed with DEET. Children should be discouraged from bathing in leech-infested waters. People should not drink from natural water sources and drinking water must boiled.

Snake bite

Most parts of the world have venomous snakes. In W Africa, S Asia, New Guinea, and Latin America, snakes maim or kill many farmers and children. Medically important groups are elapids (e.g. cobras, mambas), vipers, pit vipers, and burrowing asps. Although there are 100s of different species, you need only know about the dangerous ones where you live and work.

Clinical features (depending on the species involved)

- Local swelling, bruising, blistering, regional lymph node enlargement, and tissue damage (necrosis). Occur with vipers, pit vipers, burrowing asps, and some cobras.
- Incoagulable blood, shown by 20 min clotting test (see opposite), spontaneous bleeding from gums, nose, skin, gut, GU tract; persistent bleeding from wounds. Occurs with vipers, pit vipers, South African boomslangs, and Australasian elapids.
- Shock (hypotension) and arrhythmias. Occur with vipers, pit vipers, and burrowing asps.
- Descending paralysis (ptosis, external ophthalmoplegia, bulbar and respiratory muscle paralysis). Occurs with elapids, a few vipers and pit vipers.
- Generalized rhabdomyolysis (myalgia, myoglobinuria — black urine +ve for blood). Occurs with sea snakes, Australasian elapids, a few vipers and pit vipers.
- Acute renal failure. Occurs with sea snakes, some vipers and pit vipers.

Hospital treatment

First aid — see opposite.

Assess and observe patients carefully for at least 24 h.

- Antivenom, the only specific antidote, is indicated for any signs of systemic envenoming listed above *or* for local envenoming that is rapidly spreading *or* involves more than half the bitten limb or digits. Give an appropriate antivenom (check package insert for species covered) by slow IV injection or infusion.
- Watch for early signs of anaphylactoid reactions and treat with IM adrenaline (adult 0.5 mg, child 10 mcg/kg) and IV H_1 antihistamine and hydrocortisone 200 mg. Don't waste time with non-predictive hypersensitivity tests.
- Give a tetanus toxoid booster but antibiotics only if there is local necrosis, contaminated bite site, or abscess.
- Bulbar/respiratory paralysis requires intubation and assisted ventilation.
- Correct hypovolaemia (bleeding or extravasation into swollen limbs).
- Treat renal failure with dialysis.
- Nurse swollen limbs in the most comfortable position.
- Debride necrotic tissue but avoid fasciotomy unless haemostasis has been restored and intracompartmenal pressure >40 mmHg.

Snake bites — first aid

- reassure the patient (only ~50% of bites by venomous snakes cause envenoming, which usually takes hours to become serious).
- do not interfere with the bite site in any way (e.g. do not attempt to suck out or aspirate the poison).
- immobilize the person as far as possible, especially the bitten limb.
- transport patient to medical care by vehicle, boat, stretcher, etc.
- treat pain with paracetamol or codeine tablets (**not** aspirin or NSAIDs).
- never attempt to catch or kill the snake.
- never use traditional methods (tourniquet, incision, suction, herbs, etc).

20-minute whole blood clotting test

Put 2 ml venous blood into a plain glass test-tube. Leave undisturbed for 20 minutes, then tip once. If the blood runs out (no clot), consumption coagulopathy has occurred and antivenom is indicated. Repeat 6 h after giving antivenom. If the blood remains incoagulable, give another dose.

If negative, can be repeated hourly if envenoming is suspected. Recovery will take 6 h after effective administration of antivenom since *de novo* synthesis of clotting factors is required.

Pressure-immobilization method

Only for bites by suspected elapids whose venom can cause rapid paralysis: bind the bitten limb very firmly with long stretchy (crepe) bandages, from the digits to axilla/groin, incorporating a splint. Loosen if the limb becomes painful or if the peripheral pulse is occluded.

Prevention of snake bites

- avoid all snakes and snake charmers.
- never disturb, corner, attack, or handle snakes — dead or alive.
- if a snake is cornered, remain motionless until it has escaped.
- never walk in undergrowth or deep sand without proper leg/footwear.
- always carry a light at night.
- be careful collecting firewood with bare hands.
- never put a hand or push sticks into burrows or holes.
- avoid climbing trees or rocks covered with dense foliage.
- when climbing, don't put hands on ledges that cannot be seen.
- never swim in vegetation-matted rivers or muddy estuaries.
- avoid sleeping on the ground use a hammock or camp bed, a tent with sewn-in ground sheet, or a mosquito net tucked under a sleeping bag.

Scorpion sting

The most dangerous scorpions inhabit deserts or hot dusty terrains in North Africa, the Middle East, South Africa, the Americas, and S Asia. They likely cause more than 100,000 medically significant stings each year. Most deaths occur in children.

Clinical features: stings are excruciatingly painful. Systemic symptoms reflect release of autonomic neurotransmitters: acetylcholine (causing vomiting, abdominal pain, bradycardia, sweating, salivation) and then catecholamines (causing hypertension, tachycardia, pulmonary oedema, and ECG abnormalities).

Management: for pain, infiltrate local anaesthetic at the site, ideally by digital block if the sting is on finger or toe. Powerful opiate analgesia may be required. For systemic envenoming (difficult to distinguish from pain and fear in children), antivenoms are available for dangerous African/ Middle Eastern and American species. Hypertension, acute left ventricular failure, and pulmonary oedema may respond to vasodilators such as prazosin (0.5 mg PO q3–6 h).

Prevention: scorpions hide in cracks, crevices, and under rubbish. Encourage people to not walk around in bare feet, to sleep off the ground under a permethrin-impregnated bed net, and to always shake out boots and shoes before putting them on.

Spider bite

The most dangerous spiders are the black/brown widows (*Latrodectus*) in the Americas, southern Europe, Southern Africa, and Australia; wandering, armed, or banana spiders (*Phoneutria*) in Latin America; funnel web spiders (*Atrax* and *Hadronyche*) in Australia; and brown recluse spiders (*Loxosceles*) in the Americas. Spiders cause few deaths.

Clinical features: bites happen when people brush against a spider that has crept into clothes or bedding. *Latrodectus*, *Phoneutria*, and *Atrax* are neurotoxic causing cramping abdominal pains, muscle spasms, weakness, sweating, salivation, gooseflesh, fever, nausea, vomiting, alterations in pulse rate and blood pressure, and convulsions. *Loxosceles* is necrotic. Rarely, *Loxosceles* cause systemic effects such as fever, scarlatiniform rash, haemoglobinuria, coagulopathy, and renal failure.

Managment: is mostly symptomatic. Antivenoms are available in South Africa, Australia, and Brazil where bites are an important medical problem.

Hymenoptera sting anaphylaxis

Stings by bees (*Apidae*), wasps, hornets and yellow jackets (*Vespidae*), and ants (American fire ants *Solenopsis*, Australian jumper ants *Myrmecia*) are a very common nuisance in most countries. However, 2–4% of the population become allergic, developing massive local swelling or potentially lethal anaphylaxis if stung. In tropical countries, mass attacks by bees and wasp-like insects are not uncommon. In the Americas, Africanized 'killer' bees have killed many people.

Clinical features: symptoms of anaphylaxis including urticaria, angioedema, shock, bronchospasm, and GI symptoms.

Management: give adrenaline.

Prevention: desensitization is effective but time-consuming. Self-injectable adrenaline ('Epi-Pen' or 'Ana-Pen') is the best first aid.

Fish stings

Stinging fresh and salt water fish (stingrays, cat fish, weevers, scorpion, and stone fish) have venomous spines on gills, fins, or tail. Most commonly, they sting when trodden upon on the ocean or river bed.

Clinical features: immediate excruciating pain is followed by local swelling and inflammation. Rare systemic effects include vomiting, diarrhoea, sweating, dysrhythmia, hypotension, and muscle spasms. Stingrays' barbed spines can inflict fatal trauma (pneumothorax, penetration of organs). Spines left embedded in the wound with their venomous integument will cause infection unless removed.

Management

- *First aid:* agonizing local pain is dramatically relieved by immersing the stung part in hot (<45°C) but not scalding water which will cause a full thickness scald. Alternatively, local anaesthetic can be infiltrated or applied as a digital block.
- *Antivenom:* Australia produces an antivenom for the most dangerous species stone fish (genus *Synanceja*).
- *Infection:* all fish wounds can become infected with lethal marine pathogens including *Vibrio vulnificus*).

Prevention: advise people to shuffle or prod the sand ahead of them with a stick to disturb ground-lurking fish, to avoid handling dead or live fish, and to keep clear of fish in the water, especially in the vicinity of tropical reefs. Footwear protects against most species except stingrays.

Jelly fish stings

Common jelly fish (*Cnidarians/Coelenterates*) that sting include: Portuguese men o' war (blue bottles), sea wasps, box jellies, cubomedusoids, sea anemones, and stinging corals. Tentacles are studded with millions of stinging capsules (nematocysts) that fire their venomous stinging hairs into the skin on contact. Lines of painful blisters and inflammation result. Allergy may cause recurrent urticarial rashes over many months. Notorious Northern Australian and Indo-Pacific box jellyfish (*Chironex fleckeri* and *Chiropsalmus* spp.) and *Irukandji* (*Carukia barnesi*) can kill.

Clinical features: severe musculoskeletal pain, anxiety, trembling, headache, piloerection, sweating, tachycardia, hypertension, and pulmonary oedema may evolve.

Management: remove the victim from the water (prevent drowning). Inhibit nematocyst discharge by applying commercial vinegar or 3–10% aqueous acetic acid (ONLY *Chironex* spp. and other cubozoans including *Irukandji*) or a slurry of baking soda and water (50% w/v) (*Chrysaora* spp.). Don't use sun tan lotion or alcoholic solutions! Ice packs relieve pain. Antivenom for *C. fleckeri* is available in Australia.

Sea urchin stings

Long, sharp, venomous sea urchin (Echinoderm) spines become deeply embedded in the skin, usually of the sole of the foot, when the animal is trodden upon.

Management: soften the skin with salicylic acid ointment and then pare down the epidermis to a depth at which the spines can be removed with forceps. Most sea urchin spines are absorbed rapidly provided they are broken into small pieces in the skin. If they penetrate a joint or become infected, surgical removal may be necessary.

Immunization

Section editors   **Matthew Snape**
                      Andrew Pollard

Introduction

Both the achievements and shortcomings of vaccines in preventing disease in tropical countries are extraordinary. It is estimated that more than 2 million childhood deaths were averted by immunization in 2003. The number of polio cases fell by 99% between 1988 and 2005. The polysaccharide–protein conjugate vaccines offer the hope of a 'new wave' of vaccines with the potential for a dramatic reduction in diseases such as meningococcus, pneumococcus, and *Haemophilus influenzae* type B (Hib).

And yet 1.4 million children died from vaccine-preventable diseases in 2002. In 2004, measles resulted in 454,000 deaths — the majority of them in children. Many vaccines still require cumbersome mechanisms such as maintenance of a cold chain and IM injection, with the entire infrastructure these demand. It is because of the enormous potential of vaccines that these issues need to be addressed. Initiatives such as the Global Alliance for Vaccine and Immunization (GAVI) offer the hope that the populations most in need will benefit from the potential that vaccinology offers.

Expanded Programme on Immunization

Guidelines of the Expanded Programme on Immunization (EPI) for childhood vaccination are given on ￼ p 811. However, the epidemiology of the diseases which the EPI aims to combat will differ between different countries. To reflect this variation, policy needs to be made at national or regional level to decide which vaccines should be included in the country's infant and childhood immunization schedules. These national policies will take precedence over the EPI guidelines presented here and can be written on ￼ p 809. A summary of national guidelines can be accessed at the WHO website:

http://www.who.int/immunization_monitoring/en

Abbreviations for particular vaccines

BCG	Bacille-Calmette-Guerin vaccine
dT	Combination tetanus toxoid and low-dose diphtheria toxoid vaccine for use in individuals over 7 years of age
DT	Combination diphtheria toxoid and tetanus toxoid vaccine for use in children less than 7 years old
DTP	Combination diphtheria toxoid, tetanus toxoid, and pertussis vaccine
DTaP	Combination diphtheria toxoid, tetanus toxoid, and acellular pertussis vaccine
HepB	Hepatitis B vaccine
Hib	Haemophilus influenzae type B vaccine
MMR	Combination measles, mumps, and rubella vaccine
MR	Combination measles and rubella vaccine
IPV	Injected polio vaccine (salk vaccine)
OPV	Oral polio vaccine (sabin vaccine)
TT	Tetanus toxoid vaccine

National/regional recommendations*

Age	Vaccines
Birth	
6 weeks	
10 weeks	
14 weeks	
6 months	
9 months	
Birth	

* National/regional recommendations for infant immunization may be written here. See 📖 p 811 for WHO recommended infant immunization schedule.

Immunization strategies and schedules

Immunization schedule design

The timings of the vaccines recommended by the EPI are based on a compromise between:
- The desire to immunize as early as possible, thereby protecting the child before he/she becomes exposed to the infectious agent, and
- The requirement to wait both for the infant's immune system to mature and for maternally-derived antibodies that crossed the placenta prenatally to wane, so that the immunization will be effective.

In general, vaccines are recommended for the youngest age group that is at risk for developing the disease and whose members are able to receive the vaccine safely and develop an adequate response. Many vaccines require more than one dose and it is recommended that these doses be separated by at least 4 weeks. Increasing the intervals between doses, as is recommended in developed countries, enhances the immune response to the vaccines but results in the child being susceptible to the disease for a longer period of time.

Optimization of vaccine uptake

The most common reason for children dying from a vaccine-preventable disease is that they have not received the vaccine. Optimization of vaccine uptake is crucial and can be facilitated by:
- Offering immunizations as often as possible.
- Administering all vaccines for which a child is eligible simultaneously at a single visit.
- Routine screening of immunization status of all women and children.
- Awareness of true and false contraindications for immunizations (📖 p 815).
- Maintenance of adequate vaccine delivery.
- Appropriate utilization of multi-dose vials (📖 p 812).

Administration of vaccines

Recent data from industrialized countries has highlighted the importance of using the appropriate needle length (i.e. 25 mm) when administering intramuscular vaccines in order to reduce reactogenicity and, potentially, increase immunogenicity. Data addressing this question in developing countries are not yet available. Intramuscular vaccines should be administered to infants in the lateral aspect of the thighs, while children above the age of 12 months should receive their vaccines in the deltoid muscles. Vaccines administered on the same limb should be separated by at least 2.5 cm. With the exception of OPV, if 2 live vaccines (see 📖 p 816) are to be administered, they should be administered either at the same time or at least 1 month apart. Due to an increased risk of lymphadenopathy, no vaccine should be administered into an arm used for BCG administration for 3 months after receipt of BCG. In the case of an interruption to an immunization schedule, the schedule should proceed as if no interruption had occurred i.e. there is no need to 'restart' an immunization schedule.

WHO recommended infant immunization schedule

Age[1]	Vaccines	Hepatitis B[2]		
		Scheme I	Scheme II	Scheme III
Birth	BCG, OPV-0[3]		HepB-1	HepB-1
6 weeks	DTP-1, OPV-1, Hib-1	HepB-1[4]		HepB-2
10 weeks	DTP-2, OPV-2, Hib-2	HepB-2	HepB-2	HepB-3
14 weeks	DTP-3, OPV-3, Hib-3	HepB-3	HepB-3	HepB-4
9 months	Measles[5] ± yellow fever[6]			
Variable	Japanese encephalitis[7]			

1. Babies born prematurely should be vaccinated at exactly the same times after birth as babies born at term.

2. Scheme I may be used in countries where perinatal transmission is less frequent (e.g. sub-Saharan Africa); scheme II or III, incorporating a birth dose of HepB, are recommended where perinatal transmission of HepB is common (e.g. South-East Asia).

3. In polio-endemic countries.

4. HepB administered beyond the perinatal period can be given as either a monovalent vaccine or in combination with DTP ± Hib.

5. Where there is a high risk of mortality from measles under the age of 9 months (e.g. HIV-infected infants), measles vaccination should be carried out at both 6 and 9 months.

6. In countries where yellow fever poses a risk (see 📖 p 821).

7. In endemic countries (📖 p 820); variable schedules from 9 months of age.

Booster doses

Recommended for the following vaccines:

Vaccine	Recommended boosting schedule
Tetanus*	A total of 3 further doses to be given at: • 4–7 years of age (DTP or dT according to local policy) • 12–15 years of age (dT) • early adulthood (dT)
Pertussis	1 further dose at 1–6 years
Measles	1 further dose, either as part of routine schedule or in mass immunization campaigns

* Maternal immunization is a highly effective method of controlling neonatal tetanus. Recommendations vary according to previous immunization status.

Transport and storage of vaccines

The vulnerability to extremes of temperature of the majority of vaccines used in the EPI schedule means that maintenance of an adequate 'cold chain' (to ensure vaccine transport at optimum temperatures from manufacture to the point of use) is essential to an effective immunization programme. To this end, the following innovations have been introduced:

- Cold chain monitor — detects excessive temperatures during shipment.
- Vaccine vial monitor (VVM) — for the cumulative heat exposure of an individual vial.
- Freeze watch™ monitor — for exposure of vaccine shipments to temperatures below freezing point.
- Stop!Watch™ — combining the indicators from the cold chain monitor and the Freeze watch™ monitor.

Detailed guidance on the use of these devices and the maintenance of cold chain is available at:

http://www.who.int/vaccines-documents/DoxGen/H5-CC.htm

In order to reduce vaccine wastage, the use of already opened multi-dose vials at subsequent immunization sessions has been condoned by the WHO for the following vaccines: OPV, DTP, TT, DT, HepB, and liquid formulations of Hib. Multi-dose vials of these vaccines can be used for a period of up to 4 weeks after the opening of the vial provided that:

- The cold chain has been maintained, the VVM has not reached the 'discard point', and the vaccines are within their 'use by' date.
- The rubber vaccine vial septum has not been submerged in water (e.g. by melting ice).
- Aseptic technique has been used to withdraw all doses.

Needle use and disposal

More than 1 billion immunizations are injected annually in developing countries. Without adequate safety mechanisms, each one of these episodes creates the potential for transmission of blood-borne infections to both vaccine recipients (through re-use of disposable needles) and health care workers (through needle-stick injuries). To minimize these risks, the WHO advocates:

- All immunizations requiring injection be administered via single-use auto-destruct (AD) needles.
- No vaccines are administered without access to safety boxes to dispose of used needles.
- Disposable syringes can be used to reconstitute lyophilized vaccines, but must not be recapped.
- Safety boxes should be sealed when ¾ full.

Disposal of the safety boxes remains problematic in many areas and is most commonly performed by incineration.

Adverse reactions

Although modern vaccines are extremely safe, some vaccines may lead to adverse reactions. It is difficult to prove that a vaccination causes a specific event. Instead, population studies are required to look for an association between the vaccination and an adverse event (e.g. clustering of cases after receipt of vaccine or a higher incidence in vaccinated compared to unvaccinated groups).

Adverse reactions may be caused by
- *Inappropriate administration:* e.g. abscesses after poor mixing of vaccines or use of non-sterile needles or syringes; disseminated disease in immunocompromised patients after inappropriate administration of BCG or measles vaccines.
- *Properties of the vaccines:* e.g. reactions caused by either the immunizing agent itself or by other components of the vaccine such as antibiotics, adjuvants, or preservatives.
- *The immune response to the vaccine:* e.g. allergic reactions.

Mild adverse events are common (e.g. 20–50% of DTP recipients experience mild local reactions, while 5–15% of measles vaccine recipients experience fever and rash 6–12 days after immunization). These do not constitute contraindications to further immunization.

Severe adverse reactions are extremely rare. Reports of association of DTP with many adverse events have been made, but comprehensive studies have failed to link it to almost all of these. Reactions such as febrile convulsions or anaphylaxis do occasionally occur; however, for all EPI recommended vaccines, any vaccine-associated adverse events are much less common than the severe complications caused by the diseases prevented by the vaccines.

Misconceptions about vaccines
There have always been concerns about the safety of immunization programmes — this is only appropriate for an intervention in which a biologically active agent is given to large numbers of healthy children. Unfortunately, even after a vaccine's safety has been demonstrated, some misconceptions may persist. Recent examples include concerns that the oral polio vaccine caused infertility or was responsible for the spread of HIV infection. The resurgence of polio in regions rejecting the polio immunization as a result of these erroneous beliefs has demonstrated the ability of misinformation to undermine immunization programmes.

More information about common vaccine misconceptions and information that can be used to reassure parents and community leaders can be obtained from the WHO at: *www.who.int/immunization_safety/aefi/ immunization_misconceptions/en/*

Contraindications to vaccination

There are few absolute contraindications to vaccination. Every opportunity to vaccinate a child or woman of child-bearing age should be taken. There is a high risk that delaying vaccination until the child has recovered from a mild inter-current illness will result in that child not getting their full complement of vaccinations.

True contraindications to immunization include:

- Illnesses severe enough for the child to be hospitalized — if the child is vaccinated but dies from the pre-existing illness, the vaccine may be thought (erroneously) to have contributed to the child's death. However, immunize as soon as the child's general condition improves.
- For *live* vaccines (see opposite), immunodeficiency diseases, or immunosuppression due to malignant disease, therapy with immunosuppressive drugs or irradiation. HIV/AIDS is a special case — see below.
- A severe adverse event (anaphylaxis, collapse or shock, encephalitis, encephalopathy, or non-febrile convulsions) to a vaccine contraindicates further doses of that vaccine. If the adverse reaction occurred following a dose of DTP vaccine, then either omit the pertussis component and continue with the DT vaccine or use a vaccine containing acellular pertussis (if available).
- For vaccines prepared in egg (e.g. influenza, yellow fever), a history of anaphylaxis following egg ingestion. Vaccines prepared in chicken fibroblast cells (e.g. measles, MR, MMR) are safe for such individuals.

In general, *live* vaccines should not be given to pregnant women and pregnancy should be avoided for >1 month following immunization. Immunization in pregnancy may be considered where there is a high risk of exposure and the need for vaccination outweighs any possible risk to the foetus (e.g. yellow fever vaccine and OPV).

Immunization of HIV-infected persons

Immunization of HIV +ve persons needs special consideration because of:
- Increased susceptibility of individuals with AIDS to severe illness from vaccine-preventable infections such as TB and measles.
- Impaired response to vaccines in the advanced stages of AIDS (but most HIV +ve adults and children will mount a good vaccine response).
- Potential risk of live vaccines in immunocompromised individuals (e.g. disseminated BCG infection following administration of BCG vaccine).

As a general rule, *asymptomatic* HIV +ve individuals should receive all recommended EPI vaccinations as soon as possible, while symptomatic HIV +ve individuals can receive all immunizations except BCG and yellow fever (see WHO/UNICEF guidelines opposite). As for any severely ill child, severely ill HIV +ve children should not be vaccinated. Children who are at risk of, or have acquired HIV through vertical transmission should receive the recommended immunizations at the same ages as other children.

Live vaccines

- BCG
- Measles
- Mumps
- Rubella
- MR
- MMR
- OPV
- Yellow fever
- Oral typhoid

Conditions which are NOT contraindications and MUST NOT prevent a child from being vaccinated

- Minor illnesses such as URTI or diarrhoea, with fever < 38.5°C.
- Allergy, atopic manifestations, asthma, hay fever, or 'snuffles'.
- Prematurity, small for dates infants, or jaundice after birth.
- Malnourished child or child being breastfed.
- Family history of convulsions.
- Treatment with antibiotics, low-dose corticosteroids, or locally acting (e.g. topical or inhaled) steroids.
- Dermatoses, eczema, or localized skin infection.
- Chronic diseases of heart, lung, kidney, and liver.
- Stable neurological conditions e.g. cerebral palsy/Down's syndrome.

WHO/UNICEF recommendations for the immunization of HIV-infected children and women of child-bearing age

Vaccine	Asymptomatic HIV infection	Symptomatic HIV infection
BCG	Caution[1]	No[1]
DTP	Yes	Yes
OPV[2]	Yes	Yes
Measles[3]	Yes	Yes
Hepatitis B	Yes	Yes
Hib	Yes	Yes
Yellow fever	Yes	No[4]
TT	Yes	Yes

1. In regions with high rates of TB, BCG vaccine should be given to all infants for whom there is no known contraindication, including those whose HIV status is unknown due to limited diagnostic resources. However, in view of reports of disseminated BCG in HIV-infected children, the vaccine should probably be avoided in those who are known to be HIV infected. Where health services allow, infants of indeterminate status born to HIV-infected mothers should be closely monitored and tested to exclude HIV infection before BCG vaccine is administered.

2. IPV can be used as an alternative in symptomatic HIV-infected children.

3. Because of the risk of severe early measles infection, HIV+ve infants should receive measles at 6 months and as soon after 9 months as possible.

4. Pending further studies

EPI recommended vaccines

Always consult the manufacturer's data sheet before using a vaccine. See 📖 p 815 for general contraindications.

BCG

A freeze-dried preparation of a live attenuated strain of *Mycobacterium bovis* given as a single ID injection. Early administration recommended as it is most effective in preventing TB meningitis and miliary TB, diseases that are more common in infancy. The duration of protection beyond 10–15 years is uncertain; booster doses are not recommended by the WHO. Hypersensitivity should be excluded by a negative tuberculin skin test if BCG is administered after the neonatal period. BCG also protects against leprosy. *Contraindications:* confirmed HIV or other forms of immunocompromise. *Side-effects:* a small swelling forms 2–6 weeks post vaccination that may progress to a benign ulcer. Local abscesses may occur, particularly after incorrect administration (e.g. SC rather than ID). BCG lymphadenitis and osteomyelitis may occur.

Hepatitis B vaccine

A suspension of inactivated hepatitis B surface antigen (HBsAg) adsorbed onto aluminium salts. It is given by intramuscular injection (as per guidelines on 📖 p 810). Booster doses are not recommended. It is available both as a recombinant and plasma-derived product — both are equally safe and effective and can be used interchangeably. The vaccine is available either as monovalent HepB or in combination with DTP ± Hib or DTaP ± Hib; only the monovalent vaccine should be used for immunization at birth. Neonatal vaccination provides immunoprophylaxis against perinatal infection. The use of hepatitis B immunoglobulin at birth for prevention of perinatal transmission is not recommended by WHO.

Pertussis vaccines

Available in 2 forms — whole-cell vaccine (containing killed pertussis bacteria, commonly used in developing countries) or acellular vaccine (containing inactivated pertussis toxin in combination with 1–4 other immunogenic components). Both are given by IM injection, normally as part of DTP or DTaP vaccine. Primary immunization in infancy is essential as pertussis mortality occurs predominantly in this age group. A booster dose is recommended between the ages of 1 to 6 yrs; duration of protection following this is estimated at 6–12 yrs. Adolescents and adults can, therefore, be infected and transmit pertussis to susceptible infants.

Side-effects: 10–50% infants experience mild reactions such as local swelling, fever, and irritability after whole cell vaccine. Prolonged crying occurs in <1%; seizures and hypotonic episodes occur much less commonly. These reactions are less common after acellular pertussis. Following a severe reaction to DTP, it is appropriate for whole cell pertussis to be omitted from subsequent immunizations, by using either DT or acellular pertussis containing combination vaccines. No association between whole cell pertussis and chronic encephalopathy has been found.

Tetanus toxoid vaccine

A formaldehyde-inactivated preparation of tetanus toxoid adsorbed onto aluminium salts that can be given by IM or deep SC injection. It is normally administered to infants as part of DTP (but can be administered as DT if pertussis is contraindicated).

WHO recommended schedule: 6 doses of vaccine — 3 in infancy, a booster at 4–7 years, another at 12–15 years, and a final dose in adulthood. In addition, the administration of tetanus toxoid to a pregnant woman induces antibodies that can cross the placenta and prevent neonatal tetanus. The optimal schedule depends on the immunization history of the woman, as outlined in Table 22.1. Supplementary mass immunization campaigns are recommended in countries of high risk for neonatal tetanus and aim to immunize all women of child-bearing age.

Table 22.1 Tetanus immunization schedules in adults and pregnant women

History	dT 1	dT2	dT3	dT4	dT5
Adolescents and adults with no previous immunization	As early as possible	At least 4 weeks later	At least 6 months later	At least 1 year later	At least 1 year later
Pregnant women with no/uncertain previous immunization	As early as possible in first pregnancy	At least 4 weeks later	At least 6 months later e.g. in next pregnancy	At least 1 year later e.g. in next pregnancy	At least 1 year later e.g. in next pregnancy
Pregnant woman with 3 childhood DTP doses	As early as possible in first pregnancy	At least 4 weeks later	At least 1 year later		
Pregnant woman with 4 childhood DTP doses	As early as possible in first pregnancy	At least 1 year later			
Supplementary immunization activities in high risk areas	During round 1	During round 2, at least 4 weeks after round 1	During round 3, at least 6 months after round 2	At least 1 year later e.g. next pregnancy	At least 1 year later e.g. next pregnancy

Diphtheria toxoid vaccine

A formaldehyde-inactivated preparation of diphtheria toxin, adsorbed onto aluminium salts to increase immunogenicity. It is normally given combined with tetanus toxoid and pertussis (DTP), but can be given as DT if pertussis is contraindicated. The vaccine does not prevent infection but rather inhibits or neutralizes the toxin's effects, preventing systemic illness. A low-dose vaccine (combined with tetanus: dT) should be used in individuals >7 yrs to reduce the risk of reactions to the vaccine.

Haemophilus influenzae type b (Hib) vaccines

Consists of Hib polysaccharides conjugated to diphtheria toxoid, tetanus toxoids, or the meningococcus outer-membrane complex in order to stimulate a T-cell response. The vaccine is given intramuscularly either alone or in a combination vaccine with DTP ± HepB. Hib causes a substantial proportion of global meningitis, septicaemia, and pneumonia. However, the disease burden is often underestimated due to the difficulty of laboratory identification. Booster doses of vaccine are currently used in the majority of industrialized countries, but are not recommended in the EPI schedule.

Japanese encephalitis vaccines

Exist in 3 forms — 2 formalin inactivated vaccines (grown in either mouse or guinea pig brain) and 1 live attenuated vaccine. The mouse brain derived vaccine is the only vaccine that is internationally licensed; the guinea pig derived vaccine is produced in China and is now being replaced by the live attenuated vaccine. The mouse brain vaccine is routinely used in many Japanese encephalitis endemic countries in Asia, with variable immunization schedules. Most schedules recommend 2 toddler doses administered 2–4 weeks apart, with up to 2 subsequent booster doses in late childhood. The dose is 0.5 ml (for 1–3-year-olds) or 1 ml (for >3-year-olds). An immunization schedule of a total of 3 doses (at 0, 7, and 30 days) is recommended for travellers to endemic regions who will spend extended periods in rural areas.

Side-effects: allergic reactions (e.g. urticaria and angio-oedema) occur in ~0.6% of immunized travellers. As this reaction may be delayed for up to 10 days, it is advised that the last dose of vaccine be given at least 10 days prior to departure. Concern over an association with acute disseminated encephalomyelopathy has led to the suspension of routine immunization in Japan; a WHO review did not support such an association. Difficulties in large-scale production and expense limit the vaccine's role in large-scale immunization campaigns.

A live attenuated vaccine (SA-14-14-2) with 98.5% effectiveness 1 year after a single dose has been introduced in China. This vaccine has the potential for large-scale production at a lower cost than the inactivated vaccines, and is currently being assessed for international licensure.

Poliomyelitis vaccine

Available in 2 forms — a live attenuated oral vaccine (OPV, Sabin vaccine) and an injectable killed virus vaccine (IPV, Salk vaccine). Both vaccines contain poliovirus types 1, 2, and 3. The EPI recommends OPV because of its low cost, ease of administration, superiority in conferring intestinal protection, and potential for infecting household and community contacts, thereby boosting secondary immunity. Unfounded reports that OPV causes infertility have resulted in reduced immunization coverage in countries such as Nigeria, with a resultant increase in poliomeyclitis.

Cautions: patients with diarrhoea and vomiting require a further dose after recovery. IPV rather than OPV should be administered to immunocompromised individuals *and their household contacts.*

Side effects: OPV-associated poliomyelitis is extremely rare: 2–4 cases per million doses.

Measles vaccine

A live attenuated virus given by IM or SC injection. Measles may be given as a monovalent vaccine or in combination with rubella ± mumps (MR, MMR). It is normally given at 9 months of age but can be given at 6 and 9 months to those at high risk and should be offered to susceptible children within 3 days of exposure to infection. All children should receive 2 doses of measles vaccine.

Side-effects: a mild measles-like illness may occur in 5–15% of children 6–12 days after immunization. Convulsions and encephalitis are rare complications.

Yellow fever vaccine

Consists of a freeze-dried preparation of live attenuated virus strain (17D strain) that is grown in egg embryos and given by SC injection. Yellow fever is endemic in 33 countries in sub-Saharan Africa (where by far the greatest burden of disease lies) and 11 countries in South America. In these countries, infant immunization at the same time as measles immunization is recommended. Protection afforded by a single dose of vaccine appears to last at least 30 years. However, international travel regulations require evidence of immunization within the previous 10 years prior to arrival in endemic countries (or travel from endemic countries to countries at risk for endemic disease).

Contraindications: anaphylactic reaction to egg, immunocompromise, and age <6 months (but can be given at 6–8 months if at high risk of disease).

Side-effects: minor reactions (e.g. headache, myalgia) occur in 10–30% of recipients. Uncommon reactions include encephalitis (more common in infants), hypersensitivity, and multiple organ failure (~1 in 10 million, but possibly more common in elderly).

Other vaccines

Cholera vaccine

The parenteral cholera vaccine has poor efficacy and is no longer recommended. Two oral cholera vaccines have been developed: one is a killed whole-cell vaccine combined with a recombinant B subunit of cholera toxin (rCTB-WC), the other a live attenuated vaccine (CVD 103-HgR; not currently in production). The rCTB-WC dosing schedule is 2 doses 1 week apart in adults and 3 half doses 1 week apart in children 2–6 years of age. The vaccine is not licensed for children <2 years of age. The immunization course should ideally be completed 1 week before potential exposure to cholera. A booster dose is recommended by the manufacturers after 2 years (for adults) and after 6 months (for children aged 2–6 years). The WHO recommends that cholera vaccine be used pre-emptively in populations at risk of cholera epidemics (e.g. refugee camps), along with other cholera preventative measures. Travel immunization is only recommended for relief and disaster workers, or travellers to remote areas in which epidemics are occurring. rCTB-WC does not protect against Vibrio cholerae 0139, an emerging serotype in South Asia.

Side-effects: rCTB-WC is well tolerated, with mild gastrointestinal symptoms being the most common side-effect.

Hepatitis A vaccines

Exist in 5 variations; 4 inactivated and 1 live attenuated (produced and used only in China). Antibodies persist for at least 2 years after a single dose of inactivated vaccine. However, current recommendations suggest these vaccines are administered as 2 doses 6–18 months apart. No vaccine is licensed for use in infants <1-year-old. Hepatitis A vaccine is also available combined with Hepatitis B vaccine in a formulation to be administered as 3 doses as a 0, 1, and 6-month schedule. The high prevalence of hepatitis A in developing countries results in a predominance of asymptomatic childhood infections. Therefore, these vaccines are not recommended for use in these settings. Travellers from industrialized countries to these regions should be immunized.

Side-effects: the vaccines are well tolerated and no serious adverse effects have been attributed to the vaccine.

Influenza vaccines

Consist of 3 inactivated influenza virus strains (2 influenza A, 1 influenza B) that have been grown in eggs. The haemagglutinin (H) and neuraminidase (N) antigens used in the vaccines are determined by the WHO each year according to the anticipated prevalent strains. In addition, H5N1 vaccines are currently being developed in preparation for the potential of pandemic influenza associated with H5N1 strains.

Meningococcal vaccines

Two forms of meningococcal vaccines exist. The plain polysaccharide vaccines consist of the serogroup specific meningococcal polysaccharide capsules. These are available either as themonovalent serogroup A vaccine or as combination vaccines i.e. A and C; A, C, and W-135; or A, C, Y, and W-135. These vaccines are used in outbreak control. However, protection wanes after several years and, for serogroups other than serogroup A, are poorly immunogenic in infants.

Glyco-conjugate meningococcal vaccines are available in which meningococcal polysaccharide capsules are conjugated to tetanus toxoid, diphtheria toxoid, or CRM-197 (a diphtheria toxoid variant). Monovalent serogroup C glyco-conjugate vaccines are routinely used in many industrialized countries. The vaccine is given as 2 or 3 infant doses or a single dose at 1 year of age; a booster dose is required after infant immunization. A tetravalent meningococcal serogroup A, C, W-135, and Y vaccine is recommended in the USA for young people >11 years of age and for 'at risk' groups. Development of affordable glycoconjugate vaccines for prevention of serogroup A disease in sub-Saharan Africa is ongoing.

The poor immunogenicity of the meningococcal serogroup B polysaccharide capsule renders this unsuitable for use in a glyco-conjugate vaccine. An outbreak-specific meningococcal serogroup B vaccine, based on subcapsular proteins, is used in New Zealand, but is not suitable for use elsewhere. Development of a more broadly protective meningococcal serogroup B vaccine is ongoing.

Mumps vaccine

Consists of a live attenuated strain of the virus grown in chick embryo cells in chick culture. It is normally given by IM injection with measles and rubella vaccines in the MMR triple vaccine at 12–15 months and again at 3–5 years.

Pigbel vaccine

An inactivated preparation of toxin from Clostridium perfringens type 3 that is given by IM injection. It is effective in infants and has been given routinely to children in Papua New Guinea at 2, 4, and 6 months of age since 1980. Protection lasts for 2–4 years.

Pneumococcal vaccines

Like meningococcal vaccines, these exist in 2 forms. The plain polysaccharide vaccine contains capsular polysaccharide antigens from 23 different serotypes of Streptococcus pneumoniae. Unfortunately, these antigens do not induce a protective response in children <2 years of age and protective immunity in older individuals may be limited or short-lived. The vaccine is recommended for those >2 years of age who are at high risk for severe infection: sickle cell disease, chronic renal failure, immunosuppression, CSF leaks, HIV infection, asplenia, diabetes mellitus or chronic liver, heart or lung disease. If possible, the vaccine should be given >2 weeks before either splenectomy or chemotherapy. **Contraindications:** pregnancy, breastfeeding, during acute infection. **Side-effects:** hypersensitivity reactions may occur. These are more common following re-immunization within 3 years.

The 7 valent pneumococcal glyco-conjugate vaccine (a conjugate of the polysaccharide from 7 pneumococcal serotypes with CRM_{197}) is immunogenic in infancy and induces immunological memory. In the USA, a 75% decline in invasive pneumococcal disease in children less than 5 years of age was observed in the 4 years following the vaccine's introduction into the routine immunization schedule in 1999. The vaccine is given as 2 or 3 primary doses in infancy followed by a booster dose at ~1 year of age. Two doses 2 months apart are recommended in older children. Vaccines of higher valency (including serotype 1; a major cause of disease in many developing countries) are in development. Studies in sub-Saharan Africa revealing pneumococcal bacteraemia in 597/100,000 of under-5-year-olds presenting to hospital, and a clinical trial in the Gambia of a 9 valent pneumococcal vaccine showing a 16% reduction in mortality in pneumococcal vaccine recipients, highlight the enormous potential of these vaccines if they can be made affordable for the developing world.

Rabies vaccine

Available as a freeze-dried inactivated preparation of virus grown in either sheep brain or cultured human diploid cells. The former vaccine is still used but, due to immune responses to sheep brain antigens that contaminate the vaccine, is associated with unacceptably high rate of severe neurological complications (~1:1000). The cultured vaccine is far safer but more expensive. Its use around the world is increasing, however, particularly as novel cheaper ways of administering the vaccine (e.g. by intradermal injection) are developed.

Rotavirus vaccines

Two live oral vaccines have recently been licensed against this virus, responsible for up to a half of diarrhoea-related hospital admissions in Africa. A live attenuated vaccine (RIX 4414) has been licensed for use in Latin America and Europe. This vaccine is administered at 6–14 weeks of age, with a second dose at least 4 weeks later. A re-assortant vaccine based on a bovine rotavirus strain and incorporating capsid proteins for 5 common human serotypes has been licensed in the USA. This vaccine is administered as 3 doses commencing at 6–10 weeks of age and given at 4–10 week intervals. Large-scale studies of both vaccines have shown both to be safe and highly effective against severe rotavirus disease. Importantly, neither vaccine has been shown to be associated with intussusception, a side-effect that was responsible for the withdrawal of an earlier rotavirus vaccine (Rotashield).

Rubella vaccine:

A preparation of the live Wistar strain of the virus. It is given by deep SC or IM injection in industrialized countries, either as part of the triple MMR vaccine or as a monovalent vaccine to girls between 10 and 14 years of age. The purpose is to reduce the incidence of primary infection in pregnant women and, thus, reduce the incidence of congenital rubella syndrome in their offspring. Universal recommendation is not recommended by EPI at present as incomplete immunization is likely to increase the age at which infections occur, thereby increasing the risk of infection in childbearing women. *Contraindications:* avoid immunizing women in early pregnancy. Advise women to avoid pregnancy for 1 month following immunization. However, there is no evidence at present that the vaccine is teratogenic.

The future of vaccines in tropical countries

Funding initiatives

As a result of increasing recognition of the cost effectiveness of vaccine programmes, new funding initiatives have been developed to realize the potential of immunization in tropical and developing countries. Most prominent among these is **GAVI** (the Global Alliance for Vaccines and Immunizations). This alliance between key immunization stakeholders such as developing and donor governments, the World Bank, the WHO, UNICEF, the pharmaceutical industry, research institutes, non-government organizations, and the Bill and Melinda Gates Foundation (one of the major funders) has brought focus and unprecedented resources to the goal of optimizing immunization uptake and the development of new vaccines.

Further information is available at:
www.who.int/immunization_supply/financing/en/

Vaccine specific initiatives

Funded in part by GAVI, new vaccine-specific advocacy groups have been developed to promote the introduction of existing vaccines in developing countries. Examples include **The Hib Initiative** and **PneumoADIP**, the latter being an advocacy group for the pneumococcal glyco-conjugate vaccines. A primary role of organizations such as these is the gathering of accurate data on the (often hidden) disease burden due to the relevant organism. These data can then be used in arguing for vaccine introduction to health care policy makers.

New vaccines — under development and required

While 1.4 million of the global childhood deaths in 2002 were vaccine preventable, many more were due to infectious diseases that are not yet vaccine preventable, but may one day become so. More vaccines, including those against the diseases listed below, are required and are currently in development:
- Dengue.
- Enterotoxigenic *E. coli*.
- Hepatitis C.
- HIV (*www.iavi.org*).
- Malaria (*www.malariavaccine.org*).
- Meningococcal serogroup B.
- Para-influenza virus.
- Respiratory syncitial virus.
- Shigella.
- Schistosomiasis.

Similarly, work is ongoing to develop alternative, more effective vaccines against diseases such as TB, for which sub-optimal vaccines already exist.

Typhoid vaccine

3 forms of typhoid vaccines are currently licensed: a killed parenteral whole-cell vaccine (now largely superseded due to its reactogenicity), a plain polysaccharide ('Vi') parenteral vaccine, and a live attenuated oral vaccine. The polysaccharide vaccine is administered as a single dose by IM or SC injection and is immunogenic above the age of 2 years. Duration of protection is uncertain, however booster doses are recommended every 3 years. The live attenuated vaccine requires 3 oral doses administered 2 days apart (travellers from the USA are advised to have a fourth dose). In addition to the enteric coated capsule formulation of the vaccine (licensed for use only over the age of 6), a liquid preparation is now available, suitable for use from the age of 2 upwards. Re–immunization is recommended every 3 years for those living in endemic regions. Antibiotics and proguanil should be avoided during the three days before and after vaccination as they will inactivate the vaccine; similarly, avoid mefloquine for 12 h (and preferably 3 days) either side of immunization.

A vaccine consisting of the Vi polysaccharide conjugated to a carrier protein is currently in development and offers hope for vaccine protection of those under 2 years of age.

Appendix: websites

CDC Health topics A to Z
http://www.cdc.gov/health/default.htm
A superb site giving information suitable for doctors or the public on most infectious diseases, parasitic diseases, and non-infectious conditions.

CDC Parasitic diseases
http://www.dpd.cdc.gov/dpdx/
Another superb site giving details on parasites, life cycles, diagnostic methods, and an image bank.

Atlas of medical parasitology
http://www.cdfound.to.it/HTML/atlas.htm
Useful images of parasites, life cycles, and some clinical pictures.

CDC Division of Tuberculosis elimination
http://www.cdc.gov/nchstp/tb/default.htm
The starting point for many links to TB information.

CDC Health Information for International Travel
http://www.cdc.gov/travel/contentYellowBook.aspx
Advice on travel health and immunizations from the CDC.

Malaria Resource (TDR/WHO)
http://www.wehi.edu.au/MalDB-www/who.html
Teaches and tests microscopy skills for malaria diagnosis.

Immunization against infectious diseases 'The Green Book'
*http://www/dh.gov.uk/en/Policyandguidance/Healthandsocialcaretopics/
Greenbook/DH_4097254*
The UK guidelines on immunization.

UK malaria guidelines (2007)
http://www.hpa.org.uk/publications/2006/Malaria/Malaria_guidelines
Detailed guidance on malaria prophylaxis and stand-by treatment.

AIDS images
http://members.xoom.virgilio.it/Aidsimaging/contents.htm
Clinical pictures, microscope pictures, and X-rays of opportunistic infections in HIV.

Index